Dunn & Haimann's Healthcare Management

Ninth Edition

Dunn & Haimann's
Healthcare Management

Ninth Edition

Rose T. Dunn

AUPHA
Chicago, Illinois

Your board, staff, or clients may also benefit from this book's insight. For more information on quantity discounts, contact the Health Administration Press Marketing Manager at (312) 424–9470.

14 13 12 11   5 4 3

Library of Congress Cataloging-in-Publication Data

Dunn, Rose.
  Dunn and Haimann's healthcare management / Rose T. Dunn. — 9th ed.
     p. ; cm.
  Other title: Healthcare management
  Rev. ed. of: Haimann's heathcare management / Rose T. Dunn.
  Includes bibliographical references and index.
  ISBN 978-1-56793-358-1
  1. Health facilities—Administration. I. Haimann, Theo. II. Dunn, Rose. Haimann's
heathcare management. III. Title. IV. Title: Healthcare management.
  [DNLM: 1. Health Facilities—organization & administration. 2. Personnel
Management. WX 150 D923d 2010]
  RA971.H22 2010
  362.11068—dc22

                                                        2010010949

The paper used in this publication meets the minimum requirements of American National Standard for Information Sciences—Permanence of Paper for Printed Library Materials, ANSI Z39.48-1984.™

Acquisitions editor: Eileen Lynch; Project manager: Eduard Avis; Cover designer: Marisa Jackson; Layout: Putman Productions, LLC

Found an error or a typo? We want to know! Please e-mail it to hap1@ache.org, and put "Book Error" in the subject line.

For photocopying and copyright information, please contact Copyright Clearance Center at www.copyright.com or at (978) 750–8400.

Health Administration Press
A division of the Foundation of the American
   College of Healthcare Executives
One North Franklin Street, Suite 1700
Chicago, IL 60606–3529
(312) 424–2800

Association of University Programs
   in Health Administration
2000 North 14th Street
Suite 780
Arlington, VA 22201
(703) 894–0940

*This edition is dedicated to the memories
of my and my husband's parents,
the last of whom we lost this year.
We thank those working at the bedside
and behind the scenes in healthcare organizations
today for the many heroic measures taken
and the caring touch you provided
for our parents in their final years.*

CONTENTS IN BRIEF

CONTENTS IN DETAIL

PREFACE

The challenges facing the healthcare industry today will require fine-tuned managerial skills. Healthcare managers must keep pace with revolutionary and sophisticated breakthroughs in medical science and technology, transparency of service outcomes and charges, an educated customer base, an aging population, and federal regulations growing exponentially.

At the center of all these changes is the supervisor, who has to bring and hold together the human resources, physical facilities, professional expertise, technologies, and other support systems necessary to provide care and monitor services rendered. In addition, these tasks have to be accomplished within the fiscal constraints of a more efficient healthcare system. Therefore, healthcare managers and supervisors must understand the complexities of the organization, generational motivational differences, regional healthcare demands, and the industry as a whole.

The 21st century healthcare organization is much different than the one that existed when Theo Haimann first coached new supervisors in the early 1970s. However, his belief then remains accurate today—the hardest job in any organization is clearly that of the supervisor. The supervisor is responsible for motivating the team to achieve organization goals set by the board of directors or senior leadership. The supervisor must be able to translate the goals into understandable and achievable terms for his or her team members and gain their buy-in; without the buy-in, the organization could fail.

Many first level and middle management team leader positions, such as department managers, supervisors, and group leaders, are filled by individuals with excellent technical skills who have limited or no formal education or training in administration, management, and supervision. This book is intended for these individuals.

The book is introductory in that it assumes no previous knowledge of the concepts of supervision and management. As such, this book also is written for students taking an introductory course in management and will acquaint them with their future roles in any organization (healthcare or otherwise). It can be used in any course in which managerial, supervisory, and leadership concepts are studied.

Because this book is intended to aid people with their supervisory tasks, it serves as a reference to those individuals who already hold managerial positions. Its purpose is to demonstrate that proficiency in supervision better equips them to cope with the ever-increasing demands of getting the job done. Because non-healthcare entities have had success dealing with change and implementing efficient and effective practices, this book draws on many sources for its content to permit the supervisor to apply lessons learned by others, regardless of whether they were experienced in a healthcare environment.

To create a framework in which management knowledge can be organized in a practical way, I have chosen to use the functions of management as the primary framework: planning, organizing, staffing, influencing, and controlling. Each function is thoroughly dealt with by breaking down and explaining its relationship to the material already presented. This approach allows new knowledge, from behavioral and social sciences, quantitative approaches, or any other field, to be incorporated at any point.

The supervisor's job—to get things done with and through people—has its foundation in the relationship between the supervisors and the people with whom they work. For this reason, the supervisor must have considerable knowledge of the human aspects of supervision—that is, the behavioral factors and generational stimuli that motivate employees. This book attempts to present a balanced picture of such behavioral factors in the conceptual framework of managing.

This ninth edition of this book is sure to be a welcome addition to any manager's library. In this edition, much new material has been added, but the book retains the basic concepts and the emphasis on the five managerial functions. I have attempted to respond to each of the recommendations offered by readers and text reviewers while preparing this edition.

At the end of each chapter, the reader will find reference to additional readings should he or she desire to further study some of the concepts in the chapter. Guidance from management theorists that has surfaced during the last two decades was added to chapters 1, 2, 20, and 26. Content related to ethics and ethical decision making was added to chapters 3 and 6. Chapter 6 includes references to e-discovery and medical identity theft. The Parity Principle was added to chapter 11 and Role Theory to chapter 12.

Tools were incorporated into several chapters. For example, a partial table of contents for policy and procedure manuals and a policy and procedure template were added to chapter 9; a sample meeting agenda and minutes format were added to chapter 15; and telecommuting agreement and flex time policy were added to chapter 23. Many figures were updated as well.

The discussion on diversity was expanded in chapters 18 and 21. Chapters 27 and 28, dealing with labor unions and grievances, respectively, were updated by our respected and experienced labor attorney, Marc Leff,

Esq. However, as a reminder, neither chapter is intended to be a substitute for legal advice from an organization's legal council.

With the many changes taking place in healthcare today, I was not at a loss to find new management challenges to discuss and use as the basis for the last chapter, which traditionally has discussed emerging influences.

Instructor resources for this book are available online. Materials include discussion questions, PowerPoint slides, and a test bank. For instructions on how to access this information, e-mail hap1@ache.org.

In writing this edition, I attempted to retain the enthusiasm for effective management exhibited by Theo Haimann, the professor for whom this book is named. Haimann served as the Mary Louis Professor of Management Sciences at Saint Louis University until his death in November 1991. He always incorporated current management issues into his teachings. By doing so, he was able to keep the students' attention. This edition attempts to carry on the Haimann tradition.

No book is ever the product of one person's efforts. Many individuals contributed to its development, editing, formatting, and publishing. I was fortunate to have some of the best working with me on this edition. Eileen Lynch, acquisitions editor for Health Administration Press, provided oversight for the project and managed the development of the instructor's manual. Eduard Avis thoroughly reviewed the manuscript and offered many valuable suggestions, kept the production running smoothly, and with the assistance of Joyce Dunne, Helen Lynerd, Dojna Shearer, and Jane Calayag, ensured all Ts were crossed and Is dotted. Benjamin Burton, RHIA, JD (of First Class Solutions) was a tremendous asset in compiling the instructor's manual. Finally, several clients of First Class Solutions allowed me to reproduce documents, policies, and other figures from their healthcare organizations. For these and those readers who submitted suggested changes for this edition, I extend special thanks.

As always, I welcome your comments—good or bad—so that I can make the tenth edition better.

Rose T. Dunn, MBA, RHIA, CPA, FACHE
Chief Operating Officer
First Class Solutions, Inc.^{sm}
Maryland Heights (St. Louis), MO
Rose@FirstClassSolutions.com
800-274-1214

STEPPING INTO MANAGEMENT

THE SUPERVISOR'S JOB, ROLES, FUNCTIONS, AND AUTHORITY

Chapter Objectives

After you have studied this chapter, you should be able to do the following:

1. Provide an overview of the rapidly changing healthcare environment and the challenges it poses for managers and supervisors.
2. Discuss the dimensions of the supervisor's job.
3. Review the aspects of the supervisor's position and the skills necessary to be successful.
4. Discuss the managerial role of the supervisor.
5. Enumerate and discuss the meaning, interrelationships, and universal nature of the five managerial functions.
6. Discuss the concept of authority and its meaning as the foundation of the formal, organizational, and positional aspects of authority.

The Healthcare Perspective

The need and demand for high-quality, flexible, and energetic management in all healthcare delivery settings are intensifying. The market is demanding new delivery methods. For example, in the past, patients came to the healthcare facility; now, healthcare services are conveniently located near patients' homes and are accessible through satellite outpatient services, discount retailers, pharmacies, mobile screening units, and health fairs at the grocery store. Today's managers are challenged to effectively supervise their department operations and staffs in this decentralized environment.

Other trends affecting healthcare managers include a rapidly changing reimbursement environment that affects the amount of resources available to pay for new technologies and staff. The growth in managed care contracting seems inevitable, and many healthcare organizations are lacking the data they need to succeed in this area. Medical practice managers also are feeling the pain of reimbursement declines. The traditional **fee-for-service** arrangements have been replaced with **pay-for-performance** fee schedules and **capitation** agreements.

fee-for-service
A system that pays clinicians based on the number of services they perform.

pay-for-performance
A system that pays clinicians based on their ability to meet specified quality and efficiency measures.

capitation
A system that pays physicians, or healthcare organizations, a fixed monthly amount for each individual in a plan, regardless of whether they are treated or not.

prospective payment system
A system that pays physicians and healthcare organizations a fixed amount for every episode of care. For example, treatment for a particular injury is reimbursed at a flat rate regardless of the length of stay in the hospital or the number of physician visits related to the injury.

Finances are being affected by regulations as well. The various **prospective payment system** (PPS) regulations have resulted in significant cuts in reimbursement for services, compensation for capital expenditures, and teaching programs. These cuts have forced healthcare organizations to better manage services to streamline operations without compromising the quality of care. The Health Insurance Portability and Accountability Act (HIPAA) regulations have imposed major changes in the operations of information technology, patient financial services, compliance, health information management, and other areas.

New breakthroughs in science and technology (including robotics) are likely to change key services, such as in the fields of cardiology, oncology, orthopedics, neurology, and women's health. Insurers are channeling those they insure to a few hospitals to receive high-tech care such as lung, heart, and pancreas transplants. Hospitals, in turn, are creating centers of excellence to focus limited resources on the growth of more profitable service areas and niche markets.

Faced with a shortage of nurses, whose expertise and assistance are crucial to high-quality healthcare, providers are training other staff to perform many of the nonregulated functions previously performed by nurses. These individuals—sometimes called multiskilled professionals, nurse extenders, or certified nurse assistants—record temperatures; pass medications; draw blood; collect specimens; and perform some patient care services such as turning, exercising, and assisting patients when ambulating. These individuals are more abundant than nurses, and their hourly rates are lower, thus reducing labor costs. Employing these individuals has led to unionization activities by nursing professionals at some organizations. A shortage of nurses, low unemployment rates, and work attitudes of Generation Xers[1] have hampered the hiring efforts of many providers.

critical access hospital
A designation that allows a hospital to receive Medicare reimbursement based on its actual costs, which is generally more than typical Medicare reimbursement. The designation was designed to help hospitals in underserved areas.

In addition to these factors, many other changes from all directions are affecting healthcare delivery. Challenges such as those considered below will continue to impose constraints on healthcare services and set higher expectations.

To pool labor, clinical, and capital resources and expertise, many facilities are merging with nearby hospitals, prior competitors, or other strategically located facilities. Mergers, in some cases, have closed facilities. In fact, according to the Centers for Disease Control and Prevention (CDC 2008), the total number of short-stay, nonfederal hospitals dropped to 5,747 in 2006; this is more than 1,000 fewer hospitals than existed in 1975 (see Exhibit 1.1). Many closures were smaller rural hospitals, a situation that has been stemmed to some degree by the reclassification of these hospitals as **critical access hospitals**.

Mergers and closures are not limited to hospitals. Physicians, laboratories, and home health agencies have seen similar consolidations. When mergers occur and new entities are created, extensive and sophisticated long-range

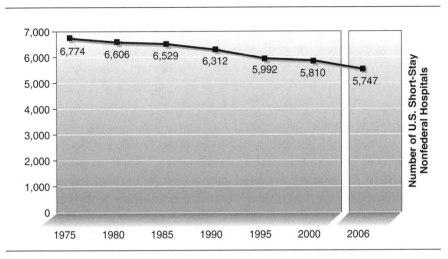

Exhibit 1.1

Number of U.S. Short-Stay Nonfederal Hospitals

SOURCE: *Health United States, 2008*, National Center for Health Statistics.

planning and good control over internal affairs are necessary. Thus, the radical reshaping of the healthcare field calls for more and better management. Managers, from chief executive officers (CEOs) down to first-line supervisors, are needed to help implement these changes and make their organizations function effectively.

The organization is the culmination of the management process. The organization is the incubator that brings resources together to provide a service, create a product, or both. Management is the process by which healthcare organizations fulfill this responsibility. The manager is responsible for acquiring and combining the resources to accomplish the goals. As scientific, economic, competitive, social, and other pressures change, it is not the nurse or the technologist on whom the organization depends to coordinate the resources necessary to cope with the change; it is the manager. Management has emerged as a potent force in our society and has become essential to all healthcare endeavors.

Today's health services are almost exclusively delivered in organizational settings.[2] Only an organizational setting can bring together the physical facilities, professional expertise, skills, information systems, technology, and myriad other supports that today's health services delivery requires, whether these services are curative, rehabilitative, or preventive. However, the physical confines in which healthcare employees work are changing. In the past, all staff came to a physical location to work. Today, many tasks are performed remotely using the Internet and high-tech hardware and software. For example, some radiology interpretations (teleradiology) and some physician evaluation services (telemedicine) are handled long-distance or through robots, while non–patient-care functions such as billing, information systems, financial services, and purchasing are often housed in facilities that are not on the same campus as the hospital or may be serving more than one organization. In addition, clinical coding and transcription are often performed at home (telecommuting). Those involved in the delivery of healthcare services and those managing the remote functions must understand the complexities of organizational life (behavior, development, and climate) and the importance of expert administration.

Because the delivery of healthcare largely means providing a service, which is by nature people intensive, approximately 57 percent of the total expenditures in the field are for wages and benefits (PriceWaterhouseCoopers 2005). Therefore, it is not surprising that employee productivity is often scrutinized, and leaders are increasingly interested in outsourcing and off-shoring services. Many feel the United States needs better administration throughout the healthcare industry. Frontline management—departmental supervisors, regardless of titles and nature of work—is responsible for the department functioning smoothly and efficiently. It is essential, therefore, that effective supervisors are developed in all areas of the healthcare field.

The Demands of the Supervisory Position

The supervisory position within any administrative structure is difficult and demanding. You probably know this from your own experience or by observing supervisors in the healthcare organizations in which you work. The supervisor, whether a manager of printing and mail services or a chief technologist in the clinical laboratory, can be viewed as the person in the middle of a pyramid structure. He or she serves as the principal link between higher administration (the top of the pyramid shown in Exhibit 1.2) and the employees (the base of the pyramid).

The job of almost any supervisor, regardless of whom or what he or she supervises, involves four major dimensions, or four areas of responsibility.

First, the supervisor must be a good boss, a good manager, and a team leader of the employees in the unit. This includes having the technical, professional, and clinical competence to run the department smoothly and see that the employees carry out their assignments successfully.

Second, the supervisor must be a competent subordinate to the next higher manager: in most instances, this person is an administrator, a center executive, or a director of a service. Ultimately, the supervisor's boss reports to owners of the organization or the board of directors or trustees.

Third, the supervisor must link the administration and the employees. For example, employees such as laboratory scientists, ultrasound technicians, and clerical support staff see their supervisor—who is perhaps the

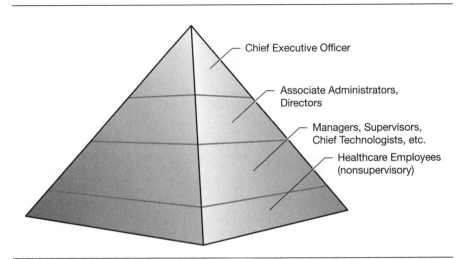

EXHIBIT 1.2
The Administrative Pyramid

Chief Executive Officer

Associate Administrators, Directors

Managers, Supervisors, Chief Technologists, etc.

Healthcare Employees (nonsupervisory)

chief technologist—as the "administration." The employees communicate their concerns to the administration through the supervisor, and the supervisor communicates the goals and policies established by senior administration. The supervisor filters the employees' concerns into categories (i.e., those that the supervisor should address, those that the supervisor's boss should address, and those that should be pushed further up the ladder and may represent concerns shared by employees outside of the department). Similarly, the supervisor receives information from multiple levels in the hierarchy and decides which information should be passed on to immediate subordinates and to those working on the front line. Goal and policy communications must be shared with all staff because the supervisor must make certain the work gets done to achieve those goals.

Fourth, the supervisor must maintain satisfactory working relationships with the directors, leaders, and peer supervisors of all other departments and services. The supervisor must foster a collegial relationship and coordinate the department's efforts with those of other departments to reach the overall objectives and goals of the institution. The supervisor must help the organization provide the best possible service and patient care regardless of which department or service gets credit.

The four dimensions of the supervisor's job are shown in Exhibit 1.3. The supervisor must succeed in vertical relationships downward with subordinates and upward with his or her superior. In addition, the supervisor must skillfully handle horizontal relationships with other supervisors.

Henry Mintzberg (1973) depicts these dimensions as roles common to the work of all managers. A role is an organized set of behaviors, and Mintzberg categorizes the roles into three groups: interpersonal, informational, and decisional.

EXHIBIT 1.3
Four
Dimensions
of the
Supervisor's
Job

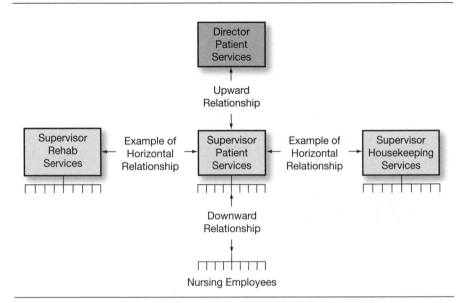

interpersonal role
A supervisor's behavior, such as relationships with other supervisors, that links all managerial work.

informational role
A supervisor's behavior that ensures that information is received and processed.

decisional role
A supervisor's behavior that uses information to make decisions.

The **interpersonal roles**, such as relationships with other supervisors, link all managerial work. This role group includes serving as a leader and liaison and maintaining effective communication with peers, subordinates, superiors, and individuals outside of the organization.

The **informational roles** ensure that information received is processed. In this capacity the manager collects information during monitoring activities, filters information received from others, and displays and disseminates information to others. Further amplification of this role is given in Drucker and Collins's book, *Management*, where the authors suggest you must ask yourself what information you need to do your job and where you will find it. Related questions are what information you *owe* others and what they *owe* you (Rosenstein 2008).

The **decisional roles** make use of the information for decision making. In this area the manager or supervisor may implement change based on the information he or she receives or collects. Doing so allows the manager to act in an entrepreneurial manner, according to Mintzberg. Alternatively, the information could be used as an alert to recognize when the organization may be threatened, when employees are disgruntled, or when work disruption may be imminent. In this situation, the role being played, according to Mintzberg, is one of "disturbance handler." The final two roles of the decisional group include resource allocator and negotiator. In both, the manager is using information to determine where resources can be best utilized and how to most economically and effectively obtain and use these resources.

Because of the complexity of these relationships, the role of the first-line supervisor in any organization is commonly acknowledged to be the most difficult. It is even more difficult for supervisors within the healthcare field, because their actions are directed by their facility's administrator as well as medical staff members. Additionally, their actions and the services provided by their departments affect patients, the quality of patient care, the people within the department, and the smooth overall functioning of the institution. In addition to their many professional obligations, healthcare supervisors must always bear in mind the needs and desires of patients and their relatives, who may be physically drained and emotionally upset. Thus, the supervisor should be informed of any concerns of his or her staff, the medical staff, and patients. All these considerations make the job of the healthcare supervisor particularly demanding and challenging.

For example, consider the long list of demands made on a charge nurse of a nursing unit. The charge nurse's duty is to provide for and supervise the nursing care rendered to the patients in the unit. She delegates some of her authority for the care of patients and the supervision of personnel to subordinate nursing team leaders, but she still must plan, direct, and control all activities within the nursing unit. She must make the rounds with medical and nursing staff. She also makes rounds to personally observe the safety, condition, and behavior of patients and to assess the need for and quality of nursing care. She may even have to assume general nursing functions in the care of patients who have complex problems or when vacancies exist.

Furthermore, the charge nurse must interpret and apply the policies, procedures, rules, and regulations of the facility in general and of nursing services in particular. She must provide 24-hour coverage of the unit by scheduling staff properly at all times. She is to communicate and report to her immediate patient care services superior all pertinent information regarding patients in her unit. She must orient new personnel to the unit and acquaint them with the general philosophies of the institution. She is also responsible for continued in-service education in her unit, teaching personnel new patient care techniques and patient safety initiatives. She also participates in the evaluation of her subordinates.

In addition, it is part of the charge nurse's job to coordinate her patient care with the care and therapeutic procedures of the various departments throughout the institution. Furthermore, she is involved in the design and regular reevaluation of the budget. She serves on a number of committees, in addition to attending all patient care management meetings. She may also be expected to help in the supervision and instruction of student nurses and medical **housestaff** when necessary. Many additional duties are often assigned to a charge nurse, depending on what the particular healthcare facility specifies in its description of this demanding position.

Although it is difficult, if not impossible, to forecast when and how a new scientific or technological event will affect the supervisory position, every

housestaff
Physicians who serve in a hospital during their internship or fellowship.

supervisor must keep abreast of changes affecting his profession. It is important that supervisors prepare themselves and their employees professionally, scientifically, technologically, and psychologically for changes that occur in the delivery of healthcare. In addition to the medical and scientific breakthroughs, increased automation and its concomitant benefits and challenges will continue to affect all supervisors. Use of electronic health records and wireless handheld units such as personal digital assistants (PDAs) has continued to expand. Supervisors and their staffs have to be familiar with these technologies. While the infusion of technology into our day-to-day activities helps us to treat patients and do our jobs more efficiently, it also provides an avenue for misuse for personal purposes. Access to the latest information on virtually any subject is just a click away on the Internet. Supervisors, however, must be attentive to the time that subordinates spend on the Internet, as they could waste valuable work time or use the Internet for personal purposes.

With a growing, complex society and increasing demands for more sophisticated and better healthcare, the job of any supervisor in the field is likely to become even more challenging. This is true whether her title is health information manager, operating room supervisor, decision support analyst, plant operations foreman, or food service supervisor. The one factor that helps the supervisor cope with all of this responsibility is the continued advancement of her knowledge and skill in the managerial part of the job.

This supervisory position is usually the first in a long career of administrative positions that require increasingly advanced management skills. For instance, a programmer analyst or software engineer may begin his ascent into management as applications manager. After serving in this capacity for some time, he is promoted to network administrator, then to information technology associate administrator, and eventually to the organization's vice president or chief technology officer (CTO).

One may also move up the ladder in a less traditional way. For example, consider the staff nurse selected to manage the preregistration and scheduling activities. After serving successfully in this capacity for some time and establishing good relations with a managed care company, the staff nurse is recruited by a managed care organization to oversee the precertification unit and is given the title of precertification manager. She is then promoted to director of benefit determinations and eventually to assistant vice president for customer service and medical management.

Most of the tens of thousands of managerial positions in healthcare today are filled by healthcare professionals who have not had any formal administrative training or studied management or administration. Therefore, it is essential that the supervisor, department head, or leader learn as much as possible about being a competent first-line manager because that position is likely his first step in the climb up the managerial and administrative ladder.

The Managerial Aspects of the Supervisory Position

The job of a supervisor can be viewed in terms of three essential skills (Katz 1974). First, the good supervisor must possess technical skills, to ensure that she understands the clinical and technical aspects of the work to be done. Next, the supervisor must possess human relations skills, which concern working with and motivating people and understanding individual and group feelings. Finally, the supervisor needs conceptual skills, which enable her to visualize the big picture and to understand how all parts of the organization contribute and coordinate their efforts. The relative degree of importance of all three skills depends on the level of the position within an organization; however, all levels of management require these skills at one time or another.

More recently, other authors have published articles proposing leadership competencies that use the Katz skills as a foundation. Perra (2001) proposed an integrated leadership model promoting staff participation whereby the leader's characteristics included shared vision, participation, communication, and the ability to facilitate change. Contino (2004) identified organizational management, communication, strategic planning, and creative skills as key competencies. Finally, Longest (1998) listed conceptual, technical, interpersonal, and political skills. Each of these authors also identified other skills, but there continues to be a correlation today with those skills Katz defined more than a half century ago.

Let us consider how the skills and roles we have been discussing may apply to the performance of two supervisors. John, a supervisor at Hometown Hospital, often appears harassed, disorganized, and overly involved in doing the job at hand; he muddles through his day and is constantly knee-deep in work. He puts in long hours and never fears doing anything himself. He works exceedingly hard but never seems to have enough time left to actually supervise. Jane, a supervisor at Upstate Hospital, is on top of the job, and her department functions smoothly and in an orderly fashion. She finds time to sit at her desk at least part of each day and keep her desk work up to date. Why is there such a difference between John and Jane?

Some supervisors are more capable or proficient than others. If you compare John and Jane to discover why Jane is on top of her job and John is constantly fixing things himself, you will probably find that Jane understands her job better and has developed subordinate staff to whom she can safely delegate assignments. Assume that both are equally good professionals, both have graduated from reputable health administration programs in the same community and have similar staffing ratios and technology available, and the conditions under which they perform are similar. Jane's results are significantly better than John's because she is simply a better manager. She is able to supervise the functions of her department in a manner that allows her to get the job done through and with the people of her department. The difference between a good supervisor and a poor supervisor, assuming everything else is equal, is the difference in each person's managerial abilities.

However, the managerial aspect of the supervisor's position has long been neglected. Instead, the emphasis has been placed on clinical and technical competence. Many new managers are appointed from the ranks of one of the various professional, clinical, or technical services or trades. As a result of their ingenuity, initiative, and personal drive, they are promoted to the supervisory level and are expected to assume the responsibilities of managing the unit. Little is probably done, however, to acquaint them with these responsibilities or to help them cope with the managerial aspects of the new job. More or less overnight, they are made a part of administration without having been prepared to be a manager. These new managers are oriented by their predecessors, and they learn more from other managers, but some problems are likely. These may be dealt with by a better understanding of the supervisory aspects of the job so that the managers are running the department instead of the department running them.

The aim of this book is to teach individuals to be successful healthcare managers. This does not mean that one can neglect or underestimate the actual work involved in getting the job done. Often, the supervisor is the most skilled individual in the department and can do a more efficient and quicker job than anyone else. He must not be tempted, however, to step in and take over the job, except for purposes of instruction, during extended vacancies, or in case of an emergency. Rather, the supervisor's responsibility is to ensure adequate staffing and to see that the employees can do the job and do so properly. As a manager, the supervisor must plan, guide, and supervise.

The Meaning of Management

The term *management* has been defined in many ways. A meaningful definition for our purposes is the process of getting things done through and with people by directing and motivating the efforts of individuals toward common objectives. You have undoubtedly learned from your own experience that in most endeavors one person alone can accomplish relatively little. For this reason, people have found it expedient and even necessary to join with others to attain the goals of an enterprise. In every organized activity, the manager's function is to achieve the goals of the enterprise with the help of subordinates, peers, and superiors.

Achieving goals through and with people is only one aspect of the manager's job, however; creating a working atmosphere—that is, a climate or a culture in which subordinates can find as much satisfaction of their needs as possible—is also necessary. In other words, a supervisor must provide a climate conducive for the employees to fulfill such needs as recognition, achievement, and companionship. If these needs can be met on the job, employees are more likely to strive willingly and enthusiastically toward the achievement of departmental objectives as well as the overall objectives of the institution. Thus, we must add to our earlier definition of management: the manager's job is getting things done through and with people by enabling them to find as much satisfaction of their needs as possible, and motivating them to achieve both their own objectives and the objectives of the institution. The better the supervisor performs these duties, the better the departmental results are.

You may have noticed by this time that the terms *supervisor*, *manager*, and *administrator* have been used interchangeably. The exact meaning of these titles varies with different institutions, but the terms *administrator* and *executive* are generally used for top-level management positions and *manager*, *leader*, and *supervisor* usually connote positions within the middle or lower levels of the institutional hierarchy. Some theoretical differences may be considered, but for the purposes of this book, these terms are used interchangeably. Furthermore, the use of gender terms—he or she—are not used to the exclusivity of the other.

As you read this book you will discover that the managerial aspects of all supervisory jobs are the same. This is true regardless of the supervisor's department, section, or level within the administrative hierarchy. Thus, the managerial content of a supervisory position is the same whether the position is director of case management, head of environmental services, chief engineer in the maintenance department, or lead clinical dietitian. By the same token, the managerial functions are the same for the first-line supervisor, mid-level manager, or top administrator. In addition, the type of organization in which you work does not matter; managerial functions are the same for a commercial or industrial enterprise, not-for-profit or for-profit organization, professional association, government agency, and hospital or other healthcare facility. Regardless of the activities of the organization, department, or level, the managerial aspects and skills are the same. The difference is in the extent to which or frequency of which a supervisor performs each of the tasks.

Managerial Skills and Technical Skills

Managerial skills must be distinguished from the professional, clinical, and technical skills that are also required of a supervisor. As stated before, all supervisors must also possess special technical skills and professional know-how in their field. Technical skills vary between departments, but any supervisory position requires both professional technical skills and standard managerial skills. Mere technical and professional knowledge is not sufficient.

It is important to note that as a supervisor advances up the administrative ladder, she will rely less on professional and technical skills and more on managerial skills. Therefore, the top-level executive generally uses far fewer technical skills than those who are employed under her. In the rise to the top, however, the administrator has had to acquire all the administrative skills necessary for the management of the entire enterprise.

Consider the following real-life example; the real name of this supervisor has been disguised. John Andrews, an English major in college, taught junior high school. When his teaching salary became inadequate to support his growing family, John joined an insurance company as a claims adjudicator (a base-level position). He noticed abnormalities in some claims from some providers and researched these for his superior. Eventually he was promoted to the fraud investigations unit and ultimately directed that operation until he was promoted to oversee all claims and investigations functions. John interacted well with physicians and insurance representatives alike. As he gained more experience, he began negotiating arrangements with physician groups and hospitals for preferred provider organizations (PPOs) and health maintenance organizations (HMOs). He was selected to be CEO of a national HMO, and was very successful. At each step of his advancement, John built on prior experience and knowledge, but he did not need to personally perform all activities to ensure the success of the HMO. He left the details to his proficient subordinates.

Similarly, the CEO of a healthcare system is concerned primarily with the overall management of hospitals and affiliated clinics, diagnostic centers, and other entities within the system. His functions are almost purely administrative. In this endeavor, the chief executive depends on the administrative, managerial, and technical skills of the various subordinate administrators and managers, including all the first-line supervisors, to get the job done. The CEO, in turn, uses managerial skills in directing the efforts of all these subordinate executives toward the common objectives of the hospital.

How does a supervisor acquire these important managerial skills? First, she must understand that standard managerial skills can be learned. Although good managers, like good athletes, are often assumed to be born, not made, this belief is not based in fact. We cannot deny that people are born with different physiological and biological potentials and that they are endowed with differing amounts of intelligence and many other characteristics; a person who is not a natural athlete is not likely to run 100 yards in record time. Many individuals who are natural athletes, however, have not come close to that goal either.

A good athlete is made when a person with some natural endowment develops it into a mature skill by practice, learning, effort, sacrifice, and experience. The same holds true for a good manager; by practice, learning, and

HOSPITAL LAND

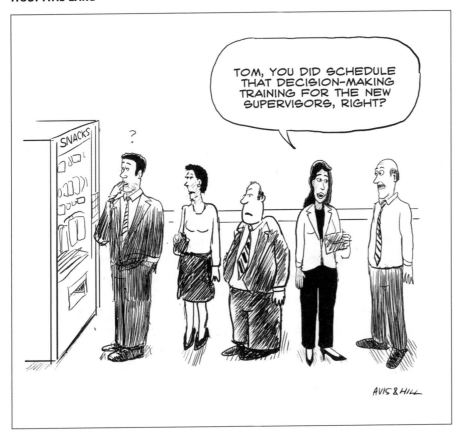

experience she develops this natural endowment of intelligence and leadership into mature management skills. One can learn and practice the skills involved in managing as readily as the skills involved in playing tennis.

If you are an advanced student of healthcare management, or you currently hold a team leader or supervisory position, you likely have the necessary prerequisites of intelligence and leadership and are now ready to acquire the skills of a manager. Developing these skills takes time and effort; they are not acquired overnight.

The most valuable resource of any organization is the people who work there, or the human resources. The first-line supervisor is the person to whom this most important resource is entrusted in the daily working situation. The best use of an organization's human assets depends greatly on the managerial ability and understanding of the supervisor, as manifested by his expertise in influencing and directing them. The supervisor's job is to create a climate of motivation, satisfaction, leadership, and continuous further self-development and self-improvement. This is a challenge to every supervisor, because it means he must also continue to develop as a manager.

Managerial Functions and Authority

The supervisor's managerial role rests on two foundations: managerial functions and managerial authority. **Managerial functions** are those that must be performed by a supervisor for him to be considered a true manager. The concept of authority inherent in the supervisory position is briefly discussed later in this chapter and more extensively throughout the book.

Five managerial functions are described in this book: planning, organizing, staffing, influencing, and controlling the resources of the organization. The resources include people, positions, technology, physical plant, equipment, materials, supplies, information, and money. (The labels used to describe managerial functions vary somewhat in management literature; some textbooks list one more or one less managerial function. Regardless of the terms or number used, the managerial functions are interrelated and goal driven and constitute one of the two major characteristics of a manager.) A person who does not perform these functions is not a manager in the true sense of the word, regardless of title. The following explanation is introductory; most of the book is devoted to the discussion, meaning, and ramifications of each of these five functions.

Planning

Planning involves developing a systematic approach for attaining the goals of the organization. This function consists of determining the goals, objectives, policies, procedures, methods, rules, budgets, and other plans needed to achieve the purpose of the organization. In planning, the manager must contemplate and select a course of action from a set of available alternatives. In other words, planning is laying out in advance the goals to be achieved and the best means to achieve these objectives.

You may have observed supervisors who are constantly confronting one crisis after another. Much like a statement in *Alice in Wonderland*, "If you don't know where you are going, any path will get you there," the probable reason for these crises is that the supervisors did not plan or look ahead. It is every manager's duty to plan; this function cannot be delegated to someone else. Certain specialists may be called on to assist in laying out various plans, but as the manager of the department, the supervisor must make departmental plans. These plans must coincide with the overall objectives of the institution as laid down by higher-level administration. Within the overall directives and general boundaries, however, the manager has considerable leeway in mapping out the departmental course.

Planning must come before any of the other managerial functions. Even after the initial plans are laid out and the manager proceeds with the other managerial functions, the function of planning continues in revising the course of action and choosing different alternatives as the need arises.

Therefore, although planning is the first function a manager must tackle, it does not end at the initiation of the other functions. The manager continues to plan while performing the organizing, staffing, influencing, and controlling tasks.

Organizing

Once a plan has been developed, the manager must determine how the work is to be accomplished—that is, arrange the necessary resources to carry out the plan. The manager must define, group, and assign job duties. Through organizing, the manager determines and enumerates the various activities to be accomplished and combines these activities into distinct groups (e.g., departments, divisions, sections, teams, or any other units). The manager further divides the group work into individual jobs, assigns these activities, and provides subordinates with the authority needed to carry out these activities.

In short, to organize means to design a structural framework that establishes all of the positions needed to perform the work of the department and to assign duties to these positions. Organizing encompasses the following elements:

- *Specialization*: a technique used to divide work activities into easily managed tasks and assign those tasks to individuals based on their skills.
- *Departmentalization*: a technique used to divide activities and people according to the needs of the organization or its customers.
- *Span of management*: a concept that defines the optimum number of subordinates a supervisor can effectively manage.
- *Authority relationships*: a set of theories concerning individuals' rights to make decisions, make assignments, direct activities, and so on regarding managing people, materials, machinery, expenses, and revenues.
- *Responsibility*: the obligation to perform certain duties.
- *Unity of command*: the concept that each individual should have one person to report to for any single activity.
- *Line and staff*: the theory of authority that defines whether one has the authority to direct (a line capacity) or advise (a staff capacity).

These and other factors are discussed throughout the book. The result of the organizing function is the creation of an activity-authority network for the department, which is a subsystem within the total healthcare organization.

Staffing

Staffing refers to the manager's responsibility to recruit and select employees who are qualified to fill the various positions needed. The manager must also remain within the budgeted labor amount for the department.

Besides hiring, staffing involves training employees, appraising their performance, counseling them on how to improve their performance, promoting them, and giving them opportunities for further development. Staffing also includes compensating employees appropriately. In most healthcare institutions, the department of human resources helps with the technical aspects of staffing. The basic authority and responsibility for staffing, however, remain with the supervisor.

Influencing

The managerial function of influencing refers to issuing directives and orders in such a way that staff respond to these directives to accomplish the job. Influencing also means identifying and implementing practices to help the members of the organization work together. This function is also known as leading, directing, or motivating.

It is not sufficient for a manager to plan, organize, and staff. The supervisor must also stimulate action by giving directives and orders to the subordinates, then supervising and guiding them as they work. Moreover, it is the manager's job to develop the abilities of the subordinates by leading, teaching, and coaching or mentoring them effectively. To influence is to motivate one's employees to achieve their maximum potential and satisfy their needs and to encourage them to accomplish tasks they may not choose to do on their own.

Thus, influencing is the process around which all performance revolves; it is the essence of all operations. This process has many dimensions such as employee needs, morale, job satisfaction, productivity, leadership, example setting, and communication. Through the influencing function, the supervisor seeks to model performance expectations and create a climate conducive to employee satisfaction while achieving the objectives of the institution. Much of a manager's time is spent influencing and motivating subordinates.

Controlling

Controlling is the function that ensures plans are followed, that performance matches the plan, and that objectives are achieved. A more comprehensive definition of controlling includes determining whether the plans are being carried out, whether progress is being made toward objectives, and whether other actions must be taken to correct deviations and shortcomings. Again, this relates to the importance of planning as the primary function of the manager. A supervisor could not check on whether work was proceeding properly if there were no plans to check against. Controlling also includes taking corrective action if objectives are not being met and revising the plans and objectives if circumstances require it.

The Interrelationships of Managerial Functions

It is helpful to think of the five managerial functions as the management cycle. A cycle is a system of interdependent processes and activities. Each activity affects the performance of the others. As shown in Exhibit 1.4, the five

EXHIBIT 1.4
Cycle of
Supervisory
Functions

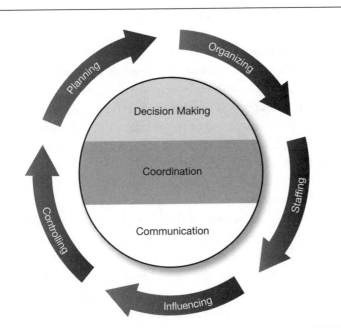

functions flow into each other, and at times there is no clear line indicating where one function ends and the other begins. Because of this interrelationship, no manager can set aside a specific amount of time each day for one or another function. The effort spent on each function varies as conditions and circumstances change. The planning function, however, undoubtedly must come first. Without plans the manager cannot organize, staff, influence, or control. Throughout this book, therefore, we shall follow this sequence of planning first, then organizing, staffing, influencing, and controlling.

Although the five managerial functions can be separated theoretically, in the daily job of the manager these activities are inseparable. The output of one provides the input for another, all as elements of a system.

Universality of the Managerial Functions and Their Relation to Position and Time

Whether as chair of the board, president of the healthcare center, vice president for patient care, or supervisor of the telephone operators, a manager performs all five functions. This idea is known as the principle of *universality of managerial functions*. The time and effort that each manager devotes to a particular function vary, however, depending on the individual's level within the administrative hierarchy.

The CEO is likely to plan, for example, one year, five years, or even ten years ahead. A supervisor is concerned with plans of much shorter duration. At times, a supervisor has to make plans for six or twelve months ahead but more frequently just makes plans for the next month, the next week, or even the next day or shift. In other words, the span and magnitude of plans for the supervisor are smaller.

The same is true of the influencing function. The CEO normally assigns tasks to subordinate managers, delegates authority, and depends on those managers to accomplish tasks. She spends a minimum of time in direct supervision. A first-line supervisor, however, is concerned with getting the job done each day, so he has to spend much time in the influencing or directing function. Similar observations can be made for organizing, staffing, and controlling (Exhibit 1.4).

Managerial Authority

managerial authority
The legal or rightful power of a manager to act or direct others.

The second major characteristic of the managerial position is the presence of authority. Authority is the lifeblood of any managerial position; a person in an organizational setting cannot be a manager without it. Why is authority the primary characteristic of the managerial position? Briefly, **managerial authority** is legal or rightful power—the right to act and to direct others. It is the power by which a manager can ask subordinates to do, or not to do, a certain task that he deems appropriate and necessary to realize the objectives of the department.

One must realize that this kind of organizational authority is part of the formal position a manager holds and is not given to the manager as an individual. This concept of authority must also include the possession of power to impose sanctions when necessary. Without such power to enforce an order, the enterprise could become disorganized and chaos could result. If a subordinate refuses to carry out the manager's directive, managerial authority includes the right to take disciplinary action and possibly to discharge the employee.

This aspect of authority obviously has many restrictions, including legal restrictions; organized labor contracts; organizational policies; and considerations of morals, ethics, social responsibility, and human behavior. For example, legal restrictions and organizational procedures require fulfilling many disciplinary and documentation steps before an employee can be dismissed. Also, every successful manager must take into consideration human behavior in the workplace: to influence and motivate subordinates to perform required duties, it is best not to depend on formal managerial authority but to use other persuasive ways and means to accomplish the job. In other words, it is far better not to depend on the negative aspects of dominance and authority.

In practice, most managers do not speak of authority at all; they prefer to speak of the responsibility, tasks, or duties they have. Such managers are right in saying that they have the responsibility for certain activities instead of saying that they have the authority to get the job done. For a supervisor, however, having authority means having the power and right to issue directives. Once you accept responsibility to oversee a certain project and achieve a certain outcome, you can delegate authority to lower-level staff to complete the project, but you cannot delegate the responsibility. The responsibility lies with you to accomplish the task through proper planning, organizing, staffing, influencing, and controlling.

The discussion in Part IV on the meaning and various other bases of authority sheds additional light on this concept. It examines how subordinates and workers react to authority and how authority is delegated. Delegation of authority means the process by which a supervisor receives authority from the superior manager as well as the process by which some of the authority assigned to this position is delegated to subordinates. Just as authority is the foundation of any managerial position, delegating authority to the lower ranks within the managerial hierarchy makes it possible to build an organizational structure with effective managers on every level.

Authority is discussed more fully throughout this book because it plays such an important role in supervisory management. This concept of formal positional authority eventually becomes a part of an entire spectrum of influence and power. At this point, however, you need only remember that authority is one of the basic characteristics of the managerial job. Without authority, managerial functions and the supervisor–subordinate relationship are weakened and become meaningless.

Expect Surprises

New managers always find challenges and surprises, but even new and seasoned CEOs experience surprises. This text will better prepare both. One need not look further than the role of the U.S. president to see the paradox that the more power you have, the harder it is to use due to the complexity of gaining the support of those who must support your vision (Porter, Lorsch, and Nohria 2004).

New supervisors will find that they cannot single-handedly run their department without the department workers' cooperation. A supervisor does not have enough time to do everyone's job, so he must rely on his employees to do theirs. We will learn in later chapters the art of giving directives or orders and the messages that are received by employees when a directive is given to them. The key to giving orders is to recognize that unilaterally giving orders may trigger resentment and result in demoralization (Porter, Lorsch, and Nohria 2004).

As noted earlier, the supervisor must utilize information he receives to determine next steps. The supervisor who nurtures information channels from peers, subordinates, and superiors will experience fewer surprises.

Finally, supervisors are expected to serve as role models. Those new to their position may find that news about the slightest misstep will spread throughout the department.

Regardless of the challenges and workload that confront you, the new supervisor must balance work and personal needs. The focus of this text is to help you understand your role and provide you with some tools to work through these day-to-day challenges.

Benefits of Better Management

The benefits a supervisor derives from learning to be a better manager are obvious. First, he is given many opportunities to apply managerial principles and knowledge. Good management by a supervisor makes a great deal of difference in the performance of the department: it functions more smoothly, work gets done on time, budget objectives are met, and team members or subordinates enthusiastically contribute to the ultimate objectives.

The application of management principles puts a supervisor on top of her job, instead of being "swallowed up" by it. She also has more time to be concerned with the overall aspects of her department, and in so doing, becomes more valuable to those to whom she is responsible. For example, she is more likely to contribute significant suggestions and advice to her superiors, perhaps in areas about which she has never before been consulted but which ultimately affect her department. In these times of rapid change and facility mergers and acquisitions, she may also find that she sees more easily the complex interrelationships of the various departments and organizations throughout the evolving healthcare system. This, in turn, helps her work in closer harmony with her colleagues who are supervising other departments. In short, she is able to do a more effective supervisory job with much less effort.

In addition to the direct benefits of doing a better supervisory job for her healthcare organization, she may gain other benefits. As a supervisor applying sound management principles, she will grow in stature. As time goes on, she will be capable of handling more important and more complicated assignments. She will advance to better and higher-paying jobs. She will move up within the administrative hierarchy and will naturally want to improve her managerial skills as she advances.

As stated earlier, an additional, satisfying thought is that the functions of management are equally applicable in any organization and in any managerial or supervisory position. That is, the principles of management required to produce memory chips, manage a retail department, supervise office work, or run a repair shop are all the same. Moreover, these principles are applicable not only in the 580,000 healthcare organizations in the United States but in other parts of the world as well (Bureau of Labor Statistics 2008). Aside from local customs and questions of personality, it would not matter whether a supervisor works in a textile mill in India, as a chief chemist in a chemical plant in Italy, as a department foreman in a steel mill in Pittsburgh, or as a supervisor of the patient-focused care unit for trauma care in a hospital in San Francisco. Being a manager means being more mobile in every direction and in every respect.

Therefore, there are great inducements for learning the principles of good management. Again, however, do not expect to learn them overnight. A supervisor can only become a good manager by actually managing—that is, by applying the principles of management to her own work. The supervisor will undoubtedly make mistakes occasionally but will, in turn, learn from those mistakes. The principles and guidelines of management discussed in this book can be applied to most situations, and efforts to become an outstanding manager will pay substantial dividends. As managerial competence increases, many of the errors and difficulties that make a supervisory job a burden instead of a challenging and satisfying task can be prevented.

Summary

The demands on good management in healthcare activities are increasing rapidly, making the role of the supervisor most challenging. To employees in the department, the supervisor represents management. To supervisors in other departments, he is a colleague, coordinating efforts with theirs and sharing information to achieve the organization's objectives. The supervisor must possess technical, human, and conceptual skills; he must have the clinical and technical competence for the functions to be performed in the department and at the same time must manage that department. Good managers are made; they are not born.

Management is the function of getting things done through and with people. The way a supervisor handles the managerial aspects of the job makes the difference between running the department and being run by the department. The managerial aspects of any supervisory job are the same, regardless of the particular type of work involved or the position on the administrative ladder. As a supervisor climbs this ladder, the managerial skills increase in importance and the technical and professional skills gradually become less important. The five managerial functions of planning, organizing, staffing, influencing, and controlling compose the first of the two benchmarks of the manager's job. Each blends into another, and each affects the performance of the others. The output of one provides the input for another. These five functions are universal for all managers, regardless of position in the managerial hierarchy and the nature of the enterprise. The time and effort involved in each function vary, depending on the manager's position on the administrative ladder.

The second benchmark of the managerial job is authority; it makes the managerial position real. This organizational, formal authority is delegated to positions within the organization, permitting those who hold it to make decisions, issue directives, take action, and impose sanctions. To be successful, a manager must recognize that this is a new environment and there will be surprises. However, by embracing the managerial functions and using the authority she has been given, a manager will be able to achieve the goals for which she is responsible. A supervisor benefits greatly both professionally and personally if she takes the time to study and acquire managerial expertise and excellence.

Notes

1. Members of Generation X (born 1965–1979) have embraced free agency over company loyalty. Ambitious, technologically adept, and independent, Gen Xers strive to balance the competing demands of work, family, and personal life (*Holiday Inn Express Navigator* 2000/2001).
2. Organizational settings include any healthcare-related entity, including but not limited to hospitals, nursing homes, clinics, surgical centers, urgent care centers, group model HMOs, physician offices, rehab centers, and home care programs.

Additional Readings

Advisory, Conciliation and Arbitration Service (ACAS). 2008. "Role of the Supervisor." [Online booklet, retrieved 12/27/08.] www.acas.org.uk/index.aspx?articleid=805.

McCrimmon, M. 2008. "The Manager's Role in Modern Business." [Online article; retrieved 9/5/08.] http://businessmanagement.suite101.com/article.cfm/the_managers_role_in_modern_business.

THE THEORIES AND HISTORY OF MANAGEMENT

Chapter Objectives

After you have studied this chapter, you should be able to do the following:

1. Identify the major schools of management theory.
2. Discuss the impact of the Industrial Revolution on management and employee relations.
3. Discuss the features and benefits of organizational development.
4. Distinguish among rational authority, positional authority, and charismatic authority.

Chapter 1 discussed the definition of management as getting activities efficiently accomplished through people. "Efficiently" implies using the least amount of resources to achieve the goal. Chapter 1 encouraged new supervisors to learn as much about management as possible. Although much learning will occur while on the job, some advantages can be gleaned from studying various schools of management thought. This chapter provides an overview of some significant management theories.

These theories touch on each of the five managerial functions: planning, organizing, staffing, influencing, and controlling. New theories are introduced every day, and each serves as a building block for the next. Because of this, management theory will continue to evolve to meet the needs of society. However, management is not a new theory. Egyptian leaders managed thousands of laborers to build the great pyramids. The Chinese built the Great Wall, and the Romans built aqueducts. To be achieved, these projects each required planning, organizing, staffing, influencing, and controlling.

Industrial Revolution (1700s–1800s)

No two countries were more responsible for the Industrial Revolution than the United States and England. In his article, "The Two Countries That Invented the Industrial Revolution," Curt Anderson (2001) points out that during the eighteenth and nineteenth centuries, England had no shortage of skilled labor. When machines were invented to automate certain tasks, few English workers lost their jobs. Instead, the machines made work more precise. By contrast, in the sparsely populated United States, the needs of a new nation required rapid and simple means of production. Machines augmented the scant workforce. Whereas in England machines served to make talented artisans better, machines in the United States served to make entrepreneurs more productive.

The Industrial Revolution changed the manager's job from owner-manager to professional, salaried manager (Robinson 2005). This 18th century phenomenon transformed the United States from an agricultural society to one that manufactured goods at small mills, shops, and factories. The shops became our early organizations—that is, two or more people working together in a structured, formal environment to achieve a common goal. As the 20th century opened, many small shops grew into factories as the inventions, machines, and processes used to manufacture goods advanced, division of labor concepts were applied, and electricity and the internal combustion engine were developed. Ford Motor Company, the Radio Corporation of America (RCA), Bell Telephone and Telegraph, and many other companies emerged during this era.

The church and the military served as models for the management and organization structures of these new entities. Today's managers can find terms (e.g., superior, subordinate, strategy, hierarchy, and mission) in the Bible and in ecclesiastical and military writings that date back to the late 1500s.

Raymond E. Miles's (1978) book, *Theories of Management: Implications for Organizational Behavior and Development*, states that the U.S. management theory evolutional model includes three schools of management theory: classical, human relations, and human resources.

Classical School (1800s–1950s)

The *classical school* of management thought began in the late 1800s and continued through the 1950s. It included such theorists as Henri Fayol, Mary Parker Follett, Henry Gantt, and Max Weber. These theorists believed in structured management approaches, and that money motivates employees. During this era, the concept of "economic man" surfaced. This management school focuses on efficiency and includes bureaucratic, scientific, and administrative management. According to Allen (2000), "Bureaucratic management relies on a rational set of structured guidelines, such as rules and procedures, hierarchy, and a clear division of labor. Scientific management focuses on the 'one best way' to do a job." Fayol, the author of *General and Industrial Management* (1916), is the founder of the classical school of management, which emphasizes "command and control" (Robinson 2005).

Henri Fayol

The man known as the father of modern management was Henri Fayol (1841–1925). Fayol defined *administrative management*, which describes how to structure an organization for high performance and flourished from the early 1800s to the 1920s. Theo Haimann, the original author of this textbook, embraced Fayol's management theory and structured his textbook around it. While other theorists were studying the worker, Fayol was studying the manager. Fayol identified five functions of management: planning, organizing, commanding, coordinating, and controlling. He further categorized the features of management into 14 principles:

1. division of work/labor through specialization,
2. authority and responsibility (including expertise and ability to lead),
3. discipline,
4. unity of command,
5. unity of direction,
6. subordination of individual interests to the organization's needs (pursue only work-related activities at work),
7. employee compensation (Hoffman 2005, 107),
8. centralization (authority based on experience),
9. scalar chain (line of authority),
10. order (all materials and personnel have a designated location)(Hoffman 2005, 107),
11. equity (fair, impartial treatment),
12. personnel stability,
13. initiative (acting without direction from a superior), and
14. esprit de corps (shared devotion to a common cause).

Scientific Management (1890–1940)

Several large industrial organizations had emerged by the turn of the 20th century. Often they included an assembly line method for manufacturing products. *Scientific management* focuses on the relationship between workers and machinery and defines how to organize tasks for people. It was believed that organization productivity would increase by increasing the efficiency of production processes or the production line. Scientific management attempts to create jobs that economize time, human energy, and other productive resources. Jobs are designed so that each worker has a specified, definitive task for which he is responsible and that can be performed as instructed. Workers are not expected to "think," but rather to follow the specific procedures and methods for each job with no exceptions. This school of management theory includes four well-known theorists: Frederick Taylor (1856–1915), Frank (1868–1924) and Lillian (1878–1972) Gilbreth, and Henry Gantt (1861–1919).

Several of the theorists from the classical school became known for their refined management theories.

Frederick Taylor

"Sigmund Freud would have had a field day with Frederick Winslow Taylor. From an early age, he was obsessed with control, and with planning, scheduling and self-regimenting" (Robinson 2005, 32). Many of Taylor's studies were performed at Bethlehem Steel Company in Pittsburgh, Pennsylvania. To improve productivity, Taylor examined the time and motion details of a job; developed a better method for performing that job; scientifically selected, trained, and developed the worker to perform the job (specialization); supported the premise that management and worker would cooperate; and divided work and responsibility equally between managers and workers. Furthermore, Taylor offered piece rates, incentives, and bonuses to increase workers' production.

Taylor (1856–1915), known as the father of scientific management, published *Principles of Scientific Management* in 1911. In his book, he delineated the roles of management and worker and wrote of his method for improving procedures: break a job down into its smallest constituent movements, time each one with a stopwatch, and then redesign the job with a reduced number of motions. Various incentives, including rest periods and a differential pay scale, were recommended to improve output. He also supported the need to develop specialization. Specialists in a task would perform the same duties every day and throughout each day, giving rise to dramatic productivity increases.

His blatant statements about workers, such as "You are not supposed to think. There are other people paid for thinking around here," gained him the reputation as the "enemy of the working man" and caused him to have to defend his system approach before a committee of the U.S. House of Representatives (Robinson 2005).

Frank and Lillian Gilbreth

Frank and Lillian Gilbreth also studied motions used in work. Utilizing motion picture technology, they studied the elemental motions, the way these motions were combined, and the time each motion took. They believed it was possible to design work processes for which times of completion could be estimated in advance (Robinson 2005). Frank Gilbreth is probably best known for his experiments in reducing the number of motions in bricklaying. While Frank Gilbreth captured the title "Father of Time and Motion Studies," his wife Lillian Gilbreth garnered the title "The First Lady of Engineering." The Gilbreths focused on waste—time and movements—and believed that there was only one best way to perform a process. This belief was later refuted by an administrative management theorist, Mary Parker Follett, whose Law of the Situation emphasized that there is no one best way to do anything, but that it all depends on the situation.

From the Gilbreths came the concept *motion study*. In a motion study, work is divided into its most fundamental elements, which are studied separately and in relation to one another. From these examinations, methods of least waste are designed. The Gilbreths also developed *time study*. This is a scientific analysis of methods and equipment used or planned in doing a piece of work, development in detail of the best way of doing it, and determination of the time required.

When the Gilbreths designed a task, they depicted with symbols 17 hand motions (e.g., select, grasp, transport, hold) associated with the task. These symbols were called *therbligs* ("gilbreth" spelled backwards). Interestingly, unions resisted some of Gilbreths' efforts, leaving their union members to use the old, more fatiguing approaches to completing their work.

Henry Gantt (1861–1919) is best known for having developed a scheduling approach that allowed management to view overlapping tasks that needed to occur over a given time. The chart that evolved from this approach became known as a **Gantt chart**. However, Gantt also was associated with Frederick Taylor. Working with Taylor during the time when Taylor was advocating piece payment systems, Gantt's management approach focused on motivating employees with rewards for good work through a base salary coupled with incentive and bonus systems. He also believed in quality leadership and effective management skills—he posited that the organization would benefit as a result of motivated employees and skilled leaders working together.

Henry Gantt

Gantt chart
A chart featuring horizontal bars, each representing the time allotted for a different task of a given project. Seen together, the bars reveal tasks that can be done simultaneously contrasted with those that must be done sequentially.

Bureaucratic Management Theory (1930–1950)

This theory focused on hierarchical structures, assignment of authority, and control. An offshoot of scientific management, the focus was on the structure rather than the employee. Max Weber (1864–1920), known as the father of modern sociology, analyzed bureaucracy as the most logical and rational structure for large organizations. He defined three types of authority: (1) **rational authority** is based on law, procedures, and rules; (2) **positional authority** of a superior over a subordinate stems from legal authority; and (3) **charismatic authority** stems from the personal qualities of an individual. Weber believed that efficiency in bureaucracies came from the following (Allen 2000):

- clearly defined and specialized functions,
- use of legal authority,
- hierarchical form of the organization,
- written rules and procedures,
- technically trained bureaucrats,
- appointment to positions based on technical expertise,
- promotions based on competence, and
- clearly defined career paths.

rational authority
Authority based on law, procedures, and rules.

positional authority
Authority of a superior over a subordinate.

charismatic authority
Authority stemming from the personal qualities of an individual.

Many of these principles are discussed further in the chapters that follow. In summary, both Fayol and Taylor were task- and thing-oriented. The Gilbreths were process-oriented, and Weber focused on structure and rules. Little attention focused on the needs of people—that is, the workers (Hoffman 2005).

Human Relations Movement (1930–Present)

This school of management theory, also known as behavioral management or neoclassical organization theory, emerged in the 1920s and emphasized how managers should behave and recognized workers as "social men." The Hawthorne Studies were undoubtedly the catalyst and most significant contribution to the *human relations movement*. The Hawthorne studies were conducted from 1924 to 1933 at the Hawthorne plant of the Western Electric Company in Cicero, Illinois (Allen 2000).

Hawthorne effect
The phenomenon that people change their behavior when they know they are being studied.

The Hawthorne studies are important to today's management because they emphasize the effect that other humans have on worker productivity. These studies were conducted by several Harvard Business School researchers, including T. N. Whitehead, Elton Mayo, George Homans, and Fritz Roethlisberger. It was Elton Mayo who identified the **Hawthorne effect** as the change that occurs when people know they are being studied.

The studies included interviews with the workers to determine the effects that various working conditions might have on productivity. One decision was to raise the level of lighting; this indeed resulted in an increase in productivity. However, for the control group of this study, the level of lighting was decreased, which resulted in an increase in productivity as well. The conclusion was that the lighting had no influence on productivity whatsoever. Instead, the increased attention from the interviewers to the employees was the catalyst for the increased productivity.

Other studies were pursued with varying degrees of interviewing, direct supervision from the research team, team projects, and involvement of the employees in the design of the activities to be studied, leading to similar conclusions that essentially defined worker attitude as a key element in productivity. Giving attention to employees is much more effective for increasing productivity than changing the working condition. The studies also showed that informal leadership exists and that work groups informally establish acceptable output levels for all workers within the group, regardless of monetary incentives offered. These findings encourage supervisors to recognize the informal organization within the formal organization and to listen to employees' complaints as they are probably a symptom of some underlying problem on the job, at home, or in the person's past. In short, Elton Mayo discovered through the Hawthorne studies that the informal organization and sentiments of the group determine work behavior.

Interestingly, H. A. Simon (1997, originally published 1945) made an important contribution to these experiments when he proposed a model of "limited rationality." The theory states that workers respond unpredictably to managerial attention, which indeed they did to the Hawthorne researchers.

Another human relations theorist, Chester Barnard (1886–1961) is best known for his acceptance theory and strategy planning emphasis. Barnard taught that the three top functions of the executive were to (1) establish and maintain an effective communication system, (2) hire and retain effective personnel, and (3) motivate those personnel. His **acceptance theory of authority** states that managers only have as much authority as employees allow them to have. This suggests that authority flows downward but depends on acceptance by the subordinate, which depends on four conditions: (1) employees must understand what the manager wants them to do, (2) employees must be able to comply with the directive, (3) employees must think that the directive is in keeping with organizational objectives, and (4) employees must think the directive is not contrary to their personal goals (Allen 2000).

acceptance theory of authority
The theory that managers only have as much authority as subordinates allow them to have.

Human Resources School (1950–Present)

Beginning in the early 1950s, the introduction of the *human resources school* of management theory represented a substantial progression from the human relations, or behavioral, school. The behavioral approach did not always increase productivity. Thus, motivation and leadership techniques became a topic of great interest. Abraham Maslow's studies were inspired by this school of thought and his research into human behavior illuminated the relationship between human needs and motivation. The human resources school understands that employees are creative and competent and that much of their talent is largely untapped by their employers. Unlike the perception Taylor had of employees, this school believed that employees want meaningful work; they want to contribute; and they want to participate in decision making and leadership functions (Allen 2000). The notion that there is a reciprocal relationship between organization prosperity and worker prosperity served as the impetus for human resources departments in many organizations.

Both the human relations and human resources theories were encouraged by unions and government regulations that reacted to the rather dehumanizing effects of the earlier scientific management and bureaucratic theories. These later theories spawned further schools based on McGregor's Theories X and Y, and Theory Z, which are discussed in further detail in chapters 11, 22, and 24. Briefly, these theories hold the following beliefs:

Theory X: People are lazy and irresponsible, inherently dislike work, must be controlled to do work, and prefer to be directed.

Theory Y: People are responsible, enjoy work, view it as natural as play and rest, exercise self-direction, seek responsibility, and work well if rewarded.

Theory Z: People will be productive when the work environment encourages group consensus and decision making, there are assurances of long-term employment, and there is a continued emphasis on quality improvement.

Contemporary Management Theories (1940s–Present)

Four contemporary management theories developed during the latter half of the 1900s due to the rapidly changing nature of organizational environments. They are the *contingency theory* offered initially by Mary Parker Follett and more recently by Alfred Chandler, Paul Lawrence and Jay Lorsch, Geert Hofstede, and Fred E. Fielder; the *systems theory* by Ludwig von Bertalanffy; *management as a discipline* defined by Peter Drucker and Henry Mintzberg; and the *chaos theory* touched upon by Tom Peters and discussed by Judy Petree.

Contingency Theory (mid-1960s)

This theory's roots are from the Classical School era, and it is espoused by Mary Parker Follett's Law of the Situation, which states that there is no one best way to do anything, but that the best method depends on the situation. Mary Parker Follett (1868–1933), a political scientist, folded her beliefs of democracy into her management thinking and advocated for jointly shared power in society and the workplace (Graham 1995).

Somewhat related to the contingency theory is Geert Hofstede's cultural differences theory. Hofstede's research suggests that management approaches vary across the world. His observations indicate that in Japan a group management approach is preferred and in the Dutch countries, a consensual relationship is dominant. Additionally, managers are selected for different traits in different countries. For example, in Germany, the technical qualifications of the individual are considered first and foremost, whereas in the United States, a cultural hero is preferred (Robinson 2005). With these variations, Follet's premise that workplace management options depend on the circumstances appears accurate.

Alfred Chandler, a Harvard Business School professor, studied four large U.S. corporations and proposed that an organization would naturally evolve to meet the needs of its strategy—that is, form follows function (Walonick 2009). A contemporary version of the "It Depends" theory is the *contingency theory*. Argued by Fred E. Fielder in 1965, management uses contingency theory when it selects an approach that takes into account all aspects

HOSPITAL LAND

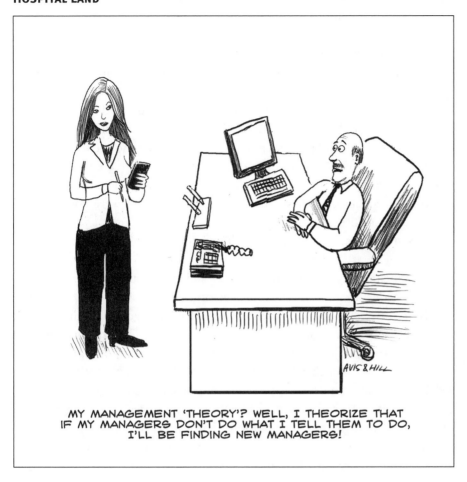

MY MANAGEMENT 'THEORY'? WELL, I THEORIZE THAT IF MY MANAGERS DON'T DO WHAT I TELL THEM TO DO, I'LL BE FINDING NEW MANAGERS!

of the current situation and factors faced by the organization. These factors or variables include organization size, task complexity, environmental uncertainty, and individual differences. Paul Lawrence and Jay Lorsch (1967) studied highly volatile industries and noted the importance of giving managers at all levels the authority to make decisions over their domain, contingent on the current situation. Still today, some call the contingency theory the "It Depends" theory.

Systems Theory (1940–Early 1990s)

The **systems theory** depicts the organization as a collection of open systems that constantly interact with the external environment and receive resources and inputs from that environment, transforming them into goods and products or services that are put back into the environment for consumption. Systems provide feedback to the inputs, processes, outputs, and outcomes. A functioning automobile, for example, is a system. The engine's spark plugs create a spark that ignites the gasoline. This ignition creates an explosion,

systems theory
The concept that an organization is a collection of open systems that constantly interact with the external environment.

which pushes the piston down, propelling the various components that create the movement of the vehicle. The failure of any of these actions serves as "feedback" to the driver as well as to the automobile "system." Thus, a car that has no gasoline cannot operate.

Applying this scenario to the healthcare environment, we find many systems to consider, such as the emergency department. Patients arrive in the emergency department, register for services, are triaged based on their condition, and are treated. If registration or triaging (inputs) are delayed, treatment (output) is delayed, and the patient's condition may deteriorate (outcome). If the registration information does not pass correctly to triage (process), the triage (process) cannot occur. Patients return to the registration desk and complain (feedback), or physicians complain that patients were not appropriately triaged (feedback).

Systems theory was first developed in the 1940s by the biologist Ludwig von Bertalanffy (1951) and served as a foundation for more advanced theories, including general systems theory and cybernetics. *Cybernetics* studies the flow of communication within a complex organization. Systems theory also is closely related to chaos theory, which may have gotten its launch from a systems theory cousin known as catastrophe theory. *Catastrophe theory* is a branch of mathematics that deals with dynamical systems and originated with the work of the French mathematician Rene Thom in the 1960s (Thom 1972). It studies and classifies phenomena characterized by sudden shifts in behavior that arise from small changes in circumstances, analyzing how the qualitative nature of equation solutions depends on the parameters that appear in the equation. For example, the timing and magnitude of a landslide are seemingly unpredictable (Parker 2008).

management by objective (MBO)
A performance measurement approach whereby the manager and his/her superior establish objectives and departmental targets. The manager's performance is evaluated on his/her department's success in achieving the targets or producing the results.

Management as a Discipline Theory (1940s–Present)

Two well-known present-day theorists dominate this space—Peter Drucker (1909–2005) and Henry Mintzberg (1939–).

Peter Drucker, widely known as the "father of modern management," held a visible position in the field of management theory for more than 60 years. Unlike Fayol, he was not a command and control proponent, rather he supported simplification and decentralization. In his book *Concept of the Corporation*, he asserted that management was not a rank or a title, but a responsibility and a practice (Robinson 2005). He stressed management fundamentals such as strategic planning and **management by objective (MBO)** or by results and asserted that management is a discipline, not a science. His concept of MBO should be credited for some of the emphasis on quality improvement because it established objectives or targets for employees to achieve measurements or matrixes often tied to performance. It kept people focused on producing results (Hoffman 2005, 122). His 1999 book,

Management Challenges for the 21st Century, clarified management's role: "One does not 'manage' people." Management's task is "to lead people. And the goal is to make productive the specific strengths and knowledge of each individual" (Geldart 1999).

Chaos Theory (1960s–Present)

The roots of **chaos theory** are found in the study of astronomy and mathematics circa 1850. Management theorists, such as Tom Peters, picked up the thoughts of these early times in the 1960s. Chaos theory recognizes that the world is unorganized and filled with unpredictable events; therefore, organizational events cannot always be controlled and managers must recognize that they will be faced with unusual challenges. Consider what healthcare managers faced when Hurricane Katrina devastated the Gulf Coast. Chaos theory depicts the organization as a living adaptive system of highly random movements that are robust and interact in a narrow space between stability and disorder, or poised at "the edge of chaos" (see, for example, Fitzgerald and Eijnatten 2002).

> **chaos theory**
> The theory that the world is unorganized and events are unpredictable; thus, managers must recognize that events cannot always be controlled.

Chaos theory is also known as "sensitive dependence." The environment is sensitive to changes in initial conditions. Just a small change in the conditions in which people work or live may result in drastically different long-term behavior of a group of employees or a community. Many long-term employees who lived in New Orleans, Biloxi, and other Gulf Coast communities never returned to work, but instead left the area permanently to find a safer environment for themselves and their families. Chaos theorists suggest that systems naturally go to more complexity, and as they do so, these systems become more volatile and must expend more energy to maintain that complexity. As hospitals attempted to reopen and rebuild following Katrina's disaster, these facilities were not only faced with huge capital outlays but also human resources replacement.

Under chaos theory, as organizations or systems expend more energy, they seek more structure to maintain stability. This trend continues until the system splits, combines with another complex system, or falls apart entirely. Sound familiar? This trend is what many see as they go through life, in organizations, and the world in general (McNamara 1999).

Consider the energy that is being spent on airport and building security post September 11, 2001, when the World Trade Center in New York and the Pentagon in Washington, DC, were attacked with hijacked airplanes. The increased efforts have been implemented to maintain the sense of security that Americans enjoy and expect. Unfortunately, the level of security in the United States prior to 9/11 failed with devastating results, creating chaos. This led to increased security measures (imposed by both citizens and the federal government), causing chaos of a different kind—that which comes with a change in procedures.

According to Judy Petree (2001), "For thousands of years humans have noted that small causes could have large effects and that it was hard to predict anything for certain." Because chaos theory is so broad and can be applied to situations every day, supervisors must recognize that even slight changes to a work environment may create chaos. Consider this real experience: A small rural hospital needed additional space for its growing surgical services. The solution was to scan all of the paper medical records, thus freeing up significant square footage to accommodate the relocation of staff and create an additional surgical recovery and prep area. The health information clerk who for 12+ years was responsible for maintaining the paper files, including retrieving them and refiling them, had limited computer skills. Several weeks prior to and after the change, the clerk was disoriented, had several days of absence, and was ill. Adapting to this change was difficult and created "chaos" for the clerk and her coworkers who had to pick up her duties during her absences. Similarly, the replacement or modification of a computer application (such as the installation of a new electronic records management system) can create challenges.

Chaos theory has a direct relationship with Bowen's family theory. Managers must recognize that employees establish "families" at work. Employees often spend more waking time with their coworkers than with the significant other they chose or their biological families. Hence, the coworkers become the "away from home" family. According to Murray Bowen, M.D. (1913–1990), the connectedness and reactivity make the functioning of family members interdependent. A change in one person's functioning is predictably followed by reciprocal changes in the functioning of others. Families differ somewhat in the degree of interdependence, but it is always present to some degree (The Bowen Center 2008). Referring back to both of the examples above, we can see how the familial ties can contribute to chaos in the workplace.

Organizational Development (Late 1950s–Present)

Organizations bring two or more people together in a formal, structured environment to achieve a common goal. By bringing individuals together, the organization serves as a social system wherein its participants use technology and work processes to achieve the goals of the organization. Thus, the long-term health and performance of the organization is directly related to enriching the environment and lives of the organization's participants. As a result, the participants are encouraged to provide input and suggestions on how to improve the environment.

organizational development
A process that seeks to increase the "health" of social and technical systems such as work processes, communication, and shared goals.

Organizational development (OD) works by increasing the "health" of social and technical systems such as work processes, communication, rewards, and shared goals. The key to the OD focus is the organization culture: shared beliefs, values, and behaviors (Zatz 2004). OD focuses on people issues, because people drive systems and systems affect people. Consider the motivation level of an employee who takes drive-up orders at a fast-food restaurant, the communications system of which is malfunctioning, crackling, and squawky. Will that employee be motivated to provide superior customer performance when the systems he has to work with are inadequate?

Characteristics of the OD approach include using a systems viewpoint; emphasizing the culture; and using methods that increase motivation, encourage removing obstacles, and help staff deal with change. OD allows people to influence systems that influence them. Employee suggestions are encouraged and implemented, often dramatically increasing quality by changing the system and allowing the individual to reach optimal effectiveness. Younger workers who were raised in an environment that encouraged participation in decision making about what to wear, what kinds of gifts are desired, where to go on vacation, and so on will continue to expect this approach in their work environment. OD accommodates the younger workforce by nurturing participation. Furthermore, OD helps organizations in the following ways (Zatz 2004):

- empowering leaders and individual employees,
- creating a culture of continuous improvement and alignment around shared goals,
- making change easier and faster,
- putting the minds of all employees to work,
- enhancing the quality and speed of decisions,
- making conflict constructive instead of destructive, and
- giving leaders more control over results by giving employees more control over how they do their jobs.

The outcomes of organizational development may include increases in the following (Zatz 2004):

- profits (or cost reduction for nonprofit organizations);
- innovation;
- customer satisfaction;
- product and service quality;
- cost effectiveness;
- organization flexibility;
- personal feelings of effectiveness; and
- job, work, and life satisfaction.

Many theorists have contributed ideas to enhance the understanding of the role of manager. Later chapters explore these and other schools of thought. Events will vary and the needs of the organization will guide you to select some components of one theory and some components of another to address different situations you face during your career.

Entrepreneurial Theory (1970s–Present)

Throughout the workday, a supervisor encounters many different personalities and situations. The healthcare supervisor needs to apply the contingency theory approach to management, possibly applying scientific management to one situation while using chaos theory to address another. A supervisor should not assume that he must use just one of these theories all the time—that will not work.

With the age range of today's worker, a department may have a 17-year-old and a 60-year-old working side by side. The younger employee may enjoy working within a self-directed team, while the older worker may prefer to do her job as she has loyally done for many years.

When we discuss the traits of our X, Y, and millennial generations, we see greater appreciation of teams and self-recognition. This is why the concept of a learning organization surfaced in the 1990s and continues today. The learning organization focuses on problem solving by teams, where employees routinely share ideas and information. When larger firms fail to provide opportunities for autonomy or to reward individual contributions, the organizations lose some of their best thinkers and workers. These individuals seek the intimacy of teams (Stine 2008); break away from the mold of "we've always done it that way"; and establish their own, smaller, innovative subcultures within the organization or their own entities outside the organization. Enter the entrepreneurial school of management.

entrepreneurial theory
The concept that individuals or small groups of individuals who are "ahead of the curve" should be rewarded and encouraged to work autonomously.

My definition of **entrepreneurial theory** may differ from others who espouse this theory, such as C. B. Handy or W. H. Bergquist. I base my description of this theory on experience and tend to side with F. A. Lins. My work with healthcare organizations for 30 years has shown that there is always one (or more) individual who is slightly ahead of the curve. Ignored by his superiors, the individual has two choices—conform with the status quo or break away. I have seen too much talent lost by healthcare organizations that are not willing to consider a new approach.

In the 1980s, I met a gentleman who thought the then quality assurance rage was a waste of time because it monitored what had happened and then retrospectively studied trends, rather than demanding excellence and requiring an explanation as well as modification of the process when excellence was not achieved. The process might have been chicken-or-egg, but the reaction was, "we're human, we can't expect excellence." His position was that we should expect excellence because we are human, allowing us to think before blindly doing. Of course, today, the Six Sigma approach to quality is exactly what my 1980s gentleman was espousing. Today's employees do not blindly follow. If management is to be successful, management must seek new approaches and establish flexible organizations that can rapidly change through support relationships in order to survive.

Within all organizations are entrepreneurs waiting to be heard. When they are not, they may leave and create privately owned organizations with an environment marked by personal interaction and brainstorming. They will not be held back by complex bureaucracies. In healthcare, we see this happen when clinicians get frustrated with burdensome scheduling processes. Rather than continue to deal with it, they join together and open their own facility, such as clinician-owned surgery centers or MRI services. Talented supervisors quit their jobs to start billing and consulting companies. Tired of not being listened to, these individuals take the entrepreneurial leap and are often successful at doing so.

So what does entrepreneurial management theory tell us? It suggests that we encourage team building but not necessarily force its development; foster sharing and testing of new ideas; listen to our customers, which include our employees; and recognize that we must be willing to accept and possibly financially support some of these ideas or find ourselves buying the services from former employees in the future.

Summary

The Industrial Revolution changed the way we work and live; it brought together technology and people. By doing so, organizations were created. As organizations developed, so did their structures and their members' roles.

The classical school of management thought began in the late 1800s and focuses on efficiency, including bureaucratic, scientific, and administrative theories of management. Bureaucratic management relies on a rational set of structured guidelines, whereas scientific management focuses on the "one best way" to do a job. Administrative management emphasizes the flow of information within the organization.

The human relations and human resources schools of management recognize the need to involve employees in decision making; those employees must also have talents that should be tapped to further the organization's goals. Ironically, these schools spawned opposite theories (Theory X and Theory Y) of the worker's attitude toward work.

Contemporary management theories recognize the rapidly changing environment in which organizations do business and that these organizations may cross multiple continents, many cultures, and various languages, all of which must come together to keep the system functioning. As these organizations expand, a manager must understand that by bringing individuals together, the organization serves as a social system in which its participants use technology and work processes to achieve the goals of the organization. Organizational development has been successful in recent times because management and employees improve work processes, communicate, participate in rewards, and share goals. However, if organizations become so large that their bureaucracy stifles innovation, the innovators will leave and seek smaller, less complex environments within which they can achieve intimacy and incubate new ideas.

Additional Readings

McNamara, C. 1997–2008. "Very Brief History of Management Theories." [Online information; retrieved 12/27/08.] Authenticity Consulting LLC. http://managementhelp. org/mgmnt/history.htm.

Tanz, J. 2003. "A Brief History of Management." [Online article; retrieved 12/27/08.] CNN Money.com. http://money.cnn.com/magazines/fsb/fsb_archive/2003/ 10/01/353427/index.htm.

CONNECTIVE PROCESSES

DECISION MAKING

Chapter Objectives

After you have studied this chapter, you should be able to do the following:

1. Discuss the importance of decision-making skills.
2. Discuss how problem solving and decision making are the essence of all managerial activities.
3. Explain the difference between programmed and non-programmed decisions.
4. Discuss five basic steps of the decision-making process.
5. Describe different decision-making approaches.

If practicing managers were asked to define in one or two words the essence of their jobs, they probably would reply "making decisions." Decision making is the core of all managerial activities; in fact, it is a substantial part of everybody's daily activities. All of us have to solve problems at one time or another; decision making is a basic human activity that begins in early childhood and continues through life.

Decision making can be defined as the process of selecting one choice from a number of alternatives. Decisions are an integral part of all five managerial functions, but they are most closely associated with the planning function. Although the manager acts within an organizational environment, in this book managerial decision making is considered an individual process.

At the heart of this process is the individual manager, whose decisions are influenced by many other people; various departments; the total organization; and a multitude of other factors such as the economy, the technology available, governmental requirements, and politics. Considering all of these influences, the manager uses decision making to connect planning with his organizing efforts, and organizing efforts with staffing determinations. The manager then uses a variety of approaches to motivate the staff to achieve what was originally intended by the decisions, modifying the plan as necessary during the controlling process.

Programmed and Non-Programmed Decisions

programmed decisions
Decisions that pertain to repetitive, structured, and routine problems that have fixed answers and standardized operating procedures, methods, rules, and regulations.

Many decision-making situations that confront us in our daily lives are not difficult to resolve because we are familiar with the issues and have a standard solution for them. These decisions are called **programmed decisions** because they refer to repetitive, structured, routine problems that have fixed answers and standardized operating procedures, methods, rules, and regulations.

For instance, a staff nurse finds that a patient in the postoperative care unit has an elevated temperature. To verify this, the nurse measures the temperature again with a different thermometer. The thermometer registers the same temperature. The nurse knows that in this situation, protocol dictates that she check the patient's temperature again after a period of time; she does so, and the results come up the same. Next the nurse determines whether the attending surgeon left orders to cover this problem; if not, she automatically decides to consult the physician for further action or use the designated treatment protocol for such a situation. The staff nurse has made several decisions up to this point—programmed decisions based on standard procedure.

operations research
The use of mathematical models, analytical methods, or structured inquiry to analyze a complex situation and identify the optimal approach.

For many decision-making situations, operations research has greatly aided in developing programmed decisions. **Operations research** is closely aligned with systems analysis and is defined as the use of mathematical models, analytical methods, or structured inquiry to analyze a complex situation and identify the optimal approach. For instance, an operations researcher investigated the supplies purchasing procedures of a medical center, from the point an item was used by a clinician to the point the replacement was purchased and restocked. Based on this information, the researcher developed a computer program that identified the ideal reorder point for each item the hospital uses, and the appropriate quantity to reorder. In an advanced organization, the actual human purchasing agent may not even be involved with this order; it may be electronically transmitted to the preferred vendor or to a vendor that offers the lowest current bid price.

However, supervisors are frequently confronted with new or unusual problems—decision-making situations for which no standard solutions exist and no program or protocol has been designed. These new problems, the dimensions and ramifications of which are not known or obvious, call for the making of **non-programmed decisions**. Although programmed decision situations occur more frequently than non-programmed problems, the supervisor is constantly called on to come up with a solution for each.

non-programmed decisions
Decisions pertaining to situations for which no standard solutions or protocols exist.

In all instances, the manager should use a logical, rational, and consistent decision-making process. When the problem being presented could affect other departments or areas, the supervisor should involve colleagues from those areas, if time permits for such team decision making. The following discussions are directed to these non-programmed decision-making situations.

The Importance of Decision-Making Skills

Problems arise when an unexpected occurrence takes place. Supervisors are called on to find practical solutions to problems that are caused by changing situations or unusual circumstances. Normally they are able to arrive at a satisfactory decision; they probably became supervisors because they made many more correct decisions than wrong decisions during their careers.

All managers at all levels make decisions. Decisions are not made in a vacuum because each one can affect the entire system. Consider the CEO of a large healthcare system who has seen the system grow and add a broad array of services—a comprehensive continuum of care—only to find his system experiencing significant losses as a result of new prospective payment systems and government auditing initiatives. He (and his board of trustees and administrative team) must now make some difficult decisions under the axiom "better shed than red" (Gee 2000, 152). Many executives in many industries made similar decisions during the recession years of 2008 and 2009.

All managers go through the same process of decision making, though the decisions made at the top of the administrative hierarchy are usually more far reaching and affect more people and areas than decisions made by a first-line supervisor. Decision making is an essential process that permeates the entire administrative hierarchy and all five managerial functions (planning, organizing, staffing, influencing, and controlling). This is why it is included in this section on connective processes (see Exhibit 1.4).

As with managerial skills, decision-making skills can be learned and, once learned, provide great benefits for the manager. Moreover, a manager's job involves not only making decisions herself but also seeing that members of her team make and understand decisions effectively.

Obviously, a supervisor cannot make all the decisions necessary for running the department. Thus, he delegates much of the daily decision making to team members who are closer to the work and have more intimate knowledge of the processes than he has. This requires him to teach his team members the process of making decisions.

Steps in the Decision-Making Process

The decision-making process involves several steps, which must be taken in the following sequence:

1. Define the problem.
2. Analyze the problem.
3. Develop alternatives.
4. Evaluate the alternatives, and select the best.
5. Take action, and follow up.

Decision making is a continuous process. Each manager learns something new from each decision made. Each decision opens up a wide array of new factors and questions that managers can stow away in their "programmed" databases for use in making the next decision.

Define the Problem

You may have heard a supervisor say, "I wish I had the answer." Instead of seeking an answer, however, the supervisor should be looking for the real problem.

The first task in decision making is always to define the problem; only then can one work toward the solution or the answer. As the saying goes, "There really is nothing as useless as having the right answer to the wrong question." In most cases, defining the problem is difficult. What often appears to be the problem might be merely a symptom; in those cases, one must dig deeper to locate the real problem. Consider a supervisor confronted with a problem of two employees who often quarrel and cannot get along. It appears that the employees simply suffer from a personality conflict. Upon examination, however, the supervisor finds that the problem is not one of personalities, but rather that the functions and duties of each employee have never really been defined or delineated. Only after the true nature of the problem has been realized can the supervisor do something about it. In the case of the quarreling coworkers, the chances are good that once the activities and duties of the two employees are delineated, the friction between them will stop.

Here's another scenario: A supervisor in a hospital's health information management (HIM) department notices that many patient records are not being properly updated when new reports and test results arrive. When she studies the situation, however, she discovers that the improper updating is simply a symptom of several conditions: (1) many reports automatically print to the patient care areas but are simultaneously replicated in the electronic health record (EHR); (2) the unit staff have not been trained to distinguish between those documents that are and are not stored in the EHR so they hesitate to file any; and (3) the reports lack any status indication, such as "original—file in patient record" versus "this file already stored online."

In this scenario, the supervisor needs to take a three-pronged approach to resolve the problem:

1. Inventory the reports that print to the floor, and determine which simultaneously go into the patient EHR.
2. Meet with information systems to develop a header or footer message that alerts the patient care unit staff which reports are not replicated in the EHR, so they know that they must file those.
3. Meet with the patient care staff to ensure they understand which records need to be filed and which do not need to be filed.

Defining a problem such as this may be a time-consuming chore, but it is time well spent. The process of decision making cannot proceed further until the problem or problems are clearly defined. Clearly defining the problem cannot always be done from an office. Supervisors need to query staff and study processes to identify the problem completely.

After the problem, not just the symptoms, has been defined, the manager can analyze it. The first step in this analysis is to assemble the facts. The supervisor decides how relevant the existing data are and what additional information may be needed. The supervisor then gathers as much of that information as possible. In the HIM example, the supervisor may need to receive and review all improperly updated reports for a period of time to determine the source of each piece (e.g., patient care units; ancillary service areas; external sources such as physician offices, other hospitals, home health agencies) before deciding on a pathway for correction.

Analyze the Problem

Many supervisors complain, however, that they never have enough facts. This complaint is often just an excuse to delay a decision, because a manager can never have all the facts. Therefore, supervisors must make decisions using the available facts.

It is also wise to consider the behavioral impact on problem definition and to remember that what is believed to be a fact may be colored by subjectivity. As much as we may want to exclude prejudice and bias, we are only human, and subjectivity creeps into any assessment, especially because employees are involved. Of course, we should make an effort to be as objective and impersonal as possible.

This process of analysis, however, requires the supervisor to think not only of objective considerations but also of intangible factors. These factors are difficult to assess and analyze, but they play a significant role, especially in healthcare institutions. Such intangibles may be factors of reputation, quality of patient care, morale, discipline, perception, or ethics. It is hard to be specific about such factors, but they should nevertheless be considered in analyzing the problem. The HIM scenario displays an excellent example of intangible factors. If a blood test was run on a patient and the results from the outside laboratory were sent to the patient care unit but not posted on the record, the physician would be unable to find the results, forcing him to re-order the test. The patient would be stuck twice with a needle, the lab would incur twice the cost, care would be delayed, and the payer would be charged two times. Worse yet, under the Office of the Inspector General's (OIG) compliance initiative this occurrence could be considered "waste" and result in a fine to the organization.

You should understand that no one person can have all the answers; you will be wise to seek input from others such as peers, subordinates, and your boss. "Top performance demands the joint effort of many people, working together toward a common goal. When an individual works together with others, effectiveness grows, creating greater productivity for everyone involved," says Gemmy Allen (2000) in her writings on consensus building. This approach to making decisions is imperative, especially when the decisions may affect another department.

Develop Alternatives

After defining and analyzing the problem, the manager's next step is to search for and develop alternative courses of action and solutions. An absolute rule is to develop as many alternatives as possible. Always bear in mind that the final decision can only be as good as the best of the alternatives you have considered. Any given situation should offer at least several alternatives. These choices may not always be obvious, but it is the duty of the decision maker to search for them. Also, some of the alternatives may not be desirable, but the manager should not decide this until all of them have been carefully considered. If this is not done, an either-or style of thinking may prevail. The type of manager who thinks this way is too easily inclined to see only one of two alternatives as the right one to follow.

Consider the following situation. A surgi-center's patient billing policy states that accounts with a balance of $15 or less will be written off after 90 days, and three notices will be sent to the patient asking for payment. Balances in excess of $15, however, will be turned over to a collection agency after the 90-day/three-notice course. A patient with a balance of $15.02 receives an aggressive call from a collection agency and in response calls the surgi-center's CEO. Even in this unpleasant dilemma, several alternatives exist, although none of them is completely desirable.

First, the surgi-center could insist on having the patient cooperate with the collection agency to pay the bill, although this would further irritate the patient. Second, a payment arrangement could be developed that requires the patient to pay the center directly, possibly causing a rift with the collection agency. Third, the center could write off the charge and implement a process to review accounts within a certain window of the collection agency referral threshold, say 10 percent, and handle these with a personal call before transferring them to the collection agency.

It is not enough for you as a supervisor to decide among the various alternatives presented by subordinates. The alternatives your staff suggest may not include all the possible choices. It is your job as a manager to think of more, and possibly better, alternatives. Even in the most discouraging situations several choices exist, and although none of them may be desirable, the manager still has an obligation to find the best solution.

Brainstorming is a tool often used to increase creativity in problem solving. If the problem is particularly vexing and if time permits, a brainstorming session with other supervisors or employees is a good method for coming

HOSPITAL LAND

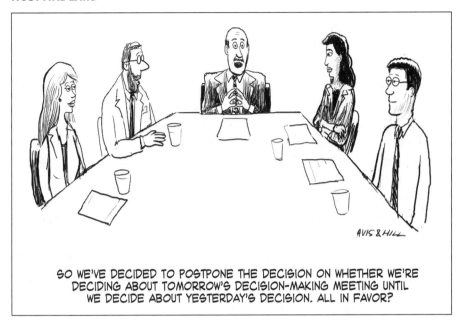

SO WE'VE DECIDED TO POSTPONE THE DECISION ON WHETHER WE'RE DECIDING ABOUT TOMORROW'S DECISION-MAKING MEETING UNTIL WE DECIDE ABOUT YESTERDAY'S DECISION. ALL IN FAVOR?

up with as many alternatives as possible. This session is likely to result in novel, unusual, and unorthodox alternative solutions.

Brainstorming is discussed later in this book. Note, however, that in any brainstorming session the participants must feel free to contribute as many alternatives as possible, no matter how extreme and wild they may seem. Even the wildest idea may have a grain of usefulness; the participants can build, or "hitchhike," on ideas presented by others. Criticism and ridicule, or even the appearance of that, cannot be allowed; such negative actions can kill a brainstorming session.

This creative problem-solving process is likely to increase the number of alternatives. The process also encourages dialogue among coworkers, which may build team spirit and gives credence to the old adage, "two heads are better than one." Even a supervisor alone can mentally brainstorm a problematic situation to find additional alternatives.

An alternative to brainstorming in person is using the Internet. Many discussion groups and forums exist on the Internet and enrollment in such groups is easy. Peers throughout the United States and around the world actively participate in discussion groups by sharing their experiences and outcomes to inquiries. Many organizations, including the American College of Healthcare Executives, the Healthcare Financial Management Association, and American Health Information Management Association, operate online discussion groups. The advantage of using this resource is that alternative points of view are obtained from a variety of backgrounds.

Evaluate the Alternatives, and Select the Best

The purpose of decision making is to select from various courses of action the one that can provide the greatest number of desired consequences and the smallest number of unwanted consequences. The manager should test each alternative by imagining that it has already been put into effect, and then determining whether it is feasible and what the consequences would be.

Once the supervisor has thought through the alternatives and appraised them, she is in a position to select one. While deciding, the supervisor should bear in mind the degree of risk involved in each course of action. No decision is without risk; one alternative will simply have more or less risk than another. It is also possible that the time factor makes one alternative preferable to another. For example, imagine you need to decide whether to invest in a new x-ray machine that is available today, or wait six months and invest in an x-ray machine that uses newer technology. The six-month wait will cost you business, but the efficiency of the newer technology may make the wait worthwhile.

While evaluating alternatives, the supervisor should also bear in mind the available resources, facilities, know-how, equipment, and data. Lastly, the manager should judge the alternatives on economy of effort—in other words, which action yields the greatest result for the least amount of effort and expenditure.

The decision must be acceptable to the group affected by it. If the alternative the supervisor thinks is best is not acceptable to the group, its effectiveness will be diminished. The group may only grudgingly carry out the action, or even quietly sabotage it. In such a situation, the supervisor may decide to choose a course of action that he feels is not the best choice, but which will be more acceptable to the affected group. Acceptability is an important consideration in this process of choice.

Ethics also play a role when a supervisor evaluates alternatives. Most organizations are sensitive to business ethics—that is, what is morally right and wrong as applied to executive behavior and decision making (Valasquez 1988; Munson 1992). In evaluating the alternatives, the manager must make certain that he complies with established corporate and professional ethical codes.

Using the criteria of feasibility, risk, timing, acceptability, ethics, resources, and economy, the manager often can see that one alternative clearly provides a greater number of desirable consequences and fewer unwanted consequences than any other. In such cases, the decision is relatively easy. The best alternative, however, is not always so obvious; occasionally, two or more alternatives may seem equally desirable. The choice then becomes simply a matter of the manager's personal preference. On the other hand, the manager also may believe that no alternative outweighs the others. In this case, it might be advisable to combine two of the better alternatives and come up with a compromise solution.

What about a situation in which the manager finds that none of the alternatives is satisfactory? You may someday face a situation in which the undesirable consequences of all the alternatives are so overwhelmingly bad that they paralyze any action. You might think the only available solution to the problem is to take no action at all. Such a solution, however, is unsatisfactory—a good manager does not leave a situation hanging. In such cases, you should search for new alternatives. Make sure all the steps of the decision-making process have been followed. Has the problem been clearly defined? Have all the pertinent facts been gathered and analyzed? Have all possible alternatives been considered? Has the department tried brainstorming? Chances are that some new alternatives will come up. However, if a good solution does not present itself at this point, you should use your experience and intuition to select the least undesirable solution, and then monitor the results carefully.

Experience

The manager's selection from the alternatives is frequently influenced by experience (this is called **experiential decision making**). No manager should underestimate the importance of the knowledge gained by experience, but it is dangerous to follow experience blindly.

experiential decision making
The practice of making decisions based on experience.

Experiential decision making is often seen in medicine. For example, a person appears at a urologist's office with lower back pain, and the urologist may initially suspect a bladder infection. An orthopedist looking at the same problem may consider it a spur on a lumbar vertebra, while a neurologist may consider it a pinched nerve. Each physician bases this initial impression on his or her experience. Before proceeding, however, the physician gathers more facts because he or she knows that blindly accepting the first impression could result in a misdiagnosis.

Similarly, when a manager uses experience to choose among alternatives, she should examine the situation and conditions that prevailed at the time of the previous decision. Current conditions may be similar to that of the previous occasion. More often than not, however, conditions from one case to the next differ, and the underlying circumstances and assumptions are no longer valid.

Experience can also be helpful if the manager is called on to substantiate the reasons for making a particular decision. Experience is a good defense tactic, and many superiors use it as valid evidence. When contemplating experience, the underlying circumstances of the past, present, and future must be considered. Only within this framework is experience a helpful approach to selecting an appropriate alternative.

Hunches and Intuition

Managers sometimes base decisions on hunches and intuition, and certain managers seem to have an unusual ability for satisfactorily solving problems by intuitive means. A deeper examination, however, usually discloses that the "intuition" on which the manager thought a decision was based is actually experience or knowledge. The manager is recalling similar situations from the past that are now stored in his or her memory.

No superior looks favorably on a subordinate who continually justifies decisions based on intuition or hunch alone. These factors may come into play occasionally, but they must always be supplemented by more concrete considerations.

Experimentation   Experimentation, or testing, is a valid approach to decision making in the scientific world; reaching conclusions through laboratory tests and experimentation for many types of decisions is essential. In management, however, experimenting is often inappropriate, costly, and time consuming. Moreover, it is difficult to maintain controlled conditions and to test various alternatives fairly in a normal work environment. There may be certain instances, however, when a limited amount of testing is admissible, as long as the consequences are not too disruptive. For example, a supervisor might decide to test different work schedules or different locations for a new desktop computer. In this small, restricted sense, experimentation may at times be valid. In a supervisory situation, however, experimentation usually is not an ideal way of reaching a decision.

Scientific   During the last five decades, a new group of highly sophisticated tools has
Decision Making   been available to aid the manager in decision making. These tools are quantitative, involving linear programming, operations research, probability, model building, and simulation. They are mathematical techniques applied by mathematicians, statisticians, programmers, systems analysts, and other
scientific decision   scientists. The overall process is known as **scientific decision making**, or op-
making   erations research. A full discussion of these tools is beyond the scope of this
The practice   book, and a short description could not do justice to this important, large,
of making   and well-documented field of scientific decision making. To gain additional
decisions based   information, one can visit many sites on the Internet as well as read journals
on quantitative   and texts.
data.
         Only certain types of management problems lend themselves to this manner of quantitative analysis and solution. In a healthcare situation, for example, it could be applicable to situations such as scheduling to minimize patient waiting times or maximize use of operating room resources; optimizing inventory stocking levels; and evaluating outcomes data to define the most effective clinical pathway. Often these analyses are performed to assist in reengineering a process, in the context of an operational or performance improvement activity. Such scientific problem solving is complicated and may be costly; however, when the magnitude of a problem warrants considerable effort and expenditure, it may be the best solution.

         The problems confronting a line supervisor usually are not of this magnitude. If a major problem is affecting the entire organization, however, or if similar problems are found in several departments, it may be advisable for top management to employ the quantitative approach.

Take Action,   Effective execution of the decision is as important as making the decision.
and Follow Up   Decision making is not complete without an evaluation of the effectiveness of the decision. This is the manager's control function. If the results are as

expected and satisfactory, the supervisor has reached his or her goal. If the results are not as expected or if unanticipated consequences arise, the supervisor should look at the situation as a new problem and go through all the steps of the decision-making process from a new point of view.

Action and follow-up are impossible without two other essential processes—communication and coordination. Unless a decision is clearly communicated to the people who must carry it out and unless it is coordinated with other decisions and other departments, it is meaningless. Thus, these two additional connective processes, discussed in the next two chapters, are vital to management's overall task of getting things done.

Avoid Unethical Decisions

Over the last several years we have seen too many examples of unethical practices in healthcare that have resulted in the imprisonment of executives and the demise of well-regarded healthcare facilities. These include healthcare executives squandering funds on personal luxuries, physicians prescribing medications from pharmaceutical companies that pay them, unnecessary surgeries, paying indigents to receive care so that false Medicaid claims can be filed, and many others. Supervisors and their frontline employees often observe these decisions occurring in the workplace and are critical to initiating an ethical response. One way to report an unethical situation is to call the compliance hotline in the facility or at the U.S. Office of Inspector General.

Bad ethical decisions are made by managers for many reasons. Some feel pressured to succeed, and others feel entitled. Others believe the rules do not apply to them. Some lack resources. None of these is reason enough to make unethical decisions. "Unfortunately, denial and rationalization have become useful forms of ethical amnesia" (Hofmann 2004, 40). Ethical behavior starts with a good model. If demonstrated by the most senior leaders, the behavior will be modeled in each echelon of management and staff. But lack of a senior model does not preclude you as a first-level supervisor from exemplifying ethical decision-making practices.

Summary

Selecting the best alternative by facts, study, and analysis of various proposals is still the best way to make a managerial decision. If an objective, rational, systematic method is used in this selection process, the manager is likely to make better decisions. The first step in such a method is to define the problem; the second step is to analyze it. The third step is to develop all the alternatives you possibly can, think them through as if you had already put them into action, and consider the consequences of each. By following this method, you will likely select the best alternative—that which has the greatest number of desired consequences and the least number of unwanted consequences.

Not only can you learn this sound method of decision making, but you, as a supervisor, can teach the same systematic approach to your subordinates. In doing so, you are assured that whenever subordinates are confronted with a decision, they can also arrive at a solution in a systematic and rational manner. Although this process is not always a guarantee for arriving at the best decisions, it is likely to produce more good decisions than would otherwise be the case.

Scientific decision making, or operations research, is an approach to problem solving that involves quantitative analysis, models, and computer applications. If the problem is of sufficient magnitude to warrant such an expensive effort, sophisticated scientific decision-making techniques that involve mathematicians, statisticians, systems analysts, or other specialists should be used.

Decision making conducted in an ethical manner is expected of all who work in healthcare. The failure to make ethical decisions has resulted in the demise of several reputable healthcare facilities and the imprisonment of managers, executives, and physicians.

Additional Readings

Harvard Business Essentials. 2005. *Decision Making: 5 Steps to Better Results.* Boston: Harvard Business Press.

McNamara, C. Authenticity Consulting. 1997–2008. "Basic Guidelines to Problem Solving and Decision Making" [Online article; retrieved 1/27/10.] http://208.42.83.77/prsn_prd/prb_bsc.htm.

Rappeport, A. 2008. "Game Theory Versus Practice." *CEO* 24 (7): 35–36.

Termini, M. J. 2007. *Walking the Talk: Pathways to Leadership.* Dearborn, MI: Society of Manufacturing Engineers.

4

COORDINATING ORGANIZATIONAL ACTIVITIES

Chapter Objectives

After you have studied this chapter, you should be able to do the following:

1. Explain the increasing need for coordination as a result of increased work specialization and fragmentation of patient care.
2. Define the meaning of coordination as linking together a multitude of activities.
3. Differentiate between cooperation and coordination.
4. Discuss the obstacles inherent in achieving coordination.
5. Discuss how managers should not treat coordinating as a separate managerial function but as a by-product of the five managerial functions.
6. Discuss the importance of good decision making and communication in achieving coordination.
7. Describe the internal and external dimensions of coordination.

Division of work, or **work specialization**, means to break down a job into smaller, more specialized tasks. Division of work and specialization, which will be discussed in Chapter 12, involves separating employees into departments, divisions, units, sections, and so on based on their shared expertise. This method of work specialization is particularly common in the healthcare field. Having many specialized departments leads to large and complex organizational structures. This proliferation of specialties is necessary to ensure the best possible care of patients as well as high standards of medical expertise. However, specialization creates problems for the management of healthcare facilities and even more difficulties within an integrated healthcare system—namely, the need for coordination, the process of linking together the activities of all units and ensuring consistency in services delivered by the same departments in each of the affiliated organizations.

The reason for coordination is that all these healthcare entities depend on each other for services, resources, information, and communications. Patient care data are created and exchanged among patient service areas (e.g., from blood bank to surgery, from surgery to intensive care, from intensive care to radiology) and between affiliated entities to ensure continuity of care (e.g., from the hospital to the home health agency, from the home health

work specialization
The process of breaking down a job into smaller, more specialized tasks.

agency to the durable medical equipment company, from the primary care physician's office to the consulting specialist). When many different specialized areas are interdependent on patient care data, more attention must be devoted to coordination.

Coordination of information in non–patient-care areas is as important as in patient care entities. If data are not accurately captured, reported, and assessed by management, workflow and support of patient care services are negatively affected and goals are not achieved.

The Meaning of Coordination

Supervisory management was defined earlier as the process of getting things done through and with people by directing their efforts toward common objectives. Thus management involves coordination of the efforts of all the members of an organization. Some authors have even defined management as the task of achieving coordination (Sisk 1977; Mowll 1989; Robbins et al. 2006) or, more specifically, of achieving the orderly synchronization of employees' efforts to provide the proper amount, timing, and quality of execution so that their unified efforts lead to the stated objectives. Other management experts have preferred to look at coordination as a separate managerial function.

coordination
The linking together of the activities in the organization to achieve the desired results.

Organization, as defined earlier, is two or more people working together in a structured, formal environment to achieve a common goal. **Coordination**, then, is the linking together of the activities in the organization to achieve the desired results. It is the connective process by which entities, departments, and tasks are interrelated to reach the objectives.

Thus, for the purposes of this book, coordination is viewed not as a separate function of the manager nor as the defining characteristic of management, but as a process by which the manager achieves orderly group effort and united action in pursuit of the common purpose. The manager does this while performing the five basic managerial functions of planning, organizing, staffing, influencing, and controlling. The resulting coordination should be one of the goals that the manager keeps in mind when performing each of the five managerial functions. Coordination, therefore, is a by-product of the appropriate execution of the five managerial functions; it is a part of everything the manager does.

The task of achieving coordination is much more difficult at the top administrative level than at the supervisory level. The CEO must achieve the synchronization of efforts throughout the entire organization, whereas the supervisor of a department only has to be concerned with coordination primarily within her own department and regarding its relation to other divisions. However, a supervisor should also keep coordination at the forefront of her mind whenever she plans, organizes, staffs, influences, and controls. Finally, she should recognize that those activities that affect other departments result in a more complex maze of coordination efforts.

Coordination and Cooperation

The term coordination must not be confused with cooperation. *Cooperation* merely indicates the willingness of individuals to help each other. It is an informal action that requires no structure or planning, and authority is retained by each party in the process. Coordination is more inclusive, requiring more than the mere desire and willingness of the participants. It is formal, requiring some planning and delineation of roles and relationships.

For example, consider a group of people attempting to move a heavy object. They are sufficient in number, willing and eager to cooperate with each other, and trying to do their best to get the job done. They are also fully aware of their common purpose. In all likelihood, however, their individual efforts are of little avail until one of them, the manager, gives the proper orders to apply the right amount of force at the right place and time. Only then will the group's efforts be sufficiently coordinated to move the object. This example introduces a third concept—**collaboration**, whereby individuals who see different aspects of a problem work together to achieve a common goal. Collaboration requires both cooperation and coordination to build substantive agreement.

collaboration
The act of individuals working together to achieve a common goal.

Ensuring timely and accurate billing is a common activity in healthcare that requires not only cooperation among several units but also, primarily, coordination of data. Clearly, if correct insurance and patient-identifying information is not collected at the time of admission or registration, the final billing function is hindered. Regardless of the accuracy and completeness of the reports prepared by the physician and the coding applied by the health information coding staff, if this information links to an incorrect insurance number or patient name, the bill may not be paid. The coordination of information gathering is dependent on each cooperating party performing his or her function with precision and transmitting the results to those other parties who rely on the information to achieve the intended goal.

To help differentiate between coordination, cooperation, and collaboration, Dave Pollard (2005) created Exhibit 4.1.

It is possible that, by coincidence, mere cooperation can bring about the desired result, but no manager can afford to rely on coincidence. Although cooperation is always helpful and its absence can prevent all possibility of coordination, its presence alone does not necessarily yield results. Coordination is therefore superior to cooperation in order of importance. Coordination is a conscious effort to tie activities together.

EXHIBIT 4.1 Coordination, Cooperation, or Collaboration?

	COORDINATION	**COOPERATION**	**COLLABORATION**
Examples	Project to implement off-the-shelf IT application; traffic flow regulation	Marriage; operating a local community-owned utility or grain elevator; coping with an epidemic or catastrophe	Brainstorming to discover a dramatically better way to do something; jazz or theatrical improvisation; cocreation
Appropriate tools	Project management tools with schedules, roles, critical path (CPM), PERT and Gannt charts; "who will do what by when" action lists	Systems thinking; analytical tools (root cause analysis, etc.)	Appreciative inquiry; open-space meeting protocols; four practices; conversations; stories
Degree of interdependence in designing the effort's work products (and need for physical colocation of participants)	Minimal	Considerable	Substantial
Degree of individual latitude in carrying out the agreed-on design	Minimal	Considerable	Substantial

SOURCE: Dave Pollard, *Meeting of Minds*, Innovation Consultants. Published March 25, 2005 in *How to Save the World* weblog. Used with permission.

HOSPITAL LAND

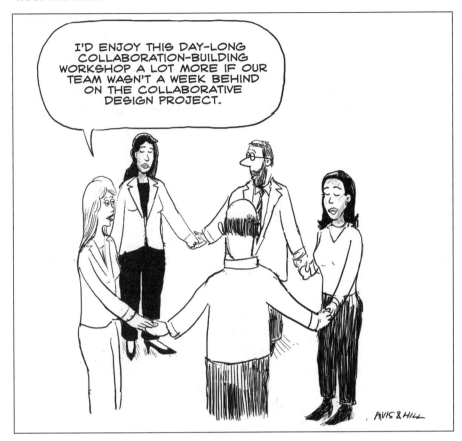

Difficulties in Attaining Coordination

Coordination is not easily attained, and it is becoming increasingly difficult as the various duties in the healthcare field become more complex. As an organization grows and more departments become decentralized, the task of synchronizing daily activities becomes more and more complicated. As the number of employees grows, rotates shifts, and telecommutes, the need for coordination and synchronization to secure the unified result increases. Not only can specialization cause problems of coordination, but human nature can present problems as well. Your employees may be hesitant to coordinate with others while performing their jobs as they are generally preoccupied with their own work because their evaluations are based on how they perform their jobs. They may be reluctant to take on additional duties, even temporarily, as it may hinder their personal schedule. Finally, they may assume that working with others as an additional assignment entitles them to additional compensation.

Coordination can be both hindered and helped by the use of automation. Perhaps you have experienced difficulties with the installation of a new computer system that did not interface adequately with existing systems. Equally devastating is when an organization has become reliant on a proprietary information system sold by one manufacturer that does not permit the integration of new technologies from another manufacturer. The organization's investment is substantial, and it cannot walk away from the asset, but it also cannot afford to do without the new technologies that may result in labor or other resource savings. This may be why **open architecture systems** are preferred; they allow different yet compatible (nonproprietary) systems from a variety of manufacturers to be used without causing a loss of coordination of data.

open architecture system
A system that allows different, nonproprietary systems from a variety of manufacturers to work well together.

Coordination and Managerial Functions

Coordination cuts through each of the managerial functions. The manager's planning stage is the ideal time to incorporate coordination. A supervisor must see that the various plans within the department are properly interrelated. These plans and alternatives should be discussed with the employees who are to carry them out so that they have an opportunity to express any doubts, objections, or suggestions for improvement. Furthermore, if the plans affect other departments, it is imperative the plans be discussed with those departments' supervisors. Including employees and colleagues in the process while plans are still flexible increases the chances for effective coordination and collaboration.

The same concern for coordination should exist when the manager organizes. Indeed, the whole purpose of organizing is to ensure coordination. Thus, whenever a manager groups activities and assigns them to various subordinates, coordination should be on her mind. By placing related activities that need to be closely synchronized within the same administrative area, coordination is facilitated.

Moreover, in the process of organizing, management should define authority relationships in such a way that coordination will result. Often poor coordination is caused by lack of understanding of who is to perform what, or by the failure of a manager to delegate authority and exact responsibility clearly. Such vagueness can easily lead to duplication of efforts instead of synchronization.

Coordination should also be an aspect of the staffing function. Having the right number of employees in various positions is important to ensure that the functions are properly performed. Equally important, the manager should see that all staff have the proper qualifications and training.

When a manager directs and influences, he is also concerned with coordination. The purpose of giving instructions, coaching, teaching, and supervising subordinates is to coordinate activities so that the overall objectives of the institution are reached in the most efficient way. As some experts have stated, coordination is that phase of supervision devoted to obtaining the harmonious and reciprocal performance of two or more subordinates' responsibilities.

Finally, coordination is directly connected with the controlling managerial function. By checking whether the activities of the department are proceeding as planned and directed, the supervisor can discover and immediately correct discrepancies to ensure coordination. Frequent evaluation and correction of departmental operations help synchronize the efforts of employees and the activities of the entire organization. Thus, by its nature, controlling is the last process to bring about overall coordination.

Coordination and Decision Making

Because the process of decision making is at the heart of all managerial functions, achieving coordination must be foremost in every manager's mind whenever she is making decisions. When choosing from the various alternatives, the manager must never forget the importance of achieving synchronization of all efforts. At times, a certain alternative taken by itself may seem to constitute the best choice. A second choice, however, may result in better coordination. This is why Chapter 3 stresses the importance of the solution's acceptability in the supervisor's consideration of alternatives. The supervisor is better advised to follow the second solution because achieving coordination is an important, if not overriding, objective.

Coordination and Communication

In all coordination efforts, good communication is imperative. It is not enough for a manager to make decisions that are likely to bring about coordination; having decisions carried out effectively is at least as important. To achieve successful execution, the supervisor must first communicate the decisions effectively to subordinates so that they understand them correctly (the importance of this is discussed in Chapter 5).

Personal, face-to-face contact is probably the most effective means of communicating with others to obtain coordination. Other means, however, such as written reports, minutes, procedures, rules, and newsletters or electronic methods such as faxes and e-mails also ensure the speedy dissemination of information to employees. Many organizations use e-mail or other Web-based technology, allowing immediate response in written form and often facilitating communication between divisions that are geographically separated. Intranets assist geographically dispersed healthcare systems to communicate within seconds new policies, services, and reports to all locations. Remote access to e-mail or intranet permits individuals at home or out of town to co-ordinate activities without delay.

Internal Communication in Healthcare Centers

The proliferation and specialization of medical sciences and technologies has generated a need for more and better coordination. Because of specialization, however, the synchronization of daily activities has become extremely complicated and coordination has become harder to attain. As the number of positions in a department or facility increases and as more specialized and sophisticated tasks are performed, the need for coordination and synchronization grows.

The process of bringing about total coordination of all divisions and levels within a healthcare facility is ultimately the concern of the chief administrator. The CEO must deal with the fact that each department, and each facility within a system, is likely to favor one route over another, depending on its particular functions and experience. Considerable thoughtfulness and understanding are required of all managerial and supervisory personnel to coordinate the working relationships of the groups above, below, and alongside each department. Even with cooperative attitudes, self-coordination, and self-adjustment by most members of the healthcare organization, duplication of actions and conflicts of efforts may still result unless administration carefully synchronizes all activities. Only through such coordination can management bring about accomplishment that exceeds the sum of the individual parts. Although each part is important, the result can be of greater significance if management achieves coordination. Good communications act as necessary lubricants in all these processes.

Dimensions of Coordination

The need for coordination exists in three directions: vertically, horizontally, and diagonally.

Vertical Coordination

vertical coordination
Coordination between different levels of an organization, such as between the CEO and a vice president.

Coordination between different levels of an organization can be considered **vertical coordination**, such as between the CEO and the vice president of facilities or between the vice president of facilities and the director of housekeeping. Vertical coordination is achieved by delegating authority, assigning duties, and supervising and controlling. Although authority carries great power, effective vertical coordination is better achieved by performing the managerial functions wisely instead of relying on the weight of formal authority (see Exhibit 15.2).

Horizontal Coordination

Horizontal coordination exists among persons and between departments on the same organizational level. Horizontal coordination helps solve problems that affect different areas. For example, one goal of many healthcare facilities is to achieve a shorter average length of stay (ALOS). Identifying a patient's diagnosis-related group (DRG) during the admission process has been identified as one solution. To make such an early diagnosis, arrangements have to be made among the various managers of the activities affected. The access registrar, health information management coding specialist, case manager, patient care manager, chief of diagnostic services, skilled nursing unit manager, and home health coordinator—all of whom are on the same organizational level—try to coordinate their activities to achieve this goal (see Exhibit 4.2).

Each individual involved manages his own department and has no authority over other managers. Horizontal coordination obviously cannot be

horizontal coordination
Coordination between departments on the same organizational level, such as between the emergency department and the radiology department.

EXHIBIT 4.2
Shortening ALOS Project

DEPARTMENTS/SERVICES	ACTIONS
Access	Registrar checks list of targeted conditions usually requiring discharge planning
Health Information Management	Coding specialist assigns working DRG for case manager
Case Management	Selects appropriate clinical pathway for condition and begins discussions with patient care, alternative care facilities, and attending physician relative to the anticipated services for this DRG, the DRG's average LOS, and reimbursement
Medical Staff	Places orders for treatment, discusses needs with family, places orders for alternative care
Diagnostic Services	Expedites scheduling to diagnostic testing and ancillary services
Patient Care	Ensures testing is completed and patient is informed and cared for
Skilled Nursing Unit	Identifies bed availability for patient care to expedite transfer
Home Health Agency	Coordinator confers with SNF and physician to provide services at home post-discharge

NOTE: SNF = skilled nursing facility; ALOS = average length of stay; DRG = diagnosis-related group ordered by any one of them. It is achieved by a policy stating that when necessary, the departments must interact, cooperate, and adjust their activities to achieve coordination. If coordination cannot be achieved, the problem must be referred to a higher level in the managerial hierarchy with authority over all these departments. In all likelihood, this is the CEO or COO (chief operating officer), who will issue the necessary directives to facilitate a solution. Obviously, if those who must deal with the problems on a daily basis can gain consensus on the solution, its implementation and future coordination will be enhanced.

Diagonal Coordination

diagonal coordination
Coordination that cuts across organizational arrangements, ignoring position and level.

Diagonal coordination cuts across the organizational arrangements, ignoring positions and levels. In a small day-surgery center, for example, close working relationships and short lines of communication make diagonal coordination easier than in a large organization. Even in this case, expectations must be reasonable. For instance, all departments in any organization need access to the engineering and maintenance department, a centralized service. However, engineering cannot be everywhere at once. This access has to be coordinated by negotiations between the users and the provider (see Exhibit 4.3). Furthermore, coordination cannot be accomplished simply by referring the problem up the chain of command. If that is done too often, tension may build between the two departments and eventually higher executives will question why the departments are unable to work together toward a harmonious solution.

The techniques and methods used in an organizational setting vary with the dynamics of the environment and the degree of specialization. If the manager cannot achieve coordination because of the dynamic nature of the environment or the breadth of a project (e.g., construction of a new hospital), an individual in a liaison role may be called on to facilitate and coordinate. Some organizations engaged in high-performance and dynamic industries use an entire coordinating department.

Because the task of securing harmonious action and internal coordination within a healthcare center belongs primarily to those in managerial positions, the task should not be assigned to a specialist such as a coordinator. The managers are in a better position than a specialist to view the various functions and to determine how they should be coordinated to bring about the desired objective, and the managers carry the authority to get the job done. Again, all managers must coordinate as they perform their five managerial functions. While some industries have found the coordinator or liaison position helpful, it is questionable whether the task of securing internal coordination within the healthcare center can be shifted or assigned to a special department or a number of individuals (Lawrence and Lorsch 1969).

EXHIBIT 4.3
Diagonal
Coordination

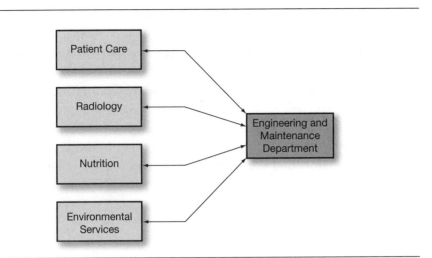

The Coordinator as a Misnomer

Some healthcare entities do have positions labeled "coordinator"; often, however, these are traditional managerial and supervisory jobs and should have been named as such. In these cases, the title "coordinator" is a misnomer. For instance, instead of having a professional known as performance improvement manager, the position may be called "performance improvement coordinator." This position, regardless of the title, is likely to be managerial to the extent that the coordinator manages some staff and activities that cut across many levels of the organization. Some healthcare centers simply prefer the word coordinator to that of supervisor—for example, shift coordinator. Information systems departments often have coordinator positions, such as clinical systems coordinator. While this position may not manage staff, it does manage resources—clinical systems. On the other hand, some staff professionals who are advisory in nature carry the title coordinator and rightly so.

Coordination with External Entities

Coordination with entities external to the institution also is needed. A special coordinator or liaison may be used in situations in which a hospital is trying to coordinate some activities with other healthcare institutions (e.g., joint venture between the hospital, long-term healthcare facility, surgical center, home health agency) or with external funding or regulatory agencies (e.g., division of family services, social security administration, worker's compensation, health maintenance organization, Medicaid). Such persons should be thoroughly familiar with the conditions and thinking of their institution and be able to explain them to others and communicate the findings and intentions back to their institution. The coordinator may or may not be granted authority to commit the institution to action. However, in most instances, the person responsible for coordinating with external factions must check with an administrator or other executive to determine how far the institution will go to support the chosen action. In this situation, the coordinator is not a manager as defined in this book.

Nevertheless, the importance of such external coordination should not be underestimated. The greater the degree of coordination among healthcare centers and related institutions, the better the overall healthcare system is. Indeed, much is being said today about improving healthcare through regional health information organizations and comparative profiling.

Summary

Coordination, the orderly synchronization of all efforts of the members of the organization to achieve the stated objectives, plays a part in every function of a manager. It is not a separate managerial function but cuts across each of the five functions and is a by-product of these functions. Coordination should not be confused with cooperation: cooperation is always helpful in achieving coordination, but coordination is more encompassing.

As a supervisor plans, organizes, staffs, influences, and controls, she must remember that the ultimate goal is to achieve coordination of all efforts. The same thought should be foremost in the manager's mind whenever he makes decisions and communicates them to the employees. Achieving coordination is a valid consideration for all managers, regardless of their position, level within the administrative hierarchy, or type of enterprise in which they work. Proliferation and specialization of the medical sciences and technologies have made coordination more difficult.

Coordination with entities external to the institution, such as government agencies, local health councils, users, and other provider groups, is also important. To achieve external coordination, facilities can use a liaison or special coordinator to provide the necessary contacts between the institution and outside entities.

Additional Readings

In Context. 2008. "Moving 'Up One Level': Preparing for Service and Supervisory Roles Through Cross-Functional Skills." [Online article; retrieved 12/28/08.] www.incontext.indiana.edu/2008/january/2.html.

Denise, L. 1999. "Collaboration vs. C-Three (Cooperation, Coordination and Communication)." *Innovating.* [Online article; retrieved 12/27/08.] www.zsr.org/results-framework-resources-2/collaborationvstheothercwords.pdf.

5

COMMUNICATING

Chapter Objectives

After you have studied this chapter, you should be able to do the following:

1. Describe the communication model and the roles of the senders and receivers.
2. Discuss how communication affects organizational performance.
3. Identify and discuss communication networks, channels, and barriers.
4. Describe how managers can ensure more effective communication by overcoming roadblocks.
5. Explain the operation of the grapevine and its importance.

From the manager's point of view, communication is the process of exchanging information in such a way that mutual understanding is achieved between two or more people about work-related issues. In general terms, it is a psychological process of sharing information to achieve a common understanding between ourselves and others. Communication is the third process that serves to link the managerial functions in an organization (see Exhibit 1.4). Employees look for and expect communication because it is a means of motivating and influencing people and changing behavior.

During uncertain times such as the recession experienced in 2008 and 2009 or when an organization's fiscal condition has critically deteriorated, employee anxiety heightens. Employees' concerns with job security, compensation reductions, and inflation drive the apprehension meter. Even more than during times of prosperity, during challenging times management must overcommunicate to calm employees and help them understand the conditions being encountered, and to seek employee input about the options management is considering to keep the organization afloat.

According to Larkin and Larkin (1994), 92 percent of American employees prefer to hear about changes from their supervisor rather than from higher levels of management. A supervisor can use her communication skills to enlist the support for change from her employees, which makes her a critical part of an organization's ability to initiate change. Communication is vital to getting a job done, and also for purposes of social satisfaction. Thus, the communication process fulfills institutional needs and human needs. Fundamentally, it is a process of pulling together the employees of the department.

Aristotle wrote, in 350 B.C., if communication is to change behavior, it must be grounded in the desires and interests of the receivers. Understanding the receivers' frame of reference (FOR) is essential to gaining their attention and interest. "FOR is colored by one's discipline, history, and desired results. To truly communicate with someone, it is essential to understand his or her FOR—the lens through which he or she is viewing the issue. The key is, you don't have to *agree* with another person's FOR, but you have to *understand* it" (Levin 2004).

Almost all daily managerial activities involve communication—that is, giving and receiving information. Because communicating involves two or more people, behavioral processes such as motivation, attitudes, perception, leadership, experience, and feelings play important roles. When the supervisor sends a message by speaking, by writing, or by electronic means, he encodes a message from a unique perspective. The perspective is influenced by perceptions of the sender's world, with the sender making assumptions about the receiver's perspectives and how the message will be received. Backgrounds, perceptions, attitudes, values, and other factors may differ widely among the individuals involved, all of which make achieving a mutual understanding of others' ideas difficult.

As with all organizations, valid information is needed by a healthcare facility to function effectively. Communication provides the key to this important resource. A hospital devotes much activity to gathering and processing information from the moment the patient enters the facility until the patient is discharged. Serious consequences can arise when communications are insufficient, become misunderstood, break down, or do not exist.

You already know that a supervisor's job is to plan, organize, staff, influence, and control the work of the employees and to coordinate their efforts for the purpose of achieving departmental objectives. To accomplish these goals, the supervisor must articulate plans and organize the arrangement of the work, give directives, describe to each subordinate what is expected, and speak to each regarding performance. All this is done by communicating.

A supervisor's skill in communication often determines his success. Communication is the most effective tool for building and keeping a well-functioning team. Communication is the only means a supervisor has to take charge of and train a group of employees, direct them, motivate them, and coordinate their activities. This ability to communicate is the essence of leadership. Is there any area of responsibility within a supervisor's job that can be done without communicating? No. Without effective communication, the organizational structure cannot survive.

HOSPITAL LAND

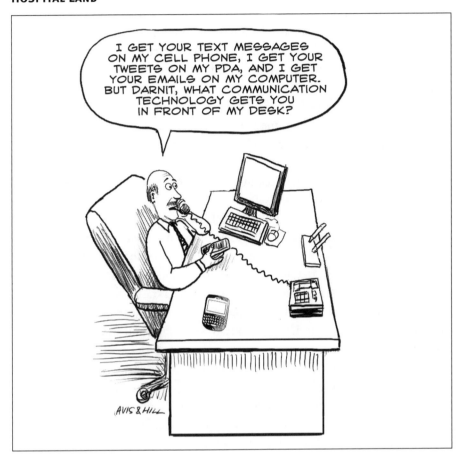

The Nature of Communication

Fundamental and vital to all managerial functions, communication is a means of transmitting information and making oneself understood by another or others. The exchange is successful only when mutual understanding results. Agreement is not necessary as long as the sender and receiver have successfully exchanged ideas and understand each other and the message received represents the meaning the message intended.

Supervisors spend most of their time either sending or receiving information. One cannot assume, however, that real communication is occurring in all of these exchanges. Also, being constantly engaged in encoding and decoding messages does not ensure that a supervisor is an expert in communicating.

Communication always involves two people: a sender and a receiver. One person cannot communicate. For example, a person stranded on a deserted island who shouts for help does not communicate because no one receives the message. This example may seem obvious, but think of the manager who sends out a large number of e-mail memos. Once a memorandum has been sent, many are inclined to believe that communication has occurred. However, communication does not occur until information and understanding have passed between that manager *and* the intended receivers.

Making oneself understood then is an important part of this definition of communication. A receiver may hear a sender but still may not understand what the sender's message means. Understanding is a personal matter between people, and different people may interpret messages differently. If the idea received is not the one intended, communication has not taken place; the sender has merely spoken or written.

Dietitian Carol M. Coughlin (2000) states that "people remember 10% of what they read, 20% of what they hear, 30% of what they see, and 70% of what they see, hear, and read." Supervisors who use only one form of communication are not as effective in sending messages as those who communicate the same message in a variety of ways. Take the staff meeting, for example. This method of communicating allows attendees to hear your voice inflections, have eye contact, and engage in two-way communication because questions can be posed and comments can be made. However, if the messages communicated at the meeting are not written down and posted in the form of minutes, they may easily be forgotten. To take this example even further, consider employees who have special needs, such as those who are deaf and may not read lips. For these employees, communication during a staff meeting does not occur at all without written material that covers the points of the meeting or without a sign language interpreter. Perhaps you hold the meeting in English and several of the attendees only speak Spanish; again, communication does not occur.

Similarly, some staff may lack the capability to read and understand memoranda or minutes. According to the National Adult Literacy Survey, 42 million adult Americans cannot read and 50 million can recognize few printed words. The number of functionally illiterate adults is increasing by approximately 2.25 million persons each year, including people who drop out of school before graduation; legal and illegal immigrants; refugees; and high school graduates (National Right to Read Foundation 2005). These individuals require oral communication in a language or media they understand. Others may find both the written and oral methods difficult to understand or retain. For these individuals, pictures, graphs, and charts may be a more meaningful method of communication. In summary, supervisors must try communication alternatives and use more than one method to ensure maximum communication.

Only through effective communication can policies, procedures, and rules be formulated and carried out. Furthermore, only with such communication can misunderstandings be ironed out, plans be achieved, and activities within a department be coordinated and controlled. The success of all managerial functions depends on effective communication. The discussion that follows focuses on the methods of communication in more detail.

Communication Network

Organizational structure affects organizational communications. Chapters 11 through 16 discuss the formal organizational structure, and Chapter 17 demonstrates that every organization also has an informal structure. The communication network in each of these structures has distinct but equally important formal and informal channels; the informal channel is usually called the **grapevine**. Each channel carries messages from one person or group to another in downward, upward, horizontal, and diagonal directions (see Exhibit 5.1).

grapevine
The informal channel of communication in an organization.

Formal Channels

The formal channels of communication are established by the organizational hierarchy and formal reporting relationships. These channels follow the lines of authority from the chief administrator to the employees. You are probably familiar with the expression that messages and information "must go through proper channels." This refers to the formal flow of communication through the organizational hierarchy.

Downward Communication

The downward flow of communication begins with someone at the top issuing a message and the next person in the hierarchy passing it along to those who report to him, and the flow goes on down the line. The downward direction is the one that management relies on most for its communication. Management devotes much time to communicating with subordinates through e-mails, memos, posters, meetings, and letters to explain objectives, policies, plans, and so forth. Supervisors send messages about these to their subordinates; they instruct employees through directives; they inform them about work methods, procedures, and rules; and they give feedback about performance and performance expectations. Generally, **downward communication** starts action by subordinates; that is, its content is mostly of a directive nature. The manager's position of higher authority requires effective downward communication. The manager should transmit the right amount of information, neither too little nor too much.

Reading a manager's communication focus takes some practice. Managers typically communicate in one of two ways—they are either "thing"

downward communication
Communication that flows down the hierarchy of an organization, such as when a vice president tells a line supervisor about a new initiative, and the line supervisor tells her employees.

EXHIBIT 5.1

The Directions of Information Along Formal Communications Channels

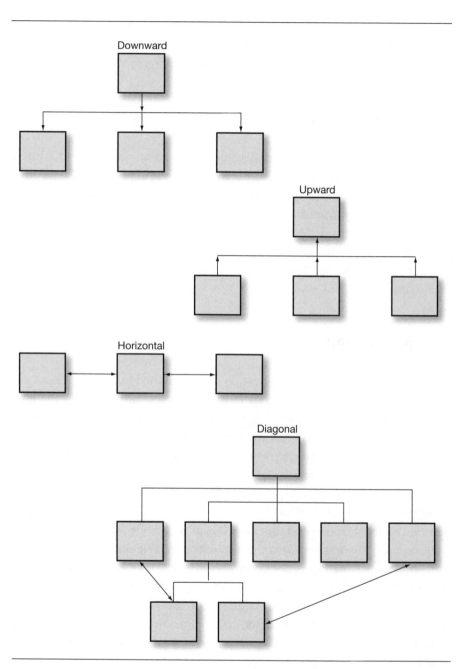

focused or "people" focused. An e-mail from your manager that asks, "How is the conversion coming?" differs in style from the query, "How is your conversion team doing?" Knowing whether a manager is thing-oriented will allow his employees to focus and structure their communications to him on "things" rather than people. Employees should study how their manager reacts under stress to gauge his coping limits. By doing so, they find out when, how often, and specifically what should be communicated to him when stressful situations arise.

Downward communication helps tie the levels of the organizational structure together and coordinate activities. Effectively utilizing first-line supervisors to communicate important changes to the frontline employees and engaging their support will aid the coordination of activities throughout the organization.

Upward Communication: Initiated by the Subordinate

Upward communication is a second and equally important direction in which messages flow through the official network—it goes from subordinates to supervisors. Any person charged with supervisory authority also accepts an obligation to keep the superior informed. Subordinates must feel free to convey their opinions and attitudes to their superior and to report on activities and actions regarding their work. Usually, employees report on work progress, activities, and problems they have encountered during their shift; air complaints; and provide responses to inquiries. Much of this exchange is predetermined and routine. Management should encourage a free flow of upward communication because this is the only means by which supervisors can determine whether their messages have been transmitted and received properly and whether appropriate action is taking place. In addition to following prescribed reporting procedures, an effective manager develops additional systems to encourage an upward flow of information.

> **upward communication**
> Communication that flows up the hierarchy, such as when a nurse tells the nursing shift supervisor about a problem with a patient.

As a supervisor, you should encourage and maintain upward communication channels and pay proper attention to the information transmitted through them. You must show that you want the facts and want them promptly. Unfortunately, the reaction of many managers to upward communication may be reluctance; after all, ancient tyrants executed the bearer of bad news. In your supervisory capacity, you must make a deliberate effort to encourage upward communication by (1) showing a genuine desire to obtain and use the ideas and reports of your subordinates, (2) being approachable, (3) truly listening, and (4) recognizing the importance of upward communication. Lack of an effective upward flow throttles the will of your employees to communicate, leads to frustration, and ultimately causes them to seek different outlets such as the grapevine, complaint lines, human resources, or union organizers.

Upward Communication: Initiated by the Supervisor

As stated at the outset of this book, supervisors are the people in the middle. They are not only responsible for providing good communication downward to their employees, they are also responsible for stimulating good communication upward from their workers and then passing this and other information to the next higher level in the administrative hierarchy. However, most supervisors agree that it is much easier for them to "talk down" to their subordinates than to "speak up" to their superior. This is especially true when supervisors have to tell their boss that they did not meet a deadline or that they forgot to carry out an order.

Nevertheless, it is the supervisor's job to keep his superior informed of the department's activities and climate. Here are some tips (see Appendix 5.1 for an example of a poorly written memo):

- Be brief.
- If you are writing a memo or e-mail, express your conclusion, findings, or recommendation on the first line.
- Do not use jargon.
- Use short paragraphs.
- Be timely.

The supervisor should inform the superior of any significant developments as soon as possible after they occur, even if the information reveals errors. Recall the discussion in Chapter 1 of the dimensions of supervision—the supervisor must be a competent subordinate. If the boss hears bad news about a department from someone other than the supervisor of that department, she will assume the supervisor intentionally withheld information or is simply incompetent. Failing to communicate negative information is one of the fastest ways for a manager to lose credibility in the eyes of a superior. One of management's unwritten rules is, "Never allow your boss to be surprised." Superiors have a right to complete information because they are ultimately responsible if anything goes wrong.

Your superiors may have to act on what you report. Therefore, they must receive the information at a time and in a format that enable them to take the necessary action. As a supervisor, you must assemble all facts that are needed and check them carefully before passing them on to your boss. Bear in mind that upward messages are subject to more distortion than are downward messages. Choose your words wisely, and try to be as objective as possible. This may be difficult at times because subordinates want to look good in the eyes of their boss. Although you may want to soften the information so that facts do not look as bad as they are, you must remember that sooner or later the full extent of the problem probably will be discovered. When difficulties arise, it is best to report the event to your superior completely, even if it means admitting mistakes. Remember that your boss depends on her supervisors for upward communication, just as you depend on your employees to pass along information to you.

horizontal communication
Communication across departments or among peer managers, departments, and coworkers in charge of different activities.

Horizontal Communication

Horizontal, sideward, or lateral communication is concerned mainly with communication across departments or among peer managers, departments, and coworkers in charge of different activities. **Horizontal communication** is frequently used to coordinate activities, inform others on the same level, and persuade others. Horizontal communication occurs more among managers than among nonmanagerial personnel. For example, lateral communication for an admission from the emergency department (ED) often occurs between the recovery room supervisor and the head nurse on the surgical floor or between the ED physician and the floor physician. This lateral channel is necessary to ensure coordination and to avoid misunderstandings. Horizontal communication also plays an important role in matrix and project organizations, as discussed in Chapter 13.

Diagonal Communication

Diagonal communication is the flow of information between positions that are on different lateral planes and activities of the organizational structure (Exhibit 5.1). For example, diagonal communication occurs between nursing personnel and the human resources department; or between nursing management and nonmanagerial members of other departments, such as the food service tray delivery person or the phlebotomist. To achieve coordination among the various functions in any organization, especially in a healthcare organization, a free flow of diagonal communication is essential. Without it, good patient care is difficult to achieve. The "Shortening ALOS Project" example (Exhibit 4.1) shows how important horizontal and diagonal communication are.

Horizontal and diagonal communication also apply to communication with patients. The language of medicine is complex and not easily understood by the public; approximately 36 percent of the public is challenged by healthcare terms (National Assessment of Adult Literacy 2006). This means that supervisors and staff must take care to communicate in terms that are understandable by patients.

Communication Media

The media used most frequently for communication are verbal (oral and written words), visual media (graphs, charts, pictures), and nonverbal (action and behavior). Although spoken and written words are the most widely used media, the power of visuals and nonverbal communication cannot be underestimated.

Verbal Communication

Words are the most effective and most widely used tools of communication. Verbal communication can be a real challenge to the supervisor because words can be tricky, and messages that mean one thing to one employee can have a completely different meaning to another. The confusion that can sometimes result from verbal communication relates to the issue of semantics. **Semantics** is concerned with the multiple meaning of words and phrases and how they are used in the context of messages. Supervisors must be aware of the many possibilities of misunderstanding that can occur because of people's different

semantics
The study of language, particularly the multiple meanings of words and phrases and how they are used in the context of messages.

semantic habits. You may have heard the story about the maintenance foreman who asked a new worker to paint the porch behind the clinic. When the foreman checked on the job an hour later, he found that the clinic physician's Porsche had been painted.

Oral Communication

The most prevalent form of communication in any organization is oral communication. Oral communication with subordinates is more effective than written communication because the recipient can hear the tone, pace, volume, and articulation of the speaker. Oral communication also usually saves time and achieves better understanding. This is true of both face-to-face and telephone communication. In daily performance, face-to-face discussions between the supervisor and subordinate are the principal means of two-way communication. Such daily contacts are at the heart of an effective communication system. Face-to-face discussions are the most frequently used channel for the exchange of information, points of view, instructions, and motivation. Some cautionary guidance is provided in Appendix 5.2.

Oral communication is simple and can be done with little preparation and without pencil, paper, or computer; therefore, effective supervisors use this medium more than any other. They know that subordinates like to see and hear their boss in person. Also, oral communication is usually well received because most people prefer talking with their supervisor to ensure that they understand what is being said and to express themselves more easily and completely.

Aside from these factors, the greatest single advantage of oral communication is that it provides immediate feedback, even if the feedback is only an expression on the listener's face. By merely looking at the receiver, the sender can often judge the reaction to what is being said. Oral communication thus may enable the sender to find out immediately what the receiver is hearing or not hearing. Oral communication also allows the receiver an opportunity to ask questions immediately if the meaning is not clear. Then the sender can explain the message more thoroughly and clarify unexpected considerations. Moreover, the manner and tone of the human voice can endow the message with meaning and shading that even long pages of written words often cannot convey. The manner and tone create the atmosphere of communication, and the response is influenced accordingly.

There are some minor drawbacks to oral communications. No permanent record of what has been said exists. The sender may forget part of the message, or some noise or random disturbance may interfere. The many benefits, however, far outweigh these shortcomings.

Voicemail

Voicemail generally provides an effective means with which to communicate to others. It has replaced "pink-slip" telephone messages and the staff who once relayed those messages. In addition, it allows the caller to call any time—day, night, or weekend—and leave a message. However, it can also be a barrier to effective communication. Voicemail can be frustrating, especially if the system is poorly configured. Some supervisors use voicemail as a screening tool and never answer a call directly. Hiding behind voicemail is annoying to callers, staff, and superiors. Following are six rules for the supervisor's effective use of voicemail:

1. If you are not in the office, make sure your voicemail is activated.
2. If you are in the office and not involved in a meeting or another call, answer your telephone.
3. Always acknowledge a call received on voicemail.
4. Leave enough information in your voicemail messages to others so that the receiving party knows why you are calling and can prepare in advance for returning your call.
5. Do not forward a caller's message to another person's voicemail without the caller's knowledge.
6. Always repeat your return telephone number and clearly enunciate the numbers.

Written Communication

Regardless of the speed and effectiveness of oral communication, a well-balanced communication system includes both written and oral media. Although oral communication is used more frequently, written messages are indispensable and are especially important in healthcare activities. Often, detailed and specific instructions are lengthy and cumbersome; they must be put into writing so that they can be studied over a longer period. The written medium is especially useful for widespread dissemination of information that may concern a number of people. Furthermore, a degree of formality, as well as legality, is conveyed by "putting it in writing." However, care must be taken in writing memos and letters to ensure that the recipients do not misinterpret the intended meaning.

Letters are appropriate for external correspondence. Allen (2000) and Kelleghan (1999) suggest the following guidelines for written communication:

- Written communication should be used when the situation is formal, official, or long term or when the situation affects several people in related ways.
- Interoffice memos are internal communication tools used for recording information, inquiries, or replies.
- Letters are formal in tone and addressed to an individual. They are used for official notices, external correspondence, formally recorded statements, and lengthy communications.
- Reports are more impersonal and more formal than a letter. They are used to convey information, analyses, and recommendations.

Communication formalities have lessened with the rising use of e-mail. A supervisor should remember, however, that writing leaves an impression with the receiver. Regardless of how lax your organization may be, you should always try to use the spell-check function on your word processing program and reread your e-mail for correct grammar and sentence structure as well as appropriate word usage before clicking on the send icon. E-mail can be dangerous because it only takes a simple click to send a message to many, leaving the sender with no "out basket" from which to retrieve a hastily prepared response.

If you get an e-mail that irks you, take a few minutes to gather your thoughts; research the facts to support your position; choose the right words to convey your response; and determine if the response should be handled via e-mail, over the phone, or in person. If you draft a response e-mail in haste, do not send it until you have had a chance to reread it the next day. Time tends to temper responses.

Written messages have many advantages. They provide a permanent record that can be referred to as often as necessary. The spoken word, in contrast, generally exists only for an instant. Written communications are typically more accurate. The sender can take the necessary time to choose precise terminology, reread, and revise. Written communication is preferable when important details are involved and a permanent record is needed, perhaps literally as "evidence" to confirm a discussion or directive, such as in the following:

```
MEMO
Date: 12-20-01

To: John Smith, CEO

From: Helen Harpin, Human Resources Director

Per our hallway conversation, I will issue a merit
increase for Ned Warner, Nuclear Medicine Manager,
even though you have not yet had a chance to
finish his evaluation. The increase will be 4.2
percent as instructed. Please advise me if I've
misunderstood your instructions. Thank you.
```

Applying the guidance given in Appendix 5.2 will enhance your written communication skills.

Visual Media

Sometimes managers also make use of visual aids to help them communicate. Pictures are particularly effective when used with well-chosen words to complete a message. Even without any words, however, visual media help convey messages. Many enterprises make extensive use of the pictorial language in such forms as blueprints, charts, graphs, models, posters, cartoons, PowerPoint presentations, and overhead projections.

Coughlin (2000) shares an illustration of the benefit of visual media in the following exercise: Two people sit back to back and are given five wooden blocks. The person on the left builds a structure from the blocks and then verbally instructs the person on the right to build the same structure. Working merely from the verbal instructions, the person on the right has difficulty duplicating the structure. However, if the person on the right were given a visual aid, perhaps a drawing of the design, this would be an exercise in simplicity.

Furthermore, Coughlin (2000) adds, "visuals can make your presentation more clear, colorful, and interesting. When done properly, visual aids will clarify information, emphasize your major points, and help people visualize concepts.... Watch speakers at continuing professional education meetings. The most enjoyable presentations do not have notes: they have great slides."

Visuals are often useful when discussing quantitative information such as changes in patient volumes. It is simply easier to interpret a graph than numbers. Bulletin boards also serve as a visual communication tool. For example, Baptist Health Care abides by a "no-secrets-and-no-excuses" philosophy. Every department has a communication board, which is organized around the organization's five pillars of excellence: People, Quality, Service, Financial, and Growth. Information posted on the communication boards includes the department's financial performance, data from surveys on service or quality, and information about the organization as a whole (Bolster 2007). Sharing information that all employees can see sets the stage for a trusting relationship between staff and leadership. It also opens the door for questions to the supervisor. Supervisors who use visual aids find that they are 43 percent more likely to succeed in persuading their staffs to take a desired course of action, according to a survey (Hanke 1998).

Nonverbal Communication

Purposeful silence, gestures, a handshake, a shrug of the shoulder, body movements, eye contact, a wink, interpersonal distance, a smile, or a frown can all carry a lot of meaning. These are examples of nonverbal communication or body language. Communication is affected by facial expression, inflection, and tone of voice. By the same token, a manager's inaction also is a way of communicating, just as an unexplained action can often communicate a meaning that was not intended. Suppose, for example, that a piece of equipment was removed from the laboratory for overhaul, the testing normally performed on the equipment was temporarily outsourced, and no explanation was given to the employees. The technologists, who may be apprehensive of a staff reduction, may interpret the action to mean layoffs are imminent, even if the supervisor did not intend to convey that message.

Supervisors must not forget that everything they do may be interpreted as symbolic or seen as a model by their subordinates, and those actions often say more about their expectations than the words they speak. What message is sent when employees see the supervisor surfing the Internet for travel locations and reading joke e-mails while her work is delegated to subordinates? The employee may receive the message that spending company time and using the organization's resources (in this case, the computer and Internet access) to conduct personal business is acceptable when in fact it is not. Because of their managerial status, all observable acts communicate something to employees, whether supervisors intended them to or not. Employees often mimic the actions of their supervisors, especially if they see positive results. A supervisor who deals with a loud, unhappy customer by speaking softly, using an apologetic approach, and eventually ending the conversation with a smiling customer provides the perfect example for staff on how to diffuse this kind of situation.

The setting for the communication also can play a role as a nonverbal medium. For example, consider the manager sitting in a reclining, comfortable office chair behind his desk and the receiver of his communication either standing up or sitting in a stiff, unyielding chair across the desk; this setting displays the power and control of the supervisor. The manager's body position and facial expression also convey meaning, whether the expression used is accessible and accommodating or closed off and condescending. Managers who wish to convey "equality" meet around a table, over lunch in the cafeteria, or at the employee's cubicle where the turf is neutral.

The supervisor must remember that nonverbal communication reinforces or contradicts what is expressed verbally. These hidden messages are often subtle and ambiguous and must be read with caution. They are, however, an important medium for the communicator.

The Manager's Role in Communication

Organizational effectiveness largely depends on its communication network functioning successfully. Most organizational structures today have many levels of supervision and long lines of communication. Breakdowns and distortions of communication can occur at any level of supervision.

We have all seen the confusion, friction, and inconvenience that arise when communication breaks down. These breakdowns are not only costly in terms of money, but they also create misunderstandings that may hurt teamwork, morale, and even patient care. Indeed, many managerial problems are caused by faulty communication. Moreover, most human relationship problems grow out of poor or nonexistent communication.

The way a supervisor communicates with his subordinates is the essence of the relationship. Managers should always remember that no communication occurs until and unless the meaning *received* by the listener is as close as possible to the meaning the sender intended to *convey*. The effective communicator realizes that the speaker and the listener are two individuals with separate backgrounds, experiences, values, attitudes, and perceptions. Both live in different worlds, and many factors can interfere with the messages that pass between them.

Barriers to Communication

Barriers to effective communication are sometimes referred to as "noise in the system." The more important barriers can be grouped into three general categories: language barriers, status and position barriers, and resistance to change barriers.

Language

Normally, words serve us well and we generally understand each other. Sometimes, however, the same words suggest different meanings to different people. In those cases, the words themselves create a barrier to communication (see Appendix 5.2). This can result in the feeling that two people "are just not speaking the same language," although both participants are conversing in English. The term **language barrier** here does not refer to a difference in native tongue but a breakdown in communication as a result of the communicator not speaking in terms, or in a style, the receiver understands. A supervisor should use plain, simple words and direct, uncomplicated language to ensure a message is understood.

language barrier
A hindrance to communication that occurs when a person speaks in a manner another person is unfamiliar with. A language barrier can exist when two people speak different languages, or if they speak the same language but use different terminology or style.

In the healthcare field, concern about the language barrier is heightened. Because there are many levels of unskilled and skilled positions in a healthcare facility, the range of language styles is broad. All employees must communicate in an understandable language to ensure patient care is delivered effectively.

Using a common, understandable language is difficult at times because many English words have several meanings, and sometimes meanings vary among different groups of people. This problem is one of semantics. For example, the word *stay* to some people means "remain in place," whereas others use *stay* to indicate their primary residence, as in "I stay in the Bridgeport neighborhood." The difference between these uses of *stay* is subtle, but could lead to a misunderstanding. Applied to the healthcare setting, when administration speaks of "increased productivity," these words have a positive, goal-oriented meaning for the manager, whereas some employees may hear, "more work ahead." When using words that can carry such different semantic understanding, the communicator must clarify the exact meaning intended. The sender should not just assume that the receiver will interpret the word in the same way she does.

Many words in the English language have similar meanings, but they convey different messages, as shown in the following lists (adapted from Altman, Valenzi, and Hodgetts 1985):

List A	List B
Firm	Unreasonable
Aggressive	Mean
Compassionate	Weak
Detail-oriented	Nit-picky/Anal
Confident	Cocky
Easygoing	Unconcerned
Selective	Unfair
Respects line of authority	Bureaucratic
Independent	Rebellious
Direct	Rude

For most people, the words in List B convey a less favorable message than those in List A. When describing someone you care for, you are likely to use the words in List A. However, the listener tends to listen and interpret the language based on his own experience and frame of reference, not yours.

Workplace Diversity

Healthcare organizations often employ individuals from different cultures, backgrounds, lifestyles, educational levels, and experiences. An organization's workforce often reflects the community it serves. Taking advantage of diverse citizenry may serve an organization well. Having individuals with bilingual skills facilitates communication with patients. However, with this diversity comes the possibility that some employees may not fully understand or may be unable to read English. To accommodate these barriers, managers must alter their communication approaches and, if needed, use a translator or use words or examples that are familiar to all. For some instructions, the supervisor may be able to show the individual how to do the task or draw a picture. A supervisor's ability to communicate in these environments and accommodate workplace diversity while still focusing on producing results contributes to his success.

Status and Position

An organizational structure and its administrative hierarchy create a number of different status levels. Status refers to how the members of an organization regard a particular position and its occupant. A difference in status certainly exists between the level of the president and that of the supervisors and between the level of the supervisors and that of their employees. This difference in status or position often creates barriers that distort the sending and receiving of messages.

For example, when employees listen to a message from the supervisor, several factors come into play. First, the employees evaluate what they hear in relation to their own position, background, and experience; then they take the sender into account. It is difficult for a receiver to separate what she hears from the feelings she has about the person who sends the message. Therefore, the receiver often adds nonexistent motives to the sender, which may alter the message received. For example, union members may be inclined to interpret a statement coming from administration in a negative manner because they are convinced management is trying to undermine the union. Often, union members consider a hospital's newsletter the administration's propaganda mouthpiece, and its contents are viewed with suspicion.

The supervisor who is trying to be an effective communicator must realize that these status and position differences influence the feelings and prejudices of the employees and thus create barriers to communication. Moreover, not only might the employees evaluate the boss's words differently, but they might also place undue importance on a superior's gestures, silence, smile, or other nonverbal expressions. Simply speaking, the CEO's words are not just words—they are words that come from the boss. This is how barriers caused by status work in the downward flow of communication.

Similar obstacles related to status and position also arise in the upward flow of communication, as all subordinates are eager to look good in their boss's eyes. Therefore, employees may conveniently and protectively screen the information that is passed up the line. A subordinate, for example, may tell the supervisor what the latter likes to hear and may omit or soften what is unpleasant. Similarly, supervisors anxious to cover up their own weaknesses when speaking to a person in a higher position may fail to pass on important information because they believe that such information would reflect unfavorably on their own supervisory abilities. After two or three selective filterings by different echelons of the administrative hierarchy, you can imagine that the final message may be considerably distorted.

Resistance to Change

Resistance to change can constitute another serious barrier to communication because messages often convey new ideas to the employees—things that may change work assignments, positions, daily routines, working environments, or social networks. Most people prefer things as they are and do not welcome changes. There are many reasons for resistance to change, but the most common is that many employees feel that keeping the existing environment in its present state is safer. (See Chapter 22 for further discussion of the reasons for resistance to and facilitation of change.)

Ultimately, everyone finds a niche in an organization. An employee's work area—a locker, a cubicle, a chair—all become part of this small workplace world, even in a large department. Many employees may be suspicious of a message that threatens to change their niche or their routine. They filter what they hear, rejecting new ideas that do not conform with the status quo. Sometimes these filters work so efficiently that the receivers do not listen at all. Even if they hear the entire message, they either reject the part of the message that conflicts with their beliefs or they find some way of twisting its meaning to fit their preconceived ideas. In the end, the receivers hear only what they wish to hear. If they are insecure, worried, or fearful in their position, this barrier to receiving communication becomes even more impermeable.

This filtering process can become a barrier to progress. Joel Barker (1993), a well-known speaker and author on this subject, uses the example of the Swiss watchmakers who, in 1970, rejected a digital watch proposal from one of their colleagues because they thought no one would want a nontraditional watch—one without a face, hands, and gears. Texas Instruments and Seiko then recognized the idea as a breakthrough in technology, and of course, capitalized on the new type of watch. Unfortunately, the Swiss were locked "in gear" and unable to progress past their own watch paradigm.

Supervisors are sometimes confronted with situations in which their subordinates appear to only half-listen to what they say. Perhaps their employees are so busy and preoccupied with their own thoughts that they only pay attention to the ideas they like. The information they do not care for, does not immediately apply to their situation, or seems irreconcilable is conveniently brushed aside, not heard at all, or explained away. This selective perception of information constitutes a serious barrier to a supervisor's communications, particularly when the message is intended to convey a change, a new directive, or anything that could conceivably interfere with the employees' routine or working environment.

Additional Barriers

In addition to the barriers already mentioned, many other roadblocks to communication arise in specific situations. For example, obstacles are caused by emotional reactions such as deeply rooted feelings, biases, and prejudice (no one is without biases). The subordinate's perception of the sender as not being trustworthy is also likely to cause distortion. Other obstacles result from physical conditions such as inadequate telephone lines, overloaded bulletin boards, lack of a private place to talk, temperature conditions, or noise. A supervisor who will not or does not take the time to listen is his own worst barrier to communication. Indifference, complacency, or the "they don't care" attitude that can be held by both supervisors and subordinates may also impede communication.

Unless managers are familiar with all barriers to communication, they are in no position to overcome them. Supervisors should not assume that the messages they send are received as intended; in fact, it may be more realistic, although discouraging, to assume the opposite. Because the effectiveness of the supervisory job depends largely on the accurate transmission of messages and instructions, managers must do everything possible to overcome these barriers to improve their communication effectiveness.

Overcoming Barriers to Improve Communication Effectiveness

Supervisors can prevent and overcome major communication barriers through adequate preparation, credibility, feedback, direct language, effective listening and sensitivity, appropriate actions, and repetition. Becoming familiar with and using these techniques increases your likelihood for successful communication.

Adequate Preparation and Credibility

Do not initiate communication before you know what you are going to say and what you intend to achieve. According to data from OfficeTeam (1999), employees waste 14 percent of every 40-hour work week as a result of unclear communication; that adds up to seven weeks per year.

For example, if you want to assign a job, be sure that you have analyzed the job thoroughly so that you can explain it properly. Only if you understand your ideas can you be sure that another person will understand your instructions. If you are searching for facts, decide in advance what information you need so that you can ask intelligent, pertinent, and precise questions. If your discussion entails disciplinary action, be certain that you have sufficiently investigated the case and have enough information before you reprimand or penalize.

If supervisors are not a reliable source of information for their team members or senior leadership, problems of credibility may arise. If, however, communicators are well prepared and honest, credibility is not a problem. Supervisors must overcome the barriers inherent in their position and those that may distort the interpretation of the message intended. The supervisor should anticipate possible reactions and questions that may arise.

Feedback

Probably the most effective tool for improving communication is feedback. It is the link between receiver and sender that makes certain that effective communication has taken place. Managers must always be alert for some signal or clue indicating that they are being understood. Merely asking the receiver if she understands and getting a simple "yes" is not usually enough. Affirmation is required to make sure that the message is received as intended and that understanding is actually taking place. The medium used in the communication affects the type of feedback you may receive.

The simplest way to obtain such reassurance is to observe the receiver and judge the responses by nonverbal clues such as a facial expression of understanding or bewilderment, a raised eyebrow, or a frown. This form of feedback is only possible in face-to-face communication, of course, which is one of the advantages of speaking to someone in person.

Another way of obtaining feedback in any oral communication is for the sender to ask the receiver to repeat in her own words what the sender has just said. If the receiver can restate the content of the message, the sender knows what the receiver has heard and understood. At the same time, the receiver may ask additional questions that the sender can answer immediately.

Additional feedback can be obtained by observing whether the receivers behave in accordance with the communication. If direct observation is not possible, the senders must watch for responses, reports, and, ultimately, results. If these are as expected, the sender can assume the message was received correctly.

Direct Language

Another helpful way to overcome blocks in communication is for the manager to use words that are as understandable and simple as possible. Although the supervisor should not "speak down" to the employees, long, technical, complicated words, acronyms, and jargon should be avoided unless both the sender and the receiver are comfortable with them. The sender should also be aware of the possible different meanings that words can have for different receivers, as discussed earlier. Again, the single most important question is not whether the receiver *should have* understood it, but if he or she *did* understand it.

Effective Listening and Sensitivity

Carefully and completely listening to the other party is also essential to communication. Good listening means more than a mere expression of attention. It means putting aside biases, listening without a fault-finding or correcting attitude, and paying attention to the meaning of the idea rather than to only the words. Atchison (2006) defines three types of listening:

1. Hearing and reacting (selective listening)
2. Engaging and focusing (active listening)
3. Accepting and supportive (reflective listening)

The supervisor who pays attention and listens to what the subordinate is saying learns more about the employee's values and relationship to the working environment (reflective listening). Understanding, not agreement, is essential. The supervisor may state occasionally what he believes has been expressed

Effective Listening Guide

1. *Stop talking!* You cannot listen if you are talking.
2. *Put the talker at ease.* Help a person feel free to talk. This establishes a permissive environment.
3. *Show a talker that you want to listen.* Look and act interested. Do not read your e-mail while someone talks. Listen to understand, rather than to oppose.
4. *Remove distractions.* Do not continue to read e-mail, tap, or shuffle papers. Will it be quieter if you shut the door?
5. *Empathize with talkers.* Try to see the other person's point of view.
6. *Be patient.* Allow plenty of time. Do not interrupt a talker. Do not start for the door or walk away.
7. *Hold your temper.* An angry person takes the wrong meaning from words.
8. *Go easy on argument and criticism.* These put people on the defensive, and they may clam up or become angry. Do not argue; even if you win, you lose.
9. *Ask questions.* This encourages a talker and shows that you are listening. It helps to develop points further.
10. *Stop talking!* This is first and last, because all other guides depend on it. You cannot listen effectively while you are talking.
    - Nature gave people two ears but only one tongue, which is a gentle hint that they should listen more than they talk.
    - Listening requires two ears, one for meaning and one for feeling.
    - Decision makers who do not listen have less information for making decisions.

SOURCE: Adapted from K. Davis and J. W. Newstrom. 1985. *Human Behavior at Work: Organizational Behavior,* 7th ed., 413. New York: McGraw-Hill Book Company. Reproduced with permission of The McGraw-Hill Companies.

by asking, "Is this what you mean?" The receiver must patiently listen to what the other person has to say, even though it may seem unimportant. Such listening greatly improves communication because it reduces misunderstanding.

Furthermore, being sensitive is necessary for effective communication. This means being aware and respectful of the other's perspective and position, and possibly even expressing empathy. Careful listening and sensitivity allow a speaker to adjust the message to fit the responses and world of the receiver. This adjustment opportunity is another advantage of oral communication over written messages.

Once an atmosphere of trust has been established through the use of reflective listening, engaging the individual in some problem solving may be appropriate. Asking nondirective and focused questions (see Chapter 20) about the problem demonstrates your interest and helps to identify one or more solutions to the concern that triggered the discussion.

Davis and Newstrom's 10 recommendations on effective listening and the use of active and reflective listening techniques (sidebar, page 87) will help prevent selective listening. When a supervisor selectively listens and then reacts without thoughtful processing of the issues and the emotions of the individuals involved, disaster is the result. Staff will think of the supervisor as a reactionary, let her make all decisions without their input and insight, lose trust in her leadership ability, and allow her to fail.

Appropriate Actions

As discussed earlier, supervisors communicate by actions as much as by words. In fact, actions usually communicate more than words. Consider the accounting supervisor who preaches that all staff must be at their desks and working by 8:00 a.m. but who arrives routinely somewhere between 8:20 and 8:40. Managers who fail to bolster their talk with action fail in their job as communicators, no matter how capable they are with words. Whether supervisors like it or not, their superior position makes them the center of attention for the employees. The boss communicates through all observable actions, regardless of whether that communication is intended.

Verbal announcements backed up by appropriate action help the supervisor overcome barriers to communication. If the supervisor says one thing but does another, sooner or later the employees will "listen" primarily to what the boss does. For example, the director of central supply services who says she is always available to see a subordinate undermines the verbal message if her office door is kept closed or if she becomes irritated whenever someone comes in. Regardless of what may or may not be written in your position description, you as a supervisor serve as a role model for your staff, and your staff mirror your actions.

Repetition

At times it is advisable for a supervisor to repeat a message several times, preferably using different words and means of explanation. A certain amount of redundancy is especially helpful when the message is important or when the directives are complicated. As mentioned earlier, adults remember 70 percent of a message that they hear, read, and see. For example, a supervisor may use multiple and overlapping tools to communicate a complex instruction for how to use a new computer application: (1) orally discuss the instruction; (2) read aloud written instructions, inserting additional comments or pointing to fields or icons on the screen to reinforce the written instructions; (3) demonstrate how to use the application, referencing the written document; and (4) watch the employee use the application once or twice to ensure the process is understood.

The degree of redundancy depends on the content of the message and the experience and background of the employee. The sender must be cautioned, however, not to be so repetitious that the message may be ignored because it sounds overly familiar or that the listeners feel patronized by the constant reminder. If in doubt, a degree of repetition is safer than none.

The Grapevine: The Informal Communication Network

Although developing sound formal channels of communication is essential, the dynamics of organizational life tend to create additional channels. This informal communication network among people in an organization is commonly referred to as the *grapevine*. Every organization has its grapevine—a network of spontaneous channels of communication. Informal communication is a logical and normal outgrowth of the casual groupings of people, their social interaction, and their natural desire to communicate with each other. People exchanging news through the grapevine should be considered a perfectly natural activity. It fulfills the subordinate's desire to be kept posted on the latest information. The grapevine also gives the members of the organization an outlet for their imagination and an opportunity to relieve their apprehensions in the form of rumors.

Attempts to eliminate the grapevine will be in vain. An efficient manager acknowledges the grapevine's presence and may even put it to good use. An informal communication network also enables the manager to surreptitiously feed some information into this channel and obtain some valuable information from it. For example, by learning who the key sources of information are, the manager can sound out employee reactions to contemplated changes before making a decision. Being attuned to the grapevine gives the supervisor excellent insight into what the subordinates think and feel.

Operation of the Grapevine

Sometimes the grapevine carries factual information and news, but most often it passes on inaccurate information, half-truths, rumors, private interpretations, wishful thinking, suspicions, and other various bits of distorted information. The grapevine is active 24 hours a day and spreads information with amazing speed, often faster than most official channels. The telephone, voicemail, e-mail, cell phones and PDAs, text messaging, weblogs, and Twitter help news travel quickly and reach many people at the same time. The grapevine has no definite pattern or stable membership, is present at all levels of an organization, and carries information in all directions. The news is carried in a flexible, meandering pattern, ignoring organizational charts. Its path

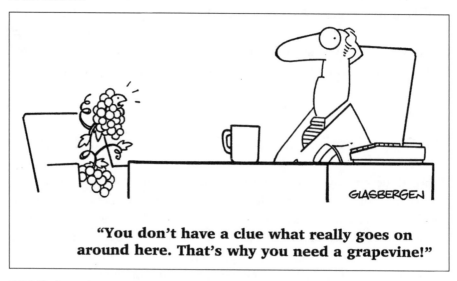

"You don't have a clue what really goes on around here. That's why you need a grapevine!"

SOURCE: Cartoon by Randy Glasbergen. Reprinted with permission.

and behavior cannot be predicted, and the path it followed yesterday will not necessarily be the same today or tomorrow.

Most of the time only a small number of employees are active contributors to the grapevine. Most employees hear information through the grapevine but do not pass it along. Any person in an organization is likely to become active in the grapevine on one occasion or another. However, some individuals tend to be more active than others. They believe that their prestige is enhanced by providing the latest news, and thus they do not hesitate to spread the news or even augment its "completeness" and "accuracy." These active participants in the grapevine know that they cannot be held accountable, so it is understandable that they exercise a considerable degree of imagination whenever they pass information along. The resulting rumors give them, as well as other members of the organization, an outlet for discussing their apprehensions.

During periods of insecurity, upheaval, and anxiety, the grapevine works overtime. In general, it serves as a safety valve for the emotions of all subordinates, providing them with the means to say freely what they please without the danger of being held accountable. Because everyone knows that tracing the origins of a rumor is nearly impossible, employees can feel quite safe in their anonymity as they participate in the grapevine.

Uses of the Grapevine

Because the grapevine often carries a considerable amount of useful information, it can help clarify and disseminate formal communication. Informal communication often spreads information that could not be disseminated through the official channels of communication. For instance, the COO "resigns" suddenly. Although top administration does not want to say publicly how the resignation came about, it does not want to leave the impression that she was treated unfairly or discriminated against. In such a situation, someone in administration may tell someone in the hospital, who "promises" not to spread further what really happened.

Supervisors who deal effectively with the grapevine are attuned to it and learn what it is saying; normal grapevine listening is not unethical behavior by supervisors. They must look for the meaning of the grapevine's communication, not merely for its words. They must learn who the key participants are and who is likely to spread the information. By feeding facts to the grapevine, supervisors can counter rumors and half-truths, using the grapevine's energy in the interest of management.

Rumors can be caused by several different factors such as wishful thinking and anticipation, uncertainty and fear, or even malice and dislike. For example, employees who want something badly enough commonly start passing the word that their wish is fact. If they want a raise, they may start a rumor that management will be giving everybody an across-the-board pay increase. No one knows for certain where or how it started, but this story spreads like wildfire. Everyone wants to believe it. Of course, building up hopes in anticipation of something that will not happen is bad for a group's morale. If a story is spread that the supervisor realizes will lead to disappointment, the manager should move vigorously to debunk it by presenting the facts. Toward this end, a straight answer is almost always the best answer. If the supervisor has been able to build a climate of trust, the employees will believe her.

The same prescription applies to rumors caused by fear or uncertainty. If, for example, the patient volumes decline and a reduction in force must occur, stories and rumors quickly multiply. In such periods of insecurity and anxiety, the grapevine becomes more active than at other times. Usually the rumors are far worse than what actually happens. Here again, giving the facts is better than concealing them. In many instances, much of the fear and anxiety can be eliminated by maintaining open communication channels. Continuing rumors and uncertainty are likely to be more demoralizing than even the most unpleasant facts. Thus, it is usually best to explain immediately why employees are being laid off. When emergencies occur, when new procedures are introduced, or when policies are changed, management should explain the reasons. Otherwise, subordinates make up their own explanations, which are often incorrect.

Other situations may arise, however, in which a supervisor does not have the facts or the facts are so confidential that they cannot be revealed. In such instances, the supervisor should let his superior know what is bothering the employees. He should ask the superior for specific instructions on what information to share, how much he may tell, and when to tell it. The supervisor should next meet with his assistants and lead employees, and give them the story and guide their thinking. Then they can spread the facts before anyone else can spread the rumors.

Although this procedure may work with rumors caused by fear or uncertainty, it might not be appropriate for rumors that arise out of dislike, anger, or malice. Once again, the best prescription is for the supervisor to be objective and impersonal and to come out with the facts, if possible. Sometimes, however, a supervisor finds that the only way to stop a malicious rumor peddler is to expose her personally and reveal the untruthfulness of the statement. If employees believe in the supervisor's fairness and good supervision, they quickly debunk any malicious rumor once he has exposed the person who started it or has given his answer to it. Thus, although there is no way to eliminate the grapevine, even its most threatening rumors can be counteracted to the management's advantage. Every supervisor, therefore, should listen to the informal channels of communication and develop the skill for dealing with them.

Summary

Communication is the process of transmitting information and making oneself understood by another or others. As long as two people understand one another, they have communicated. Agreement is not necessary for communication to be successful. To perform the managerial functions, a supervisor must realize the crucial importance of good communication.

Throughout every organization are formal and informal channels of communication. These channels carry messages downward, upward, horizontally, and diagonally. The formal channels are established mainly by the organizational structure and authority relationships. The supervisor plays a strategic role in the communication process in all these directions.

Although the spoken word is the most significant medium of communication, one must not overlook the importance of nonverbal language. In addition, action is a communication medium that often speaks louder than words. In the healthcare field, the written word is a major medium of communication. Of all media, however, oral, face-to-face communication between supervisors and employees is still the most widely used and the most effective because it provides immediate feedback.

Messages frequently become distorted or are not accurately received for many reasons. The manager must be aware of the major barriers to effective communication and how to overcome them; some barriers can be attributed to the sender, the receiver, the interaction of the two, or the environment.

In addition to the formal channels, an informal network exists, usually referred to as the grapevine. This is the personal network of information among employees fostered by social relationships; it is a natural outgrowth of the informal organization and the social interactions of people. The grapevine serves a useful purpose in every organization. Instead of trying to eliminate it, the supervisor should accept it as a natural outlet and at times participate in it for the benefit of the organization.

New communication technologies such as social media and texting have affected how business is being done. However, regardless of these new technologies, one must follow the fundamental concepts of successful communication.

Additional Readings

Group Works. 2008. "Getting Things Done in Groups." Effective Communication Bulletin 6103, August. [Online article; retrieved 12/28/08.] www.umext.maine.edu/onlinepubs/htmpubs/6103.htm#1.

Nichols, R. G., L. A. Stevens, F. Bartolome, and C. Argyris. 1999. *Harvard Business Review on Effective Communication*. Boston: Harvard Business Review Paperback Series.

Thielst, C. B. 2007. "Weblogs: A Communication Tool." *Journal of Healthcare Management* 52 (5): 187.

APPENDIX 5.1

Poorly Written Memo

Memo to: The Boss

From: The Subordinate

Re: Today's Events

Three days ago, Joe Hansen, the BME, noticed some seepage from wall 5E. The seepage continued, so Joe contacted the evening TL to periodically check the seepage and see if it could be repaired. The TL, Tim Walters, determined the water source was from the outside. After some investigation, he found it might involve the Water Company. He sent an e-mail to the Water Company. The Water Company sent out a man to check out the situation, and he determined that they had a water main leak in the ground next to 5E. They came out again today to repair the main, but in doing so, the main burst. This caused flooding in the boiler room, and it destroyed one of our boilers. The Water Company said they would pay the repair bill. We have issued a PO to have an emergency replacement installed. Just thought you ought to know about this.

Well-Written Memo

Memo to: The Boss

From: The Subordinate

Re: Boiler Destroyed

The Water Company's water main, located on our exterior wall, broke today, causing flooding of the boiler room and destruction of one of our boilers. The Water Company is paying for the replacement boiler that we ordered today on an emergency purchase order.

One of our boiler maintenance employees noticed the seepage three days ago and advised the Team Leader, Tim Walters. Tim contacted the Water

Company to take care of the situation, but, unfortunately, the main was so weak that when they started to work on it, it burst.

Just thought you'd like to know about this. Let me know if you need further information.

APPENDIX 5.2

Guidance for Better Communication

by Roger P. Holland, MD, PhD

Language

Language used properly is incredibly compelling. We want to compel them [physicians/readers] to act quickly and in the direction that we think they should go. Let's gaze at some incredibly powerful words.

But

The most consequential word to avoid in any discussion is "but." If I were visiting you at your hospital to provide an educational in-service, what would you think if I began the exit session as follows: "Ms. Smith, you have a well-managed, quiet department, with an extremely friendly staff that gave me every assistance in performing this chart review, but. . . ." Now, quickly, what are you thinking? Did you remember all the nice things I just said about your department and staff? No, you're waiting for the other shoe to drop. You're waiting for what? Bad news! It doesn't really matter what I say next because all you're waiting for is bad news. In fact, you'll actually be uncomfortable or confused if I don't say something bad. What have I accomplished by using the word "but"? First, all my preceding compliments at best will be forgotten and at worst will be now regarded with suspicion. Second, you're bracing yourself for the bad news. I've placed you in a defensive posture. Anything I hope to convey to you after the "but" will be blunted.

Rather than "but," the word I should have employed is "and." Reread my sentence, this time replacing the "but" with "and." Don't you feel better? Now, instead of bad news, you're probably anticipating some good news. Even if I'm going to give you bad news ("and your DRG coders have a problem coding cancer records"), you'll keep smiling because your brain is programmed to receive good news. I recommend that you try this on your spouse and children. Avoid "but" at all costs. (See Table I for a list of other words like "but" that should be avoided. See Table II for a list of words like "and" that should be used.)

You

Let's say I walk into your office and begin a conversation with, "You. . . ." To some people, this immediately triggers a defensive posture. Perhaps you are querying a physician and your query begins, "You said that this patient was admitted with pneumonia. . . ." Many physicians will feel threatened. Yes, it's not a rational response. We are creatures of emotion. Words can trigger, amplify, and blunt any emotion. Now the physician is waiting for you to drop the other shoe. So, let's drop it.

"You said that this patient was admitted with pneumonia, but the x-ray indicates. . . ." Now your physician is subconsciously thinking all sorts of negative things, not only about him, but of you as well. The lesson here is this: do not use pronouns that center on the physician. It doesn't matter what is going to be said next. He's already thinking of something mean to either say to you or an act of violence toward the piece of paper he's holding in his hand. This time, let's rephrase it: "This patient was admitted with pneumonia and the x-ray indicates. . . ." Isn't that better?

If a pronoun is necessary with the query, try to use plurals such as "we," "us," or "they." Don't use "you."

There are many words that elicit a defensive response. "Always" and "never" are among them. Even if you and Coding Clinics are correct, telling a physician, "According to Coding Clinics, you can never code unstable angina as the principal diagnosis in the setting of an acute myocardial infarction" is worse than waving a red cape in front of an angry bull. You can imagine the response you'll receive from most physicians! Personally, if I used either of these two words with my spouse, her immediate response is, "Always?!" or "Never?!"

The "Because" Clause

Contrary to what you may have been taught as a child, the most powerful word in the English language is not "please." It is "because." Sentences that begin with "because" get answered positively more often than any other kind of sentence. Just as "but" evokes an immediate and strong negative response, "because" evokes a very strong positive response in the mind of the listener or reader. Scientific studies have demonstrated how powerful this word is.

TABLE I Words to Avoid			
but	still	further
yet	except	as well as
however	likewise	

TABLE II Words to Use			
and	also	moreover
in addition	plus	

"Because" puts our brain into a state of positive expectancy. When the brain hears the word "but," it immediately ignores everything that came before and braces itself for something different. It's in a state of negative expectancy. When the brain hears "because" it tends to ignore everything that comes after and rushes on to, "Of course, I agree."
Example:

```
Dear Dr. Jones:

Did this patient have atrial fibrillation and did
you address it during the patient's stay?

Sincerely,
Susie Smith, DRG Coder
```

First, what's right with this query? You didn't use the words "but," "always," or "never."

And what's wrong with this query? First, it asks the physician to think. He is going to have to review the medical record. Second, you've worried him. Now he's thinking: "Did this patient have atrial fibrillation? Did I address it? Did I treat him appropriately? Didn't I transfer that patient? Didn't I already see that patient in my office for follow-up? Don't these medical record people have anything better to do than to hound me? I've got better things to do with my time. Here's what I think of their query. Swish. Three points."

Let's try again:

```
Dear Dr. Jones:

Because this patient was admitted with an acute
myocardial infarction and because the patient's
atrial fibrillation, noted on the rhythm strips of
7/17 and 7/18, was successfully addressed with
Digoxin, may we include a secondary diagnosis of
atrial fibrillation because it more completely
characterizes the patient's care?

Sincerely,
Susie Smith
```

Getting to Yes

Most people want to agree with you. When you query physicians [others], most of the time you know what the answer is that you want. Your mission is getting physicians [others] to answer in the affirmative and making it painful for them to answer in the negative.

I've noticed two things wrong with query sheets that facilities use. First, the query ends with "Yes" and "No." Try changing this to "Agree" and "Disagree." It's hard to say "No" and it's harder still to say, "I disagree." The former has no object toward which the "No" is directed; the latter implies that I—a human being with feelings—disagree with you. Nobody likes to consistently disagree with another human being. Make it hard for the physician [reader] to disagree with you.

Second, the query gives too much space for the physician to answer the query. All that space transmits a not-so-subtle message: "Doctor, I want an explanation from you. I want you to think. Fill up all the empty space!"

Think back to when you were in school and were taking a test. There, all alone on an otherwise blank sheet of paper was this question: explain the reasons that led to the war between the States.

How did you feel? Did you feel threatened with all that blank white paper facing up at you? Would you not have felt better if there were only two inches of paper or half a dozen lines for you to respond within? Doctors are people who also went through decades of schooling and who are called on every day to write essays in the form of history and physicals and discharge summaries. They hate it, but they feel compelled to do it just the same.

Paradoxically, by leaving them only a few lines in which to respond, they will feel more kindly toward the query. Looking at a few lines sends another message: the correct answer to this query is "Agree." "If I disagree, I'm going to have to explain myself and in such little space and all for no remuneration!" What's the easiest (and least painful) thing to do? To simply agree!

Roger P. Holland, MD, PhD, FAAFP, is president of Utilization PRO, Inc., and provides physician-assisted reimbursement training for health information management, utilization management, and physician advisor personnel. He can be reached at (918) 649–1100 or rph2750@hotmail.com. This exhibit is excerpted with permission by *For the Record Newsmagazine* (September 6, 1999, Vol. II, No. 18).

6

LEGAL ASPECTS
OF THE HEALTHCARE SETTING

The following individuals have contributed to this chapter: Pamela Marshall, formerly of the American College of Healthcare Executives; Brian L. Andrew, JD, of TLCVision; and Carolyn A. Haimann, JD, and Lynne Morgenstern, JD, formerly of the law firm of Lewis, Rice, and Fingersch.

Chapter Objectives

After you have studied this chapter, you should be able to do the following:

1. Understand basic information on legal issues affecting the healthcare environment.
2. Outline the basis of institutional responsibility for healthcare rendered to patients.
3. Recognize key causes for liability.
4. Identify employee litigation issues.
5. Understand the key concepts of major regulations affecting management.

Enormous pressures on the healthcare industry continue to create a legal environment of change and uncertainty. Because of unscrupulous behavior by some healthcare executives and clinicians as well as bad outcomes from services, courts have demonstrated an increasing willingness to adopt new theories of liability for healthcare institutions, both as providers of medical services and as employers. Government agencies continue to issue regulations that constrain hospitals and other healthcare provider activities in an attempt to meet two distinct and possibly conflicting goals: holding down healthcare costs and improving the quality of care.

An unbelievably growing number of federal and national regulatory entities govern healthcare organizations (see Exhibit 32.3). Healthcare institutions have lost their traditional role as charitable providers of medical care. Instead, hospitals, integrated delivery systems, home health agencies, managed care organizations, and a host of ancillary providers and payers are now recognized as business entities that, tax-exempt or not, must maintain a bottom-line profitability to survive. These providers can no longer escape the legal liability that general business has had to cope with for decades. Any advertising and marketing projects developed to address the present competitive climate in the industry must reflect their legal implications.

To function effectively in today's litigious atmosphere, everyone involved in healthcare delivery—from members of the board to physicians to administrators at all levels—unquestionably must be aware of the legal considerations that may arise from their activities and decisions and the actions of their subordinates.[1] This is the fourth of the connecting processes discussed in this text.

This chapter provides general and basic information in nonlegal language and should not be used in place of the advice of or consultation with legal counsel. The purpose is to give department heads and supervisors an overall perspective on some of the legal aspects of their positions. Be aware that issues of healthcare liability evolve from state and federal statutes and also from court decisions based on principles of common law and that they can vary between jurisdictions. As with all aspects of law, health law and court decisions applying these principles evolve and change on a continuous basis.

doctrine of charitable immunity
The legal concept that the assets of charitable organizations, such as nonprofit hospitals, will not be jeopardized by lawsuits.

For example, for a long time the courts protected hospitals and other charitable institutions from lawsuits that might infringe on their assets. This was generally known as the **doctrine of charitable immunity**. Currently, however, as discussed later in this chapter, nearly every state has established the doctrine that charitable organizations are obliged to compensate for injuries they cause.

Liability

liability
The potential of a lawsuit.

Liability is a problem that is familiar to administrators, supervisors, and employees in healthcare organizations. Individual liability primarily relates to torts and related actions (e.g., a nurse administers the wrong intravenous medication to a patient), as distinguished from liabilities associated with the organizational aspects of a healthcare entity (e.g., antitrust, tax, fraud and abuse, insurance, or regulatory issues). A **tort** is a legal wrong or an act or omission of acting that results in injury to another. Managers and employees at all levels are constantly being reminded of the potential for liability and its resulting costs to the institution. The need for in-house legal counsel, risk managers, consent forms, incident reports, and numerous requirements for documentation are reminders of the litigious environment within which the healthcare team works. Liability is on everyone's mind, and the growing number of multimillion-dollar judgments against institutions and their staffs has become a hindrance to management and physicians.

tort
An action or omission of action that results in injury to another.

Just as charitable institutions were able to avoid liability that was traditionally applied to general business corporations, so too have managed care entities been able to avoid the liability concerns that were pervasive throughout the healthcare industry. However, a growing number of courts have applied traditional vicarious liability doctrines to managed care entities, particularly to HMOs. **Vicarious liability** is a concept that one party may be held responsible for the actions of another even though the original party was not involved in the act. For example, the ambulatory surgery center has vicarious liability for the anesthesiologist who overdoses the patient because the center allows the anesthesiologist to practice there. Vicarious liability, in contrast to a tort, is based on a relationship between two or more individuals or entities rather than on the conduct or actions of the individuals or entities. The relationship is often that of independent contractor–contracting agent rather than employer–employee.

vicarious liability
The concept that one party may be held responsible for the actions of another even though the original party was not involved in the act.

HMOs, a hybrid between health insurers and healthcare providers, are subject to the same liabilities as a traditional healthcare provider, including negligence and **ostensible agency** actions. To establish a healthcare organization's liability for an independent contractor's medical malpractice based on ostensible agency, a **plaintiff** (individual or entity that believes it was wronged) must show that (1) he or she had a reasonable belief that the contractor (physician, therapist, temporary employee) was the agent or employee of the hospital, (2) such belief was generated by the organization holding out the individual as its agent or employee or knowingly permitting the individual to hold himself or herself out as the organization's agent or employee, and (3) he or she justifiably relied on this "appearance" of authority. This includes an HMO being liable for the medical malpractice of a physician if it creates the appearance that the physician is its employee, regardless of his or her actual status. Thus, all of the discussion in this chapter of potential legal concerns to healthcare providers and institutions apply to managed care organizations as well. The following section addresses various aspects of liability for the healthcare institution, the supervisor, and the employee.

ostensible agency
An organization that appears to employ an individual, even if it does not actually employ that individual.

plaintiff
The individual or entity that sues another.

The Institution's Direct Responsibility

Although liability is frequently imposed on institutions for negligence resulting in injuries to visitors and employees, most lawsuits filed against healthcare facilities involve patient injuries and allegations of negligent care. Therefore, this discussion focuses on the institution's liability for injuries to its patients and its responsibility for the medical care rendered by its physicians.

The law states that any organization that the public relies on for its safety has a duty to exercise ordinary care to prevent injury. Even before the Institute of Medicine published *To Err Is Human: Building a Safer Healthcare System* (Kohn, Corrigan, and Donaldson 2000), the emphasis on patient safety by healthcare providers and accrediting agencies was growing. The law also serves as one of the bases for the Bush administration's and Obama administration's push for electronic health records. In most jurisdictions a hospital owes a duty to provide its patients the degree of skill, care, and diligence that would be provided by a similar hospital under the same or similar circumstances. More specifically, a hospital has a legal duty to provide its patients with, among other things, premises kept in a reasonably safe condition, appropriately trained and skilled staff, reasonably adequate equipment, and proper medications. Whether a hospital has breached any of its duties to the patient in a particular situation is usually decided by a jury. If a jury finds that a hospital has failed to meet the various standards of care owed to its patients, thereby breaching its duty, the hospital can be found negligent.

negligence
An action or nonaction that results in an injury by an individual who is not acting as a "reasonably prudent person" would under the same circumstances.

For the purpose of this book, assume that any time one does not follow the healthcare organization's policies and procedures, her action(s) or lack of action may cause injury and could therefore result in a claim of **negligence** for which the entity and possibly the employee will be held liable. Negligence is when an injury occurs as the result of an action or nonaction by an individual who is not acting as a "reasonably prudent person" would under the same circumstances. Often "reasonably prudent persons" are those who are of the same profession and working within the same region of the country.

What are some examples of torts that could occur and result in a claim of negligence? One obvious example is the environmental services worker who wet-mops the floor and fails to post the stand-up signs notifying visitors or others that the floor is wet. A visitor comes along and slips, cracking a hip and fracturing a wrist. The environmental services employee committed a tort. The facility is responsible for the employee's negligence. Consider the plant engineering department that neglects to change the air filters in the air conditioning units of the pediatric floor. Suddenly a rise in infections occurs in pediatrics. The infection control committee investigates to determine the cause of the infection increase and discovers that the filters were not changed as scheduled. Even if the patient chose not to sue the facility, the failure to follow protocol would result in increased cost to the patient or patient's insurer. Some of these conditions would be considered **hospital acquired** and, as such, the expenses incurred to treat the affected patients would not be reimbursed by third-party payers.

hospital acquired
An adjective describing an injury or infection that occurred due to negligence by a healthcare facility.

Respondeat Superior

Not only is an institution directly responsible for its actions in relation to the patient, but it is also indirectly liable for patient injuries. It is legally responsible for the actions of those persons, employees, and staff over whom it exercises control and supervision. This vicarious liability arises from the doctrine of **respondeat superior**. Under this doctrine, the institution-employer is legally responsible for the negligent or wrongful acts or omissions of the employee even though the facility itself committed no wrong; the negligence of the employee is imputed to, or placed on, the employer. If an employee commits a negligent act that is the direct cause of injury to a patient, the employer

respondeat superior
The legal doctrine by which an employer is responsible for the actions or omissions of its employees.

may be liable for the damages awarded to the injured party. The doctrine of respondeat superior applies only to civil actions (between private individuals and tied to civil law); thus, an employer is not responsible for the criminal actions (violations of penal law such as blackmail) of its employees.

For an institution to be liable under respondeat superior, the employer must have the right to control the actions of employees in the performance of their duties (i.e., the method, time, and manner of work performance). If the jury determines that this is the case and that the employee (or agent) was acting within the scope and course of employment, the institution will be found liable. An act is generally considered within the scope of employment when the employee is acting on behalf of (or perceives himself or herself to be acting for) the benefit of the institution.

The doctrine of respondeat superior, however, does not release the employee from liability for his wrongful act. The employee as well as the employer may be found liable in damages to an injured third party. Under the law, the employer may pursue indemnification or recovery from financial loss from the employee when his actions caused the facility to be responsible for the loss. This occurs infrequently because the adverse effect on employee morale outweighs the benefit of attempting to collect monies from the employee. The following example illustrates the application of respondeat superior.

Assume Joe Smith has been employed by Hospital X for the past five years as a full-time registered nurse on its medical floor. He has a good job record with no incidents of poor performance or poor exercise of nursing judgment. While Joe is on duty during his assigned shift on his assigned floor, he is responsible for passing evening medications to the patients. One day Joe fails to carefully check the order for patients Ms. Jones and Ms. Brown and administers the medication ordered for Ms. Jones to Ms. Brown. As a direct result of the wrong medication being administered to her, Ms. Brown suffers a severe, sudden drop in blood pressure that results in shock. Ms. Brown recovers, but not until after an extended hospital stay in the intensive care unit. She then sues the nurse and the hospital for negligence. The jury finds the nurse liable for negligence and finds the hospital vicariously liable because it was the employer. The jury awards a single sum of money, $50,000, against both the hospital and the nurse jointly, even though the nurse was negligent and the hospital's responsibility was based solely on the theory of respondeat superior. The hospital pays the $50,000 to Ms. Brown and, in accordance with its policy, does not exercise its right of indemnification; that is, it does not ask Joe to pay the hospital $50,000.

In this example, the employer–employee relationship existed; Joe was a salaried employee whose hours of work, types of duty, and procedures for carrying them out were all controlled by his employer. Furthermore, the wrongful act, giving the wrong medication to the wrong patient, occurred while Joe was on his assigned shift performing his assigned duties; thus, the act was "within the scope and course of his employment."

Just as the hospital in this example was found responsible for the acts of its nurses, it is also responsible for the acts of all other employees, professional and nonprofessional. Thus, an institution will be liable for the negligent acts of technicians, orderlies, transporters, housekeepers, food service personnel, and so forth.

borrowed servant doctrine
The doctrine that a hospital employee is under the direct supervision of a physician when the employee is aiding the physician. In this cases, respondeat superior liability falls on the physician, not the institution.

The **borrowed servant** theory and the related **captain of the ship doctrine** are often mentioned in connection with the principle of respondeat superior. The borrowed servant doctrine applies in certain situations in which a private physician has "borrowed" the employee from the hospital to aid him or her, and thus the physician has assumed the right to control and direct the employee in the performance of a duty or task. Here, the physician and not the facility-employer is liable for that employee's negligent acts.

captain of the ship doctrine
The doctrine that a surgeon directly supervises all personnel assisting an operation; thus respondeat superior liability falls on the surgeon, not the institution.

The captain of the ship doctrine, a narrower concept than the borrowed servant theory, applies in the operating room setting. Under this doctrine, the surgeon is considered the "captain of the ship"; that is, he has complete and total control and supervision over the personnel assisting him. Therefore, the surgeon is responsible for the employee's negligent acts that occur during the procedure. The captain of the ship doctrine does not apply outside the operating room setting. This doctrine has been increasingly rejected by the courts in various jurisdictions. The current trend is to hold the institution, rather than the surgeon, responsible under respondeat superior for the actions of its operating room personnel.

In both the borrowed servant and captain of the ship situations, the key element is the extent and right of control the physician has over the employee whose acts caused the alleged injury. Courts carefully examine and juries decide whether an employee truly has become the borrowed servant of the physician before liability can be imposed on the physician for the employee's negligent acts. Generally speaking, in non–operating-room settings, a physician is not liable for negligence of an institution-employed nurse who carries out the physician's order in the regular course of the nurse's duties. If a physician issues a medically inappropriate order, a court may apportion a measure of the liability to the nurse, and therefore to the institution, if another nurse possessing the same skill and training would have questioned the order rather than carried it out.

hospitalist
A physician who practices solely in a hospital instead of in private practice, and who is employed by the hospital.

The concept of respondeat superior also plays an important role in the question of the institution's responsibility for actions of certain members of its medical staff. The facility is liable under respondeat superior for the actions of those physicians who are employed by the facility or are under its direct control and supervision. Interns and residents in a training program, for example, are considered hospital employees. **Hospitalists**, who are physicians who practice solely in hospitals instead of in private practice, also are employed by hospitals. All of these individuals are salaried by the hospital to render care to its patients; they do not have private patients; and they are under the control and supervision of the hospital, usually through a chief physician who is a hospital employee. Because of these factors, hospitals are almost always held liable for their actions.

In the past, hospitals (and other healthcare institutions) were not held liable for the actions of their private physicians practicing in the hospital or for other physicians who act as independent contractors and over whom the hospital exercises no direct control. The private physician was considered an independent contractor because she has an independent relationship with the patient apart from the hospital. The private physician made independent judgments regarding care of the patient and was not compensated by the hospital for patient care services. She was merely making use of the institution's facilities and support staff for the benefit of the patient. The facility exerted no control over the patient's choice of physician and had no right of control over the physicians' actions regarding their patients. However, liability has increased as a growing number of individuals fraudulently posing as physicians have been admitted to healthcare organizations' medical staffs through faulty credentialing practices. This has occurred for a number of reasons, one of which is the perception by the public that the healthcare organization is responsible for using reasonable care in the selection of members of its medical staff to serve the patients treated at the facility. Credentialing failures have been widely publicized since the Swango experience.[2]

> **ostensible agency**
> The principle that a hospital can be held liable for actions of private physicians who are not employed by the hospital.

Ostensible Agency

A clear trend has emerged in which the hospital has been held vicariously liable for the actions of an independently contracted private practice physician when no employer–employee relationship exists. In these situations, several courts have held that if the hospital caused the patient to believe that the physician rendering care to him was a hospital employee or agent and if the patient did not choose the physician, the hospital was responsible for the physician's acts under the theory of ostensible agency.

This principle is most often applied in circumstances in which a group of private physicians has contracted with the hospital to render special services such as anesthesiology, pathology, radiology, or emergency department coverage. These physicians are considered independent contractors, not hospital employees. Some courts have held, however, that patients who come for treatment to the emergency department of a hospital that uses these contracted services do not know, and are not expected to know, that the physicians are not hospital employees; furthermore, the patients do not choose which physician they want to attend them. In fact, the courts hold that it appears to the patient that the physician is the hospital's employee. The same applies when a hospitalized patient is taken for tests to a radiology department staffed by private physicians who have contracted with the hospital to provide services. In most cases, the patient does not select an individual radiologist to conduct the test; the patient accepts treatment from the radiologist assigned. Although the radiologist is a private physician and an independent contractor, she appears to the patient to be a hospital employee who was provided by the hospital to render care. The courts that have adopted this doctrine have made it clear that the patient cannot be expected to know or understand the specific contractual relationship between the hospital and the treating physician.

Because hospitals routinely contract with outside entities to provide services formerly rendered entirely by hospital departments, the risk of this type of exposure is great in those states that have adopted this doctrine. A carefully drawn contract can afford moderate protection for the institution, although a contract's provisions cannot absolutely ensure that a court will not find the institution liable for the acts of an independent contractor.

The courts have found a variety of factors that determine whether vicarious liability or ostensible agency exists. Any combination (although not necessarily all) of the following factors may result in a court determining liability:

- The healthcare entity invites patients to use its services.
- A patient receives treatment at the hospital by a physician provided by the hospital without specific selection by the patient.
- The hospital fails to advise the patient that the emergency department (ED) physician or another hospital-based physician is not an agent or employee of the hospital.
- The hospital arranges for a specific group of physicians to exclusively provide certain types of medical service.
- The hospital directly bills patients for services of the ED or the hospital-based physician.
- The hospital undertakes to collect the accounts receivable of the ED or the hospital-based physician.
- The hospital shares the ED, radiology, anesthesiology, or pathology collections with physicians or guarantees them a minimum compensation level.
- The ED or another hospital-based physician is prevented by a contract with the hospital from conducting a private medical practice or from practicing at any other hospital.
- The hospital owns the equipment and operates the department used by ED or hospital-based physicians.
- The hospital through its employees indicates that the physician is an agent of the hospital (e.g., referring to the physician as "our" doctor).
- The hospital's management controls the appointments of physicians.

Healthcare institutions should take steps to address these factors if their entities are located in a jurisdiction favoring the ostensible agency doctrine.

Institutional Responsibility for Medical Care and Treatment

As mentioned earlier, nonprofit, tax-exempt healthcare institutions (most often hospitals) were traditionally not considered legally responsible for the negligence of private physicians chosen by the patients themselves and therefore were protected by the doctrine of charitable immunity. The hospital was considered to be merely the provider of the physical premises where physicians carried out their work. The hospital did not "practice medicine"; only the physicians did. The hospital's legal responsibility for the quality of care rendered by private physicians in its facility, however, has expanded greatly in recent years and now falls under the category of corporate negligence.

The **corporate negligence** doctrine is primarily the result of case law beginning in 1965 with the Illinois Supreme Court case of *Darling v. Charleston Community Memorial Hospital.* In this landmark case, the plaintiff sustained a fracture in his leg during a football game and was taken to Charleston Community Memorial Hospital for treatment. There the leg was casted, but severe complications arose, resulting in the eventual amputation of the plaintiff's leg. The plaintiff brought suit against the physician and the hospital. The Illinois Supreme Court held the hospital liable for the patient's injuries and held that the hospital owed a direct duty of care to the patient. This was a landmark decision because it imposed on the hospital the duty to monitor the quality of patient care.

corporate negligence
The doctrine that a corporation is legally responsible for actions of associated individuals, even nonemployees.

The Darling case has been cited, followed, and expanded on by courts in most other states, and the implications of the Darling decision for hospitals have been widely debated. The general trend since the decision has been toward holding the institution directly responsible for the medical care rendered to its patients. The court in this case said (*Darling v. Charleston Community Memorial Hospital* 1966):

> The conception that the hospital does not undertake to treat the patient, does not undertake to act through its doctors and nurses, but undertakes instead simply to procure them to act upon their own responsibility, no longer reflects the fact. Present-day hospitals, as their manner of operation plainly demonstrates, do far more than furnish facilities for treatment. They regularly employ on a salary basis a large staff of physicians, nurses, and interns, as well as administrative and manual workers, and they charge patients for medical care and treatment, collecting for such services, if necessary, by legal action. Certainly, the person who avails himself of "hospital facilities" expects that the hospital will attempt to cure him, not that its nurses or other employees [sic] will act on their own responsibility.

Clearly at this point, although the hospital is not legally responsible for the negligent acts of its private physicians acting as independent contractors, a hospital has a legal duty to monitor the quality of patient care and the care given by its private physicians. A hospital is usually held directly liable under the corporate negligence doctrine for failing to (1) select and retain only competent physicians on its medical staff; (2) regularly and routinely review the activities of its physicians; (3) formulate, adopt, and enforce adequate rules and policies to ensure quality care; and (4) take necessary action against those physicians when the hospital has knowledge or reason to know that they are not performing according to set standards, are incompetent, or are endangering patient welfare.

In fact, state and federal legislation (e.g., the Health Care Quality Improvement Act of 1986) has imposed peer review responsibilities on hospitals that include reporting disciplinary actions and lawsuits against physicians on the hospital's staff to government agencies (e.g., through the National Practitioner Data Bank). Some states have extended the reporting requirements to include nurses and other clinicians.

Liability exposure has also resulted from changes in reimbursement for healthcare services, primarily as a result of increased managed care products. The principal method used to manage healthcare under a health benefit plan is utilization review; a medical insurance company, for example, designates a specified number of days for hospitalization of a plan enrollee. If complications develop and the patient requires a longer stay, the physician must seek third-party payer approval for the additional time. If that request is denied, the hospital is not paid for the extended stay. These developments have given rise to the perception, whether or not it is true in practice, that patients are being prematurely discharged. Suits for injuries caused by premature discharge may not only be brought against hospitals but against physicians and third-party payers as well.

Thus, in those situations in which hospitals act as the managed care entity, concern is increasing about potential liability for medical treatment decisions that may arise out of adverse payment determinations. The notable California Appellate Court case known as *Wickline v. State of California* (1987) held that third-party payers could be held liable to a patient if their prior authorization programs were administered in such an arbitrary or negligent manner so as to injure the plaintiff. However, in this case, the court absolved the payer from liability, ruling that the responsibility for deciding the course of the medically necessary treatment, including when to discharge a patient from the hospital, belonged to the treating physician rather than to the third-party payer. In those situations in which hospitals have significant oversight of physician practices, it is incumbent on the hospital to ensure that the physicians use to the extent possible all appeals and other grievance mechanisms set forth by the payer.

The growth of sophisticated information systems and the increased demand for data mean that more outsiders have access to patient-specific information. Because of breaches of information systems (e.g., recent cases involving Maria Shriver, George Clooney, and Britney Spears in California as well as others), regulations (see discussion on HIPAA later in this chapter) have been imposed to protect patient information regardless of whether it is maintained in an electronic or paper format. As maintaining the confidentiality of patient records becomes increasingly difficult for healthcare entities, providers, and payers alike, patients are becoming more concerned with the release of what they consider to be personal information. In turn, as more healthcare entities install electronic health records, information becomes increasingly accessible to providers, payers, employers, and other organizations. Federal and state initiatives toward electronic health records and health information interchange (such as regional health information organizations [RHIOs]) require greater attention to the confidentiality and security of patient records. Although it is the institution's responsibility to develop security and confidentiality procedures, it is a supervisor's responsibility to make employees aware of these procedures and to monitor compliance.

Negligence and Malpractice

Malpractice is a term often used synonymously with negligence in reference to the actions or wrongful acts of physicians, nurses, and other healthcare professionals. In fact, these terms are not identical but are similar. *Negligence* is defined in *Black's Law Dictionary* (West Publishing 1979, 930) as follows:

> The omission to do something which a reasonable man, guided by those ordinary considerations which ordinarily regulate human affairs, would do, or the doing of something which a reasonable and prudent man would not do.

Malpractice is the term for negligence of professional persons. Malpractice is defined in *Black's Law Dictionary* (Garner 1999, 959) as follows:

> Professional misconduct or unreasonable lack of skill ... is usually applied to such conduct by doctors, lawyers, and accountants. Failure of one rendering professional services to exercise that degree of skill and learning commonly applied under all the circumstances in the community by the average prudent reputable member of the profession with the result of injury, loss, or damage to the recipient of those services or to those entitled to rely upon them. It is any professional misconduct, unreasonable lack of skill or fidelity in professional or fiduciary duties, evil practice, or illegal or immoral conduct.

Any individual can be negligent, such as when one drives carelessly and strikes another vehicle or when a homeowner fails to rope off a hole in his front walk that is not easily visible. Only a professional person such as a physician, however, can commit malpractice.

To determine what constitutes negligence, the law has developed a measuring scale called the *standard of care*. Generally speaking, this is determined by what a "reasonably prudent person" would do under similar circumstances. This reasonably prudent person is, more specifically, a hypothetical person with average skills, training, and judgment and represents the yardstick for measuring what others should do in similar circumstances. If someone's performance fails to meet the standard, negligence has occurred. Also, if it was foreseeable that failure to meet that standard would cause injury and if the negligence was the direct and proximate cause of injury, liability is imposed.

A number of elements are necessary to maintain an action for negligence: (1) there must be an injury to someone, (2) a duty must be owed to the injured person, (3) a breach of that duty must occur, and (4) the breach of this duty must have been the proximate cause of the injury. If any one of these elements is missing, a negligence claim theoretically cannot be maintained successfully. The standards of care that medical professionals must meet are higher than those imposed on laypersons. The following is an example of how these elements of negligence apply in the hospital setting in reference to a professional person.

Assume Jane Doe is a registered nurse in a jurisdiction that permits recovery against nurses for malpractice. Jane is assigned to give medicine to Mr. James, a patient under her care. She misreads the order, which is for 40 milligrams (mg) of the antibiotic gentamicin, and instead gives him 400 mg of gentamicin. This drug is extremely potent, and Jane knows that an excessive dose can cause renal (kidney) problems. Mr. James suffers renal shutdown and has to be hospitalized for several more weeks. Applying the elements as previously outlined, Jane has a duty to the patient to possess that degree of skill and learning ordinarily possessed by nurses. She also has the duty to meet the standard of care for nurses in this same situation—that is, to act as a reasonably prudent nurse would have acted. In this case, to meet that requisite standard of care, she should have given the ordered medication to the right patient, in the ordered dose, at the ordered time, and by the ordered mode of administration. Jane deviates from the standard of care (breaching her duty) by failing to give the correct dosage and is thus negligent. If her negligence is the proximate cause of harm to the patient, she is liable for damages. The burden is on the plaintiff to prove the standard and deviation from it. The jury must then decide whether the negligent act is the cause of the injury.

Despite the perceptions of most plaintiffs, it is important to recognize that not all bad results or unexpected outcomes come from negligence or imply liability for the person committing the act. Assume Jane gives the correct dosage of medication to the patient. Assume further that Mr. James has never taken the medication before and on inquiry has said he has no known allergies to any drugs. Five minutes after he receives the medication, he suffers a severe, unanticipated allergic reaction resulting in a cardiac arrest. In this case, although the medication causes injury to Mr. James, Jane is not liable. She meets her duty of care. She gives the correct dose to the right patient, at the right time, and in the correct manner of administration. She has no reason to anticipate that Mr. James would have an allergic reaction. Because she does not breach her duty, she is not negligent. Therefore, without committing negligence, Jane cannot be found liable.

Often the most difficult element to prove in a negligence action is causation. One may be negligent but not held liable if the negligent act is not the cause of harm to the other party. If Jane gives the wrong dose of medication to Mr. James but he suffers no ill effects, she is still negligent. Because her negligent act causes no harm, however, she probably will not be held liable for damages. Furthermore, as the time between the negligent act and the injury lengthens, the more difficult it becomes to prove causation.

Supervisor's Liability

The previous sections describe how the healthcare professional can be held personally liable for his actions. Can the healthcare professional be held personally liable for his negligent actions as a supervisor as well?

The supervisor is not liable for the acts of those supervised on the basis of respondeat superior because the supervisor is not the employer of those he supervises. The institution is the employer, and the supervisor has only administrative responsibility for those he directs. A supervisor is also not liable just because someone under his supervision acts negligently and causes injury to a third party.

Using these guidelines, a supervisor's performance may be measured against the standard of care for a reasonably prudent person in the same or similar supervisory position. If a supervisor fails to meet the standard, he as a supervisor may be held liable for the harm caused. If a supervisor permits or directs someone to perform a duty that he knows (or reasonably should know) the person is not trained to perform, the supervisor may be held liable for negligent supervision if that person causes harm.

Assume Betty Green is the director of respiratory therapy. The hospital has a provision stating that no registered therapist employed less than three months shall be allowed to do endotracheal suctioning without assistance unless the director is familiar with and has reviewed and approved the new employee's performance of that task. Wanda Burnside, a new employee, has been working under Betty's supervision for one month. Betty has observed Wanda help another therapist suction a patient and concludes that Wanda does not perform the task adequately and needs some additional in-service training. Mr. Kane, a patient, has an order to be suctioned if needed, and Betty tells Wanda to suction him. Wanda does so, but incorrectly, causing injury to the patient's tracheal wall. Betty will probably be held liable for negligent supervision. She has reason to know that Wanda by herself could not yet adequately and skillfully perform suctioning on a patient.

HOSPITAL LAND

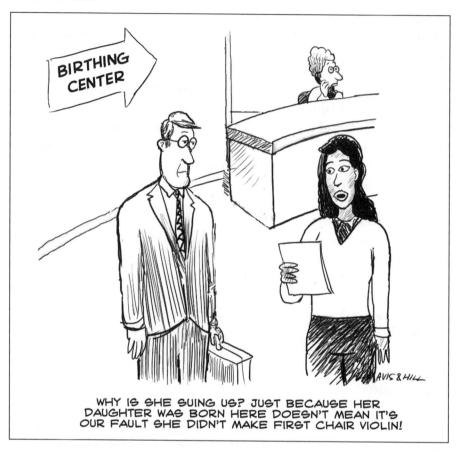

WHY IS SHE SUING US? JUST BECAUSE HER DAUGHTER WAS BORN HERE DOESN'T MEAN IT'S OUR FAULT SHE DIDN'T MAKE FIRST CHAIR VIOLIN!

Liability for nursing supervisors frequently arises as a result of the actions of nursing students under their direct control and supervision. Supervisors need to exercise particular care in not permitting nursing students and others in training to perform tasks and duties for which they are not yet trained or do not have adequate skill, information, or experience.

Remember the example given earlier in which Joe gave the medication intended for Ms. Jones to Ms. Brown? In this case, Joe had worked on his floor for five years with a good record and no incidents of poor performance or faulty nursing judgment. The head nurse, Joe's supervisor, is not liable for Joe's negligent act. Because the head nurse is not Joe's employer, she is not liable under respondeat superior. Also, she is not liable as a supervisor because she has no reason to think Joe is not able to properly perform the task of passing out medications. If, on the other hand, Joe made ten similar mistakes in the past several months and the supervisor is aware of this and takes no action to counsel Joe or make sure he is performing properly, the supervisor may be held liable for negligent supervision.

As a practical matter, legal actions against healthcare supervisors are not as common as those against healthcare professionals, primarily because the potential for injury to plaintiffs is relatively remote.

Additional Potential Causes for Liability

Many other areas of healthcare can lead to liability risks for the institution, its supervisors, and its employees. To minimize these risks, healthcare institutions must take care to obtain informed consent from patients; follow proper admission and discharge procedures to avoid charges of false imprisonment, negligent failure to render treatment, or abandonment of care; properly select and credential providers; and ensure a safe work environment for employees. Institutions and personnel must also deal with controversial issues fraught with philosophical, moral, legal, and ethical complexities such as abortion, sterilization, and the right to die with dignity. A discussion of these is beyond the scope of this chapter.

Employee Litigation

Employees are becoming increasingly aware of their legal rights, resulting in an explosion in the number of legal actions brought by employees against their current or former employers. Often these claims involve a former employee alleging unlawful discharge by the employer. This is a recent phenomenon; historically the law viewed the employment relationship as "at will"; that is, if there was no contract for a specific term, the employee or employer could terminate the employment relationship at any time and for any reason.

The first exceptions to this legal principle originated with statutory and constitutional prohibitions against discrimination based on race. More recently sex, national origin, age, handicap, and pregnancy discrimination have been prohibited by statute and regulation. Consequently, the courts in many states have begun to acknowledge other situations in which an employer cannot rely on the "employment-at-will" doctrine. Courts have recognized claims in which an employee was discharged for refusing to perform an illegal act, for whistle-blowing (**qui tam**) against the employer, or for breaching what the employee alleges to be an express or implied contract. In many states, employees have successfully claimed that employee handbooks are essentially valid written contracts or that statements made during job interviews constitute implied contracts.

Employee litigation, however legitimate, places additional burdens on supervisors because part of the responsibility of a supervisor is to treat an employee fairly, to follow institutional policy regarding discipline, and to monitor and document the employee's performance accurately. If a supervisor fails to follow proper procedures and to document incidents and the manner in which employees discharge their duties, the institution is left open to claims that an employee was disciplined for discriminatory or wrongful reasons and not for poor performance.

qui tam
A provision of the federal False Claims Act that allows a private citizen to file a suit in the name of the U.S. government.

Personnel-Related Regulations

An increasing number of new regulations are being passed by Congress and other regulatory bodies to protect employee rights and to protect them from injury. The supervisor is responsible for ensuring his or her department or work area complies with these regulations. Often the human resources department provides supervisors with instructions for these evolving regulations.

Americans with Disabilities Act

The Americans with Disabilities Act (ADA) is a comprehensive federal statute that was enacted to protect those with physical or mental disabilities. It makes it illegal for most entities to discriminate against individuals with disabilities in such areas as employment and public accommodations. The ADA has spawned a variety of novel claims that could not have been predicted even a short time ago. Therefore, expert healthcare employment relations' legal counsel should be consulted for additional information.

The act identifies a disability as a past, current, or perceived physical or mental impairment of a major life activity. Employers are prohibited under the ADA from doing any of the following:

1. limiting, segregating, or classifying a job applicant or employee with a disability in a way that adversely affects job opportunities or status;
2. participating in an arrangement that has the effect of discriminating against an individual with a disability;
3. using standards, criteria, or methods that have the effect of discriminating on the basis of disability;
4. denying equal jobs or benefits to individuals based on their relationship or association with an individual known to be disabled; or
5. using standards or tests that screen out individuals with disabilities unless the standard or test is job related and consistent with business necessity.

The ADA imposes on employers a duty to "reasonably accommodate" the ability of an individual with a disability to perform essential job functions. The Equal Employment Opportunity Commission (EEOC 2002) defines reasonable accommodation as "any change in the work environment or in the ways things are customarily done that enables an individual with a disability to enjoy equal employment opportunities." Such reasonable accommodation includes the following:

- making facilities accessible to and usable by persons with disabilities;
- job restructuring;

- modifying work schedules;
- reassigning a person with a disability to a vacant position;
- acquiring equipment or devices;
- adjusting or altering tests;
- providing training materials;
- furnishing readers or interpreters; and
- making other similar adjustments to a job.

A reasonable accommodation need not be the best accommodation available, as long as it is effective for the purpose. An individual with a disability must request a reasonable accommodation from the employer. A request can be made by a "family member, friend, health professional, or other representative" on behalf of an individual with a disability. Once a request is received, management is expected to act promptly. Not all requests are initiated by the person with a disability or his or her representative. The supervisor may see the need for a reasonable accommodation and initiate the request. For example, the supervisor for transcription of radiology reports notices that one of the transcriptionists nearly presses her nose to the monitor of her computer. After private questioning, he finds that she has a visual deficit. At this point he orders a larger monitor with larger fonts. Similarly, a plant engineering foreman may notice that one shop hand has to stretch to reach items hanging on the post board behind the workbench. The foreman may initiate an order to have the workbench height lowered or order a raised platform that the shop hand can use. Although height may not be considered a disability for many, it does cause a "handicap" when doing one's job in this situation.

An employer may not use qualification standards or selection criteria that screen out or tend to screen out individuals with disabilities on the basis of their disability unless the standard or criterion is job related and consistent with business necessity. (The standard or criterion must be a legitimate measure or qualification for the specific job for which it is being used and must relate to the essential functions of the job.) In screening applicants for positions, however, an employer is not required to lower existing production standards applicable to the quality or quantity of work for a given job in considering the qualifications of an individual with a disability if these standards are applied uniformly to all applicants and employees in that job.

Under the ADA, an employer may not inquire into an applicant's medical condition or disabilities prior to making a conditional offer of employment. An employer, however, may ask a job applicant about her ability to perform specific job functions, tasks, or duties, as long as those questions are not phrased in terms of a disability. An employer also may ask an applicant to describe or demonstrate how she will perform specific job functions if this is required of everyone applying for a job in that job category, regardless of disability. The ADA regulations have many facets. Supervisors should seek additional guidance from the human resources department.

Sexual Harassment

Organizations must strive to promote a workplace that is free from sexual harassment and should have policies against such harassment. Sexual harassment is considered a form of sex discrimination and is therefore a violation of Title VII of the Civil Rights Act of 1964 and the amendments thereto. In addition, the 1991 Civil Rights Act amended Title VII and provided for compensatory and punitive damages and jury trials.

The EEOC, the federal agency that enforces this law, has issued guidelines regarding sexual harassment. The guidelines define sexual harassment as unwelcome sexual advances, requests for sexual favors, and other verbal or physical conduct of a sexual nature when

1. submission to such conduct is made, either implicitly or explicitly, a term or condition of an individual's employment;
2. submission to or rejection of such conduct by an individual is used as the basis for employment decisions affecting such an individual; or
3. such conduct has a purpose or effect of substantially interfering with an individual's work performance or creating an intimidating, hostile, or offensive working environment.

Sexual harassment can involve individuals of the same or different sex. Examples of sexual harassment include, but are not limited to, unwelcome sexual advances whether or not physical touching is involved; sexual jokes or comments of a sexual nature whether conveyed verbally or in writing (including e-mail or voicemail messages); whistling; leering; unwanted touching; the display of sexual pictures, magazines, or photographs; or other physical or verbal conduct of a sexual nature that interferes with a person's work or that creates a hostile workplace for a person. It also includes instances in which a supervisor or coworker asks for a sexual favor (including kissing) in exchange for any term or condition of the job such as a favorable review, salary increase, or promotion.

Supervisors should pay particular attention to working relationships and conversations among employees. What some employees consider inoffensive, humorous, or harmless flirting could be offensive to others. Supervisors should remember that it is not the intent of the harasser but the impact on the other person that could potentially create a hostile work environment and create a liability for the employer. It is important that employees feel they can discuss such situations with their supervisor or the human resources department.

Any employee who believes that he has been subjected to harassment of any type should consider telling the offending party that he objects to the conduct. If the employee is uncomfortable confronting the offending party or if the conduct continues, the employee should report the incident to his supervisor or the human resources department. Guidance on acts that constitute sexual harassment can be obtained from the human resources department.

Family and Medical Leave Act of 1993 (FMLA)

This act provides up to 12 weeks of absence to eligible employees for certain family and medical reasons. Reasons for taking leave include (1) to care for a child after birth or placement for adoption or foster care; (2) to care for a spouse, child, or parent who has a serious health condition; or (3) to care for oneself because of a serious condition that makes one unable to perform one's job.

A serious condition is one that requires inpatient care in a hospital, hospice, or residential medical facility; results in a period of incapacity of more than three consecutive days that involves treatment two or more times by a healthcare provider or one occasion that results in a regimen of continuing treatment under the supervision of a healthcare provider; is a chronic condition requiring periodic treatment by a healthcare provider that continues over an extended period of time; is a permanent, long-term condition requiring supervision; or is a nonchronic condition that requires multiple treatment such as restorative surgery after an accident or cancer or kidney disease.

Guidance on the actions required by management to extend or document conditions qualifying for FMLA leave can be obtained from the human resources department.

The Occupational Safety and Health Administration (OSHA) Recordkeeping Rule

Employer recording and reporting of occupational injuries and illnesses is one method that OSHA uses to monitor workplace safety. The reporting and recording rules require employer records to include any work-related injury or illness at work and in in-home offices resulting in one or more of the following conditions:

- death,
- days away from work,
- restricted work or transfer to another job,
- medical treatment beyond first aid,
- loss of consciousness, or
- diagnosis of a significant injury or illness by a physician or other licensed healthcare professional.

Supervisors need to review the working conditions in their departments to identify potentially hazardous or other conditions that could cause a work-related injury or illness. Some of the common situations are as follows:

- lifting injuries when moving patients (nursing and therapy),
- wrist and shoulder injuries when filing records (health information),
- falling-object injuries when items are stacked high on shelves (central supply),
- falls when a floor is wet (environmental services), and
- needle sticks when needles are not properly disposed of (environmental services).

Recordkeeping rules require employers to record all needle sticks and sharp-object injuries involving contamination by another person's blood or other bodily fluids. These rules support the need for privacy by prohibiting the recording of an individual's name on reports of certain types of injuries or illnesses (e.g., sexual assaults, HIV infections, mental illnesses).

Because the hospital is open to the public, it, like other businesses, may have workplace violence (e.g., assaults, shootings, hostage situations, domestic disputes) and may be a target for terrorists. Accrediting agencies and governmental entities such as the Centers for Disease Control and Prevention (CDC) have issued recommendations to facilities to be prepared to respond to acts of physical violence and biological or chemical terrorism. Organizations have implemented educational programs and procedures to safely open mail and expand workplace security; offered additional opportunities to telecommute; and increased drug testing and criminal background checks to try to limit exposure to criminal activities.

Although OSHA monitors workplace safety, it cannot guarantee it. Guidelines to prevent workplace injuries such as back and repetitive motion injuries and needle sticks can usually be obtained from your occupational therapy or employee health departments. Emphasizing these guidelines with your staff contributes to providing a safe environment. You as a supervisor must try to see conditions that could cause injury, sense changes in employee attitudes or personalities that may erupt in violence, and keep a pulse on illnesses that may be caused by a work condition.

Other Regulations

HIPAA and Medical Identity Theft

The Health Insurance Portability and Accountability Act of 1996 (HIPAA) has several components that affect day-to-day management activities. One component of the act (portability) allows employees, after termination by an employer, to remain insured. This component is managed through the payroll and human resources department. Other components address security, privacy, and transaction issues. HIPAA affects all employees of any healthcare organization or entity.

HIPAA specifically requires healthcare providers to take precautions to protect patient-identifiable information from unauthorized release or access, tampering, or misuse. Inappropriate disclosures may result in fines up to $250,000 and prison time. With these penalties in mind, confidentiality statements and practices are more important than ever. With an increase in uninsured individuals, the value of a patient's insurance information and identity has risen, thus resulting in increased medical identity theft. Healthcare organizations are now required to comply with "red flag" regulations that include having protections in place for patient insurance, credit card, and other financial information to protect against such theft.

As a result of HIPAA and other compliance-related concerns, the use of passwords, biometrics (e.g., fingerprints, cornea scans, palm scans), and other security measures are being used to ensure that the user is (1) authorized to have access to the system or specific application and (2) authorized to have access to the data or data field. Time-outs on computers have been shortened to ensure that when one walks away without logging off the computer automatically logs off to reduce the possibility of an unauthorized user accessing confidential or proprietary data. Accrediting and licensing agencies monitor the facility's precautions in their on-floor rounds during their surveys.

However, as a supervisor, your role is to ensure that computer access is controlled and that patient-identifiable information is protected from unauthorized access and discarded in appropriate containers.

E-Discovery

Related to the explosion of patient data maintained electronically is the 2006 modification to the Federal Rules of Civil Procedure (the rules that govern civil lawsuits), specifically the rules that pertain to the discovery of electronic data, known as **E-Discovery Rules** (K&L Gates 2006). These new rules stipulate under what circumstances parties to a civil lawsuit can gain access to electronically stored information (ESI) related to a patient and/or a patient's care, regardless of where that information is stored. This expansive regulation includes allowing a plaintiff's attorney to request ESI from any electronic system including, but not limited to, voicemail, e-mail, biomedical devices (such as anesthesia equipment and other monitors), PDAs, and, of course, the organization's computer system. The supervisor's role in e-discovery is to (1) know what patient data are stored where in her department, (2) ensure staff is educated in the proper use of e-mail and voicemail systems appropriately since anything they write or say in these systems is discoverable, and (3) follow the organization's rules for retention and destruction of ESI.

E-Discovery Rules
Part of the Federal Rules of Civil Procedure that pertain to access to electronic patient records for parties to a civil lawsuit.

Ethics and Qui Tam

In recent years there have been several high-profile corporate misconduct and fraud cases. While most of these cases emanated from accounting improprieties, the results had serious negative impacts for the employees, stockholders, and public, destroying some of the world's largest companies, shattering retirement programs, and putting thousands of employees out of work. As a result, Generally Accepted Accounting Principles (GAAP) and corporate ethical behavior have changed. The Sarbanes-Oxley Act of 2002 incorporates harsher penalties for certain crimes, stipulates more independent directors, and transfers the setting of auditing standards from the private sector to the public sector (the Public Accounting Oversight Board). Federal initiatives have set minimum expectations for organizations with regard to ethical practice and compliance with regulations.

Stronger ethics policies have been initiated at healthcare organizations to address accounting, billing, coding, purchasing, and patient care practices. HealthSouth's ethics statement appears on its website (see Exhibit 6.1).

EXHIBIT 6.1
HealthSouth
Corporate
Governance
and Ethics
Statement

HealthSouth is fully committed to good corporate governance and the highest standards of business conduct. In today's culture, good corporate governance and adherence to a high ethical standard is simply good business.

We are dedicated to conducting our business with the highest level of integrity while maximizing value for its investors. In October 2003, we implemented our revised Corporate Compliance and Ethics Program to assist HealthSouth directors, officers and employees in making the right choices regarding our business practices. Our revised corporate compliance and ethics program is described in our Corporate Compliance Handbook, which includes our revised standards of business conduct.

We are also dedicated to effective corporate governance. In January 2004, the board of directors approved a number of changes in our corporate governance platform in the interest of transparency and accountability to our stakeholders. Our principles of corporate governance meet or exceed the requirements of the Sarbanes-Oxley Act of 2002 and, although we are not currently listed on the New York Stock Exchange, the revised listing standards of the New York Stock Exchange. HealthSouth's principles of corporate governance are set out in our Corporate Governance Guidelines and the various charters of the standing committees of our board of directors.

SOURCE: Courtesy of HealthSouth. 2005. [Online information; retrieved 9/11/05.] www.healthsouth.com.

The Department of Justice (DOJ) reports that after violent crime, healthcare fraud is the department's top priority. The number of healthcare fraud investigations pending at the DOJ is in the thousands. The DOJ's primary weapon in prosecuting healthcare fraud is the federal False Claims Act (FCA) of 1863 (31 U.S.C. secs. 3729–3733). The DOJ may entertain lawsuits filed by private individuals on behalf of the federal government as a qui tam claim. These claims may include charging organizations with submitting false claims to the government. The FCA rewards qui tam or whistleblowers with a share of any resulting recoveries as a bounty and protects them from discharge for filing false-claims lawsuits against their employers. In 2008, approximately 78 percent of the DOJ's $1.3 billion in settlements and judgments were for qui tam lawsuits filed under the FCA (DOJ 2008).

Managers have an obligation to make ethical decisions—do the right thing. Because managers are authorized to make purchases, they may be tempted to make inappropriate decisions when they select vendors. Many organizations have established rules related to accepting gifts from vendors or suppliers. Giving gifts is one of the principal areas that can trigger what are commonly called the "referral statutes," otherwise known as the antikickback and Stark II laws (Oak 2005). One of the basic ethical assumptions is that healthcare management and clinical decision making will be independent, objective, and focused on the best interests of the patient and proper stewardship of public funds (Oak 2005).

Supervisors are responsible for reviewing, supporting, and signing code of ethics documents and for educating their subordinates about the organization's ethical policies. At the same time, healthcare organization compliance programs encourage and often require employees at any level to report inappropriate practices anonymously to the organization's compliance "hotline." Supervisors should encourage a climate of doing what is legally and ethically right and identify any variances to the contrary.

Summary

The healthcare institution's legal responsibility for what occurs on its premises or what is done by its employees and agents is cause for concern by administrators, supervisors, and employees. The professional members of the healthcare team also are held to strict standards of care and are held liable for negligent acts.

Those practicing in the healthcare field should familiarize themselves with the various aspects of their job that could result in liability to themselves or their institution. They must be able to recognize potential legal issues, understand the practical ramifications, and exercise caution and care in the performance of their duties. A growing number of entities impose regulations on healthcare organizations and their management.

Recent fraudulent activities have resulted in closure of large organizations and imprisonment of corporate officers. These indictments combined with DOJ initiatives in false-claim submissions have encouraged expanded compliance and ethics practices, policies, and procedures at most healthcare organizations. The supervisor is in a pivotal role to set the tone for workplace safety, compliance, and fairness.

Notes

1. This chapter does not cover situations in facilities operated by the Veterans Administration, Army, Navy, Air Force, Public Health Service, or other federal agencies.
2. Michael Swango had successfully been admitted to several medical staffs across the United States and the world. Faulty credentialing practices failed to reveal a pattern of patient deaths that occurred during his assignment at different hospitals. He was indicted for murder on numerous accounts. Known as "Dr. Death," it is thought that he may have been responsible for 30 to 60 patient deaths.

Additional Reading

Harris, D. M. 2007. *Contemporary Issues in Healthcare Law and Ethics*, 3rd ed. Chicago: Health Administration Press.

PLANNING

MANAGERIAL PLANNING

After you have studied this chapter, you should be able to do the following:

1. Describe the planning function and its importance as a primary management tool.
2. Discuss the need for and extent of forecasting, which provides the background for managerial planning.
3. Recognize the value of projections and population changes in planning for the healthcare industry.
4. Discuss the various planning steps.
5. Relate goals and objectives to organizational planning.
6. Describe how management by objectives can be used to implement plans.

Planning is the most important managerial function. It is the process of deciding in advance what is to be done in the future. Logically, planning must come before any of the other functions because it determines the framework in which the other management functions—organizing, staffing, influencing, and controlling—are carried out. Today's healthcare activities operate in an environment that is always changing in ways institutions can neither control nor predict precisely. This increases the need for planning. The only way healthcare organizations can survive is to forecast the future, plan rationally, and prepare for change. Although many plans are not carried out exactly as anticipated because of changing circumstances, experience has shown that institutions that plan tend to be more successful than those that do not plan.

In planning, management is concerned with collecting the right data, formulating a strategy, establishing the objectives (critical success factors or key performance indicators) to be achieved, and determining how to achieve them. Critical success factors may include patient satisfaction, employee turnover, outcomes, and physician recruitment. When planning information is assembled, the external and internal environments are studied, planning premises are set out, and decisions to reach organizational goals are made. Some healthcare organizations have **management engineers** serve as members of their planning staff. Management engineers are competent at compiling data

management engineer
An individual who uses data and analytics to improve processes.

125

and using analytics to improve processes. This skill is integral to a function that is known today as **business intelligence**.

In 1958 Hans Peter Luhn defined business intelligence as "the ability to apprehend the interrelationships of presented facts in such a way as to guide action towards a desired goal" (Grimes 2008). In 1989 Howard Dresner (later a Gartner Group analyst) proposed business intelligence as an umbrella term to describe "concepts and methods to improve business decision making by using fact-based support systems" (Power 2007).

The decisions made in planning provide the departments (operational units) of the organization with their objectives and with the expectations (standards or metrics) against which performance is measured.

Thus, when the manager plans a course of action, she attempts to ensure a consistent and coordinated operation aimed at achieving the desired results. Stating goals or plans alone does not bring about these results; to achieve them, a manager must know the plan and what is expected of her department. Without plans, however, random activities by all managers prevail, resulting in confusion and possibly even chaos. The plan serves as the road map for managers to follow as they chart their path to the goal.

The Nature of Planning

Just as an organization's leadership must plan for the future of the organization, a department manager must plan for the proper functioning of his department. How can a manager properly and effectively organize the workings of the department without having a plan in mind? How can the department head effectively staff and supervise the employees without knowing the objectives for the department and the policies, procedures, and methods to follow? None of these functions could be performed without planning. No substitute exists for the hard thinking that planning demands. Therefore, only after having made the plans can the manager organize, staff, influence, and control.

However, planning does not end abruptly when the manager begins to perform the other functions. It should not be a process used only at occasional intervals or when the manager is not engrossed in daily tasks. Rather, planning is a continuous process. With day-to-day planning, the supervisor realistically anticipates future problems, analyzes them, determines their probable effect on activities, and chooses the actions that will lead to the desired results for the unit and for the organization.

Planning Is a Task of Every Manager

Planning is the job of every manager, whether chair of the board, clinic administrator, operating room director, or materials management supervisor. By definition, all of these people are managers and therefore all of them must plan. The importance and magnitude of the plans depend on the level at which plans are determined. Planning at the top level of administration is more fundamental and further reaching than at the supervisory levels of management, where the scope and extent of planning become narrower and more detailed.

Thus, the administrator is concerned with the overall aspects of planning for the entire healthcare organization, such as constructing new facilities, adding new services, aligning with other organizations, and enlarging outpatient services. While the chief information officer's (CIO) long-range planning may include setting objectives for achieving a paperless environment for the organization, the information systems supervisor who is knowledgeable about this plan defines priorities (i.e., which areas should be involved, what equipment is needed), writes new procedures, and determines activities to fulfill these objectives. A supervisor is more concerned with departmental plans for getting the job done promptly and effectively each day, or, as some say, "operationalizing" the plan or "making it happen," while the administrator or senior-level executive is determining what "it" will look like in the future.

Although planning is the manager's function, others should be called on for advice. Some healthcare institutions have full-time employees known as "planners," usually in a staff position. Often, these individuals work in a decision support function where they have access to and have compiled a competitive intelligence database[1] about the organization and comparative facilities. They help the CEO and others of the administrative team in their forecasting efforts, long-term strategy, and planning decisions. Most supervisors are not likely to need such planners' help. However, at times a manager may require special knowledge as he plans, such as human resources (scheduling as a result of nursing shortages), information systems (implementing an electronic medical record), accounting (procedures to record the lease of a Pyxis drug-dispensing machine), or other professional and technical aspects. In such instances, the supervisor must feel free to call on specialists within and outside the organization to help with the planning.

Forecasting Future Trends

Although the future is fraught with uncertainties, managers must make certain assumptions about it to be able to plan. These assumptions are based on forecasts that provide information essential to the planning process. Forecasting is done by scanning the external and internal environments for useful information. Because the appraisal of future prospects is inherent in all planning, the success of an enterprise greatly depends on the skill of management, first in forecasting and second in preparing for future conditions.

Forecasts as the Basis of Planning

Management typically confines its forecasting effort to factors that experience suggests are important to its own planning. Thus, chief administrators of the healthcare facility select those forecasts that have a direct material bearing on the healthcare field in the broadest sense.

In trying to make predictions, administrators consider the general economic, political, labor, and social climates in which the healthcare institution must operate during the next few years. This information comes from reviewing forecasts on government policies, legislation and regulation, government spending, merger and consolidation activities, and insurer penetration to determine how these might ultimately affect the activities of healthcare providers.

Thus, top-level administrators do not actually perform the research and statistical analysis for all their forecasts. They frequently use data published in government and trade publications or made available by hospital or healthcare organizations, healthcare system research staffs, and other experts in various fields. Administrators then try to predict the general trends for the delivery of healthcare as it affects the various providers and users in relation to cost effectiveness and other considerations.

Administrators are anxious for the data that will be yielded from the 2010 census, as they have long had to rely on projections based on data from the 2000 census. The population is growing, graying, and diversifying. The rate these demographic changes are occurring in a healthcare organization's region tells the organization's leaders which services the facility should be offering, the specialists that should be recruited, and the diversity of employees that should be hired in years to come. The breakdown of population figures by age and sex provides even more meaningful data.

EXHIBIT 7.1
Baby Boomer
Bulge

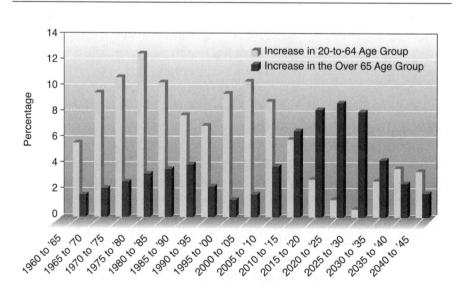

SOURCE: Originally published in *Chief Learning Officer* magazine, www.clomedia.com. Used with permission.

Exhibit 7.1 shows that the children born during the baby boom that occurred after World War II are reaching Medicare age. The boom creates a surge of 60-year-olds starting in 2010 that will place demands on the healthcare system for several decades. These demands are similar to the ones that occurred in schools in the early 1950s when the baby boomers reached kindergarten.

According to the Pew Report and the data depicted in Exhibit 7.1, the nation's elderly population will more than double in size from 2005 through 2050 (Pew Charitable Trusts 2008). A century ago, the average adult spent only 1 percent of his life in a morbid or ill state; the whopping 13 percent of our population over 65 now accounts for 44 percent of hospital care, 38 percent of emergency medical services responses, 35 percent of prescriptions, 26 percent of physician office visits, and 90 percent of nursing home use (Dychtwald 2009).

The number of working-age Americans contributing to the Medicare fund will grow more slowly than the elderly population (Passell and Cohn 2008) utilizing the fund. This growth not only affects healthcare service utilization but also tax expense for employers to fund Medicare benefits. A supervisor will likely be asked to identify processes to deliver high-quality service while using less labor and other resources for the organization.

Growth in the diversity of the population will continue as well. The Latino population, already the nation's largest minority group, will triple in size and will account for most of the nation's population growth from 2005 through 2050. Latinos will make up 29 percent of the U.S. population in 2050 (Passell and Cohn 2008). This means that healthcare organizations and our management styles need to change to address alternative medicine preferences, language barriers, family values of different cultures, signage needs, food preferences, cultural superstitions/beliefs, holy day recognition, and religious beliefs.

In addition to age and race demographics, management may monitor other information, such as unemployment rates, to forecast uninsured rates (Exhibit 7.2).

Supervisory Forecasts

Scientific and Technological Developments

When supervisors make departmental forecasts, their assumptions about the future cover a much narrower field than those of administrators. For example, the home health director might report that, according to the Bureau of Labor Statistics, there will be shortage of 553,000 home health aides by the year 2018 (Bureau of Labor Statistics 2009). A supervisor should forecast mostly those factors that may have some bearing on the future of his or her department. Supervisors should determine whether a trend is growing for more sophistication in their fields. It is important to keep abreast of the rapid and

EXHIBIT 7.2

Unemployment
Rates by State,
Seasonally
Adjusted,
November
2008
(U.S. Rate =
6.7 Percent)

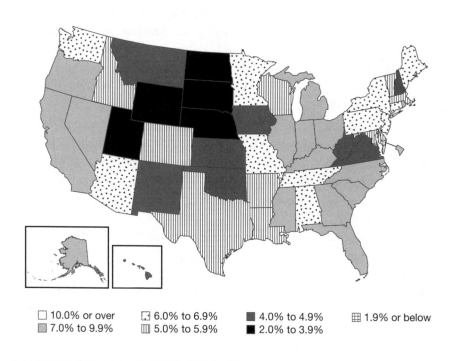

☐ 10.0% or over	☐ 6.0% to 6.9%	■ 4.0% to 4.9%	⊞ 1.9% or below
▨ 7.0% to 9.9%	▥ 5.0% to 5.9%	■ 2.0% to 3.9%	

SOURCE: Bureau of Labor Statistics Local Area Unemployment Statistics. [http://www.bls. gov/web/mstrtcr2.pdf].

often revolutionary developments in the medical field, in technology, and in automation. Of course, supervisors also have to contend with some broader assumptions such as cost containment, government involvement, staff recruitment, skill requirements, and other concerns in the healthcare field.

Based on past events, the supervisor should make some assumptions on what the future holds. In making such assumptions, she can look to the sources of supplies, available technology, and regulations specific to her functions. Supervisors can also learn by attending lectures, national meetings, and exhibitions and by joining professional organizations and reading their journals. Advances in the medical sciences and technology are progressing so rapidly that a department's functions and staff's responsibilities may significantly change year to year. Consider, for instance, the impact of further computerization and automation of equipment such as automated analyzers, which have become so sophisticated, small, and inexpensive that the technology can easily be installed at physician offices, thus reducing the demand for testing at the hospital laboratory. Such projections are essential for the planning done by supervisors in clinical laboratories: Will more, less, or about the same number of employees be needed with the same, different, or additional education or training? Should the equipment be bought or leased? The supervisor must consider these and similar questions.

Employees and Skills

Supervisors also have to make forecasts about the types of employees who will be working in the department in the future. Changes in healthcare technology will probably create a need for some employees who have been educated and trained in completely new and advanced scientific fields and are capable of coping with state-of-the-art technology and areas such as robotics, genetics, electronics, use of artificial intelligence, and neural networks.

At the same time, supervisors will be challenged with serious shortages of nurses, health technologists, home health and nursing aides, coding specialists, and even clerical staff. These positions are no longer glamorous to young people joining the workforce. Conventional full-time jobs are perceived to limit time available for family or personal activities and are going unfilled. Supervisors will not only need to grow staff from within but build schedules that accommodate more employees working part-time schedules. They will need to be more sensitive to the noneconomic demands that young people expect to fulfill on their jobs and the potential for generational clashes at the work site. Cultural and generational diversity will be a challenge for staff and leaders alike, as Generation Y 20-year-olds, raised with computers in every aspect of their lives, work side by side with 50- and 60-year-olds. Planning for the team-building efforts that may be required will be imperative for supervisors. Meeting all types of demands, such as material, psychological, and professional, will be particularly important if supervisors must find people who possess skills that up to now may not have been required in the department.

At the supervisory level, leaders will be expected to select new employees who have certain basic skills that can be built on with internal educational programs to enable them to perform multiskilled tasks. Further, they will be asked to develop educational programs to teach these individuals the many skills they will be required to master. They will need to plan both time and effort to bring existing staff up to par with a varied skill set as well as plan the educational curriculum to teach new employees. Lastly, they will need to create monitoring tools to ensure the employees have learned the skills, maintain their skills, and are performing according to expectations. The planning spectrum in this type of environment will be vast.

Benefits of Planning

Planning is a rigorous process of establishing objectives; deciding on strategies, tactics, and activities to achieve them; and formally documenting expectations. It results in purposeful organization and activities, which in turn minimize costs and reduce waste. Deciding in advance what is to be done—and how, by whom, where, and when—promotes efficient and orderly operations and reduces errors. All efforts are directed toward a desired result so that haphazard approaches are minimized, activities are coordinated, and duplications are avoided. Thus, planning has many benefits that no manager can afford to neglect.

Effective management demands optimum use of the organization's resources. Managers are entrusted with the management of both the employees and physical resources (space, equipment, tools, and materials) of the department. Determining how all these resources are used is their primary responsibility, and the basis on which their managerial performance is judged.

The Strategic Planning Process

Planning can occur at any level of an organization. Although some of this chapter focuses on upper management planning, similar steps are appropriate for the department, section, or team manager. The development of missions and visions and discussion of other concepts in this chapter are not limited to the interests of boards of trustees. As a supervisor, you will be able to apply the steps discussed to your work team's efforts.

Managers may be asked to contribute information for consideration during the strategic planning sessions typically attended by the board of trustees or directors, members of the medical staff, and senior management or administration. In addition, the strategic planning facilitator may invite external experts to guide the thinking. Such experts may include the organization's external auditors, professional or trade association leaders, bankers, and community leaders.

Long-range planning is a component of strategic planning, but the two types of planning have different intents. When leaders conduct long-range planning, they generally develop a plan for accomplishing a goal or set of goals over a period of several years, with the assumption that current knowledge about future conditions is sufficiently reliable to ensure the plan's reliability over the duration of its implementation (Alliance for Non-Profit Management 2009a). It's doubtful that anyone believes he knows enough about future conditions affecting healthcare with the surge in medical tourism, continued governmental intervention, rise in under/uninsureds, and competition among providers. On the other hand, strategic planning assumes that an organization must be responsive to a dynamic, changing environment and stresses the importance of making decisions that will ensure the organization's ability to successfully respond to changes in the environment (Alliance for Non-Profit Management 2009a).

The development of a strategic plan leads simultaneously to two very different outcomes: an actual strategic plan *document* that lays out a road map for the future and the *process* of engaging key stakeholders in strategic debate.

It is about building a coalition of supporters for whatever direction is outlined (Clark and Krentz 2006). According to Beckham (2005), throughout the strategic planning process, leaders should ask five fundamental questions:

1. What are the most important challenges we'll face in the foreseeable future? (strategic issues)
2. What do we aspire to be? (vision)
3. What are the most important things we need to do to become what we aspire to be? (strategies)
4. How do we intend to accomplish our strategies? (tactics and action plans)
5. How will we know how we're doing? (measurement)

Strategic planning is based on decision making because to answer the questions above and throughout the strategic planning process, choices must be made. The plan ultimately is no more, and no less, than a set of decisions about what to do, how to do it, and why to do it (Alliance for Non-Profit Management 2009b).

Validating the Mission

One of the first steps during any strategic planning process is to validate the organization's mission, a statement that describes what the organization does, what its purpose is, or why it exists. Golden Rule Insurance Company has a mission statement that starts with, "Golden Rule chooses to be ethical because it is right, not because it is good business practice." Generally, the mission statement is timeless; a nursing home mission statement may be, "We provide long-term, skilled nursing and rehabilitative services for individuals residing in our facility in a cost-effective and high-quality manner." The ideal mission statement is short and concise. Examples appear in Exhibit 7.3.

The mission of an organization may change if it merges with another, or the mission may change naturally over time as new services are added. Consider how the mission about providing long-term, skilled nursing services would change if this organization were acquired by either hospital in Exhibit 7.3.

Once the organization's mission is established, each department's mission can be developed; the departments should be supportive of the organization's mission. For example, the physical therapy department's mission may be, "We provide quality and effective rehabilitative services for our patients and home care clients."

As mentioned earlier, much information is needed for planning effectively. The review of this information is known as the **environmental assessment** and is not limited to internal information. Some organizations have found the *Futurescan* publication from Health Administration Press a valuable

environmental assessment
A comprehensive analysis of conditions inside and outside an organization, ranging from politics to finances.

EXHIBIT 7.3
Mission
Statements

HERMANN AREA DISTRICT HOSPITAL, HERMANN, MISSOURI

We provide quality healthcare and wellness services to all persons seeking treatment.

RUSH UNIVERSITY MEDICAL CENTER, CHICAGO

Rush University Medical Center is a multifaceted health services corporation and the foundation of the Rush System for Health. The Medical Center's primary purposes are: to provide comprehensive, coordinated health care services to people in the Chicago metropolitan area and selected tertiary services to people throughout the nation; to educate and train health professionals to meet national needs as well as those of the Rush System, with special emphasis on primary care practitioners; to advance health care knowledge by fostering basic, applied and clinical research which also serves to enhance clinical programs; to improve the West Loop and University Village communities of which the Medical Center is a member; and to foster the individual growth and satisfaction of Medical Center employees and staff.

SOURCES: Reprinted with permission of Hermann Area District Hospital, Hermann, MO and Rush University Medical Center, Chicago.

resource in gauging what may be happening externally. To be able to predict the impact of changing or adding services, linking with another organization, and so forth, one must know what is happening outside the walls of the organization specifically and in the healthcare industry in general. Therefore, the environmental assessment includes a comprehensive analysis of information about the following (Purcell 2001):

- the organization's current, past, and potential future customers;
- competitors in the region and those who may invade the region served by the organization or provide perceived better services than the organization;
- societal changes such as demographic shifts in the aged population, movement of the population, unemployment, un- and underinsured trends, or expectations from society in general of healthcare providers;
- industry indicators and comparative data (such as HealthGrades, Leapfrog, Solucient for quality and financial ratios for fiscal health);
- regulatory and accreditation changes;
- credit market conditions, to determine if the facility will qualify for the capital needed for the strategic plan; and
- how the organization is performing (e.g., financially; in terms of patient outcomes and volume; staff and patient satisfaction; licensure issues).

PESTHR analysis
An acronym that stands for political, economic, social, technological, human resource, and regulatory forces. These are all elements of an environmental analysis.

Strategic planners have an acronym for these elements of the environmental assessment: **PESTHR analysis**—political, economic, social, technological, human resource, and regulatory forces.

However, as with any planning effort, managers must balance the amount of data they prepare and present for planning purposes. Too much data can be overwhelming and time-consuming. In short, you need the right data to make informed planning decisions (Clark and Krentz 2006, 63).

Here's an example of an external environmental issue. Assume that several organizations in your community have had their accreditation survey and passed accreditation. However, your facility received "conditional accreditation." This is a problem, because the managed care companies in the area only extend contracts to those hospitals that passed and had higher Hospital Compare[2] scores. This external environment situation will force all in the organization to focus and coordinate their plans to quickly resolve the issues causing the conditional accreditation status.

The last component, the internal organization review, may include patient origin data and market share, utilization trends by clinical service, medical staff composition (age, specialty), human resource challenges (hard-to-fill vacancies, staff shortages), financial position, patient satisfaction, and outcomes of services. It is often coupled with what is known as a **SWOT analysis**. SWOT (s̲trengths, w̲eaknesses, o̲pportunities, and t̲hreats) analysis evaluates the internal organization based on its:

> **SWOT analysis**
> An examination of the strengths, weaknesses, opportunities, and threats an organization faces.

- strengths compared with regional competitors and community needs and demands;
- weaknesses compared with competitors, and patient and staff satisfaction surveys, or based on staff's perceptions of the organization's internal functions;
- opportunities for advancing ahead of competitors, serving a patient population not served or under served currently; and
- threats from external or internal competitors or agents that could stymie the organization's success.

Appendix 7.1 shows the input obtained from the managers of a healthcare facility prior to the board's strategic planning session. Appendix 7.2 displays the board's SWOT from its planning session.

Creating the Vision

Once the environmental assessment and analysis have been completed, the leadership of the organization (those participating in the strategic planning activities) formulates a vision. The vision of an organization is a statement about where the leadership sees the organization going in a designated period of time; hence, the vision is timebound (Zuckerman 2000). The vision should be clear and concise, and ideally should be a single statement (Exhibit 7.4). In essence, the vision statement is an all-encompassing strategy for the organization.

Exhibit 7.4

Vision
Statements

Littleton Regional Hospital, Littleton, New Hampshire

Littleton Regional Hospital will be the leading provider of healthcare, and the best organization in which to work.[3]

Rush University Medical Center, Chicago

Rush University Medical Center will be recognized as the standard for an academic medical center delivering the highest quality care integrated with research and education in health fields.

SOURCES: Reprinted with permission of Littleton Regional Hospital, Littleton, NH and Rush University Medical Center, Chicago.

The next planning step is to prioritize those actions indicated for the organization to continue to succeed and deliver its mission as it progresses toward its vision. To expand on our earlier example, the vision may read as follows: "Within five years Shady Oaks Nursing Home will be a system of three nursing homes to provide high-quality residential care for those needing skilled nursing and rehabilitative care, as well as one location providing residential housing for those who can care for themselves in a continuing care community located in the suburbs of our community." The strategic plan for the next year may be to open one of the skilled homes. Each department manager will be responsible for developing action plans to ensure the home is efficiently designed and constructed in a timely manner.

Determining the Critical Success Factors or Objectives

Once the vision is determined and the analysis of the environmental data completed, the board of directors and senior administration establish broad strategic thrusts to achieve the vision. (See Nickols [2000] for more definitions of strategy.) Strategic thrusts may also be called strategies, which are approaches to achieve the vision. The thrusts for our example may include (1) a fund-raising program to raise the money needed to build or acquire two additional nursing homes and the property and buildings for the residential housing, (2) lobbying the legislature or regulatory agencies to avoid any delays that would prevent the organization from achieving its vision, or (3) proposing a bond issue to support the expansion. The planning group not only sets the vision but also identifies various routes for management to take to achieve the organization's broadest goals. In effect, the strategic planning group could be perceived as sitting on the seat of a bicycle and pedaling it down a path toward the vision (Exhibit 7.5). Strategies take on value only as

EXHIBIT 7.5 Strategic Planning Model

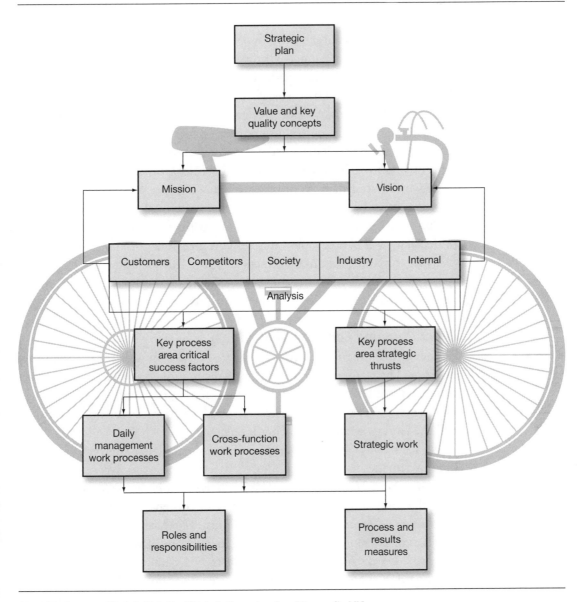

SOURCE: Courtesy of Kevin J. McArdle of McArdle Enterprises, Inc., Minneapolis, MN.

committed people infuse them with energy (Kouzes and Posner 2002) and gain the buy-in of the organization's staffs to achieve them.

In addition to the strategic thrusts, the information from the environmental assessment identifies critical success factors. These are important milestones that must be met to achieve the strategies. One may be obtaining a state certificate of approval before a competitor obtains one for a given community location or establishing an effective marketing campaign to support the fund-raising program. In some organizations, a critical success factor may be called an organization goal.

With the vision, strategic thrusts (strategies), and critical success factors (goals) defined, senior management and administration identify the objectives that support the critical success factors and bring the vision to reality. The burden of the effort to make the organization successful lies with management and staff. The full strength of this group must be marshaled to achieve the vision. As a supervisor, you will meet with your administrative leader and possibly your subordinates to define the objectives for your department, the impact of these objectives on your daily work processes, and the interdepartmental relationships that must be established or strengthened for total organizational success (Exhibit 7.6). You, your peers, and your superiors will create *operating plans* or detailed plans to accomplish the strategic goals laid out in the strategic plan (Alliance for Non-Profit Management 2009b). The operating plan may correspond to the fiscal year or grant cycles, depending on the funding source(s), and serve as a building block for the future years.

Other Planning Considerations

planning horizon
The length of time for which a manager should plan.

The length of time for which a manager should plan is called the **planning horizon**. The planning horizon is usually distinguished as long term, intermediate, or short term. The exact definitions of long-term and short-term planning depend on the manager's level in the hierarchy, the type of institution, and the kind of activity in which it is engaged.

Generally, *short-term planning* covers a period up to one year, and planning of activities to be carried out over a period of one to five years is known as *intermediate planning*. This planning horizon contains fewer uncertainties than the long-range planning, which has to contend with highly uncertain conditions of several decades hence. Thus, *long-term planning* usually involves a considerably longer horizon—generally, any plan that extends beyond five years. Because of the healthcare industry's dynamics, healthcare organization board members, CEOs, and senior executives find it difficult to plan beyond a decade. Much regulatory change is dependent on the political party controlling Congress and the potential for congressional and presidential changes every four years.

The supervisor's planning period is probably short range—that is, for one year at the most or perhaps for six months, one month, one week, or even one day. A supervisor can definitely plan some activities in certain departments three, six, nine, or twelve months in advance, such as renovating the main lobby and registration areas or implementing a case management application. On the other hand, supervisory planning often is for a shorter time—a pay period, a week, a day, or only a shift. Such short-range planning is frequently

EXHIBIT 7.6 Planning Terminology and Definitions

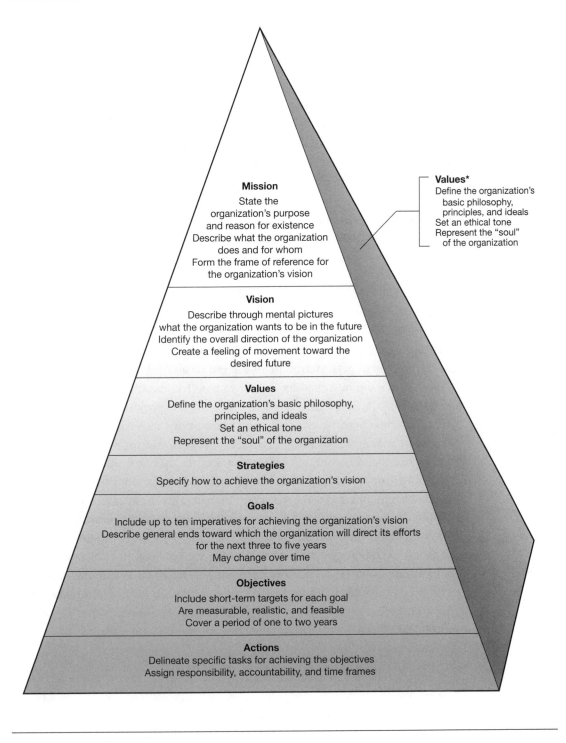

Values*
Define the organization's
basic philosophy,
principles, and ideals
Set an ethical tone
Represent the "soul"
of the organization

Mission
State the
organization's purpose
and reason for existence
Describe what the organization
does and for whom
Form the frame of reference for
the organization's vision

Vision
Describe through mental pictures
what the organization wants to be in the future
Identify the overall direction of the organization
Create a feeling of movement toward the
desired future

Values
Define the organization's basic philosophy,
principles, and ideals
Set an ethical tone
Represent the "soul" of the organization

Strategies
Specify how to achieve the organization's vision

Goals
Include up to ten imperatives for achieving the organization's vision
Describe general ends toward which the organization will direct its efforts
for the next three to five years
May change over time

Objectives
Include short-term targets for each goal
Are measurable, realistic, and feasible
Cover a period of one to two years

Actions
Delineate specific tasks for achieving the objectives
Assign responsibility, accountability, and time frames

*The values support each step equally.

SOURCE: Zuckerman (2005). Used with permission of Health Administration Press.

needed in patient care services and in other departments that have difficulty recruiting talented staff to ensure there is adequate staffing and supplies for the daily activities.

It is more desirable if the supervisor is able to make longer-range plans, but for practical purposes, proper attention must be given to seeing that the work of each day is accomplished. This short-range planning requires the supervisor to take the time to consider the nature and amount of work that is to be done each day by the department, the person(s) responsible for doing the work, and when the work has to be done. Furthermore, this daily planning, by definition, must be done ahead of time; many supervisors prefer to do it at the end of the day or shift, when they can size up what has been accomplished already to formulate plans for the following day or shift.

Occasionally, a supervisor is also involved in intermediate and long-term plans. For example, the boss may want to discuss planning for new activities for the institution. A supervisor may be informed of a contemplated expansion or the addition of new facilities, for instance a nursing home, and is then asked to propose what the department can contribute or what is needed. If a hospital plans for an enlarged outpatient surgical center, the director of nursing as well as the operating room supervisors are asked to be deeply involved. These supervisors are assigned to develop short-term measurable targets, or objectives, and then delineate the specific tasks or actions for achieving the targets. Action plans are the result of this delineation process.

As shown in Appendix 7.1, from time to time the administrator might request that the supervisor look into the future and project the long-term trend of a particular activity, especially if it is apparent that such activity will be affected by major breakthroughs in medical science and technology or by regulatory change. Certainly the plant engineering manager was involved in the planning for the selection and installation of a new roof for the facility and the IT management team was involved in preparations for installation of the electronic medical record. It is important for supervisors to participate in such long-range planning because strategic planning is ultimately about resource allocation to competitively meet the patient care needs of the community (Clark and Krentz 2006, 66). The supervisor not only needs to contribute to the plans but needs to understand that the plans may require staffing modifications or provide for new equipment, space, or technology for the department. The Economics Press, Inc. (1999) offers the following planning suggestions:

> Start your planning by asking questions about the new project: "How does the upcoming job differ from the one my team is working on now?" Even a small change, such as a tighter deadline or a change of location, could lead to big problems if you and your team are not prepared for it. Once you've decided what makes the upcoming job different from the last one, ask yourself: "What problems and mistakes are likely to occur? And what's the best way to avoid them?" If you have to coor-

dinate your efforts with another department or team, you will have to work out a joint, detailed schedule with them. If needed, materials must be obtained before the project can begin. Another question: "Will anyone need additional training?"

The long-range plans also may indicate that subordinates with completely new skills and education are needed and that a search for them must start immediately. Learning new procedures and techniques might be necessary as a result of new and different ways of diagnosing and treating medical conditions. For instance, consider the transition from a film library in the radiology department to a picture-archiving communications system with Web access for telemedicine. Even though these technologies are readily available, their implementation date is often placed in the long term because of the high cost and the time it takes to acquire the equipment (a capital expenditure). In these situations, the supervisors must participate in long-range planning to ensure adequate space, staff and user training, and so forth. On the other hand, some long-range plans may actually result in elimination of staff. The use of robotics, such as the da Vinci Surgery System, and technology such as smart capsules for endoscopic diagnostics are reducing the need for some procedures or the labor associated with the procedures.[4]

The Integration and Communication of Plans

Integrating, coordinating, and balancing long-range, intermediate, and short-range plans are essential. Therefore, the supervisor's short-range plans must support intermediate plans, which in turn should support long-range plans. Long-range planning should not be viewed as an activity separate from or contrary to short-range planning. All too often, however, there is a gap between the knowledge of top management and that of lower-level management concerning planning. This gap is often justified by the claim that many of the plans are confidential and cannot be divulged for security or proprietary reasons. Most employees know that little can be kept secret in any organization. On the other hand, supervisors should realize that some limitations to what they are allowed to know exist, and top-level administration may not wish to disclose all their plans for competitive reasons.

To the extent necessary, plans should be communicated and fully explained to subordinate managers so that they are in a better position to formulate derivative plans for their departments. Along the same line, supervisors should always bear in mind that their own employees are affected by the plans they make. Not only supervisors but their staff must clearly understand the objectives of their own department as well as how their goals support the goals and objectives of the entire institution. Because employees execute whatever has been planned, the supervisor should explain in advance the plans for the department. The manager may even want to consult his subordinate supervisors, team leaders, and line employees for suggestions because some may be in a position to make helpful contributions. The supervisor must bear in mind that the successful completion of a task depends on the full understanding of its purpose by those who have to carry it out. The supervisor should also remember that well-informed employees always are better employees. Such employees appreciate that they have not been kept in the dark. It is good management to make certain that all employees at all levels are thoroughly informed about the objectives to be achieved.

The Use of Objectives in Planning

Goals and objectives are not exactly the same thing, though they are often used interchangeably.

Goals or strategic thrusts support the vision and define results; for example, "our medication error rate will be lower than the regional average as defined by our liability carrier." *Objectives or critical success factors* set targets and describe how our goals will be achieved. One such objective may be to eliminate and/or reduce the acceptance of handwritten orders by securing 90 percent of all orders through computerized physician order entry by the end of the first quarter.

All planning has the purpose of achieving organizational goals and objectives. In this sense, objective has a broader meaning. For example, it was Barack Obama's objective to win the 2008 presidential election. In this context, objective and goal are synonymous.

Effective management is always management by objectives. This holds true for the CEO of a hospital, for the supervisor on the "firing line," and for all managers on the levels in between. Formulating objectives should therefore be foremost in every manager's mind. Once the goals have been established, additional plans, such as action steps, policies, standard procedures, methods, rules, programs, projects, and budgets, are designed to achieve the objectives.

Primary Objectives or Goals

In general, many healthcare centers have such primary objectives as providing **primary**, **secondary**, or **tertiary care**; providing healthcare at a reasonable cost; doing research; recruiting outstanding clinicians and employees; providing preventative health services; and training employees to deliver care or perform activities customarily associated with a healthcare institution. In addition to these goals, a healthcare facility can have many other objectives, such as implementing an environmental program, achieving excellent outcomes, establishing a good and caring image in the community, and maintaining fiscal viability. Some of these objectives will tie to an organization's values.

A healthcare institution also strives toward many other, less tangible objectives. In relation to its employees, for instance, its goal is to be a good and fair employer. The objective in this case is to establish the reputation of

primary care
Initial physician contact, such as in an emergency room, clinic, or physician's office.

secondary care
Patient care provided by specialists who do not normally have first contact with a patient, such as urologists or dermatologists.

tertiary care
Highly sophisticated and specialized inpatient care, normally in a healthcare facility that specializes in that type of care, such as a heart institute.

HOSPITAL LAND

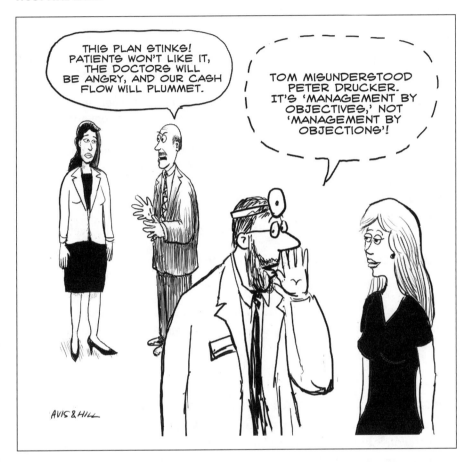

being a good place for people to work. These objectives may actually speak to the organization's values. According to Zuckerman (1998), "values define the organization's basic philosophy, principles, and ideals." A **value statement** answers the question, "what is important to this organization?" and cites the beliefs and behavioral standards that are fundamental to the organization. As shown in Exhibit 7.7, the values statement may be short or long, but should express the entity's moral and ethical basis (Purcell 2001).

value statement
A statement that defines what an organization holds important.

Most organizations have many primary objectives, and the difficulty lies in ranking and balancing them. This is especially true for healthcare facilities. If the CEO chose a single objective and excluded all the others, the effectiveness of the institution's overall performance could be jeopardized. Because healthcare activities must function in a constantly changing and increasingly challenging environment, it is necessary to continually reevaluate objectives and to add new ones that support the values of the organization and meet the needs of the communities served.

EXHIBIT 7.7
Example of
Values
Statements

CATHOLIC HEALTHCARE WEST, SAN FRANCISCO

Our Values

Catholic Healthcare West is committed to providing high-quality, affordable health care to the communities we serve. Above all else we value:

- Dignity—Respecting the inherent value and worth of each person.
- Collaboration—Working together with people who support common values and vision to achieve shared goals.
- Justice—Advocating for social change and acting in ways that promote respect for all persons and demonstrate compassion for our sisters and brothers who are powerless.
- Stewardship—Cultivating the resources entrusted to us to promote healing and wholeness.
- Excellence—Exceeding expectations through teamwork and innovation.

LITTLETON REGIONAL HOSPITAL, LITTLETON, NEW HAMPSHIRE

Values: Integrity, Respect, Compassion, Excellence.

SOURCES: Courtesy of Catholic Healthcare West, San Francisco and Littleton Regional Hospital, Littleton, NH.

Secondary or Departmental Objectives or Goals

The primary objectives of an institution are its goals. In turn, goals specific to departments can be called secondary, operative, supportive, or derivative objectives. Because each department or division has a specific task to perform, each must have its own clearly defined goals. These secondary goals and objectives of the departments must stay within and contribute to the overall framework of the organization's primary goals.

Because they are concerned with only one department, however, secondary objectives are necessarily narrower in scope. They enable departmental managers to operate at their own discretion, although, again, always within the limits of the overall institutional (primary) goals. For instance, if the stated organizational goal is, "to support research so that our clinicians are able to deliver state-of-the-art healthcare," the stated mission of the facility's decision-support department may be, "to systematically collect and maintain all patient demographic and medical data and to facilitate analysis of the data so that the resulting information benefits the user." Therefore, the departmental objectives or goals for the decision-support department may be to (1) work closely with patient financial services, health information, and accounting to obtain timely data; (2) collect, analyze, and publish various hospital and clinical comparative statistics; and (3) review and assess concurrently and retrospectively the outcomes and utilization of services.

Obviously these departmental objectives are specific, but their fulfillment contributes to the achievement of overall institutional goals. In fact, the primary objectives could not be achieved if these and all other departmental objectives were not fulfilled.

Developing Objectives

Planning is a dynamic process. Objectives must be flexible and adaptable to changes in the internal and external environments. Therefore, frequently reviewing, revising, or updating objectives is a managerial duty on all levels.

Objectives should represent measurable targets that lead to the achievement of a given goal. The acronym SMART indicates the steps to writing strong objectives—specific, measurable, attainable, result-oriented, time-limited (Allen 2000). Objectives must be established for each goal. An example of an organizational goal may be, "to expand community access to primary healthcare services." A corresponding objective may be, "to open three off-site ambulatory care clinics in the coming fiscal year at a cost not to exceed $2.5 million." For objectives to be achievable, the board and senior management must ensure that the resources are available.

Monitoring the Effectiveness of the Strategic Plan

Once management has created the strategic plan, the plan must be implemented through the efforts of all departments and staffs of the healthcare entity. Top down or bottom up, an organization's workforce implements any changes; if the staff do not respect or understand the undertaking, the plan is doomed at inception (Purcell 2001). As with any plan, knowing whether the decisions were right or wrong requires monitoring the implementation and effectiveness of the plan. This monitoring effort is known as **performance management (PM)**. PM collects data to monitor whether the **critical success factors (CSFs)** of the plan were achieved as intended. An appropriate PM may include making necessary revisions to the plan or operations to achieve corporate goals. Involving all employees in the development of CSF measurements defines what management is interested in and the results it expects. Sometimes, this process is carried out through a management by objectives approach.

Management by Objectives

To achieve specific results from setting these departmental objectives, organizations use a process called **management by objectives (MBO)**. The term and concepts were first introduced by management expert Peter Drucker (1954) in the early 1950s and have become popular.

MBO is an integrative management concept, containing elements of the planning function together with participative management, collaboration,

performance management (PM)
The process of monitoring the implementation and effectiveness of a plan.

critical success factors (CSFs)
Sub-goals of a plan. CSFs are monitored during performance management to measure progress of the overall plan.

management by objectives (MBO)
A management system in which managers and subordinates set goals and use progress toward those goals as measures of success.

motivation, and controlling. It is the process of collaborative goal setting by the manager and subordinate. The degree to which goals are accomplished plays a major role in evaluating and rewarding the subordinate's performance. MBO demonstrates the interrelationships of the managerial functions and the systems approach to management. Therefore, MBO is also discussed in other chapters of this book. This section, however, is primarily concerned with the meaning of MBO in connection with setting and achieving objectives.

When a facility begins an MBO program, top administration must communicate the reason that MBO has been adopted, must indicate that the program starts at the top of the organization, and must project the results the program is expected to produce. All managers and employees also need to be educated and informed about their role in the program. Often organizations create "dashboards" to monitor their progress.

As stated, MBO is concerned with goal setting for individual managers. In this process, a manager at any level and her immediate subordinate jointly develop departmental goals in accordance with organizational goals. Once institutional goals are clarified, the manager and the subordinate, on a one-to-one basis, develop and agree on the subordinate's goals during a stated period. The subordinate then defines the objectives to achieve the goals. To be operational, these performance objectives must be specific, measurable (quantifiable), and challenging, but they should also be realistically attainable within the time frame established. This means that each objective must provide a plan showing what work is to be done, in what time frame it is to be done, who is to do it, and what resources the individual can use to get it done. Quantitative indicators must also be established to measure what work is achieved.

To be realistic, it should be possible to carry out the activity within the time frame set—a period long enough to meet the objective, but short enough to provide timely feedback and still permit intervention if necessary. In general, the goals should meet the three criteria of specificity, conciseness, and time frame. The degree to which these goals are achieved is a major factor in evaluating and rewarding the subordinate's performance.

It is important that these goals be jointly established and agreed on ahead of time. At the end of the period, both the supervisor and the subordinate participate in the review of the subordinate's performance to see how results for the period compare with the objectives he set out to accomplish. If the goals were achieved, new goals are set for the next period. If a discrepancy exists, efforts are made to find solutions to overcome these problems and the manager and subordinate agree on new goals for the next period. MBO clearly is a powerful tool in achieving involvement and commitment of subordinates (see Exhibit 7.8).

The next three chapters explore other tools that contribute to a supervisor's planning success.

EXHIBIT 7.8
Management
Objectives

GOAL	EXPECTED DATE
Reduce by 50% the denials for inappropriate admissions	4th quarter
Capture data (by physician and payer) on inappropriate admissions	1st quarter
In cooperation with the VP Medical Affairs, develop an educational program for the medical staff	2nd quarter
Present education program for each clinical service	2nd quarter
Present one-on-one educational program for those physicians with the majority of admission denials	2nd quarter

Summary

Planning is the managerial function that determines what is to be done in the future. It is the function of every manager, from the top-level administrator to the supervisor of each department. Planning is important because it ensures the best utilization of resources and economy of performance. The planning period at the supervisory level is usually much shorter than the period at the top administrator's level. Nevertheless, the short-range plans of the supervisor must coincide with the long-range plans of the enterprise.

All planning must be done with forecasts of the future in mind. Forecasting is an art, not a science. As of yet, no infallible way of predicting the future exists; however, forecasting accuracy increases with experience. One should always remember that at the base of all forecasts lie certain assumptions, approximations, opinions, and judgments. Entitywide forecasts or assumptions are made by top-level administration, and the supervisor narrows these down to forecasts for the departmental activity.

Over time, making assumptions about the future should become a normal activity for all managers. They should exchange ideas, help each other, and supply information whenever it is available. They most likely will act as a check on each other, and their analysis of what the future holds will probably be quite reliable. Even if some of the events that have been anticipated do not materialize or do not occur exactly as forecasted, it is better to have foreseen them than to be suddenly confronted by them. Having foreseen these events, supervisors have prepared themselves and the state of the organization's affairs to be able to incorporate changes whenever they are needed. Although this task may sound formidable for supervisors, it is their job to be alert to all possible changes and trends. Based on these assumptions and forecasts, the supervisor makes plans for the department. This is the only way supervisors can prevent their own and their employees' obsolescence.

Establishing the vision is an essential step in planning. The vision guides managers to set goals and objectives. Although the overriding or primary objectives are determined by top-level administration, many secondary objectives or departmental goals must be clarified by the supervisor and must be in accordance with the primary objectives of the overall undertaking. The work of "operationalizing," or making the vision become reality, is in the hands of the managers and their staff who develop measurable objectives and action plans to accomplish the goals.

One useful technique for implementing plans is management by objectives, a process of collaborative goal setting that leads to evaluation. To be successful, this approach must establish realistic time frames and expectations that are mutually agreed on.

Notes

1. Competitive intelligence database is described by Alan Zuckerman (1998) and includes such information as annual reports, copies of websites, newspaper articles, demographic/economic indicators, technology factors, market size and characteristics, state licensure and other state filing, 990 and 10K reports, public vendors, etc.
2. Hospital Compare is a tool available through the U.S. Health and Human Services to allow the public to compare the quality of care provided by hospitals in the area. See more information at www.hospitalcompare.hhs.gov.
3. Littleton Regional Hospital was named one of the 100 Best Places to work in *Modern Healthcare's* survey of November 2008. Littleton ranked 40.
4. Readers may find the final report "Robotics in Healthcare," dated 10/3/2008, interesting. It is available online at http://ec.europa.eu/ information_society/activities/health/docs/studies/robotics-final-report.pdf.

Additional Readings

Bolster, C. J. 2008. "Planning During Turmoil—Credit Challenges and Healthcare Finance." *HFM* 62 (11): 55–62.

The Society for Healthcare Strategy and Market Development. 2010. *Futurescan 2010: Healthcare Trends and Implications 2010–2015*. Chicago: Health Administration Press.

APPENDIX 7.1

WHAT REGULATORY CHANGES ARE HAPPENING IN YOUR FIELD THAT WILL HAVE AN IMPACT ON THIS HOSPITAL, THE MEDICAL STAFF, AND/OR YOUR HOSPITAL?

REGULATORY IMPACT	POTENTIAL OUTCOMES
Nurse practitioners may be able to write controlled-substance scripts in future	Physicians and/or nurse practitioners may not support this change
Fire code changes	Additional fire prevention system installations
Privacy/security enforcement	New (locking) file cabinets in clinics
Potential radiology certification requirements	Some staff are not certified; may need to seek certification
Recovery audit contractors	Recovery of reimbursement received for observation cases and some short inpatient stays
Some states mandating the use of EMRs	Selection of a compatible system that is fully interfaced/integrated with hospital system; user resistance; cost
P4P in home health and Medicare inpatients	Additional documentation efforts; reimbursement changes
ICD-10	Massive reeducation
Mandatory MRSA screening	Operational changes, costs, no reimbursement, education needs
Medicaid does not cover patients >21 yrs	Loss of revenue; increase in nonreimbursed care
Core measures	Increased data collection efforts; lack of consistent documentation from clinicians

WHAT CHANGES ARE HAPPENING IN YOUR FIELD THAT WILL HAVE AN IMPACT ON CAPITAL NEEDS FOR YOUR DEPARTMENT? WHAT WILL YOU NEED TO ADDRESS THESE CHANGES? COST ESTIMATE?

CHANGE	COST ESTIMATE
Endoscope requested	$160,000
Smaller riding mower to mow areas with new landscaping	$1,500
New clinic building	$250,000–$350,000
New EKG machine	$4,000
EHR for clinics and hospital	$500,000–$1,000,000
Digital mammography because some physicians are referring elsewhere because we're not digital	$500,000
Dual-head power injector (for IV contrast)	<$100,000
New garbage disposal	<$2,000
Establish IT department to manage IT applications, assist users	$100,000
More advertising needed to promote services we currently offer	unknown
New PCs	$1,500 each
Telemonitoring in home health	$20,000
Ortho Blood Bank Gel System	$20,000–$30,000
Chemistry analyzer	$30,000–$40,000
Scanning of patient records and/or more space for health information management	$100,000
New dictation system (too few lines for dictation now)	$15,000–$20,000
Copier	$6,000–$8,000
Encoder	$20,000

WHAT ARE THIS HOSPITAL'S STRENGTHS?

STRENGTH	RELATED ISSUES
Hometown personal touch	Employees know too much about the patients—neighbors
Short waiting times in ED; fast test results	
Good basic services	
Community is supportive of hospital	No growth in community
Long-term management team; solid experience; highly educated	Unable to keep up with growth/changes in field
Employee empowerment	Lax; poor demeanor; dress code enforcement lacking; inconsistent discipline
Higher staff-to-patient ratio	
New patient room wing	Patients very satisfied with new area
Excellent rehab reputation	Dated facilities/equipment
Seeing younger patients	
Good skilled nursing facility (SNF) unit	
Good physicians	
Specialty services offered	Need more
Staff are kind and friendly; go above and beyond; not much "not my job"	
Our SNF is in our facility with ready access to high technology	Beautiful facility; access to therapy; close to home and family

WHAT DO OUR COMPETITORS DO BETTER THAN WE DO?

COMPETITION	WHAT WE NEED TO DO
Quality advertising/ impressive	Funding needed for billboards and radio; need more than brochures; spotlight our technology and each of our services
Radiology in each of their outpatient service areas	Do more to lessen inconvenience of patients; consider an outpatient service center where all outpatient services are located including testing capability
Greater range of services	Add derm, pain, oncology
Excellent signage	Place large sign on our building that is visible to the community and over our entrance
Broad range of physicians and specialists	Continue recruitment efforts for specialists
Competitive rehab services	Renovation/new equipment; address issue with physicians who refer elsewhere
Getting physician referrals	Educate physicians and patients—they have a choice
Availability of outpatient services—weekends and evenings	Expand clinic hours and/or establish urgent care center; must provide after-hours pediatric care

WHAT ONE OPPORTUNITY DO YOU THINK THE HOSPITAL SHOULD "JUMP ON" AT THIS TIME?

WHAT?	CONSEQUENCE/OUTCOME
After-hours clinic service	People go to our competitor and get tied into their physicians/system
Renovate physical therapy; include pool	Only one in area with pool services; reclaim market share
Acquire/open more rural health clinics	Capture greater referrals to our facility and ancillary services
Integrated hospital and clinic information system, including EHR	Effective use of labor and data for planning and treatment purposes
Add a radiologist	Improve timeliness of readings and patient care
Add a gynecologist	Reclaim women's market

APPENDIX 7.2

STRENGTHS

Board is local

History

Personalized service

"New" facility

Geographic remoteness precludes nearby competition

Good providers—high quality

Loyal community and community financial support

Strong affiliation with healthcare system

"Rural healthcare at its best"

Good cash reserves

Responsive and flexible leadership

Employees empowered

Hometown personal touch

Continued . . .

STRENGTHS *Continued*

Short waiting times in ED; fast test results

New facility gives people impression that everything is new and that we can do more

Good basic services

Location; close to home; visitor ease

Long-term management team; solid experience, highly educated

Critical access status—reimbursement

Higher staff-to-patient ratio than others

New patient room wing is beautiful

Excellent rehab reputation

Starting to see younger patients

Younger physicians—open to change

Good SFN unit; located in building and has access to acute care services and technology

New surgeon is well received

Specialty services are offered

Staff are friendly and kind; go above and beyond

WEAKNESSES

History

Location

Difficulty recruiting specialists

Community members go elsewhere

Limited resources

Lack of IT integration

Lack of effective marketing program

Limitations on anesthesia care

Need for additional staff education and cross training

Lack of 24-hour and weekend surgical service

Lack of radiology in each of our outpatient service areas

Lack a greater range of services

Not present at all community activities

Weak auxiliary

Inadequate signage

Lack of services on weekends and evenings

Competition infringing on our services and market

Lack of pediatric, orthopedic, oncology, and chemotherapy services

Need a more sophisticated website

THREATS

Reimbursement changes

Economy

New government regulations

Disaster/pandemic flu

Competition (outpatient services)

National nursing shortage

Loss of specialists

Loss of Rural Health Clinic designation/preferred reimbursement

Younger population have less loyalty to hometown hospital/clinicians

OPPORTUNITIES

Land adjacent to hospital becoming available—would be ideal for medical office building

Layoffs occurring at competitor—may allow us to fill some technical positions

Funding available to hire an experienced marketing manager

New affiliation with hospital system includes access to specialists

Improve promotions of our facilities, staff, and medical staff

Establish an urgent care center at one of our clinics; keep it open weekends and evenings

Continue renovation of our patient care facilities

Add ultrasound services

TACTICAL CONSIDERATIONS IN PLANNING

Chapter Objectives

After you have studied this chapter, you should be able to do the following:

1. Define and discuss different strategies for resource planning.
2. Recognize that planning requires attention to other elements, including timing, resource utilization, financial considerations, and safety.
3. Identify approaches to planning for the proper utilization of materials, machinery, and manpower.

While planning, supervisors must keep in mind how these plans affect others. Peers and subordinates assess the impact that plans or changes have on them or their departments first. Any perceived negative impact may result in resistance or lack of support for the initiatives. Success or failure of planning depends largely on the reaction of those involved, whether they are employees, supervisors of other departments, top-level administration, the medical staff, patients, or visitors. Thus, a supervisor plays a significant role in ensuring plans come to fruition—that of change agent.

The Supervisor as a Change Agent

If one envisions a management pyramid, the frontline supervisor is at the base of it—the broadest section of the pyramid. She must encourage the most individuals to embrace changes decided upon by the few at the peak of the pyramid. The supervisor's effectiveness as an agent of change is demonstrated by her ability to convince the employees, gain their willingness, prepare them, and mobilize them to make changes in their work environment.

To be an effective change agent, a manager must have solid communication and organizing skills. He must be able to anticipate reactions and plan how to best address the concerns that will be voiced. Typically, effective change agents identify allies who can help them facilitate the change. These allies may be peers, superiors, and often subordinates. Finally, McConnell (1993) says, the element of trust should be demonstrated by both the change agent and those affected by the proposed change. Change, he says, is a continuum of unfreezing (breaking down the barriers of how we do it now), moving (transitioning to the new approach), and refreezing (incorporating the change and tweaking it to meet the needs of the organization).

Several tactical or political strategies are at the supervisor's disposal to help minimize negative reactions and to facilitate the success of the plans. **Tactical approaches** are short term. They are a means to get to the desired end. A combination of these approaches may be used, depending on the situation at hand. For example, a plan to outsource the environmental and food services functions of an organization requires tactical considerations by the current departmental managers and the administrator for these functions. Administration may involve managers, supervisors, and possibly some of the line staff, such as lead cooks and housekeepers, to help develop some of the criteria that will be used in selecting a firm. In addition, these individuals may be part of the interview team. The goal is that by involving staff in parts of the decision, administration will gain their buy-in to the change.

tactical approaches
Short-term actions leading toward goals.

Planning Strategies

Because timing is a critical factor in all planning, the manager may choose the strategy that tells her to strike while the iron is hot. This strategy advocates prompt action when the situation and time for action are favorable. On the other hand, the supervisor may prefer to use the wait-and-see strategy, which takes the approach that time is the great moderator. This is not an endorsement of procrastination but of moving more slowly and seeing if factors take care of themselves after a short period of time.

concentrated mass offensive
A strategy of pulling together all resources and taking sudden, radical action to quickly solve a problem.

When significant changes are involved in planning, the supervisor may use the strategy known as **concentrated mass offensive**. This strategy advocates quickly pulling together all resources and taking radical action all at once to get immediate results. The creation of quasi-immediate service "hospitals" during Hurricane Katrina may be one example. Another approach may be team involvement. This strategy involves employees using various techniques such as brainstorming to solve what-if questions. This approach may be used if the organization has set a goal to improve patient satisfaction during the next year. Team involvement takes time but also provides for buy-in on plans by the employees. It also allows management to use the input of the employees as an information resource. On the other hand, the supervisor may prefer to just get a foot in the door. This approach may be used to initially introduce a pending change, such as "We will need to expand coverage of our department to seven days a week. However, we will not be able to add staff. Be thinking about this, and we'll discuss it further at next week's department meeting." This tactic implies that proposing merely a portion of the plan in the beginning may lead to gradual acceptance, especially if the program is of such magnitude that its total acceptance is doubtful.

Sometimes one supervisor's plan may involve changes that could come about more easily if supervisors of other departments participate. It may therefore be advisable to seek allies to promote the change—that is, to adopt the strategy that promotes strength in unity. For example, if a supervisor plans to propose a weekend differential for some of the employees, it may be wise to get other supervisors to join the effort in presenting a general request for a weekend differential to the management. This may involve the you-scratch-my-back-and-I'll-scratch-yours strategy. This tactic, known as **reciprocity**, is practiced in business, in political circles, and by colleagues who wish to present joint action on a particular issue.

reciprocity
A tactic that involves giving a colleague something in return for something. Also called "you scratch my back and I'll scratch yours."

The choice and application of these political tactics depend on the people involved, magnitude and urgency of the objective, timing, means available, and various other factors. These tactics are not always appropriate. Properly applied, however, they can minimize difficulties and increase the effectiveness of the supervisor's planning.

Planning the Utilization of Resources

Every supervisor is entrusted with a large number of valuable resources to accomplish his job. These resources are grouped into three categories—materials, machinery, and manpower (the 3 Ms). The supervisor has a duty to specifically plan how to use the resources available so that the work of the unit can be managed efficiently and cost effectively. This means that detailed plans must be made for the proper use of equipment, instruments, space, materials and supplies, and supervisor's and employees' time.

Because institutions make substantial investments in equipment, plans for its efficient use must be made to protect the investment. In many departments, much of the equipment's usage depends on the orders of the physicians and surgeons. However, it is the supervisor's job to ensure that employees use the equipment with care.

Patient Care Equipment and Other Machinery

Furthermore, the supervisor must ensure that the department is properly maintained. Equipment that is poorly maintained and does not function properly could lead to serious problems, perhaps even resulting in a patient's lawsuit for damages. When the supervisor discovers that a piece of equipment is malfunctioning, he should immediately determine if it is being operated properly or if a maintenance problem exists. The proper steps to remedy the malfunction should be taken at once. Supervisors should work closely with the maintenance department or biomedical services and plan for periodic maintenance checkups.

Most facilities have an established program to check equipment at regular intervals in accordance with the manufacturers' guidelines. Records of these checks should be maintained. If a piece of equipment becomes worn, these records provide the supervisor with evidence to support replacement.

HOSPITAL LAND

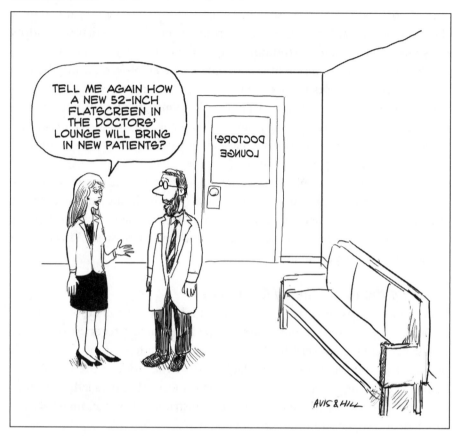

In addition, such records of maintenance, repair, and corrective action are often reviewed by regulatory and accrediting agencies at the time of facility inspections.

Also, it is the supervisor's job to determine if the equipment serves its purpose and if better options are available for doing the work. This does not mean that a supervisor must always have the very latest model available or the technology with the most "whistles"; however, the supervisor should plan to replace inefficient equipment and select equipment with features that can do the job. If the medical staff will be affected by or use the equipment, such as a new electronic signature application to sign reports and orders or a new endoscope, then the medical staff should be involved in deciding to update the equipment, participating in vendor demos, and recommending the replacement models or manufacturers. If the enterprise uses an outside biomedical service, supervisors should obtain its advice on replacement brands because the service may have encountered a more reliable model or brand elsewhere. Finally, if the system is to interface or integrate with the organization's information system, a representative from information technology services should participate in the system evaluations.

Once supervisors decide to replace old equipment or introduce new systems, they must plan such replacements carefully. In addition to consulting with the medical staff, they must read professional journals and literature circulated by hospitals and related associations, listen to sales presentations, and keep themselves abreast of current developments within their fields. Only with this type of background can the supervisor submit to her boss intelligent plans and alternatives for the replacement of the equipment. The recommended changes should be well substantiated. The proposal should include such items as projections of better patient care, utilization, cost effectiveness, community need, collaboration required, payback or return expected, customer sensitivity, and the important considerations of leasing versus buying.

Financial Considerations When Proposing the Purchase of New Equipment

Every year department managers submit requests for new equipment. The requests are often evaluated by an administrative or board committee, generally known as the capital expenditures committee. Funds for the equipment, or capital, are derived from an accounting process that sets aside a portion of monies each month or year in a fund called **accrued depreciation**.

Competition for the accrued depreciation is usually high. All managers want to update their facilities, equipment, and furnishings. Furthermore, new technologies for patient care purposes may be requested by members of the medical staff. Since the medical staff bring patients to the facility, their requests often are given greater attention.

accrued depreciation Funds set aside each moth to pay for new equipment or capital.

The final decision, however, remains with higher management. Even if the request is turned down, the supervisor has demonstrated that she is on top of the job, planning for the future. Eventually the plans for replacing equipment probably will be accepted, and the administrator will realize that the supervisor planned for the department's equipment with foresight (Exhibit 8.1).

Planning a Safe Environment

Traditionally healthcare providers have been aware of the need for safety for their patients, employees, and visitors; after all, some hospital deaths are caused by unsafe conditions within the healthcare facility. Furthermore, the emphasis by accrediting agencies, the push for computerized physician order entry, and the federal government's support of an electronic health record for every individual by 2014 make every healthcare employee doubly aware of the importance of safety.

Although most healthcare facilities have a safety committee or safety department, its existence alone cannot fulfill the institution's obligation to plan, create, and maintain a safe environment. As part of their responsibilities, managers and supervisors must diligently watch their areas and attempt to eliminate safety hazards. The recent flood of liability suits against hospitals and the publicity on medication and surgical errors have put additional emphasis on the need for safety. Most recently, Medicare's reimbursement reduction for hospital-acquired conditions has increased administration's awareness.

Exhibit 8.1

What to
Consider When
Preparing
Capital
Requests

When preparing a capital expenditure request, a manager should consider the following points:

1. Is the request supportive of and consistent with the organization's strategic plan?
2. Is the request responsive to the needs of the customers served as described by the marketing department?
3. Is the request responsive to the needs of the operating department? Will it solve an operational problem?
4. Has the request been fully justified by analysis of the benefits it will offer the organization/department?
5. Is the proposal supported by firm price quotations by vendors and contractors?
6. Is the request financially fundable?

SOURCE: Sweeny and Rachlin (1987).

As discussed in Chapter 6, a patient is entitled to expect that the healthcare facility staff follow proven protocols and that the premises are reasonably safe. Care must be taken regarding equipment, instruments, and appliances so that they are adequate for use in the diagnosis or treatment of patients. If defective equipment causes injury to a patient, the hospital may be liable. Patients have brought lawsuits against healthcare facilities and their professional staffs because of defective beds, medication errors, broken thermometers, inoperative patient call systems, improperly calibrated x-ray equipment, and improperly prepared food. These examples indicate why The Joint Commission stresses the National Patient Safety Goals and the Life Safety Code in its surveys.

Exposure to potentially dangerous materials or chemicals is common in healthcare facilities. For example, the food service and environmental staffs are exposed to cleansing agents and disinfectants, and the pathology staff are exposed to various media used to assist in evaluating tissues and bodily fluids. It is the supervisor's duty to keep his staff informed of chemical agents with which they may come in contact. When chemical agents of any type, such as detergents, correction fluid, printer toner, or laboratory chemicals, are used in the work setting, a Material Safety and Data Sheet (MSDS) should be prominently posted in the work area. These MSDSs provide staff with information such as how to treat the employee if the chemical is ingested or gets in the eyes.

Another concern supervisors must take into account today is the rise in workplace violence. Consider the following events and how you as a supervisor could have planned for security or protective measures to protect the individuals involved:

- A drunken, 50-year-old Salem man was brought to Beverly Hospital for treatment. As a nurse helped him get ready to leave, he lunged at her, grabbed her crotch, and tore through her hospital scrubs. He refused to let go. (Massachusetts Nursing Association 2005).
- "A female physician was accosted and sexually assaulted in an elevator at Bridgeport Hospital.... Police sources said [the perpetrator] may have posed as a hospital employee.... She managed to grab the elevator telephone but no one answered" (*Connecticut Post* 2005).
- An ex-boyfriend held an urgent care center employee hostage, called her three sons to tell them what he was about to do before shooting and killing her at the urgent care center where she was a lab technician (Knowles 2008).
- A former Alaska hospital worker shot two of his former supervisors, killing one, a day after being fired (D'Oro 2008).

In 2000, health service workers overall had an incidence rate of 9.3 per 10,000 workers for injuries resulting from assaults and violent acts. This rate compares to 2 nonfatal assaults per 10,000 workers in 1999 in the private sector (Washington State Department of Labor and Industries 2006; U.S. Department of Labor 2009).

No place or individual is immune from violence today. Taking training courses and reviewing publications such as the Centers for Disease Control and Prevention's NIOSH (2002) report "Violence: Occupational Hazards in Hospitals," can help identify precursors to violence, such as marital discord or depression, and prepare the supervisor to take appropriate measures if violence erupts in the workplace. The organization's safety officer and the local police department are excellent resources for prevention and safety advice.

Workplace injuries are another safety concern. Overall, the number of fatal work injuries recorded by the U.S. Department of Labor has declined. Today, however, much emphasis is placed on reducing or eliminating injuries caused by repetitive hand and finger motions, often linked to the increased use of computers and keyboards in the workplace. The U.S. Bureau of Labor Statistics (2008) reported that injuries from repetitive motion continue to be the event with the highest median days away from work—20.

Obviously, reducing or eliminating such causes of injuries among staff benefits the supervisor. Safety evaluations are not limited to at-facility work sites. Some staff, such as transcriptionists, information systems technicians, and patient financial services employees, now telecommute or work at home. The supervisor may need to inspect home offices, offer ergonomic furniture, and hold safety classes. The occupational therapy department will be able to assist in evaluating the staff's workspaces.

The true responsibility for safety lies with every manager, from the CEO down to the supervisors. The supervisor, being the person on the spot, must stress safety more than anyone else and must enforce safety procedures. Safety must be foremost in the supervisors' and employees' thoughts and must be a constant consideration in all supervisory planning. It must be integrated in all policies, procedures, methods, practices, and directives so that accidents and incidents do not occur or at least are significantly reduced.

Planning Space

Supervisors must also plan for the best utilization of space. First, they should determine whether the space assigned to the department is being used effectively. Industrial engineering or space design help, if available, may be requested to make this determination. If such help is not available, the supervisor should make a layout chart showing the square footage of the department, the location of equipment and supplies, and the work paths of the employees. Such a chart can then be studied to determine whether the allocated space has been laid out appropriately to avoid cross trafficking or whether areas need to be rearranged so that the department's workflow and work can be done more efficiently.

For example, say the chief laboratory scientist of the clinical laboratories shows that their annual workload has been increasing by approximately 10 percent, which would nearly double the workload in approximately seven years, from 40,000 to 78,000 tests. She also points out that the increased volume requires additional instrumentation that requires more square feet of room. She shows how long the laboratories have occupied the same space. The chief technologist then draws up a typical laboratory space plan, showing a layout for separate work units or technical sections—hematology, urinalysis, biochemistry, histology, serology, bacteriology, immunology, blood bank—and the support areas. At the same time, the supervisor points out that a satellite of the laboratory facilities should preferably be on the first floor near the emergency department and patient registration areas and should be easily accessible to surgery, rather than on the present upper-floor location. However, keeping in mind the cost-effective utilization of hospital space, the supervisor also discusses the feasibility of moving the remainder of the labs to an off-site location. She then presents these materials during a discussion with the administrator and the medical director of the laboratory.

Layout planning may show the need for additional space, a different location, or both. If such a request, based on thorough planning of the space currently allotted, is made to the administrator, the likelihood that it will be granted is greater. In this case, the chief laboratory scientist most likely will be competing with many other managers who probably also requested more space. Even if the request is denied, these plans will not have been drawn up in vain. They most likely will alert the chief laboratory scientist to some of the conditions under which the employees are working, and perhaps that information can be used to plan more efficient work methods under the existing conditions.

Appendix 8.1 shows sample forms and floor plans and discusses some of the intricate details a supervisor may be asked to address when planning new or expanded space.

Planning Utilization of Materials and Supplies

The supervisor must plan for the appropriate use, security, and conservation of the materials and supplies entrusted and charged to the department. Every department has some supplies that are ideal for the household and therefore lend themselves to pilferage. Items such as thermometers, file folders, trash bags, and even scrubs are examples of such supplies. It is not uncommon to experience increased supply usage—specifically, for pencils, pens, and tablets—in September, which coincides with the start of school. In most departments, the quantity of materials and supplies used is substantial. While a single item may represent only a small value, the aggregate of these items adds up to sizeable amounts in the budget of a healthcare facility. Controlling access to these items through the use of locked storage cabinets, using RFID (radio-frequency identification) tags to monitor whereabouts of small or coveted equipment (such as IV stands or wheelchairs), periodic inventorying, and minimizing the quantity on hand help to limit loss. Not all loss is intentional, as there is **pocket loss**—supplies that leave the facility (innocently) in the pockets of lab coats or uniforms. Proper planning ensures that materials and supplies are used as conservatively as possible without compromising sterility, asepsis, and sanitary requirements.

pocket loss
The accidental loss of supplies that leave the hospital in employees' pockets.

Planning Utilization of the Workforce

The employees in a department are the most valuable resource. Therefore, planning for their full utilization must be foremost in every manager's mind.

Planning for the best utilization of the workforce also entails developing methods for recruiting good employees, enhancing employee satisfaction, searching for all available sources of qualified employees, and working for their retention. Furthermore, proper utilization means conducting an ongoing search for the best ways to group employee activities and to train, supervise, and motivate employees.

Finally, effective use of workers means the continual appraisal of their performance, appropriate promotions, adequate plans for compensation and rewards, and, at the same time, fair disciplinary measures.

All these considerations play an important role when the supervisor plans for the best utilization of the department's workforce. Each of these topics is addressed in further detail later in the text. Only through such human resource planning can a situation be created in which workers willingly contribute their utmost to achieve both personal satisfaction on the job and the department's objectives. Employees, in turn, amply reward a supervisor who considers their personal satisfaction important. Planning for the best utilization of employees is at the heart of expert supervision.

Summary

Plans must be made for the full utilization of all the resources at the supervisor's disposal. More specifically, she must plan for proper use of equipment and instruments, work methods, and processes. The supervisor should plan to effectively use the space available and to maintain control of materials and supplies under his supervision. The efficient use of time also must be planned. Most important, the supervisor must plan for the best overall utilization of the employees in the unit. This means, among other things, seeing that employees are able to find satisfaction in their work.

Throughout all planning, the supervisor should be concerned with the effects of these plans on other members of the organization. At times, the manager may need to resort to various tactical considerations that are helpful in getting the department's plans accepted and effectively implemented.

Additional Readings

Johnson, S. 2002. *Who Moved My Cheese: An Amazing Way to Deal with Change in Your Work and in Your Life.* New York: Penguin Putnam Publishers.
Journal of Healthcare Management. 2008. "Interview with William Petasnick, FACHE." *Journal of Healthcare Management,* 53 (6): 352–55.

APPENDIX 8.1

Space Planning Tools

It is said that a manager needs no desk nor for that matter an office because she should be observing what is happening among the staff in their work sites. Immediate feedback should occur when something is done right and observed firsthand. Managers cannot do this in an office. Often the size of an office is proportional to the rank of an individual in an organization. Office size, therefore, may help explain positions that appear on an organizational chart. However, offices do not exist in all organizations.

The chairman of Aluminum Company of America (ALCOA) moved out of his lush executive suite into a Spartan cubicle in the mid-1990s. The chairman and other executives decided they should spend their workdays in a cluster of cubicle offices that allowed them to lean over a makeshift wall to confer rather than wait for formal meetings. Changes such as these occurred at IBM, Nickelodeon, and the American Health Information Management Association (AHIMA). Open office arrangements increase communication and possibly increase production, as individuals cannot hide inside an office to read a book or have long telephone conversations. These open office arrangements are usually less expensive and provide design flexibility, as cubicles can be easily rearranged. For departments that have staff who telecommute for part of the week, open office and cubicle arrangements allow telecommuters to use available cubicles when they are not working remotely.

At some time during his career, a supervisor will be asked to work with a design specialist to lay out new or renovated workspace. To do so, it is important to know fundamental office design practices. A typical design worksheet appears in Exhibit A. Workspace areas typically vary by position level. Directors may have enclosed offices or cubicles with higher walls to provide additional privacy for meetings and conversations. Their space may be 155 square feet to 175 square feet and include a desk, credenza, bookcase, and round meeting table. Managers may be assigned space that ranges from 110 to 144 square feet. The larger work area allows space for a small round conference table for the manager and two or three staff members to meet spontaneously in the manager's office (Exhibit B). Supervisory positions may have space allocations ranging from 64 to 100 square feet. Typically, this area includes sufficient desk and filing space for the supervisor and an extra chair for a staff member or visitor (Exhibit B). Staff members who require desk space, such as data analysts, transcriptionists, billing and collections staff, and dietitians, may be allocated 40 to 90 square feet (Exhibit B).

Some areas require extensive filing space, such as radiology, pharmacy, and the library. In these areas, the manager needs to determine whether stationary open shelving or moveable shelving (Exhibit C) meet their needs. Using moveable, condensed filing systems may reduce the floor space requirement by as much as 50 percent. To use this type of filing system, one must consider (1) whether the weight-bearing load of the floor accommodates the weight of condensed shelving, (2) the number of access aisles required, and (3) reasonable reaching height. When selecting shelving units, the items to be stored on the shelves must be measured. For example, books may require 10 inches deep by 12 inches between shelves while some radiology films may require 17 inches deep and 18 inches between shelves.

When using moveable shelving, ensure the shelves are deep enough for the item to be pushed in all the way on the shelf. If it sticks out, it may trigger a safety switch that does not allow the shelving units to move. Shelves typically have widths of 36, 42, and 48 inches. Other filing options are vertical and lateral files. A typical five-drawer vertical file cabinet provides 125 linear inches of file space and consumes 6 square feet of floor space. Lateral file cabinets that are 36 inches wide provide 204 linear inches of filing space and consume 3 square feet of floor space. Generally, lateral file cabinets are more expensive than vertical file cabinets.

Aisles between desks should be no less than 24 to 26 inches. The same holds true for work areas that have file cabinets.

This overview emphasizes the value of utilizing space planners from the organization's construction and design department or from a local architect to ensure that you do not shortchange your needs. These professionals also are able to suggest alternative arrangements and space-saving features such as overhead storage units, worklights, and portable pedestals, that help your staff work more efficiently.

Exhibit A

Farnsworth GROUP — DESIGN CRITERIA WORKSHEET

ENGINEERS
ARCHITECTS
SURVEYORS
SCIENTISTS

Date: _____

Project: _____

Project No.: _____

Department:	Room Name:	Room No.

General Requirements:

A. Floor:
- ☐ Vinyl Composition Tile
- ☐ Rubber Tile
- ☐ Sheet Vinyl
- ☐ Sheet Tile
- ☐ Seamless Flooring
- ☐ Ceramic Tile
- ☐ Quarry Tile
- ☐ Terrazzo
- ☐ Carpet Tile
- ☐ Carpet Broadloom
- ☐ Unfinished
- ☐ Sealed
- ☐ Conductive
- ☐ Patch
- ☐ Existing
- ☐ _____
- ☐ _____
- ☐ _____
- ☐ _____
- ☐ _____

B. Walls:

N	S	E	W	
☐	☐	☐	☐	Plaster
☐	☐	☐	☐	Cement Plaster
☐	☐	☐	☐	Gypsum Board
☐	☐	☐	☐	Concrete Block
☐	☐	☐	☐	Brick
☐	☐	☐	☐	Paint
☐	☐	☐	☐	Vinyl Wallcovering
☐	☐	☐	☐	Epoxy Coating
☐	☐	☐	☐	Ceramic Tile
☐	☐	☐	☐	Structural Glazed Tile
☐	☐	☐	☐	Unfinished
☐	☐	☐	☐	Borrow Lite
☐	☐	☐	☐	Folding Partition
☐	☐	☐	☐	Demountable Partition
☐	☐	☐	☐	Patch
☐	☐	☐	☐	Existing
☐	☐	☐	☐	Fire Rated
☐	☐	☐	☐	Sound Wall
☐	☐	☐	☐	_____
☐	☐	☐	☐	

E. Doors:
- ☐ Width
- ☐ Operation
- ☐ Label
- ☐ Solid
- ☐ Hollow
- ☐ Vision Panel
- ☐ _____
- ☐ _____
- ☐ _____

F. Casework:
- ☐ Steel
- ☐ Plastic Laminate
- ☐ Wood
- ☐ Corrosion Resistant Top
- ☐ Plastic Laminate Top
- ☐ Solid Surface Top
- ☐ Stainless Steel Top
- ☐ _____
- ☐ _____

C. Base:
- ☐ Vinyl
- ☐ Rubber
- ☐ Ceramic Tile
- ☐ Quarry Tile
- ☐ Terrazzo
- ☐ Structural Glazed Tile
- ☐ Seamless Integral
- ☐ Patch
- ☐ Existing
- ☐ Wood
- ☐ _____
- ☐ _____
- ☐ _____

D. Ceiling:
- ☐ Acoustical
- ☐ Lay-in
- ☐ Concealed
- ☐ Adhesive
- ☐ Plaster
- ☐ Cement Plaster
- ☐ Gypsum Board
- ☐ Unfinished
- ☐ Existing
- ☐ Patch
- ☐ Paint
- ☐ Fire Rated
- ☐ _____
- ☐ _____

G. Special Construction
- ☐ Prefabricated Construction
- ☐ X-ray Shielding
- ☐ R-F Shielding
- ☐ Neg./Pos. Pressure Room
- ☐ Isolation Room
- ☐ ICU Doors
- ☐ _____
- ☐ _____
- ☐ _____
- ☐ _____
- ☐ _____
- ☐ _____
- ☐ _____

H. Notes and Comments:

_____

_____

_____

_____

_____

_____

_____

_____

_____

_____

_____

_____

_____

_____

Continued

EXHIBIT A *Continued*

Farnsworth *DESIGN CRITERIA WORKSHEET*

Electrical Systems:	Mechanical Systems:

A. Utilities and Services:
- ☐ 110V duplex Outlets
- ☐ 220V duplex Outlets
- ☐ Wire Mould
- ☐ X-ray Outlet
- ☐ Special Outlet
- ☐ 110V Emergency Power
- ☐ 220V Emergency Power

B. Lighting:
- ☐ Fluorescent
- ☐ Compact Fluorescent
- ☐ Incandescent
- ☐ Halogen
- ☐ Mercury Vapor/Halide
- ☐ Emergency Lighting
- ☐ Surgical Lighting
- ☐ Dimmable
- ☐ Ballast
- ☐ _____
- ☐ _____

C. Communications:

Rough-in / Wiring / Equipment / Special Outlet

- ☐ ☐ ☐ ☐ Telephone
- ☐ ☐ ☐ ☐ Intercom
- ☐ ☐ ☐ ☐ Public Address
- ☐ ☐ ☐ ☐ Paging
- ☐ ☐ ☐ ☐ Music
- ☐ ☐ ☐ ☐ Nurse Call
- ☐ ☐ ☐ ☐ Central Dictation
- ☐ ☐ ☐ ☐ Physiological Monitoring
- ☐ ☐ ☐ ☐ Charting
- ☐ ☐ ☐ ☐ CCTV
- ☐ ☐ ☐ ☐ Cable TV
- ☐ ☐ ☐ ☐ Data Processing
- ☐ ☐ ☐ ☐ Internet
- ☐ ☐ ☐ ☐ Emtek
- ☐ ☐ ☐ ☐ _____
- ☐ ☐ ☐ ☐ _____

D. Notes and Comments:
_____
_____
_____
_____
_____
_____
_____
_____
_____
_____
_____
_____
_____

A. HVAC:
- ☐ Air Conditioned
- ☐ Special Environment
- ☐ Temperature
- ☐ Humidity
- ☐ 100% Exhaust
- ☐ _____
- ☐ _____

B. Utility and Services:
- ☐ Hot Water
- ☐ Cold Water
- ☐ Deionized Water
- ☐ Chilled Water
- ☐ Natural Gas
- ☐ Steam
- ☐ Sprinklers

C. Medical Gases:

Wall / Ceiling / Column

- ☐ ☐ ☐ Air
- ☐ ☐ ☐ Oxygen
- ☐ ☐ ☐ Vacuum
- ☐ ☐ ☐ Nitrogen
- ☐ ☐ ☐ Nitrous Oxide

D. Plumbing:

Handicapped / Conventional / Knee / Foot / Wrist Blade / Goose Neck / Divertor Valve / Aerator Valve / Vacuum Breaker / Hose Spray

- ☐ ☐ ☐ ☐ ☐ ☐ ☐ ☐ ☐ ☐ Lavatory
- ☐ ☐ ☐ ☐ ☐ ☐ ☐ ☐ ☐ ☐ Counter Sink
- ☐ ☐ ☐ ☐ ☐ ☐ ☐ ☐ ☐ ☐ Scrub Sink
- ☐ ☐ ☐ ☐ ☐ ☐ ☐ ☐ ☐ ☐ Clinic Sink (Flushing Room)
- ☐ ☐ ☐ ☐ ☐ ☐ ☐ ☐ ☐ ☐ Mop Receptor
- ☐ ☐ ☐ ☐ ☐ ☐ ☐ ☐ ☐ ☐ Water Closet
- ☐ ☐ ☐ ☐ ☐ ☐ ☐ ☐ ☐ ☐ Urinal
- ☐ ☐ ☐ ☐ ☐ ☐ ☐ ☐ ☐ ☐ Shower
- ☐ ☐ ☐ ☐ ☐ ☐ ☐ ☐ ☐ ☐ Floor Drain
- ☐ ☐ ☐ ☐ ☐ ☐ ☐ ☐ ☐ ☐ Drinking Fountain
- ☐ ☐ ☐ ☐ ☐ ☐ ☐ ☐ ☐ ☐ Cup Sink
- ☐ ☐ ☐ ☐ ☐ ☐ ☐ ☐ ☐ ☐ Tub
- ☐ ☐ ☐ ☐ ☐ ☐ ☐ ☐ ☐ ☐ Emergency Eyewash
- ☐ ☐ ☐ ☐ ☐ ☐ ☐ ☐ ☐ ☐ Emergency Shower

E. Notes and Comments:
_____
_____
_____
_____

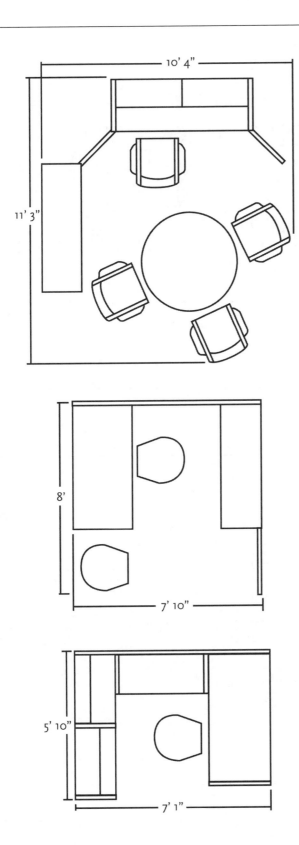

Exhibit C

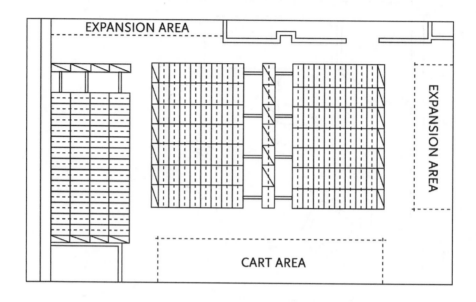

Exhibit D

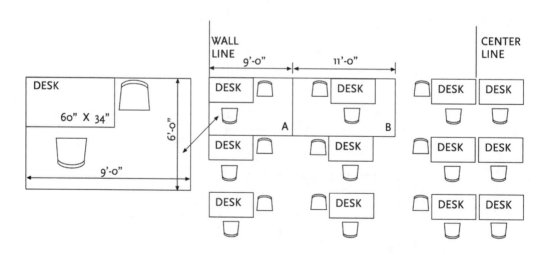

WORK STATION 3-A - 54 SQ. FT.
            3-B - 66 SQ. FT.

PLANNING TOOLS

Chapter Objectives

After you have studied this chapter, you should be able to do the following:

1. Describe the types of and distinguish between standing plans, repeat-use plans, and single-use plans.
2. Discuss the various types of standing plans and their effect on managerial decision making.
3. Differentiate policies from procedures, procedures from methods, and policies from rules.
4. Discuss the value of organizational manuals.

Once the entitywide goals are established and the objectives are determined, managers must design numerous plans necessary to achieve fulfillment of the goals. Several different types of plans are devised to implement objectives. These are policies, procedures, methods, rules, programs, projects, and budgets. These plans must be designed to reinforce one another; that is, they must be internally consistent, integrated, and coordinated. Because every manager probably has to devise or at least use each type of plan at some time, he should be familiar with the meaning of all of them. The major plans are formulated by top administration, but department supervisors have to formulate their own departmental plans accordingly. The purpose of all these plans is to ensure that the thinking and actions taken on different levels and in different departments of the institution are consistent with and contribute to the overall objectives.

These different types of plans can be divided into two major groups: repeat-use plans and single-use plans. Policies, procedures, methods, and rules are commonly known as repeat-use or standing plans. They are used for problems that occur regularly. **Repeat-use plans** are applicable whenever a problem situation presents itself that is similar to the one for which the standing plan was originally devised. **Single-use plans** are used for nonrecurring situations. These plans are no longer needed once the objective is accomplished. Within this single-use plan category are programs, projects, and budgets.

repeat-use plan
A plan that can be used whenever a situation arises that is similar to the situation the plan was originally created for.

single-use plan
A plan for nonrecurring situations.

Policies

policy
A standing plan that expresses an organization's general response to a problem or situation.

Policies are probably the most important and frequently invoked repeat-use plans a manager must depend on. Generally, they are issued and set by the top management of the organization. Policies provide managers with a general guideline for decision making, such as "all staff should wear clothing that is appropriate for a business environment and for meeting with the public." They are general statements that channel the thinking of all personnel charged with decision making. Because they are broad, policies do not have definite limitations and boundaries. Policies reflect constraints, and as long as a supervisor stays within these limitations, she will make an appropriate decision—one that conforms to the policy.

In this way, policies facilitate the job of both managers and subordinates. They ensure uniformity of decision making throughout the organization. Policies are standing plans that express the organization's general response to a problem or situation. Thus, top management directs decisions toward the achievement of the organizational goals, expressing values and ideas it deems important. Policies help to coordinate activities, and as the organization grows larger and more complex, the need for policies increases.

Policies as an Aid in Delegation

Policies cover the various areas of the organization's activities: some relate to the managerial functions (e.g., a promotion-from-within policy), others relate to operational functions (e.g., patient care, public relations, and marketing policies), and still others cover the safety and health of the employees. By issuing these policies, top-level administration sanctions or supports in advance the decisions made by subordinate managers, as long as they stay within the broad policy guidelines. Because of this expected outcome, these policies are classified as **empowerment policies**. After having set policies, a higher-level manager should feel reasonably confident that whatever decisions subordinates make fall within policy limits. In fact, subordinates probably come up with decisions comparable to those the manager would have made. Thus, policies make it easier for the higher-level manager to delegate authority to subordinates.

empowerment policy
A policy that sanctions in advance decisions made by subordinates, as long as they stay within the policy guidelines.

Policies are a great help to subordinate managers as well. They provide guidelines that help subordinates make decisions and at the same time ensure uniformity of decisions throughout the enterprise. Therefore, the clearer and more comprehensive the policy guidelines are, the easier it is for the higher-level managers to delegate authority and for the subordinate managers to exercise authority.

The Origin of Policies

Policies are determined by management, particularly by the higher administrative levels. Formulating policies is one of the most important functions of

HOSPITAL LAND

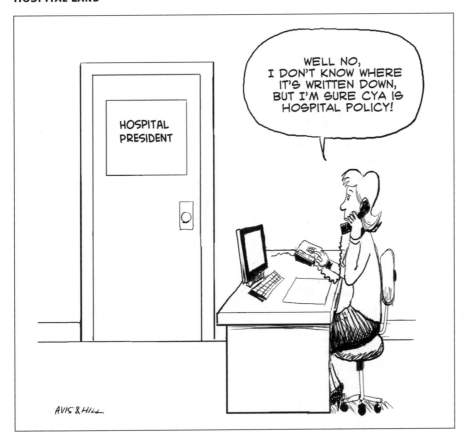

top-level management. These managers are in the best position to establish the various types of policies that help achieve the enterprise's objectives. Once the corporate policies have been set by the top-level administrator, they in turn become the guidelines for various policies covering divisions and departments, such as patient care policies. Such divisional and departmental policies are created or developed by the various managers lower in the managerial hierarchy. This type of policy formulation, originated at the top administrative level and pursued by the lower managerial levels, is the most important source of policies.

Occasionally, however, a supervisor may have a problem situation not covered by an existing policy. In such cases the supervisor should confer with the boss or human resources to (1) determine if any existing policies may be applicable or (2) jointly agree on the appropriate action until a policy is issued to cover such situations if it is likely that the current problem will recur.

For instance, suppose an employee asks for a leave of absence to care for a neighbor. To make the appropriate decision, the supervisor would prefer to be guided by policy so that the decision is in accordance with all other decisions regarding leaves of absence. The supervisor may find, however, that the administrative and FMLA (Family Medical Leave Act) policies do not apply to this situation and therefore he is in a quandary. Instead of making an ad hoc decision (a decision that pertains to this case only), he asks his department's human resources liaison to issue a policy, to which he can refer whenever leaves of absence for similar reasons are requested in the future. The supervisor probably will not have to make such a request very often because a good human resources director in collaboration with the administrative team usually foresees most of the areas in which policies are needed.

On occasion, however, the supervisor may have to appeal to his boss, stimulating the formulation of what is known as an **appealed policy**. Imagine you are a supervisor and one of your employees has been tardy three times in the same pay period. According to the human resources policy, any employee with three tardies in the same pay period will be suspended for one day. However, this employee shares with you that she is a single parent and her babysitter has car problems this week. Additionally, this employee is the only employee who works on third shift. So you appeal to your boss for an exception to the policy. According to Marriner-Tomey (2004, 220), as appeals are taken up the hierarchy and decisions are made, appealed policies are created and guide future decisions. Policies developed in this manner can be uncoordinated and inconsistent. When a number of policies are being appealed, it may be time to assess current policies for gaps or updating.

In addition to empowerment and appealed policies, some policies are externally imposed on an organization by outside factors such as the government, accrediting agencies, trade unions, and trade associations. For instance, to be accredited, hospitals and other healthcare facilities must comply with certain regulations issued by an accrediting agency. These regulations must be translated into institutional policy, and all employees must abide by them. These are called **imposed policies**.

Accrediting agencies often require hospitals to have formal written policies on patient care matters. Another body that imposes policies externally is the Equal Employment Opportunity Commission (EEOC). Unless the healthcare center was an equal opportunity employer before federal and state fair employment codes were legislated, such a policy statement can be regarded as one that was externally imposed on the institution.

appealed policy
A policy established as an exception to an existing policy. This appealed policy may be for a single instance or special circumstance or may apply to a subset of the organization.

imposed policy
A policy created to comply with outside factors, such as accrediting requirements.

Clarity of Policies

Because policies are such a vital guide for thinking and thus for decision making, it is essential that they be stated simply and clearly. (See Exhibit 9.1 for an example of a code order policy, which is common in many healthcare organizations.) An effective policy should require a manager's judgment but not complex interpretation (Finnegan and Amatayakul 1990). Policies must be communicated so that those in the organization who are to apply them understand their meaning.

EXHIBIT 9.1

Code Order
Policy
Statement

BARNES-JEWISH HOSPITAL
Nursing Policy and Procedure

Document: __C15__
Reviewed: __7/99__
Revised: __2/00__

CODE 7

I.   POLICY

A.   Upon recognition of an unconscious patient, visitor or staff member, the first responder must call for help to ensure immediate overhead code is called and delivery of the nearest defibrillator and crash cart.

B.   Any BLS (Basic Life Support) trained employee can initiate CPR. It is of utmost importance that the first BLS responder begin CPR immediately and that delays in CPR till code team arrive are unacceptable. RN's, LPN's, PCT's are to be BLS certified every two years utilizing the American Heart Association/Red Cross course.

C.   Cardiopulmonary resuscitation must be initiated on all patients unless there is a written order not to resuscitate.

D.   Designated BLS instructors for each area are responsible for providing BLS classes each year for ongoing staff certification.

E.   Each RN, LPN and PCT is responsible for maintaining a current BLS certification.

F.   Nurse managers or their designees are responsible for maintaining records of the employees' BLS certification and to provide a method to keep staff familiar with the crash cart contents.

G.   For patient safety, transport of the post-arrest patient from north to south campus of BJH must be minimized. Communications between the nursing supervisor or code team member and the ICU attending MD or charge nurse must first be made to acquire an ICU bed on the north campus for that patient (i.e., lowest acuity patient moved out to allow for post-arrest patient's ICU admission). In the event that all north campus ICU beds are completely filled with high acuity patients, transport via the link to the south campus must be arranged via the nursing supervisor. The transport of any post-arrest patient to an ICU, either between campuses or intra-hospital, must include the following: A physician and nurse familiar with the patient must physically stay with that patient until the patient is transported to an ICU and report of events is given to the accepting physician and nurse. Other personnel needed for transport may include dispatch (2–3), RT's, other RN's or physicians.

SOURCE: Courtesy of Barnes-Jewish Hospital, St. Louis, MO.

Most policies are written, which helps understanding. Other benefits of written policies include:

1. The process of writing policies requires the top-level administrator to think them out clearly and consistently.

2. Written policies are easily accessible; the subordinate managers can read them as often as they wish.
3. The wording of a written policy cannot be changed by word of mouth and therefore it can always be consulted.
4. Written policies are especially helpful for new managers who need immediate help in solving a problem.
5. Written policies can be made available electronically on the organization's intranet to enhance access for all staff.

Although these advantages are significant, one disadvantage of written policies is that once policies are in writing, management may be reluctant to change them. Thus, some enterprises prefer to have their policies communicated by word of mouth because they believe that this is more flexible, allowing the verbal policies to be adjusted to different circumstances with greater ease than is possible with written policies. The exact meaning of a verbal policy may become scrambled, however, making it difficult to apply the policy properly. For this reason, written policy statements are generally considered more desirable.

The Flexibility of Policies

Although policies must be consistent to successfully coordinate the activities of each day, they must also be flexible. Some policies even explicitly state this flexibility using such words as "whenever possible," "whenever feasible," or "under usual circumstances." For instance, one of the most widely practiced policies today is, "Our enterprise believes in and practices promotion from within whenever possible." If these qualifying clauses are built in, the manner in which the supervisor applies the policy determines its degree of flexibility. The supervisor must intelligently adapt the policy to the existing set of circumstances. Such flexibility, however, must not lead to inconsistency; policies must be administered by supervisors with regularity and continuity.

The Supervisor and Policies

Although supervisors seldom have to issue policies, they must frequently use them. Supervisors primarily apply existing policies in making their daily decisions, but they must also explain the meaning of policies to employees of their departments. Therefore, it is essential that they clearly understand the policies and learn how to apply them appropriately.

A manager who heads a major department, such as the director of patient care services, may find it necessary to write and issue policies for the department. In fact, external accrediting and licensing agencies examine such patient care policies for compliance with their regulations. All of them must reinforce and be in accordance with the overall policies of the healthcare organization. Included among these policies probably is a patient care policy stating that the welfare of the patient is the foremost concern of the patient care service and that it takes precedence over all other considerations. In all likelihood, the institution's overall policy of fairness and nondiscrimination also shows up in a patient care policy. The policy may state that patients shall be accorded impartial access to treatments or accommodations to the extent that these are available and medically indicated, regardless of the patient's race, color, creed, or national origin. The policy also may state that the patient's right to privacy shall be respected, consistent with medical needs, and so forth.

Periodic Review of Policies

Changes in the healthcare environment, accompanied by changes in an institution's own goals, require older policies to be periodically reviewed, revised, or removed, regardless of how well-thought-out the policies were when originated. Such a review may uncover policies that contradict other policies or policies that have become so outdated that no one follows them. In such cases, top-level administration must either rewrite or abandon the questionable policies because an institution cannot afford to let its various subordinate managers decide which policies are still current or whether they should still be observed.

Procedures

Procedures are repeat-use plans for achieving the institution's objectives. They are derived from policies, but are more specific. It is not uncommon for the policy statement and the procedure to be combined in the same document. Procedures are guides to *action*, not guides to thinking. Procedures specify a set of actions to be followed step by step. They outline a chronological order for the acts that are to be performed. In brief, procedures prescribe a path toward the objectives; they describe in detail how a recurring activity is to be performed and are commonly used in the daily operations. For example, recall the policy that stated, "Our institution promotes from within whenever possible." The purpose and objectives of this policy are clear. The procedure defines the steps to be taken in a chronological sequence to fulfill the meaning of the policy. These steps might be stated as follows:

procedure
A repeat-use plan that leads toward achievement of an organization's goals. Procedures explain the actions required to comply with policies.

1. Every opening in the institution must be posted on the employees' bulletin board in the employees' cafeteria for two weeks.
2. Any internal potential candidate should obtain a job description from the human resources department.
3. Potential candidates must inform their present boss before arranging for an interview.
4. An interview between the applicant and the manager in the department with the opening will be arranged by the human resources department.

There are literally hundreds, if not thousands, of procedures in a healthcare center. Just think of the number in nursing services alone, such as the procedures for administering medications, examining critically ill patients, initiating protocols without a physician order, and discharging patients. Often organizations establish a standard template for policies and procedures. If these documents are placed on the organization's intranet, the common format allows for easier searching of a given topic. See Appendix 9.1 for an example of a policy and procedure template.

Although supervisors do not have much opportunity to issue policies, they have many opportunities for devising and issuing procedures. Because supervisors are the managers of the department, they determine how the work is to be done. The difficulty is that many supervisors work under considerable pressure and find little time for this type of planning. Moreover, the supervisor is often so close to the jobs performed in the department that she believes the prevailing work methods are satisfactory and that not much can be done about them. The level of detail in written procedures may differ, depending on the skill and educational level of the staff. As educational levels increase, more freedom to act based on tested and demonstrated experience is permitted.

Some employees already have been thoroughly trained in standard practices and procedures before being hired. For example, nurses, therapists, physician practice managers, and clinical dietitians receive many years of schooling and training, during which great emphasis is placed on the proper procedures and methods for performing certain tasks. In managing a department in which such highly skilled employees are at work, the supervisor's job is simplified. One of the main concerns is to ensure that good, generally approved procedures and methods are performed in a professionally accepted way.

However, even with that training, no two healthcare institutions are likely to have identical procedures. Even after many years of good schooling and experience in other healthcare settings, new employees have to become familiar with the procedures, methods, and idiosyncrasies of the new facilities. This is the reason each healthcare organization requires employees to participate in new employee orientation. In addition to a facilitywide organization, often the department that the employee is joining provides an orientation to the department-specific policies, procedures, schedules, and job-related activities. This is often done by matching the new employee with a coworker who can serve as a mentor and resource in the early weeks and months.

Effective work procedures designed by the supervisors for the institution result in definite advantages. One of these is that the process of preparing a procedure requires analyzing the work to be done. To maintain a high level of efficiency and the best possible patient care, occasionally the supervisor must study the operations performed to be able to plan improvements. If the department begins doing something new, the supervisor has to write a complete set of new procedures and methods for this new activity. For example, if the staff begins using new laser techniques, the manager of that unit has to develop new procedures for this operation. The manager does so with the help, information, and support of medical specialists, technologists, and possibly the manufacturer of the equipment.

Moreover, once a supervisor establishes a procedure, its existence helps ensure consistent and uniform action and a predictable outcome. In addition to these benefits, procedures provide the supervisor with a standard for appraising the work of the employees. Because a procedure specifies the sequence of actions, it also decreases the need for further decision making. This makes the supervisor's job, as well as that of the employees, easier. The supervisor is also more likely to assign work fairly and to distribute it evenly among the employees.

A good supervisor spends considerable time and effort devising efficient procedures for the department. From time to time, of course, the supervisor needs to review and revise departmental procedures because some are likely to become outdated. This review can be done in collaboration with the staff members who are performing the job. Changes to the process may have occurred that were not captured in the procedure. The staff member performing the function is in the best position to identify where the procedure requires updating. The supervisor also should try to look at all of the department's operations from the point of view of a newcomer. In other words, he should look at the current operations objectively. The supervisor should ask the following questions: Is each operation really necessary? What is the reason for it? Could the procedure be combined with another operation? Are the various steps necessary? Are they performed in the best possible sequence? Are there any avoidable delays? The supervisor should also seek ideas from employees who are doing the job because they often can make valuable suggestions for improved methods and procedures. Employee teams can also be useful in developing new procedures and identifying external barriers to performing their jobs effectively. These barriers may require the supervisor to work with peer supervisors outside of his department to improve the flow of work inside.

Methods

A **method** also is a standing plan for action, but it is even more detailed than a procedure. A method may also be called a practice. Whereas a procedure shows a series of steps to be taken, a method is concerned only with a single operation, or with one particular step. The method tells exactly how this particular step is to be performed. For instance, one typical patient care procedure guides nurses step by step in how to account for controlled substances at the beginning of each shift by both the nurse going on duty and the nurse going off duty. For each step in this procedure, there exists a method. For

method
A standing plan that details one single part of a procedure.

example, one method explains exactly what is to be done in case of unavoidable spilling or accidental destruction of narcotics: the nurse involved must record what happened; the remnants must be returned to the pharmacy, if possible, or discarded altogether; and another professional nurse must verify the spill and witness the report form.

For most of the work done by the employees of a department, there exists a "best method"—that is, a best way for doing the job—and it is the supervisor's responsibility to specify to employees what that is. Indeed, a large amount of the supervisor's time is spent devising methods. However, one should not devise methods in a vacuum. The supervisor should solicit input from the staff and assess any regulatory requirements when defining methods. Once a method has been devised, it carries with it all the advantages of a procedure, such as uniformity of action, predictability of outcome, and standard for appraisal.

productivity standards
Reasonably achievable quantitative and qualitative expectations based on relevant data, benchmarks, or industry metrics.

Using established methods, supervisors also may be asked to establish **productivity standards** for their staff. Productivity standards are reasonably achievable quantitative and qualitative expectations based on relevant data, benchmarks, industry metrics, or a combination of these indicators. Creating productivity expectations takes time, because production history, methods of improving production, equipment used, and industry norms must be assessed. Supervisors must be able to define not only the quantity expected but also the quality of the activities expected. The definitions form the framework within which management establishes the standards of performance. Once the standards are established, a simple and timely reporting mechanism must be developed as a control system. (Control is discussed in chapters 27 through 29.) It is outside the realm of this book to discuss in depth the various techniques to gauge production and establish productivity standards. Supervisors are encouraged to obtain more information on these techniques before embarking on a program of establishing standards.

In determining the best method as well as establishing standards, a supervisor may occasionally need to enlist the help of another professional, such as another clinician, a human resources specialist, or a management engineer (a specialist in motion and time study), if such a person is available in the organization. Most often, however, the supervisor's own experience and the input of her team members are probably broad enough to allow her to design the best work methods.

Rules

rule
A statement that forbids or requires a certain action or inaction.

A **rule**, probably the most explicit kind of a standing plan, is a statement that either forbids or requires a certain action or inaction without variation. A rule does not provide a guide to thinking; it does not leave any discretion to the party involved. A rule is related to a procedure insofar as it is a guide to action and states what must or must not be done. A rule, however, is not the same as a procedure because it does not specify a time sequence for the particular action. Rules pertain whenever and wherever they are in effect. A no-smoking rule, for instance, is one issued by management and is probably just one of a long list of safety rules. This rule is a guide to action, or more precisely a guide to inaction. No order of steps is involved, however; it simply requires "no smoking" wherever and whenever it is in effect.

Rules develop from policy; they are not part of it. For example, the institution's safety policy is to make the facility a safe and healthy place for the patients, employees, and visitors. Safety considerations play an important role in all procedures and methods, and the no-smoking rule is just an outgrowth of the original safety policy. The same applies to the rule issued by the supervisor of the clinical laboratories that all employees are to wear gloves and impervious gowns at all times or by the chief engineer that requires his tradesmen to wear goggles when using the electric drill or grinder in the shop.

It is the supervisor's duty to apply and enforce the rules and regulations of the healthcare institution uniformly, whether they are defined by higher management or set by the supervisor. There are many occasions when supervisors have to set their own departmental rules. For example, the dress code may state that employees must come to work "appropriately attired" for their job. This general rule gives each director the right to devise a more detailed dress code to meet the needs of the department, including requiring uniforms for the food service and security staffs. The pediatric patient care manager may have a more lax dress code to allow staff to wear costumes and other paraphernalia to raise the spirits of their young patients. Because supervisors have the obligation to see that rules are observed, they should be involved in the formation of these rules. Again, these rules are developed from overall organizational policies and must reinforce and support them.

Work Simplification

This chapter points out that the supervisor is deeply involved in designing, developing, and writing procedures and methods. As noted earlier, the supervisor should continually review and, if necessary, revise procedures and make plans concerning improved work methods and processes in the department.

Much has been written on *work simplification* or methods improvement, which is "an organized approach to determine how to accomplish a task with less effort in less time or at a lower cost while maintaining or improving the quality of the outcome" (Abdelhak et al. 1996). The efforts of the Gilbreths, discussed in Chapter 2, focused on methods improvement. Ben B. Graham (2001) offers a summary of work simplification in Appendix 9.2.

According to Abdelhak and colleagues (1996), "The fundamental objectives of work simplification are (1) simplify, (2) eliminate, (3) combine, and (4) improve." For more information on work simplification process charts, review the recommended readings noted in Ben Graham's article (see reference list at the end of this chapter). Additionally, we explore this process and other approaches that focus on process improvement in Part VII.

Organizational Manuals

The *organizational manual* (also known as the administrative manual) is a helpful tool for communicating the organization's practices effectively. It provides, in comprehensive written form, the decisions that have been made with regard to the institution's structure. It defines the institution's major policies and objectives, contains organizational charts of the institution and of specific departments (see Chapter 12), and provides job descriptions. Moreover, the organizational manual is a readily available reference defining the scopes of authority, responsibilities of managerial positions, and channels to be used in obtaining decisions or approval of proposals.

One of the chief advantages of a manual is the analysis and thinking necessary before it can be written. Another advantage is that the manual is of great assistance in the indoctrination and development of managerial personnel. The manual should clearly specify for each manager what the responsibilities of the job are and how they relate to other positions within the organization. In addition, it reiterates for the individual manager the objectives of the enterprise and of the department, and it provides a means of explaining the complex relationships within the organization. Supervisors should familiarize themselves with the contents of the institution's manual, especially those parts affecting their own department. Often managers create department manuals to serve as communication tools for their staff.

Organizational manuals are valuable tools only if they are up to date. Because the manual is in written form, it is more difficult to change. Unless manuals are kept current and incorporate changes, they are more of a hindrance than a valuable aid. As stated before, another difficulty with a manual is the initial effort it takes to compile one.

Content

In the organizational manual, top-level management states the major objectives and goals of the institution. Although the content of both the organizational and departmental manuals varies from one healthcare institution to another, almost all include statements of goals, objectives, and overall policies. The manual often mentions, for example, the organizational objectives concerning the education of medical and other professionals, investigative studies, and care of the indigent. It may state an objective, "to be alert and responsive to the changing needs of the community and the environment." The administrative manual should be comprehensive enough to guide departmental managers on overall organizational issues and is often supplemented with a departmental manual that includes some items that appear in the administrative manual and department-specific detailed policies and procedures. See Exhibit 9.2 for a listing of common contents.

Contents	Organization	Department
Goals and objectives	X	X
Mission, vision, and values statements	X	X
Code of conduct and compliance policies	X	X
Policies	X	X
Scope of services	X	X
Listing of departments and description of functions	X	
Maps of the organization	X	
Listing of functions within the department		X
Contact list of directors, administrators	X	X
Descriptions of organizational executives' roles	X	X
Contact list of staff members/call tree		X
Phone and fax directory	X	X
Organization chart of the organization	X	X
Organization chart of the department		X
Position descriptions		X
Department procedures		X
Department schedule/work schedule of staff		X

Exhibit 9.2
Contents of Organizational Manuals

Programs and Projects

program
A single-use plan with a complex set of activities to reach a specific major objective.

project
A single-use plan that is smaller in scope than a program, and may be undertaken within an overall program.

A **program** is a single-use plan with a complex set of activities to reach a specific major objective. The program may have its own guidelines, such as policies, procedures, and budgets, and may extend over several years. For instance, building a new assisted living and extended care facility within a healthcare system is a major one-time undertaking. Such a program involves many derivative plans, each of which can be considered a **project**. Such plans would include selecting the architects and contractors for the new construction, arranging public information for the local community, providing information for the local medical society, and recruiting the needed personnel. Arranging the financing itself is a project. At the department level the program may be designing the new laundry department for the facility. One project for the laundry department would include evaluating and selecting new laundry equipment. The laundry manager is also expected to develop a staffing plan and budget for the new department.

A project, therefore, is similar to a program but is smaller in scope. It is an undertaking that can be planned and executed as a distinct entity within the overall program; all projects must be coordinated and synchronized so that the major program can become a reality. Programs and projects are single-use plans; once they are achieved, they are filed away. Planning a program is usually a concern for top-level administration, whereas department heads and supervisors are often involved in one of its many projects. It is also possible for a project to be initiated without a connection to a major program.

For instance, assume the new assisted living and extended care facility is located in a rather affluent community, the economy is such that unemployment in the area is extremely low, and there is limited public transportation available. As such, it may be difficult to recruit laundry workers. Therefore, the manager may need to work with the human resources department to develop both a transportation plan and compensation structure that attract individuals to commute to this community to do the job. In this situation it is not the program—the assisted living and extended care facility—that caused the shortage of staff, but rather the combination of the location of the facility and the economy.

Some projects may be quite complex. To manage these endeavors, the project manager may use Gantt or PERT charts.

Gantt chart
A bar chart that shows planned and actual activities of a project in a fashion that allows managers to see when activities are falling behind.

The **Gantt chart** was introduced by Henry Gantt (see Chapter 2). The project is displayed as a bar chart that shows the planned and actual activities. Once the manager decides which activities need to happen and the amount of time that is allotted to each of them, the manager plots them on the chart. The chart becomes a control device that allows managers to see when activities are falling behind and/or taking more time than anticipated to accomplish. This type of planning tool is useful when there are a few activities to manage and when they are independent of each other. Exhibit 9.3 provides an example of a Gantt chart.

Project Evaluation and Review Technique (PERT) is a planning tool developed by the U.S. Department of Defense, originally used to ensure that complex military projects remained on schedule. In its sophisticated form, PERT uses probabilities and three time estimates for each task involved in the project. PERT is an effective tool for scheduling complex projects and when activities are dependent on one another. The visual display allows the manager to compare what effect alternative actions have on the completion of the project or subset of activities. The steps involved in PERT planning are (1) identify each task involved in the project; (2) estimate the time required to complete each task; (3) determine the relationships among tasks—which must occur first, second, etc.; which is dependent on another; and which tasks may occur simultaneously with or independently from others; and (4) determine when the project must be completed. Once these factors are known, a graphical representation or chart is drawn, depicting one or more paths for the various tasks and linking those tasks dependent on one another's completion before the next task can occur. The time estimates are entered along the linking lines between tasks. The cumulative times for a given path represent the total time required to complete that path. If the cumulative time exceeds the "due date" for the project's completion, the project will be delayed. PERT helps managers to identify when resources have to be shifted to keep on schedule.

In the PERT diagram (Exhibit 9.4), Task C is dependent on Task A. Task D is dependent on Task C and Task E. Task E is dependent on Task B. Therefore, before Task D can begin, 16 days will elapse (Task B + Task E). Tasks A and C will have been completed before Task B is completed. Because Task D requires 11 days, the project should be completed within the 30-day timetable required.

project evaluation and review technique (PERT)
A planning tool that ensures complex projects are completed on time.

EXHIBIT 9.3
Gantt Chart Example

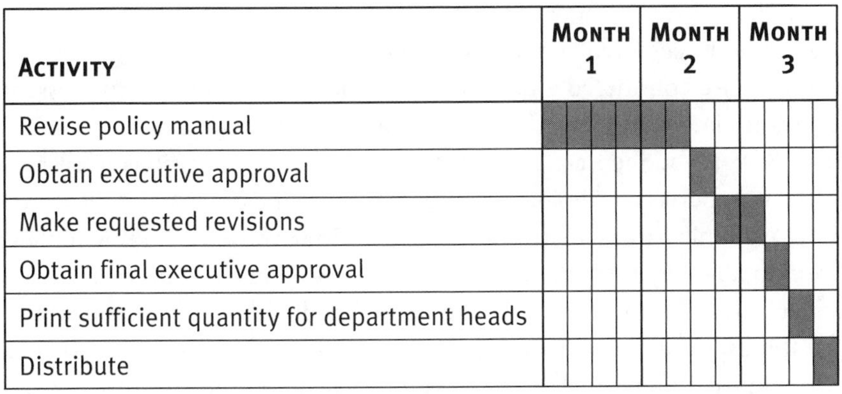

ACTIVITY	MONTH 1	MONTH 2	MONTH 3
Revise policy manual	▨▨▨		
Obtain executive approval		▨	
Make requested revisions			▨
Obtain final executive approval			▨
Print sufficient quantity for department heads			▨
Distribute			▨

EXHIBIT 9.4
PERT Chart
Example

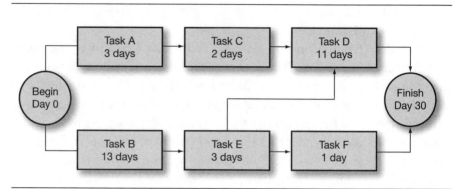

Budgets

Budgets are usually thought of only in connection with the controlling function, but this is too narrow a view. Budgets also are plans that express the anticipated activities and results in numerical terms. Such terms may be dollars and cents. However, most items start out in other measurable terms such as nursing hours, hours per patient day, or kilowatt hours; tests to be run; output; materials; computer time; inventory levels; or any other unit used to perform work or to measure specific results. Because the overall budgets for the entire institution are ultimately expressed in the one common denominator of dollars and cents, and because most values are convertible to monetary terms, all budgets are eventually translated and expressed in monetary terms. Although budgets are an important tool for controlling, developing a budget is also part of the planning function. As we know, planning is the duty of every manager. Using the budget and working within it is part of the manager's controlling function, which is in Chapter 25.

Because a budget is a plan expressed in numerical units, it has the distinct advantage of being stated in exact and specific terms instead of in generalities. The figures in a budget represent actual plans that are seen as goals and standards to be achieved. These plans are not mere projections or general forecasts; they are considered a basis for daily operations, cost effectiveness, and the bottom line. They are guidelines about the institution's expectations.

Because budgets are so important for the daily operations of every department, supervisors who have to use them should participate in their preparation. It is only natural that people resent arbitrary orders, and this applies to having to abide by budgets they see as arbitrary. Thus, it is necessary that all budget objectives and allowances be determined with the full input of those who are responsible for executing them. All supervisors should actively participate in the budget-making process for their units, and this should not be mere "pseudo participation." They should participate in what is commonly known as "grassroots budgeting," and supervisors also should be allowed to submit their own budgets.

Each supervisor has to substantiate the budget proposals in a discussion with the boss and possibly with top-level administration, where the budgets are finalized. This is what is meant by active participation in budget making, and it ensures the effectiveness of the process. Such participation, however, should not be construed to mean that the suggestion of the supervisor will prevail. The supervisor's budget should not be accepted if the higher-level manager believes it is based on plans that are inadequate, overstated, or incorrect.

Differences among budget estimates should be carefully discussed by the supervisor and higher-level manager, but the final decision rests with higher management. Nevertheless, if a budget is arrived at with the participation of the supervisors, the likelihood that the supervisors will live up to it is higher than if the budget had been simply handed down to the supervisors by their boss.

In conclusion, it is important to remember that the budget is a single-use plan. When the period is over, the budget is no longer valid. A new budget will have to be drawn up, and a new planning period will have to be established.

Summary

To reach all of an organization's objectives, different types of plans must be devised. The broad range of plans can be grouped into repeat-use and single-use plans. The first group is designed for a course of action that is likely to be repeated several times, whereas the second group is designed for a course of action that is not likely to be repeated in the future.

Policies, the major type of repeat-use plans, are guides to thinking, and most originate with the chief administrator. In most cases, the supervisor's concern with policies is primarily in interpreting them, applying them, and staying within them whenever decisions are made for the department. Although supervisors do not usually originate policies, they are often called on to design procedures, methods, and rules, which are other repeat-use plans. These plans are guides for action, not guides for thinking. Supervisors also participate in the establishment of budgets, which are single-use plans expressed in numerical terms. Occasionally supervisors are involved with programs and projects, which are two more examples of single-use plans.

It is a supervisor's duty to simplify work processes. Continual, periodic assessment of job descriptions, procedures, and methods is key to ensuring departmental efficiency.

Policy and Procedure Template

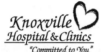

Knoxville
Hospital & Clinics
"Committed to You"

Template Title:	**Policy / Procedure Template**
Process Category:	**Organizational Management System**
Date of Revision:	2/3/09
Revision Number:	3

Instructions:

Before using this template, delete this first section. These pages record the approvals and revision history for the **template design**.

This template should be used to document all Policies and Procedures. Reference the Organizational Management System for additional instructions.

The template itself may be modified or not as directed by this table.

Section	Permissible Modifications	
Title		
Process Category		
Date of Revision	Do not modify the left field	
Revision Number	The right field is fully modifiable – an entry per field is required	
Purpose		
Overview / Description	Fully modifiable. Delete if there is no appropriate entry	
Policy Statement		
Scope		
Procedure	If there is no Procedure for this document, delete all sections pertaining to Procedures.	
Equipment / Supplies	For Equipment / Supplies - This heading is not always applicable. It is used most often in nursing, clinical or Patient areas where specific equipment and supplies are needed to accomplish a certain task. Delete if there is no entry.	
Records to be Maintained		
References	Add references. If a Policy_Procedure was created to meet a specific requirement of some licensing, accreditation or regulatory agency, that document should be referenced (e.g. State, PHICO, CLIA, OSHA, or EMTALA). OMS documents are referenced without version number if the document is required for the process addressed.	
Attachments	Fully modifiable – if there are no attachments then delete.	
Process Owner & other Department Heads Approval	• Do not modify, add to or delete from the columns of these tables • Do not delete previously approved revision entries/rows • Do delete unused rows	Use one row for department approval even if several department heads must approve
Physician or Medical Director Approval (if applicable)		Use one row for physician approval
Revision History		Use one row for the revision history

Page 1 of 5

Continued

Continued

Process Owner & Other Department Head Approval

Version	Name	Title	Signature	Date
1	Ann H	Organizational Excellence Director		
2	Ann H	Organizational Excellence Director		
3	Ann H	Organizational Excellence Director		

Physician or Medical Director Approval (if applicable)

Version	Name	Title	Signature	Date
N/A				

Revision History

Version	Date	Author(s)	Revision Description
1	8/21/2008	Ken S	To originate
2	10/7/2008	Lisa E	Changed "N/A" entries to delete the section. Deleted "Roles" section. Deleted "Example 2" of Responsibility Matrix. Changed order of items in Procedure section and clarified directions. Added a note under "Records to be Maintained".
3	2/3/09	Lisa E	Deleted Responsibility Matrix. Deleted the reference to Control of Clinical, Regulatory, and Non-Clinical Records Policy and Procedure under the Records to be Maintained section.

Review Only History with No Changes or Insignificant Wording Updates & No Content Changes – No Training Required – No Revision Change

Date	Reviewer(s)	Review / Update Description
11/12/08	Lisa E	The Review Team recommended "Exit Criteria" be changed to "End Result" for clarity. Additional documents were added to the References section instructions.

Continued

Policy / Procedure Title: (Type Policy_Procedure Title Here)

Process Category: (Type Process Title Here)
Date of Revision: (Type Date of Revision Here)
Revision Number: (Type Revision Number Here)

Purpose:

To describe the inputs, outputs, process, procedure, roles and responsibilities to execute [type process name here].

Overview / Description:

(Narrative overview and / or description of key features of the processes that is a maximum of 1 page)

Policy Statement:

(Narrative description of the Policy associated with the processes described in this document)

Scope:

(Define where and when this procedure is applicable)

Page 3 of 5

Continued

Continued

Procedure:
(Narrative description of Key features of the detailed procedure is optional. This section can be used if you have information you need to cover that has not been captured in the process overview.)

- o Inputs
  - ▪ (Type input here)

- o Outputs
  - ▪ (Type output here)

- o End Result (links back to Purpose)
  - ▪ (Type end result here)

(If process flow is being used, copy here. Otherwise delete these words and use table below. If a process flow is used, delete the table below.)

Task Description	Role	Recommended Work Products Templates and Techniques

To add more rows, place cursor in last row of Date column, press [Tab]

Equipment / Supplies:

Records to be Maintained:

Record	Responsibility	Location	Retention Period	Disposal Time
Specify in detail records to be maintained for all processes described in this policy / procedure – one line per record type	Specify who by title is responsible to maintain the records	Specify where the records are to be maintained	Specify how long the records are to be kept	Specify time allowed after the retention period to properly dispose of the records

Page 4 of 5

Continued

References:
Enter any reference documents including regulatory, governmental, accreditation, equipment manuals, internal documents such as checklists, etc.

Attachments:
Enter any attachment names or enter N/A (normal entry)

N/A

Process Owner & Other Department Head Approval				
Version	Name	Title	Signature	Date

To add more rows, place cursor in last row of Date column, press [Tab]

Physician or Medical Director Approval (if applicable)				
Version	Name	Title	Signature	Date

To add more rows, place cursor in last row of Date column, press [Tab]

Revision History			
Version	Date	Author(s)	Revision Description

To add more rows, place cursor in last row of Revision Description column, press [Tab]

Review Only History with No Changes or Insignificant Wording Updates & No Content Changes – No Training Required – No Revision Change		
Date	Reviewer(s)	Review / Update Description

SOURCE: Reprinted with permission from Knoxville Hospital & Clinics, Knoxville, IA.

APPENDIX 9.2

Work Simplification

Work simplification has generated billions of dollars through effectiveness and efficiency for organizations that focused on their people and gave them tools for continuous improvement. Since the 1960s, the glamour of electronics has seduced many organizations into treating their people as expenses rather than resources. For those organizations whose leaders truly believe that their people are their most valuable resource, the tools of work simplification are still available, and better than ever.

In 1946, the American Society of Mechanical Engineers (ASME) did something that was even then a long time in the making. They established a set of symbols as the ASME Standard for Operation and Flow Process Charts. Twenty-five years earlier, in 1921, Frank and Lillian Gilbreth had presented "Process Charts—First Steps in Finding the One Best Way" at the Annual Meeting of ASME. By the time the symbols were standardized, they had evolved into a solid set of five symbols that covered every aspect of work, in any work environment, that can be used with very little confusion. The first process charts appeared as a series of symbols strung down a page in sequential order. This was (and still is) a simple and effective way to track the flow of a person or a piece of material through a work process.

In 1932, Allan Mogensen (1989) founded work simplification, which is defined as the organized application of common sense. Mogensen used the process chart (among other tools) to organize and study work, and he drew on the common sense of the people who did the work for improvement ideas. Mogensen defended participative improvement with these words: "The person doing the job knows far more than anyone else as to the best way of doing that job, and therefore is the one person best fitted to improve it." It is this human element of work simplification that distinguishes it from most other improvement techniques. It is predicated on people who do the work being involved in improving that work. It does not treat people, products, and information as inputs and outputs, using accounting terminology. It regards people as a treasured resource, the safekeepers of the corporate (or organizational) memory, which is the most vital factor in successful continuous improvement! Mogensen described the process chart as follows: "In order to achieve measurement, tools are needed and the most important of these is the process chart. . . . The process chart is the lifeblood of work simplification. It is an irreplaceable tool. It is a guide and stimulant. It takes time to properly utilize but there is absolutely no doubt that it works" (Mogensen 1989, 44–46).

Mogensen began conducting work simplification conferences at Lake Placid in 1937 and continued them for nearly 50 years. (Lillian Gilbreth was part of the original staff, returning each year until the mid-1960s.) Ben S. Graham was a student at Mogensen's 1944 Conference. He was unique in his class in that he did not come from a manufacturing environment. He learned the methods of work simplification and adapted them to the office while directing the paperwork simplification effort at The Standard Register Company. There he developed the horizontal process flow chart to accommodate multiple information flows. He also embraced an employee team approach to process improvement, which is summarized in this statement he made in 1958: "Participation by the worker in developing the method eliminates many causes of resistance and assures enthusiastic acceptance. This is more important than all the techniques put together." Graham subsequently joined Mogensen's staff as the resident expert in paperwork simplification.

A few of the organizations that have embraced work simplification in the past include the following (Mogensen 1989):

- *Texas Instruments.* Its former CEO Pat Haggerty described work simplification as "TI's most effective program for fostering personal involvement at all levels of the organization while yielding tangible benefits to the company."
- *Maytag.* Its former CEO Daniel J. Krumm stated, "Work simplification plays an integral part in Maytag's total cost-reduction efforts and makes a significant contribution year after year."
- *Procter & Gamble.* In 1983, P&G realized nearly $1 billion in first year savings as a result of work simplification.
- *Ford.* Ford-Connersville's annual first-year savings increased from $400,000 to $10 million during 11 years of applying work simplification. Savings in administrative processes grew from $820,000 to $1.5 million in three years.
- *Standard Register.* The company introduced work simplification to the office environment, and it was the first to offer business process improvement to clients to support the sales of new information systems.
- *The U.S. Navy.* Over a period of 14 years, about 250 projects produced a typical annual return for the Navy of more than $150,000 per project.

These days, processes change so fast that many organizations have failed to keep up. Their work is undocumented and as changes are made the complexity mounts. The simple and effective approach of work simplification has more to offer than it ever had. However, its use is not widespread. It appears that many organizations are focusing their attention on purchasing solutions for their business rather than mastering their work themselves. Where the purchased solutions lead to downsizing, the corporate memory is discarded, leaving the organization dependent on those from whom it purchased its processes.

The work simplification approach utilizes the corporate memory rather than discards it. It counters increasing complexity with continuous improvement and enables the workforce to be the masters of their processes. It is on the program at many universities, and it is being applied in increasing numbers of organizations across the United States and Canada and in South America, Europe, and Australia, as these companies seek to regain control of their operations.

New methods for studying work are introduced on a regular basis. Usually they focus effectively on one or another aspect of improvement, but they often fail because they do not deal rigorously with the work itself. This is a good time to look back and discover again a simple tool that visually displays processes in a universal language that can be readily understood by anyone who wants to understand.

Today, if you are pursuing Six Sigma or Lean manufacturing, using kaisan or value stream mapping, managing your supply chain, developing a business-to-business strategy, establishing an electronic commerce presence, managing day-to-day internal operations, or documenting your processes for certification or audit, understanding the fundamental steps in your work processes will help you get those things done. Work simplification helps you get there . . . faster, cheaper, and better!

SOURCE: Adapted from Ben B. Graham, "Rediscover Work Simplification." Ben Graham Corporation website, 2001. http://www.worksimp.com/articles/bricklayer.htm.

TIME MANAGEMENT TECHNIQUES

Chapter Objectives

After you have studied this chapter, you should be able to do the following:

1. Classify how time is spent.
2. Identify tools for managing one's time.
3. Define the benefits of a time-use chart.
4. Distinguish how one may need to manage staff and plan staff's time depending on the management theory followed.

"To waste your time is to waste your life, but to master your time is to master your life" (Lakein 1989). If supervisors want more time, they have to "make" it themselves. The supervisor's own time is one of the resources for which he is responsible. Every supervisor has probably experienced days that were so full of pressures and demands that he began to feel as though all the matters that needed attention could never be resolved. (See Exhibit 10.1.) The only way to keep such days at a minimum is for the supervisor to plan for the most effective use of time. Technologies that had promised huge time savings have actually consumed more of a manager's time. The manager who in the past received 10 to 20 letters or memos a day may now receive dozens of calls or voicemails and over a hundred e-mail messages per day.

Unfortunately, problems at work come up constantly but without any order of importance or priority. Thus, the first thing the supervisor must do is determine which problems must be attended to personally and which can be assigned to someone else. The supervisor cannot delegate some matters, but most can be assigned to staff members. Every time the supervisor assigns one of her duties to an employee, time is gained to take care of matters that represent a more effective use of her time. This delegation of tasks is worthwhile even if some valuable time must be spent training one of the employees in a particular task. When in doubt, the supervisor should delegate. Doing so routinely will build the skills of subordinates, allow the supervisor to complete other tasks, and expand the supervisor's ability to take on additional subordinates or functions—a concept discussed in Chapter 11 known as span of management. Any remaining matters have to be classified according to their urgency.

EXHIBIT 10.1

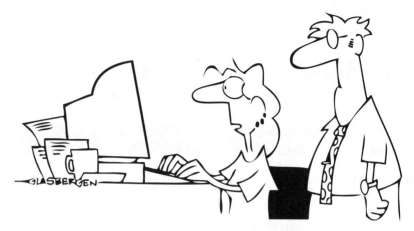

"Is there a file compression program that will help me
squeeze 12 hours of work into an 8 hour schedule?"

SOURCE: Copyright 2004 by Randy Glasbergen. Used with permission.

Use of Time

Stephen R. Covey (1989), in his popular book *The Seven Habits of Highly Effective People*, identifies four ways in which we spend time. If managers follow Covey's advice, they will work to concentrate their time preparing for the future rather than being driven by the future when it arrives as a crisis. In addition, Covey provides guidance in setting priorities. Two terms that define activities are "urgent" and "important." Urgent items require immediate attention because they act on us. For example, a ringing phone is urgent. Important items have to do with results, and those items contribute to the manager's mission, values, or goals (Covey 1989).

Unless supervisors distinguish between those matters that must be done (urgent items) and those that ought to be done (important items), they are inclined to pay equal attention to all matters before them. Consequently, planning and other more important tasks may not receive the attention they truly deserve. By distinguishing between the two, supervisors are giving priority to matters that need immediate attention. A supervisor should therefore plan his time so that the most important things appear at the top of the schedule. The supervisor must make certain, however, that free time is scheduled to enable him to attend to new urgent items. Some emergencies occur that a supervisor must deal with when they arise. Flexibility makes it possible to take care of these situations without disrupting the other activities planned.

Many techniques have been devised to help supervisors control their time schedules. One of the simplest is to use a desk calendar or computer scheduling system to schedule or make a to-do list of appointments, meetings, reports, and discussions. The supervisor should schedule these events far in advance, so they automatically come up for attention when they are due. Electronic calendars and reminder lists on your computer or personal digital assistant (PDA) can help you organize your time as long as you do not become a slave to entering items on the lists rather than completing them.

Another effective way of planning each week's work, as well as knowing what is being accomplished as the week progresses, is to keep a planning sheet. This sheet is prepared at the end of one week for the week to follow. It shows the days of the week divided into morning and afternoon columns and a list of all items to be accomplished. Then a time for accomplishment is assigned to each task by placing the task in the morning or the afternoon blocks of the assigned day. As a task is accomplished, its box is circled. This approach can be accomplished using a PDA or your computer's software in lieu of paper.

Those tasks that have been delayed during the day must be rescheduled for another time by placing them in an appropriate block on a subsequent day. Those tasks that are planned but have not been accomplished during the week (the ones that remain uncircled) must be rescheduled for the following week. Such a record shows how much of the original plan has been carried out at the end of the week and shows how the supervisor's time was spent. Based on this record, the supervisor is then able to plan the next week, and so on. Over time, the supervisor can become better at forecasting the time required to accomplish tasks and at planning his own workload. Furthermore, the accounting of time spent allows assessment of which activities were time wasters and serves as a reminder to eliminate those activities.

Markovitz and Giangrande (2006) suggest several simple time-management tips: (1) filter out low-value information, i.e. eliminate those things that have little value to managing your department, such as unsubscribing from mailing lists and newsletters you do not read; (2) do the worst first—don't put it off only to rush to finish it by the deadline; (3) deal with it now, i.e., when something comes to your e-mail, handle it or delegate it; and (4) batch similar tasks.

Regardless of whether this particular system or another is used, the supervisor must schedule the time each week and must have some method of reporting the tasks that are planned and those that have been accomplished (see Exhibit 10.2). A supervisor should build into his schedule time for unplanned and urgent events; these consume time that he may have set aside to do something else.

Depending on the number of people who report to a supervisor, she might consider setting aside a certain time period each day, say 3:00 to 5:00, when her door will be open to staff to discuss issues. According to Eileen Batchelor (2008), the scheduled time benefits staff, because they know there

Exhibit 10.2
Sample Method
for Recording
Tasks

MONDAY 10/23	TUESDAY 10/24	WEDNESDAY 10/25	THURSDAY 10/26	FRIDAY 10/27
AM	AM Work on job descriptions	AM See personnel director about Helen Talk to maintenance about new elec. outlets.	AM Arrange dates for evaluation interviews.	AM Work on dress code revisions
PM Check leave of absence policy	PM	PM Read minutes last meeting of infection Com.	PM Start work on new budget.	PM Attend management seminar

is time available for them. Of course, if something arises with a patient or physician that needs immediate attention, that will take precedence.

Many short, easy-to-read booklets on time management are available. Reading one or two of these will provide ample ideas for making the most of time.

Time-Use Chart

A manager needs to assess how his time is being used to eliminate time wasters. He can figure out how time is spent by keeping a time-use chart or a time log. Midway through and at the end of the day, or every half-hour if the supervisor chooses, he should list, on a half-hour basis, all of his activities. This log should be kept during a typical work cycle for at least two weeks. At the end of the week, a review of this log will tell the supervisor how much time he spent in counseling and instructing employees, on the phone, answering e-mail, in meetings, on personal chores, socializing, or having lunch. Then the supervisor should create some broad classifications for daily activities such as routine duties, regular supervisory duties, special duties, emergencies, and innovative thinking.

HOSPITAL LAND

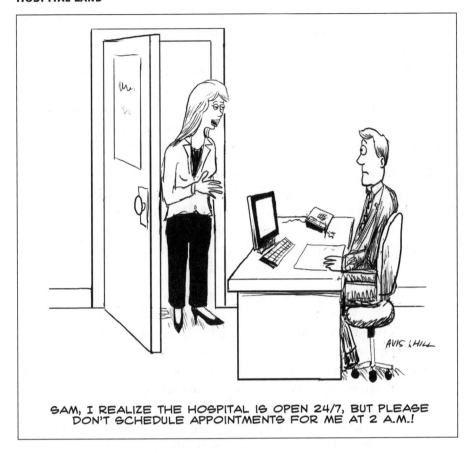

SAM, I REALIZE THE HOSPITAL IS OPEN 24/7, BUT PLEASE DON'T SCHEDULE APPOINTMENTS FOR ME AT 2 A.M.!

The supervisor may find that 20 percent of the time was spent on routine work, which could and should be assigned to some of the subordinates. A large percentage of time was devoted to regular supervisory duties such as checking performance, giving directives and instructions, evaluating and counseling employees, and promoting and maintaining discipline. These are supervisory duties that the manager alone should do. Then the supervisor should find out how much time she spent on special duties such as serving on committees, attending professional meetings, planning next year's budget, changing the dress code, and reviewing procedures. Again, all this time is probably spent wisely.

A certain amount of time also will be spent on emergencies—that is, unpredictable events that demand some of the supervisor's attention. In addition, some time should be open for creative and innovative thinking, which is essential for planning advances or changes for the department and the progress of the institution. The boss evaluates the supervisor on how well the department's job gets done, which includes the implementation of innovative changes and development of suggestions.

Studying the time-use chart illustrates how the time was spent and in which areas a supervisor can make more time. Unless the supervisor has a clear picture of this, routine tasks can creep in and reduce the time available for real supervisory duties.

This raises the question, "Who controls the supervisor's time?" Throughout our discussion, the fact that only the supervisor can control time has been emphasized, and what is done with this time is his responsibility. However, another interesting approach to managing time is suggested by Oncken and Wass (1974). They examine three kinds of managerial time:

boss-imposed time
Time used by an individual to accomplish items required by the boss.

1. **Boss-imposed time** is used by an individual to accomplish those activities that the boss requires and the supervisor cannot disregard.
2. **System-imposed time** is used by an individual to support peers and to cooperate with and coordinate activities of the organization.
3. **Self-imposed time** is used by an individual to accomplish the items the supervisor originates and agrees to do herself.

system-imposed time
Time used by an individual to support peers and cooperate with the organization.

self-imposed time
Time used by an individual to accomplish items she originates herself.

subordinate-imposed time
Time spent dealing with subordinates, such as counseling, evaluating, and providing direction.

The supervisor cannot do much about boss- and system-imposed time. She can, however, make changes in the self-imposed time. Some of the supervisor's self-imposed time is taken up by subordinates; this is called **subordinate-imposed time**. Subordinate-imposed time can be consumed by such things as counseling, idle chitchat, providing direction, evaluating situations or dilemmas posed by subordinates, and settling disputes. The latter has become a significant time consumer according to Accountemps (2008), which estimates 18 percent of a supervisor's time is spent resolving employee personality clashes. Roberts (2006) estimates that personality clashes contribute to at least 50 percent of an organization's resignations. Ramsey (2005) offers the following guidance to help reduce management's time in such conflicts:

- Encourage employees to settle conflicts themselves before bringing them to management.
- Separate the disputing parties if necessary.
- Remind employees to carefully consider both how they say things and what they say.
- Stress teamwork.
- Provide formal conflict-resolution training.
- Use appropriate progressive disciplinary steps.
- As a last resort use termination as a consequence.

The remaining time after boss-, system-, and self-imposed time is called discretionary time. To increase discretionary time, the supervisor must reduce the subordinate-imposed time by counseling employees on their issues but sending the employees back to their offices to resolve the issues rather than doing the problem-solving work for them.

Finally, new supervisors may find it beneficial to track available time by day of the week. While healthcare typically is a $7 \times 24 \times 365$ business, not all functions within a healthcare organization are open 7 days a week. That being said, when you return to work on Monday the supervisor will face messages, mail, and work that has accumulated from Saturday and Sunday. Accountemps's 2008 survey of executives found that 57 percent of the respondents identified Tuesday as their most productive day of the week (Accountemps 2008). When a supervisor identifies a day that has the least boss-imposed and system- imposed demands, that is the day the supervisor needs to block as his self-imposed day to focus on his work. One last suggestion offered by Accountemps: Taking short breaks throughout the day can help a person replenish his energy and fight fatigue.

In summary, effective time management increases the manager's discretionary time for managerial tasks and innovative thinking. Another important benefit of effective time management is the reduction and control of stress.

Managing the Employees' Time

When planning for the effective use of the subordinates' time, much will depend on the supervisor's basic managerial strategy and assumptions about human nature. Douglas McGregor (1985) states that most managers base their thinking on one of two sets of assumptions about human nature, which he calls Theory X and Theory Y. The Theory X manager believes that the average employee dislikes work, avoids work, and tries to get by with doing as little as possible. The employee has little ambition and has to be forced and closely controlled in each and every job. In these cases, the manager may require the use of specialized software, such as project management software. The manager estimates the time required for the project and expects the employee to explain any variances from that time allocation.

The Theory Y manager operates with a drastically different set of assumptions regarding human nature. She believes that most employees consider work natural and that most are eager to do the right thing, seek responsibility under the proper conditions, exercise self-control, and do not need to be constantly reminded to do their work.

If a supervisor is a Theory Y manager, she expects employees to do the right thing and to turn in a fair day's work. Because one cannot expect employees to work indefinitely at top speed, however, the plans for their time are based on a fair output instead of a maximum output. Allowances are made for fatigue, personal needs, unavoidable delays, and a certain amount of unproductive time during the workday.

In planning employees' time, as in other aspects of planning, the supervisor may be able to get assistance from a specialist employed by the facility, preferably a motion and time specialist. However, most supervisors usually can figure out what can be expected of their employees. Managers are generally capable of planning reasonable performance requirements that their employees accept as fair. Such requirements are based on average conditions and not on emergencies. These reasonable estimates of employees' time are necessary because the supervisor must depend on the completion of certain tasks at certain times. The supervisors themselves may have been given deadlines, and to meet them, they must have a reasonable estimate of how fast the job can be done.

In some situations, the subordinate's time is paced and is set by someone or something other than the supervisor because of the nature of the activity performed. For instance, the time an operating room nurse or technician spends on a case is determined by the type of surgery and the speed and skill of the surgeon. In the clinical laboratories and even in the food service dish room, the time required is set by the speed of the equipment used. Unexpected complications may add to the time normally necessary to complete the job. In these cases, average time estimates can still be made, but the time allotted must allow for the various contingencies that arise.

Because employees are a high-cost commodity, supervisors must coordinate the use of this valuable resource. In some healthcare departments, such as information systems and engineering, project management software can be used to help team leaders and team members organize tasks, track costs, and meet deadlines. However, the supervisor may need to write an action plan that captures the important steps of the process and due dates. This type of plan forces the supervisor to consider the issues that affect the process and gives staff expectations in terms of timeliness. Gantt charts may be used to display the impact of various steps in the process. Work simplification efforts help management find wasted time as a result of redundant or outdated efforts.

In addition to planning for the normal employee time, it may be necessary to plan for overtime. Overtime should be considered only as an emergency measure. If the supervisor finds that overtime or working a double shift is regularly required, plans need to be changed by altering work methods, obtaining better or more equipment, or hiring more part-time or full-time employees. The supervisor must also plan for employee absences. One cannot plan for those instances in which employees are absent without notice, but one can plan for holidays, vacations, leaves of absence, or layoffs for overhaul. Plans for these absences should be worked out in advance to ensure smooth functioning of the department.

Summary

Of the many resources a supervisor is responsible for, probably the most valuable one is time, both the supervisor's and his or her employees'. Identifying time wasters and eliminating them, whether through delegation, reassignment, or discontinuance, are necessary to accomplish one's work. The supervisor must set priorities for the unscheduled events of the day and distinguish among those items that must be done.

Several techniques and tools are available to supervisors today, including scheduling software, desk calendars, planning sheets, and time-use charts. Understanding what is consuming one's time is the first step in organizing and prioritizing it to accomplish more tasks more effectively.

Once the supervisor has identified the day(s) of the week that he is likely to have the least interruptions, he should block that time to complete his work.

Additional Readings

McGinn, P. 2004. *Leading Others, Managing Yourself*, ch. 4. Chicago: Health Administration Press.

Rasmussen, P. 2009. "Time Management: The Emergency Room Syndrome in Time Management." [Online article; retrieved 1/26/09.] www.bukisa.com/articles/ 20895_time-management-the-emergency-room-syndrome-in-time-management.

ORGANIZING

FUNDAMENTAL CONCEPTS OF ORGANIZING

Chapter Objectives

After you have studied this chapter, you should be able to do the following:

1. Discuss why organizing is an important managerial function.
2. Discuss three fundamental organizational underpinnings—authority, chain of command, and span of management.
3. Describe the common types of authority.
4. Compare and contrast line and staff departments.
5. Discuss the typical relationships between line and staff.
6. Discuss the major factors that influence the width of the span of management.
7. Review the concepts of microsystems and team management as an approach to expanding the span of management.

Planning defines the mission, goals, and objectives of the organization. An organization provides the framework to bring people and resources together to accomplish the organization's plans. The managerial function of organizing defines and arranges the resources and activities needed to accomplish the objectives and establishes the relationships among various functions within the organization. These activities and functions form subsystems that are synchronized and coordinated into a larger system, called the *formal organization*. Hence, organizing is the process of deciding how best to group and relate organizational activities and resources to achieve the organization's mission. In doing so, one determines the lines of authority and channels of communication, and develops patterns of coordination (Gratto Liebler and McConnell 2004). Fayol stated that the organization takes on form when the number of workers rises to the level requiring a supervisor (Roussell, Swansburg, and Swansburg 2006).

How the formal organization looks and works depends on the organization's overall objectives, size, geographic span, space constraints, technology, culture, and many other factors. Management must have an organizational strategy that can be adapted to a competitive and changing environment. The structure of the organization will follow that strategy and will require restructuring from time to time to accommodate the board's vision; reimbursement and regulatory changes; and demands for new services, technologies, and expertise.

All of the chapters in Part IV of this book are concerned with building an effective organization. We will discuss horizontal organization—how to divide the work into departments—and we will look at dividing the work vertically by delegating authority. As a consequence of growth and specialization, management may consider adding staff to the organization. In doing so, lateral and diagonal relationships will be created by adding line and staff relationships, other essential building blocks of the organization.

Formal Organization Theory

The managerial function of organizing is an impersonal function, because the organization is designed around its activities, not the individual personalities in place to perform them. Of course, the organization's structure must allow people to function and thrive. We discuss all these considerations in the staffing and influencing functions. When the manager designs the structure, however, it is done without thinking of specific persons.

Formal organization theory rests on several major principles:

1. Authority is the lifeblood of the managerial position, and the delegation or distribution of authority makes the organization come alive. Authority may be line or staff in nature.
2. The span of management sets limits on the number of subordinates a manager can effectively supervise.
3. The division of work is essential for efficiency. This may require designing jobs (job or work specialization).
4. The formal structure is the main network for organizing and managing the various activities of the enterprise. Often this is done through departmentalization.
5. Unity of command must prevail; that is, each person should take orders from and report to only one boss.
6. Coordinating activities and resources is a primary responsibility of management and is fulfilled by performing the managerial functions properly.

These major principles of organization are a primary concern of the senior executives of the organization, the CEO and the COO. They must translate these principles into a formal organizational structure so that the institution operates smoothly and accomplishes its objectives.

organizational structure
The formal arrangement of jobs in the organization.

Organizational structure is the formal arrangement of jobs in the organization. The structure is displayed in the organizational chart or table of organization (TOO). An organizational chart typically includes the title of each manager's position and, by means of broken or solid connecting lines, depicts who is accountable to whom, who has authority for each department, and what type of authority is held.

Because the application of these formal organizational principles involves all levels of management, it is also necessary for supervisors to understand them and know how they are used. This knowledge helps them organize their own department and coordinate its activities with those of the rest of the institution. Supervisors are frequently asked to carry out (and may even be asked to help make) decisions involving reorganization, departmentalization or division of work, the span of supervision, and the delegation of authority.

As individuals move up the managerial hierarchy, they are called on to participate in more and more organizational decisions. Some of these deal with organizational design to respond to the changing environment. **Organizational design** is a process involving decisions about such things as work or job specialization, departmentalization, chain of command, span of control, and centralization or decentralization. Thus, although the CEO or COO initially applies the formal principles to establish the overall organizational structure and activities, the department heads, supervisors, and other middle- and lower-level managers must make these principles and the resulting structure work. This is why a discussion here of the organizing process on an overall, or institutional, basis is essential before discussing it on the departmental, or supervisory, level.

The many contingencies facing management are a constant challenge, and the dynamic nature of organizing enables the manager to bring about change and absorb and accommodate change as the need arises. This enables the enterprise to pursue and achieve its objectives continuously.

Authority and Span of Control

Although organizing is a dynamic process, it rests on two fundamental concepts, authority and span of management (also known as span of control). **Authority**, the right to direct others and to give orders, is one of the bases through which the manager gets the job done. It is the underpinning of the organization. When organizing, one assigns responsibility for a piece of the organization to one or more subordinate managers. Those individuals who are given the responsibility for a function and its associated resources must be given enough authority to carry out those responsibilities. This authority–responsibility relationship is known as the **parity principle**. **Span of management** deals with another dimension of organizing: the scope of supervision, or the number of people who report to a particular manager. We will explore both of these fundamentals further in this chapter.

organizational design
A process involving decisions about such things as work or job specialization, departmentalization, chain of command, span of control, and centralization or decentralization.

authority
The right to direct others and to give orders.

parity principle
The concept that individuals who are given responsibility for a function must be given enough authority to carry out that function.

span of management
The scope of supervision, or the number of people who report to a particular manager.

Authority

In chapters 1 and 2, we referred to the importance of authority to the managerial position. That discussion of authority merely stated that it is the lifeblood of the supervisory position and one of the characteristics of a manager. In addition, we mentioned that delegating authority breathes life into an organization; without it, an organization cannot and does not exist. Therefore, we must first examine and understand the concept of authority.

Authority is the key to the managerial job; at the same time, it carries many interpretations. In a general sense, authority refers to the formal or official power of a manager to influence decisions and to obtain the compliance of the subordinate by using directives, communications, policies, and objectives. Such authority is associated with the manager's function in the organization; it is vested in organizational roles or positions, and it is legitimized by the organization. As long as an individual holds the position, she has the privilege of exercising the authority that is inherent in it.

Positions are meaningless unless they are occupied by someone. Therefore, we generally speak of the authority of the manager, the authority that is delegated to the manager, and so forth. Although it would be more precise to speak of the authority of the managerial position itself or the authority delegated to that position rather than to the person who occupies it, the difference is generally regarded as semantic. As long as we understand that authority in this sense resides in the position, we may speak rather loosely of the authority of the manager and recognize that if the manager leaves the position, he forfeits the authority that was granted to it.

Source of Nature of Authority

Max Weber (1974) expressed authority as "legitimate power" to give orders. The subordinates' compliance rests on the belief that it is legitimate for managers to give orders and illegitimate for subordinates not to obey them. This kind of authority is vested in organizational roles and positions, not in the individuals who occupy these positions. As long as an individual holds the position, she has the privilege of exercising the authority that is inherent in it. Once a manager leaves an organizational position, she loses the authority inherent in it, and the authority goes to the successor.

While examining the foundation for this organizational authority, Weber identified three bases of authority: tradition, rules and regulations, and charisma. **Traditional authority** "rests on the belief in the sacredness of the social order" (Weber 1985). For instance, in a patriarchal society, the father receives legitimacy as an authority through custom.

Rules and regulations form a second basis of authority. Subordinates are expected to comply with orders because, in a bureaucratic organization, superior–subordinate authority relationships are defined by rules and regulations.

traditional authority
Authority that arises from the subordinates' belief in social order.

While today's managers may have concerns about how younger workers comply with rules and regulations, they generally acknowledge that people who have experienced 9/11 or terrorism and dramatic advances in technology seem to want to make a positive impact in their jobs and communities and willingly work within the structure to do this.

Weber's third basis of authority, charisma, refers to a manager's ability to secure the compliance of subordinates through the power of personality. Employees willingly follow a manager with charisma, because he inspires them to succeed.

Other explanations of the meaning and sources of authority are presented by Barnard (1989). The formal authority theory and the acceptance authority theory are two contradictory theories of the source of authority. In **formal authority theory**, authority originates at the top of the organizational hierarchy and is delegated downward from superiors to subordinates. In **authority acceptance theory**, a leader's authority originates at the bottom of the organizational pyramid and is determined by his subordinates' willingness to comply with it. Each of these theories is discussed below to provide further insight.

formal authority theory
The belief that authority originates at the top of an organization and is delegated downward from superiors to subordinates.

authority acceptance theory
The belief that a leader's authority originates at the bottom of the organizational pyramid and is determined by his subordinates' willingness to comply with it.

Formal Authority Theory and Chain of Command

Formal authority is the top-down theory. It traces the flow of authority downward from top-level management to subordinate managers. This flow is known as the *chain of command*. A supervisor can trace his authority directly from his boss, who has delegated it to him. She in turn receives authority, for example, from an associate administrator, who receives authority from the administrator, who traces authority directly back to the board of directors, who receive their authority from the owners or the stockholders, or in the case of elected board members, the community. In private corporations, therefore, one may say that the actual source of authority lies in the stockholders, who are, loosely speaking, the owners of the corporation. These owners delegate their power to administer the affairs of the corporation to those they have put into managerial positions. That power flows down from the board of directors to the top executive and through the chain of command until it reaches the supervisor.

The authority that a manager has by virtue of his position in an organization is limited, either explicitly or implicitly. Some limitations stem from internal sources while others are from external sources. *External limitations on authority* include such implicit factors as our mores, community practices, and lifestyle. These are coupled with the many legal, political, ethical, moral, social, and economic considerations that make up our society. For example, laws referring to collective bargaining and resulting contractual obligations and fair

Limitations of Authority

HOSPITAL LAND

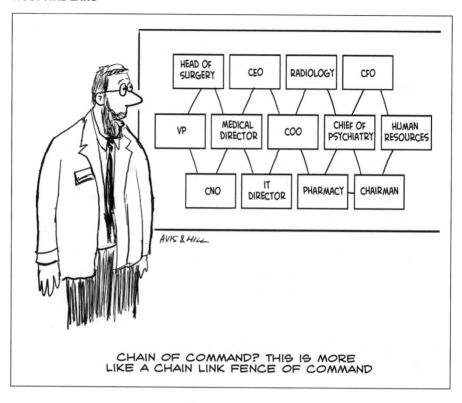

CHAIN OF COMMAND? THIS IS MORE
LIKE A CHAIN LINK FENCE OF COMMAND

employment practices are specific examples of external and explicit limitations on authority.

In contrast, *internal limitations on authority* are set mainly by the organization's articles of incorporation, bylaws, and organization policies. In addition to these overall internal restrictions, each manager is subject to the specific limitations spelled out by the administrator when duties are assigned and authority is delegated. Generally, there are more internal limitations on the scope of authority the further down one goes in the managerial hierarchy. In other words, the lower the rung on the administrative ladder, the narrower is the area in which authority can be exercised. This is known as the *tapering concept of authority*, as shown in Exhibit 11.1.

All these internal limitations are explicit, fairly obvious restrictions on authority. In addition to these, a number of more implicit limitations, such as biological restraints, exist simply because human beings do not have the capacity to do certain things. No subordinate should be expected to do the impossible. Thus, physical and psychological restrictions on authority must be recognized and accepted.

Weber (1974) summarizes authority as management's legitimate right to give orders and the employees' obligation to carry out these orders because

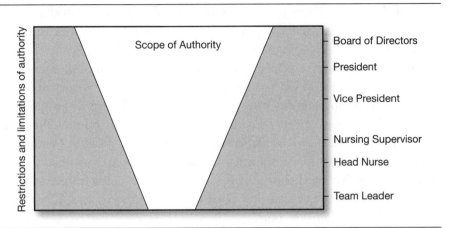

EXHIBIT 11.1
The Tapering
Concept of
Authority

the orders are derived from a legitimate power. A problem could arise, however, when such an order seems unethical to the employee or outside the limits of the job. This raises the question of whether the subordinate has some say in this matter, thus leading to Barnard's acceptance theory.

Authority Acceptance Theory

As discussed in Chapter 2, the authority acceptance theory addresses the role of subordinates in managerial authority. It is a bottom-up approach in which employees give managers their authority. In addition to Chester Barnard (1886–1961), other experts maintain that management has no meaningful authority unless and until subordinates confer it; that is, formal organizational authority is effective only to the extent that subordinates accept it. In reality, subordinates often do not have a real choice between accepting or not accepting authority. The only choice they have is to leave the job. Nevertheless, this is a worrisome consideration, indicating that there is considerable merit in looking at authority as something that must be accepted by employees.

Advocates of the acceptance theory state that in most cases a manager does not have a real problem; an employee, on accepting a job, knows that the boss of the department has the authority to give orders and take whatever appropriate action comes with the managerial position, including disciplinary action. When an employee decides to work for a healthcare institution, she agrees, within the limits of the job, to accept orders given by the organization. The decision of whether an order carries authority, however, lies with the person to whom it is addressed and does not reside in "persons of authority" or those who issue those orders, according to Barnard (1956). Furthermore, Barnard emphasizes that employees cannot accept a manager's orders if they do not understand what the manager wants them to do or if they do not have the ability or resources to comply with the manager's directive.

Formal Authority Theory Versus Authority Acceptance Theory

Differences between the formal authority theory and the acceptance authority theory significantly influence the practice of supervision, or the manner and the attitudes with which supervision is approached. This becomes more obvious with the realization that adhering to the acceptance theory does not necessarily rule out the downward delegation of authority from upper to lower levels of management. The acceptance theory can be thought of as merely another dimension to the formal concept of organizational authority. That is, in addition to having formal authority delegated from above, managers must also have such authority recognized and accepted from below. All managers must be aware that they possess formal authority and, if need be, can resort to it as a final recourse.

Today no one wants to rely exclusively on the weight of his formal authority to motivate workers to perform their jobs. At times, however, every manager has to make full use of this authority and power, but with hope that these occasions are the exceptions and not the rule. Even when the manager must invoke this authority, the manner in which it is done makes a difference in whether it is resented or accepted fully. If such actions are accepted graciously most of the time, the manager will know that the subordinates have chosen to recognize and respect the authority that superiors have formally delegated to him. View authority and power as a funnel, broad at the top and narrow at the bottom. Always assume you have enough authority and power to meet your obligations, but do not abuse your power while meeting your obligations and responsibilities (Integrated Publishing 2009).

line authority
Formal authority granted by an organization to a supervisor.

staff authority
Authority that resides in those with certain expertise who counsel or assist those with line authority. People who work in the accounting department, for example, may have staff authority and advise the department managers on financial matters.

Types of Authority

Authority can be categorized into various types. These include: line or positional, staff versus functional, and personal or charismatic.

Line authority reflects existing superior–subordinate relationships in the chain of command. It is the formal authority an organization grants a supervisor to direct the activities of those reporting to him. Also known as *positional authority,* it is based on the supervisor's position on the organization chart, vested in the position not the person, and is impersonal. Positional or line authority exists in all types of organizations. We may not like or care for a particular individual, but we recognize and accept the legitimacy of that person's position and authority.

Staff authority is resident with those who have certain expertise and are given the right to counsel or assist those with line authority. We accept their expert advice and recognize that this person is an "authority" in a particular specialty. The larger the organization, the more staff positions available to advise line managers. Staff authority is often granted to those in human resources, accounting, compliance, materials management, and plant engineering. Staff and line personnel must work closely to achieve the goals of the organization.

Closely associated with staff authority is *functional authority*. Functional authority is based on expertise and knowledge. Functional authority comes from specialization. **Functional authority** is authority restricted to a narrow area and coupled with a special right given to someone who normally would not have authority to direct or command others. This right is based on expertise in the specialized field. Although functional authority is limited to a specific area or topic, it is full authority and gives the staff member the right and power to give orders outside of normal authority lines in this limited area.

For example, an executive director decides that the human resources director's office should have the final word in cases of employee dismissal. In recent years, the laws, regulations, court decisions, and interpretations referring to fair employment practices have become an important area of managerial concern and a specialty that requires daily attention by someone in the organization. The department of human resources probably is best suited to keep up to date in this area. To avoid and minimize problems of this nature for the healthcare center, the administrator decides to confer functional authority in the special area of dismissals. Now the human resources director, rather than the line supervisors, has the authority to make the final decision relative to termination or alternative disciplinary measures. As you can see, for the line supervisor, functional authority overrides staff authority when the line supervisor "must" abide by the individual who has been granted functional authority.

Functional authority undoubtedly violates the principle of *unity of command*. This principle, as you recall, states that the subordinate is subject to orders from only one superior regarding all functions. Functional authority, however, introduces a second superior for a particular managerial duty (such as the discharging of employees, in our example above). Functional staff orders have to be carried out by the line supervisor to whom they are directed. If the line supervisor should disagree strongly, she can appeal to the superior manager up the line. However, unless these orders are changed, which is unlikely, the supervisor has to comply with them.

Functional authority is advantageous because it allows the maximum effective use of a staff specialist's expertise, leading to improved operations. It enables staff to intervene in line operations in situations designated by top-level management and provides for consistent treatment of certain situations across the organization, while still maintaining the overall chain of command. There is a price for this intervention-violating unity of command, and this may cause friction in some organizations. It is up to the administrator to weigh the advantages and disadvantages before assigning functional authority.

The Authority of Attending Physicians and Surgeons

Another line of internal authority is found only in a healthcare setting—the authority exercised by physicians and surgeons, some of whom may be employees of the healthcare organization. These are full-time chiefs of a medical

functional authority
Authority given to individuals with expertise in specialized areas and limited to particular situations. For example, a hospital's safety officer may be given the authority to send ambulances away from the emergency department—something he normally would not have the authority to do—if he feels the emergency department is dangerously overcrowded.

specialty, physicians under contract by the hospital or clinic to serve in various "director" roles, and other physicians and surgeons who are members of the medical staff.

The potential exists for tensions and misunderstandings between administration and members of the medical staff. The administration must consider the entire healthcare entity or system as an organized activity—that is, its relationships with all its employees, its financial viability, and its role in the community. The physician's interests, however, are likely to be focused on the patient and at times on the physician's own economic well-being. Members of the medical staff often wonder whether the administrative staff really understand their problems, and vice versa.

There may also be conflicts between the full-time and part-time members of the medical staff. These may relate to policies established by the full-time members that adversely affect the part-time members. For example, the full-time staff may want to exert control over the care plan of a patient that a part-time employee feels responsible for, or full-time staff may impose teaching obligations on part-time physicians, limiting the amount of time those physicians can spend with patients in their offices. In recent years, the addition of **hospitalists**, who have demonstrated positive outcomes (Dichter 2003), are being inserted between the attending physician and her patient as well as between the attending physician and the patient's nurse. In these cases the nurse or other patient care professional may find himself in a triad of command—taking orders from the immediate functional supervisor, the attending physician, and the hospitalist.

hospitalist
A physician who is employed by a hospital, rather than operating his own private practice.

In most hospitals, clinics, and HMOs, these frictions and violations of unity of command are minimal because both groups strive toward the best results for the patient and the healthcare center. In most situations, a natural partnership exists between administration and the medical staff, the first providing the necessary facilities and personnel and the latter, regardless of their staff status, providing the medical expertise.

There is little doubt that the physicians direct the care of the patients they admit to the healthcare facility or see in their offices. In this connection they have clinical/therapeutic/professional authority and exercise substantial influence throughout the healthcare entity at many organizational levels and in many functions. Physicians allowed to practice at the hospital, surgical center, or clinic, usually referred to as the medical staff, are not shown on the hospital organizational chart in any direct line or staff relationship under the CEO unless they are employees of the hospital or clinic. They are usually placed in a vague relationship to the board of directors on the chart. They practice medicine at the hospital, but they are outside of the administrative line of authority. They are "guests" who are granted practice privileges to perform certain services, but they have much authority over various people in the hospital. Their authority is exercised over the patient and especially over the nursing and patient care staff regarding medical issues. They also give orders to and expect compliance from many other employees of the hospital—for example, personnel in the nuclear medicine department, laboratories, and cardiopulmonary services.

As a second line of authority, orders from the physician or surgeon clearly violate the principle of unity of command. In fact, while in the operating room (OR), the surgeon is known as the "captain of the ship," a concept discussed in Chapter 6. This may lead to a situation in which operating room personnel in particular are accountable to two bosses; that is, they must take orders from and are responsible to their supervisor (the OR manager) and simultaneously the surgeon. This can cause difficulties when orders from the administrative source of authority (the OR manager) and the clinical/professional source of authority (the surgeon) are not consistent. Nevertheless, the physician constitutes an outside source of authority who can marshal the resources of the facility without being in the chain of command. The physician also is not responsible to the administrator, except for her professional medical conduct and for those policies, rules, and regulations governing the medical staff.

This dual command obviously creates administrative and operational problems, including communication, discipline, cost control, and coordination challenges. Moreover, dual command can cause considerable confusion in situations where authority and responsibility are not clearly defined. This may prompt attending physicians to circumvent administrative channels. Additionally, the administration may think that the physicians, through their power and authority, are interfering with administrative responsibilities. Regardless of all the complications inherent in this duality of command, it is an integral part of every healthcare organization. To avoid or minimize these challenges, positions and authority must be clearly defined for all who work on the healthcare team.

Personal Authority and Power

Thus far we have spoken of line and staff authority. Whereas positional or line authority is impersonal, functional authority in this sense is highly personal. It is associated with the individual, and it is the individual's knowledge and expertise that make him the authority. Whereas line authority can and must be delegated, functional authority cannot be delegated; it remains with the individual wherever he may be and work. Although it is highly personalized, functional authority has some aspects of positional authority because some organizations, especially healthcare centers, demand that certain positions be filled only by individuals with special skills and expertise. Many examples and applications of functional authority are found in a hospital, probably more than in any other organized activity. Functional authority rests on acceptance, but it stems from an individual's knowledge.

charismatic authority
Authority that stems from the compelling personal characteristics and charisma of a leader.

power
The ability to influence others or get others to act in a certain way.

coercive power
Power based on fear.

reward power
Power based on the ability to distribute something of value.

referent power
Power based on the personal attraction of an individual or the desire of other people to be like that person.

There is another type of authority that stems from the expertise or personality of an individual who is in neither a line nor staff position. *Personal authority* is based on an individual's characteristics, magnetism, and charisma. Some call this charismatic authority. In **charismatic authority**, the compelling personal characteristics and charisma of the leader inspire the subordinates and followers to carry out the orders. Subordinates and followers accept personal authority because their needs are consistent with the leader's goals. Personal authority motivates the followers to work willingly and enthusiastically toward the achievement of the objectives. This concept of personal authority can be equated with leadership, which is discussed in Chapter 22.

Related to personal authority is power. **Power** is the ability to influence people toward organizational objectives or the ability, as opposed to the right, to get others to act in a certain way. Power may or may not include authority. Informal leaders, through their personal authority, often have the ability to influence behavior in the absence of formal authority (Integrated Publishing 2009; Blanton 2009). French and Raven (1960) defined several types of power (excluding legitimate power or power based on one's position), including **coercive** (based on fear); **reward** (based on the ability to distribute something of value); and, as may be seen associated with personal authority, **referent** power (based on another person liking you or wanting to be like you). Individuals possessing personal authority may carry one or more of these powers and could have an influential impact on your staff's performance.

Integrated Approach to Authority

To be an effective manager in any industry, it is not enough to depend on the weight of positional authority based on legitimacy, although occasionally this may be the last resort. It is much more desirable if the manager relies on a combination of all types of authority to manage effectively. This is even more important in the healthcare field because of the occupational and professional characteristics of the people involved.

Line and Staff

We have talked about line authority and staff authority. In healthcare facilities, one usually speaks of different staffs, such as the nursing staff, medical staff, plant engineering staff, and administrative staff. In this context, the word *staff* applies to a group of people who perform similar jobs, such as nurses, physicians, and maintenance engineers. We also use the term *staff* as a verb to describe the function of selecting individuals to accomplish a task, for example, the supervisor staffs the second shift. In the general field of management and administration, however, the meaning of the term staff is different. *Staff* is spoken in connection with *line*, and both these terms refer to authority relationships as described earlier in positional versus staff authority.

Because no one, not even the CEO, could possibly have all the knowledge, expertise, skills, and information necessary to manage a modern organization, staff becomes an essential and critical part of the institution. Line managers retain the administrative and authoritative parts of the activities, whereas staff representatives supply expert advice and support—the scientific, technological, technical, and informational aspects. Without these aspects, the institution cannot function properly.

Origin of Staff

In management theory, the term *staff* has been around since the days of ancient Athens and Rome. The technical definition refers to an individual or individuals who serve in an advisory capacity to the manager(s) of an organization. Consider the president of the United States. He has many issues he must keep abreast of and does so through the use of a team of staff advisors. Staff positions may also serve in an **extender role**—that is, they may perform portions of a task or prepare pieces of a project or study for the manager when the manager cannot do everything himself or herself.

extender role
The role of an employee who takes on tasks or projects for a manager who cannot do all the work himself.

As organizations grow in size and complexity, and as the environment changes and impinges more and more on them, the duties of managers increase. Managers add subordinate managers by creating more departments and delegating authority (Exhibit 11.2). Sooner or later, however, the manager's span of management is so large that no more additional supervisors can be added because the manager cannot pay proper attention to them. At this point, personal staff is added, which means one or more assistants to do the work that cannot be delegated.

When executives find themselves in a position in which they need a personal aide (sometimes referred to as an "administrative assistant" or "assistant to" such as "assistant to the president") to help them in performing duties that they cannot delegate, a personal staff position may be created. The person in this position is a staff aide to the particular executive rather than to the organization at large; the placement of the assistant to the president in Exhibit 11.3 shows this relationship.

This person performs a variety of tasks for the executive, such as gathering information, conducting research, and relieving the executive of detail work. This position is also often used to train and develop junior managers to acquaint them with how higher-level executives function. The assistant-to position has no line authority. This individual, however, often plays a role in the channels of informal communications and in the workings of the informal organization.

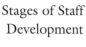

EXHIBIT 11.2
Stages of Staff
Development

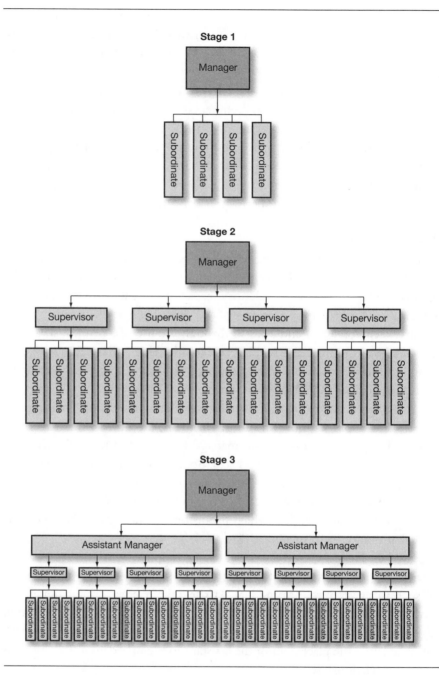

Even with assistants, however, managers eventually encounter areas they need specialized help in, such as fair employment practices, compliance regulations, and healthcare law. At this juncture specialized staffs and possibly staff departments are introduced into the institution to provide counsel and advice in various special fields to any member of the organization who needs

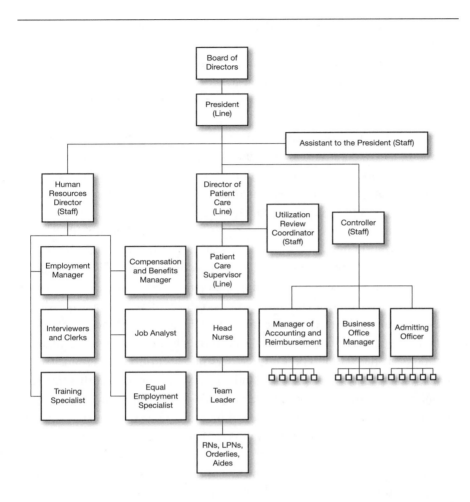

EXHIBIT 11.3
Staff's Chain of
Command
Alongside the
Line
Organization

it (see Exhibit 11.3). Today staff activities are increasing, as is the number of people working in these roles and functional areas.

Line and Staff Organization

Staff personnel are advisory in their duties, whereas **line personnel** have direct responsibility to ensure goals are achieved through their subordinates. Whereas a line manager or supervisor may seek advice from a staff advisor, the line supervisor determines the action that must be taken next and then directs the subordinates to carry it out. In Chapter 5, you will recall that we discuss staff planners, who assist the CEO in the planning function. In that situation, staff develop planning premises and may coordinate the planning activities. They probably collect data or conduct studies for management to use as the basis for decision making. But it is the line managers who make all the decisions involved in preparing the plan. The line managers define the objectives,

staff personnel
Employees who specialize in specific duties or areas of expertise, but who generally do not make important decisions that affect the organization.

line personnel
Employees with direct responsibility to ensure goals are achieved through their subordinates. Line personnel may be advised by staff personnel, but line personnel make the decisions.

allocate the resources, establish the timetable in which goals must be accomplished, and so forth.

Conflict over organizational and operational problems may occasionally arise between line and staff, regardless of how well the relationships were defined. This is because of the two types of authorities at work: positional and formal on one side, with the weight of expertise and knowledge on the other. In most organizations, line and staff work together harmoniously. Harmonious cooperation between line and staff is especially important in a healthcare institution because the input of so many specialists is necessary for the delivery of good healthcare. Much depends on the sensitivity and tact of the staff people and the clarity of organizational arrangements.

Department supervisors need to know whether they are attached to their organization in a line capacity or a staff capacity. They might be able to find this out by studying an organization chart or reading the job description or, if that does not clarify it, by asking their superior manager. Line and staff are not characteristics of certain functions; rather, they are characteristics of authority relationships. Therefore, to ultimately determine whether a department is related to the organizational structure as line or staff is to examine the intentions of the CEO. The CEO confers line authority on certain departments, usually to generate products and services, and she places others into the organizational structure as staff to serve in advisory or supportive roles for the line management. Staff positions are not inferior to line personnel in terms of authority, or vice versa; they are simply completely different in nature. As these differences are discussed, keep in mind that the objectives of the staff elements are ultimately the same as those of the line organization—namely, achievement of the institution's overall goals of delivering the best possible care.

Line Organization

line organization
The organizational structure built on a straight chain of command from the top of an organization to the bottom.

The simplest of all organizational structures is the **line organization**, which depicts the primary chain of command and is inseparable from the concept of authority. Thus, when we refer to line authority, we mean a superior and a subordinate with a direct line of command running between them. In every organization, this straight, direct line of superior–subordinate relationships runs from the top of the organization to the lowest level of supervision. Exhibit 11.4 depicts one direct line of authority running from the board of directors to the president of the institution through the vice president of patient care services, a nursing director, a head nurse, a team leader, and finally to the other nursing employees.

Unity of Command

The uninterrupted line of authority from the chairperson of the board to the team leader in Exhibit 11.4 ensures that each superior exercises direct command over the subordinate and that each subordinate has only one superior

EXHIBIT 11.4
A Direct Line
of Authority

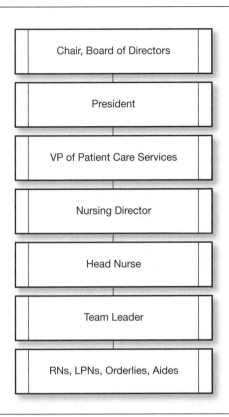

to whom he is accountable. This is known as the principle of unity of command. **Unity of command** means that each employee has a single immediate supervisor, who in turn is responsible to her immediate superior, and so on along the chain of command. Thus, everyone in the line organization knows precisely who the boss is and who the subordinates are. The individual knows exactly where she stands, to whom orders can be given, and whose orders have to be fulfilled.

It is easy to see that line authority can be defined as the authority to give orders—that is, to command. It is the authority to direct others and require them to conform to decisions, plans, policies, and objectives. The primary purpose of this line authority is to make the organization work by evoking appropriate action from subordinates. Direction and unity of command have the great advantage of ensuring that results can be achieved precisely and quickly.

This type of direct line structure, however, does not answer all the needs of the modern organization. This structure was adequate when organizations and their environments were not as complex as they are today. In most enterprises now, activities have become so specialized and sophisticated that an executive needs assistance to direct all of his subordinates properly and expertly

unity of command
The principle that states that each employee has a single immediate supervisor, who in turn is responsible to her immediate superior, and so on along the chain of command.

in all phases of their activities. Line management today definitely needs the help of others to make the right decisions.

Staff Organization

Staff are auxiliary in nature; they help the line executive in many ways. Staff provide information, counsel, advice, and guidance in any number of specialized areas to all members of the organization whenever and wherever a need may exist. However, staff cannot issue orders or command line executives to take their advice. Staff make recommendations to the line. With the exception of staff specialists who have functional authority, that advice can be accepted, ignored, rejected, or altered by the line. Because staff are expert in their specialties, the advice is usually heeded, but it does not have to be. When the line accepts the staff's suggestion and implements it, this suggestion becomes a line order. Line authority is based on superior–subordinate relationships; it is positional and managerial. Staff's authority is based on expertise; it is advisory and not managerial. Obviously, staff are not inferior to line and line is not inferior to staff. They are just different, and both are needed to complement each other to achieve objectives.

The right to command is not part of staff authority, with two exceptions. First, within each staff department there exists a line of command with superior–subordinate relationships, just as in any other department. Staff's own chain of command, however, does not extend over to the line organization. Rather, it exists alongside the line organization as shown in Exhibit 11.3. The second exception arises when staff have been given functional authority by the CEO. This important concept was introduced earlier in the chapter.

You can probably see more clearly why all supervisors must know whether their position is attached to the organization in a line or a staff capacity. They must know to understand their function and relation to the other members of the organization. If it is a staff capacity, the function is to provide information, guidance, counsel, advice, and service in their specialized area to whomever may ask for it. As far as the supervisor's own department is concerned, however, it will not matter whether the position is line or staff. Within every department the supervisor is the line manager. She is the only boss, regardless of whether the department is attached to the organization in a staff or a line capacity.

Personal Staff Versus Specialized Staff

Distinguishing Between Staff and Line It is common practice for certain activities in each organization to be undertaken as staff activities. This does not mean, however, that one can assume these are always staff activities. Line and staff, as stated before, are characteristics of authority relationships and not of functions. Thus, even a title does not offer any clue in recognizing line or staff. In many enterprises, one typically finds a vice president of engineering, a vice president of human resources, and a vice president of operations. None of these titles, however, indicates whether the position is line or staff. The little square box on the organizational chart also does not offer any help in this dilemma.

Because the reason for establishing a staff in most instances is to obtain the best current advice, however, it is usually in the interest of the line manager to follow staff suggestions. For all practical purposes, the authority of the staff lies in their expertise in dealing with problems in their field. They will sell their ideas based on their authority of knowledge, not on their power to command. A person who acts in a staff relationship must know that his task is to advise, counsel, and guide, not to give orders, except within his own department. If any of the suggestions of the staff are to be carried out, they are carried out under the name and authority of the line officer, not that of the staff person.

Span of Management

Another important element of an organization's foundation is the number of people who report to a particular manager. This defines the **span of management**, also known as *span of control*.[1] This concept deals with the number of people any one person can supervise effectively. Several factors influence the span of one's control, including the following:

1. competence/skills of the supervisor and her employees,
2. physical proximity of employees to each other and their supervisor,
3. extent of time spent by the manager performing nonsupervisory duties,
4. frequency of required interaction among employees and between the employees and their supervisor,
5. extent of standardized procedures,
6. similarity and complexity of tasks being supervised,
7. frequency of changes in process, and
8. ability to use technology to monitor performance.

Each of these factors must be considered when pondering span of control. Should it be relatively narrow, with few subordinates per manager, or reasonably wide, with many subordinates per manager?

Depending on the diversity of tasks and activities involved, organizations create divisions, departments, sections, or teams and place someone in charge of each. In doing so, the resulting organization may be *tall* or *flat*. In Exhibit 11.2, we see the organization starting as flat and eventually becoming tall—that is, with more layers. *Tall organizations* may be more expensive because more managers are required and communication may be challenging because there are additional channels through which it must pass. *Flat organ-*

span of management
The number of individuals a manager supervises. Also called *span of control.*

izations tend to have higher employee morale and productivity because there are fewer layers one must go through to speak to the top boss. However, both morale and productivity can be hindered by having too many direct reports, causing the supervisor to be spread too thin to adequately respond to employee or customer concerns.

The establishment of departments in an organization is not an end in itself. It is not desirable per se because departments are expensive; they must be headed by someone and staffed by additional employees, all of which costs large sums of money. Furthermore, creating departments is not intrinsically desirable because the more there are, the more difficulties are encountered in communication and coordination. However, departments do make the division of work possible. Some departments are too large and require further compartmentalization into sections or teams. Furthermore, with the expansion of and access to technologies that allow communications to flow not only within a single building but across multiple entities on a campus or across the country, organizational structures have become less constrained by the walls of a building. Today's healthcare environment requires the care location to be conveniently accessible for the patient and medical staff. Services that traditionally were only offered in the hospital are now dispersed and provided in stand-alone entities spread out across a community.

This decentralization can be supported by a team approach known as a microsystem (Cowen et al. 2008) consisting of a subpopulation of patients and their multidisciplinary health professionals. The groups interact with each other whenever patients and caregivers are together. Microsystems may exist within a formal structure or outside of it. They facilitate the way work is accomplished and require a management structure to communicate, plan, and coordinate the work activities. Microsystems are patient-centric systems that allow the same care team to follow and evaluate the patient through the patient's continuum of care. Thinking about the care team structure from a patient's needs forced Alegent Health to reexamine key service lines, such as cardiovascular, where patients need conveniently located diagnostic services, emergency departments when chest pain occurs, and acute care if indicated (Molpus 2009).

Regardless of the compartmentalization approach(es) selected, departmentalization allows an organization to incorporate the principle of the span of management, or the span of supervision. Regardless of teaming or other nontraditional organizing approaches, span of supervision continues to be a crucial factor in structuring organizations.

The Relationships of Span to Levels

Because no one can manage an infinite number of subordinates, the administrator must create departments, or distinct areas of activities, over which a manager is placed in charge. The administrator delegates authority to this manager. The manager in turn re-delegates authority to some subordinates, who in turn supervise only a limited number of employees. In this manner, not only are departments and subsections of the department created, but the span of supervision is established. The number of managerial levels in the organization is determined as well, because the number of superior–subordinate interactions that can be effectively handled is limited.

To examine this relationship between the span of supervision and the levels of an organization, imagine a hypothetical organization in which 81 subordinates report to one chief executive, thus representing an organizational level (see Exhibit 11.5). Few will disagree that 81 subordinates are too many people for the executive to manage. However, everyone tends to want to report directly to the boss. To ease her burden, the executive is given three associates. Under each of these three associate administrators there would now be 27 employees. By creating associate administrators, however, we have

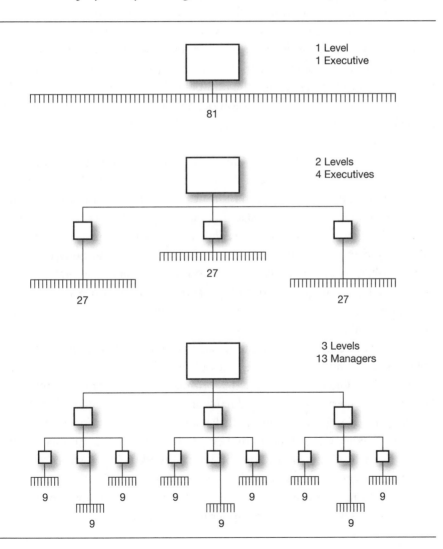

EXHIBIT 11.5

Relationship Between the Span of Supervision and the Levels of an Organization established two levels of organization and have a total of four executives. Assuming that 27 subordinates are still too many, the organization could create a third managerial level, increasing the total number of managers to 13 and reducing the number of subordinates per manager to 9. Each of the four executives on the upper two levels will have three subordinates, and each of the nine supervisors on the lowest level will have nine subordinates. The span of supervision has thus been reduced drastically from the original 81 to a maximum of nine.

This example shows what occurs when one begins to narrow the span of supervision. The narrower the span becomes, the more levels of management have to be introduced. As with departments, this is not desirable because it is expensive and may interfere with communication and coordination. Every manager costs money, not only in salaries, but in supporting expenses (offices, furnishings, educational allowances, and possibly support staff salaries). More levels will complicate communication, even distort it with omissions and misinterpretation of the messages. Finally, adding levels to an organization creates problems with morale because it increases the distance between employees and upper administration. Therefore, a constant conflict exists between the width of the span and the number of levels. The problem is whether to have a broader span of supervision or more levels, or vice versa, and it is a problem that all managers face throughout their careers and one for which a clear solution is not evident.

All of the issues discussed thus far were confirmed in two studies. The first study, conducted by Doran and colleagues (2004), sought to determine if the cost-cutting and restructuring in healthcare had an impact on nursing employee retention, patient satisfaction, outcomes, and other factors. The key findings indicate a correlation between the width of the span of control and turnover and employee and patient dissatisfaction. The second study, conducted by the College of American Pathologists on hospital clinical laboratories, does not define the ideal span of control but shows a correlation between smaller span of management and increases in productivity (Valenstein, Souers, and Wilkinson 2004).

However, attempts to quantify an optimum span of control appear in the works of Graicunas (1937), Urwick (1956), Davis (1951), and Hamilton (1921). While Graicunas developed a formula that accounted for interactions between the supervisor and subordinates and subordinates and their peers, he, Urwick, and Hamilton all indicated that five to six direct reports, at least at the executive level, is the ideal number. Davis stretched the number to 30 at the manager level, depending on the type of work being performed by the subordinates and the level of the supervisor. Thus, no definitive answer exists to the question, "How many subordinates should report to a given manager?" One can only say that there is an upper limit to this figure.

Although we do not know exactly what the upper limit should be, it is interesting that in many enterprises the top-level administrator has only five to eight subordinate managers reporting directly to him. Descending down the managerial hierarchy, the span of supervision generally increases. It is not unusual to have 15 to 20 people reporting to the supervisor. On closer inspection, the number of subordinates who can be effectively supervised by one manager actually depends on numerous different contingency factors. These factors determine not only the actual number of relationships but also their frequency and intensity. Therefore, before deciding the proper span of supervision in a particular organization, it is necessary to examine the more important contingencies that influence the magnitude of the span.

As mentioned earlier, one of the factors that influences the magnitude of the span is the competence of supervisors—that is, quality of management, experience, and expertise. Some supervisors are capable of handling more subordinates than are others. Some are better acquainted with good management practices, such as time management; others have had more experience and are simply better all-around managers. While a person who is a "good manager" may be able to supervise more employees, limitations still exist, however, on the human capacity and the amount of time available during the workday.

Factors Determining the Span of Supervision

What the manager does with this time is of utmost importance in determining the span. For example, a supervisor needs more time to make an individual decision for every problem that arises than to make initial policy decisions that anticipate problems that might arise later. Clear and complete policy statements reduce the volume of, or at least simplify, the personal decision making required of a manager and thus can increase the span of supervision. The same applies to other managerial processes that determine in advance definitions of responsibility and authority, procedures, methods, and performance standards. Predeterminations such as these reduce the number of decisions the manager has to make and likewise increase the potential span of management.

Another factor that determines how broad a span a manager can handle is the competence and makeup of the subordinates. The greater the capacities and self-direction of the employees, the broader the manager's span can be. The education, experience, and training possessed by the subordinates are also important. The more experienced they are at their jobs, the less they need their supervisor, thus freeing the manager to increase the span.

Another contingency on the manager's span is the amount and availability of help from staff specialists within the organization. If a healthcare organization has a range of experts who provide various kinds of advice, support, and service, the manager's span can be wider.

The number of subordinates who can be supervised also depends on the nature and importance of the activities the subordinates perform. If these activities are complicated, are highly important, carry critical consequences, or change frequently, the span of supervision has to be small. The simpler, less complicated, or more uniform the work, the greater can be the number of persons supervised by one supervisor.

Closely related factors that have a bearing on the span of supervision are the dynamics and complexity of a particular activity. In those departments engaged in dynamic, critical, and unpredictable activities, such as the emergency department, the span is very narrow. In those departments concerned with more or less stable activities, such as food production in the dietary department, the span of supervision can be broader.

Another factor that determines the span of supervision is the degree to which a fairly comprehensive set of standard procedures and objective standards can be applied. If enough procedures and standards exist and are available for subordinates to gauge their own progress, subordinates do not need to report to and contact their boss constantly. Objective standards and standard procedures result in less frequent interactions, freeing the manager for a broader span.

For some tasks, the use of technology to assess productivity and quality allows the supervisor to spot individual variations that may require more of her attention, rather than personally sampling all staff members' output on a daily basis. This technology or monitoring feature is usually available in organizations using workflow software applications, such as an electronic document management application or a direct dialing program for collections; or other technologies such as laundry operations where pounds are captured by the individual washer units and the laboratory where specimen counts are captured by the laboratory testing equipment. These technologies ease the oversight burden for the supervisor, thus allowing her to direct more staff. This is not to say that the supervisor should not occasionally assess the work of all staff members, but rather these tools allow the manager to focus on those who have performance variations outside the manager's expectations.

Teams and Their Impact on Span of Management

Finally, organizations have had success expanding the span of control through the use of self-directed teams. These teams further compartmentalize a department. Each team has a leader who is formally appointed or selected by the team. The team is empowered with some of the traditional supervisory duties and authority, such as assigning workloads to team members, scheduling vacations or weekend duty, checking each other's work, and even preparing performance reviews, thus relieving the supervisor of those duties (Exhibit 11.6). Team management allows authority to be shared, broadens the span of control, and encourages staff to work together rather than compete with one another. With broader spans of control, the organization also functions with fewer supervisors.

Teams are often assembled on an ad hoc or temporary basis to study a process or a complex issue. These ad hoc teams usually include individuals

Exhibit 11.6
Team Authority

Authority Worksheet Date: _____

Teams must define which member(s) have authority to take certain actions. At the beginning of any project, the team leader and the team should decide who has responsibility for each of the following authorities. Sometimes the authorities will be shared among members, with the team leader, or with other leaders or teams. Therefore, others may need to be involved in this discussion too. Each person agreeing with the delegated duties shall enter their initials in the initial column.

This worksheet should be used to make sure that all relevant authorities are defined, discussed, and agreed to by all participating parties.

1. Which team members were involved in the granting of authorities?
    a. _____
    b. _____
    c. _____

2. Were any team leaders or non-team members not involved in this decision?
    Yes: _____ No: _____

3. Who were the team leaders or non-team members who were not involved in this decision? _____

4. As a team, discuss and decide which of the following authorities are necessary to accomplish the work assigned. Discuss which authorities should be assigned to the team leader or to others outside of the team. Make notes in the blocks below or on additional paper as necessary and make sure everyone involved receives a copy of this document.

5. Identify others outside of the team who have been involved in completing this delegation of authorities: _____

Delegated Authorities for Meeting Project Needs

Authorities	Team Leader	Comments	Team Members	Initials
Define the work that is to be accomplished or mission of the team.				
Assign tasks to team members.*				
Establish and manage the project schedule.				
Routinely update administrative champion.				

Continued

with expertise or knowledge of the issue and who have an interest in improving the process. Team members typically serve on these teams because they wish to encourage cooperation among departments, divisions, or other teams. Often teams are provided training, such as meeting facilitation, problem identification, problem solving, and interpersonal skill building.

Regardless of the factors considered, management must keep in mind that the economic benefits of a broad span of control are rapidly diluted if communication is compromised, especially during poor economic times when

EXHIBIT 11.6
Continued

AUTHORITIES	TEAM LEADER	COMMENTS	TEAM MEMBERS	INITIALS
Identify potential products or services.				
Select products or services.				
Identify potential vendors, suppliers, or contractors.				
Negotiate rates with vendors, suppliers, or contractors.				
Select vendors, suppliers, or contractors.				
Eliminate or terminate the services or products of vendors, suppliers, or contractors not selected.				
Identify team members or others who should work on this project.				
Select team members or others.				
Eliminate or reassign team members or others.				
Authorize payments to suppliers, contractors, or vendors.				
Recommend how much team members are paid or if bonuses are to be issued.				
Authorize pay and/or bonuses for team members.				
Offer alternatives to achieving goals.				
Approve or disapprove alternatives offered by team members or others.				
Prepare budget.				
Approve budget.				
Approve variances to budget.				
Evaluate the team's performance.				
Summarize "lessons learned" and the team's success or failure.				

* Will this authority differ if more than one team leader is involved?

communication must be heightened and occur more frequently. Dave Ulrich in his book *The Leadership Code* suggests that a message may need to be communicated 10 times, in a variety of ways, before it will be understood by the recipient (Stern 2009). This degree of communication frequency will challenge the most talented supervisor if the span of supervision is too broad. Urwick (1956, 43) states it succinctly: "There is nothing which rots morale more quickly and more completely than poor communication and indecisiveness. ... And there is no condition which more quickly produces a sense of indecision among subordinates or more effectively hampers communication than being responsible to a superior who has too wide a span of control."

Summary

Management's organizing function is to design a structural framework that enables the institution to achieve its objectives. To do so, one must assess the organization's overall mission and objectives, its size, geographic span, space constraints, and changing environment. If an organization exists in a rapidly changing environment, it may need to restructure itself often.

Organizing defines and arranges the activities needed to accomplish the objectives of the organization. Work is divided horizontally into departments, then divided vertically by delegating authority. As the organization grows the need for staff positions increases. Staff provide expert counsel and service in a specialized field to whomever in the organization needs it. Staff are not inferior to line staff, or vice versa; rather, they represent different types of authority relationships. The line manager has the authority to give orders, whereas the staff manager usually only has the authority to make recommendations. The advice can be accepted, ignored, rejected, or altered by the line manager who requested it. Because staff represent expertise in a specialty, however, the advice is usually accepted. Staff's authority is based on expertise; it is advisory, not managerial authority.

The CEO must decide whether a department is attached to the organization in a line or in a staff capacity. Because line and staff are quite different, it is essential for every supervisor to know in which capacity he or she serves. The supervisor in a straight, direct chain of command that can be traced all the way to the top-level administrator is part of the line organization. The line organization generally follows the principle of unity of command, which means that each member of the organization has a single immediate superior.

On establishing the structure, positions within the organization are granted authority to manage resources and activities assigned to them in concert with the responsibilities assumed or in accordance with the parity principle.

Authority and span of management are two basic elements of the organizing function. Authority is the right to give orders and directives and to expect that they be carried out. Much has been said and written about the source of authority. The formal authority theory is top down; it views authority as coming from the U.S. Constitution, the recognition of private property, social institutions, owners, stockholders, boards of directors, higher management, and so on down the line to the supervisor.

The opposite view, the acceptance authority theory, views authority as coming from the bottom up. This theory states that managers have no authority unless and until the subordinates accept their authority, and subordinates normally accept only those directives they perceive to be legitimate.

Tradition, rules, and charisma are the bases of authority, which lead to three major types of organizational authority. Positional authority is based on the position in the organization; staff and functional authority are based on knowledge and expertise, but while staff authority is advisory in nature, functional is more directive; and personal, or charismatic, authority comes from the subordinates' needs being consistent with the leader's goals.

Since functional authority grants rights to override line authority in a limited area, it violates the principle of unity of command. Similarly, duality of command is created by an attending physician's clinical/therapeutic authority. These additional channels of command result from the nature of healthcare delivery. Many areas of functional authority exist in most healthcare centers.

Many factors must be considered when defining the structure of an organization and the span of control assigned to each of the managerial and supervisory positions. Too broad a span may result in lackluster performance of the staff and the supervisor, poor morale, and customer as well as employee dissatisfaction; too narrow a span may result in too many supervisors—a costly endeavor for the organization. While a definitive size for the ideal span of control has not been discovered, there has been research done in this area that indicates a consensus of 5–6 direct reports at the executive level and possibly up to 30 at the manager level.

Determining the span of supervision at each level and the number of managerial levels is important. The span of supervision states that there is an upper limit to the number of managerial levels. The actual width of this span is determined by such factors as the competence of the supervisor as well as the competence and experience of the subordinates to be supervised by one manager.

The smaller the span of supervision, the more levels of supervisory personnel are needed. This shapes the organization into either a tall, narrow pyramid or, in the case of a broad span of supervision, a shallow, wide pyramid. On the other hand, broadening the span of control or increasing the use of team management enhances the shallow pyramid or flat structure and allows employees to manage their own activities without consuming a manager's time.

Note

1. Span of management may also be called span of authority, span of supervision, or scope of supervision.

Additional Reading

Barclay, L. "Following in the footsteps of Mary Parker Follett." Emerald Insight. [online information; retrieved 2/13/09.] www.emeraldinsight.com/Insight/ViewContentServlet?Filename=Published/ EmeraldFullText Article/Articles/0010430508.html.

12

DIVISION OF WORK AND DEPARTMENTALIZATION

Chapter Objectives

After you have studied this chapter, you should be able to do the following:

1. Describe the importance and benefits of division of work—that is, job specialization.
2. Describe the advantages and disadvantages of departmentalization and departmentalization methods.
3. Explain the supervisor's goal when designing the "ideal" department.
4. Consider alternative models for displaying the organization chart.

As stated in the previous chapter, organizing means deciding how best to group the activities and resources of the organization to achieve its mission. Formal organization theory rests on several major principles. Two of these are division of work and departmentalization.

Division of work, or job specialization, means the degree to which each task of the organization is broken down into component parts. This is essential for efficiency and for the achievement of objectives.

Departmentalization, or compartmentalization, is the process of grouping activities into distinct units according to logical arrangements. Departmentalization creates the building blocks for the formal structure, the main network for managing the various activities of the enterprise.

These two major premises of organization are the primary concern of the CEO in a smaller organization or the COO in a larger one. He must translate these principles into a formal organizational structure for the institution. Because the application of these formal organizational principles involves all levels of management, it is also necessary for the supervisor to understand them and know how they are used. This knowledge helps the supervisor organize the department and coordinate its activities in concert with those of the rest of the institution. The supervisor is frequently asked to carry out, and maybe even help make, decisions involving departmentalization and division of work.

Making a Pin (Nail) Involves 18 Tasks

Without Specialization
1 worker doing all 18 tasks yields approximately 20 pins a day.
20 workers make 400 pins a day.

With Specialization
20 workers make 100,000 pins a day.
1 worker makes approximately 5,000 pins a day.

SOURCE: Smith, A. 1776, 1967. *The Wealth of Nations.* Chicago: Henry Regnery.

Division of Work or Job Specialization

job specialization
Breaking down a task into smaller parts, and having each part or step of the task performed by a different individual.

Division of work is an age-old practice. Consider the division of work in early tribal societies: women planted and maintained the gardens and washed clothes, while men hunted for food and protected the tribe. **Job specialization** is breaking down a task into smaller parts, and having each part or step of the task performed by a different individual. Thousands of years ago, human beings divided work in this manner because they realized a group of people, each performing a small specialized part of the overall job, could accomplish more than the same number of people each doing the whole job alone. Adam Smith's oft-cited example from 1776 of job specialization in a pin (nail) factory confirms this advantage (see box).

Furthermore, with specialization, each individual learns how to do her task exceptionally well and allows high-skilled workers to concentrate on tasks that require high skills while lesser-skilled workers perform less-complicated tasks. Additionally, teaching an individual a single task makes employee replacement easier. In other words, the division of work results in greater efficiency and higher production. Industrial mass production in the United States during the 20th century expanded largely because of specialization. However, excessive specialization can lead to employee boredom. Adam Smith, known as the Father of Economics, stated, "The man whose life is spent in performing simple operations . . . has no occasion to exert his understanding. He generally becomes as stupid and ignorant [as] is possible for a human creature to become" (Box et al. 1999).

Healthcare organizations utilize the specialization and division of work theory. Continuous advances in medical sciences and technology result in greater specialization of healthcare professionals, facilities, and equipment and

HOSPITAL LAND

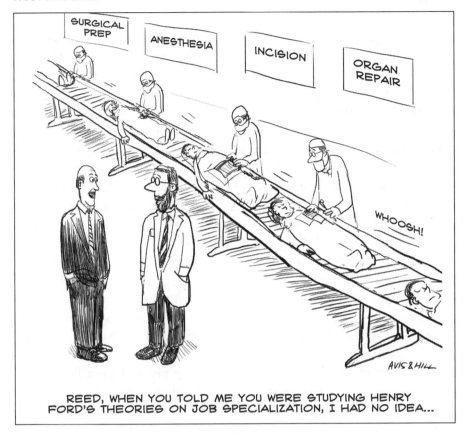

REED, WHEN YOU TOLD ME YOU WERE STUDYING HENRY FORD'S THEORIES ON JOB SPECIALIZATION, I HAD NO IDEA...

increased fragmentation of the delivery of care. For example, ophthalmologists have foundational specialty training in ophthalmology, but some specialize in retinal conditions while others specialize in surgical techniques such as Lasik surgery. One home care agency may specialize in serving newborns, while another agency specializes in serving the geriatric population. Because of the proliferation and specialization of medical sciences and technologies, healthcare centers have become large and complex organizations.

This proliferation of specialties helps healthcare providers offer state-of-the-art care. However, this specialization creates administration problems, because various organizational structures are needed to coordinate the specialties. It also inconveniences those patients who prefer to go to one physician for everything that ails them.

In essence, as the healthcare industry becomes more sophisticated, higher degrees of expertise are required, forcing specialization of its professionals and staff. In light of Adam Smith's concern, the impact specialization may have on motivating employees is discussed in Part VI of the book.

Departmentalization

When the organization grows and a single person can no longer personally supervise all personnel in the organization, additional managers are employed and assigned specific functions or departments and employees to supervise. Almost every healthcare organization must departmentalize, because division of work into specialized tasks produces a more efficient operation. As stated, **departmentalization** is the process of grouping various activities into natural units by logical arrangements. A department, by definition, is a unit; it is a distinct area of activities over which a manager or supervisor has been given authority and for which he has accepted responsibility. The terminology may vary and a department may be called a division, service, section, unit, office, or similar term, but it still represents a closely related set of activities. Departmentalization relies on specialization, which is the core determinant. By departmentalizing the organization, a horizontal and vertical grouping of specialized activities is attained.

departmentalization
The process of grouping various activities into natural units by logical arrangements.

The top-level executive of an organization groups the various activities into departments. Some departments established this way are small and require no further subdivision; others are so large that managers have to subdivide their departmental staffs into smaller units, sections, or teams to create an effective span of control. For this reason, every manager must become acquainted with the various alternatives available for grouping activities.

The process of departmentalization can be done on the basis of (1) functions, (2) process and equipment, (3) territory (location), (4) customer (patient), (5) time, or (6) product.

Functions

The most widely accepted practice of departmentalizing is grouping activities according to functions[1] or common tasks. All activities that are alike or similar and involve a particular function are placed together into one department under a single chain of command. This is depicted for nursing or patient care services in Exhibit 12.1. In a functional organization, all patient care services are placed under the chief nurse executive. Other common functional alignments are finance, compliance, and support services.

As an institution grows and undertakes additional work, often new duties are added to the already existing departments. For instance, an addition of an outpatient surgical center may logically be assigned to the surgical services director. However, when we study product- or customer-oriented organizations, this function may be more appropriately placed under the ambulatory services director. Regardless, expansion of service offerings and the concomitant additional patient volume require adding more employees and levels of supervision within the functional departments. Occasionally, however, new services require adding a new department; for example, a rural

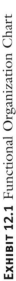

Exhibit 12.1 Functional Organization Chart

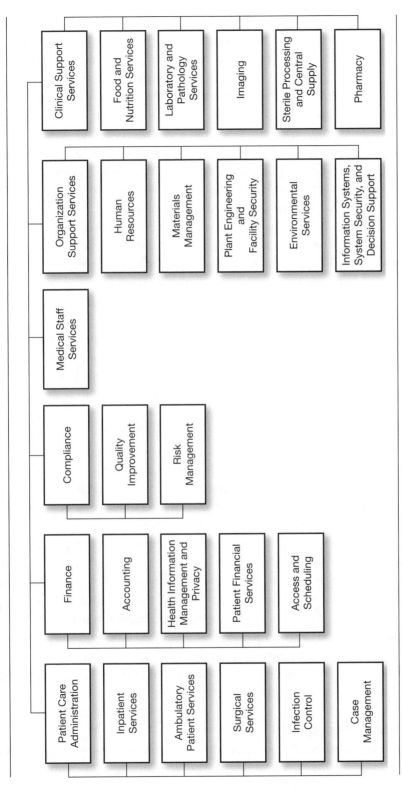

hospital that purchases several physician practices and a rural health center may need to establish a physician practice management department.

Departmentalizing by function is a natural, logical way of arranging various activities. This kind of departmentalization takes advantage of specialization by combining the functions that belong together and that are performed by experts in that functional field with the same type of education, background, equipment, and facilities. The experts for each function are brought together under a supervisor for the area where they can share their common expertise and participate in technical problem solving. Each functional supervisor is concerned with only one type of work and concentrates all of her energy on it. This leads to an efficient use of resources.

Functional departmentalization also facilitates and enhances coordination because one manager is in charge of one type of activity throughout the entire organization. Coordination is easier to achieve this way than it would be if the same function were performed in several different divisions. Another advantage of functional departmentalization is that it makes the expertise and skills of one or a few individuals available to the enterprise as a whole.

Functional design also facilitates in-depth skill development and allows for clear career paths. For example, an employee may start out at the Technician I level and after a year move up to the Technician II level. If the technician has three or more years of experience, he may qualify for the team leader position; after five years, the day supervisor position; and so forth. Eventually, the individual becomes an expert in each of the tasks performed by the department. Because functional departmentalization is a simple and logical method and has all these advantages, it is the most widely used way of setting up departments.

Some disadvantages to functional departmentalization have arisen in large organizations, especially when the undertaking grows in size. It may limit the staff's ability to see the complete process, emphasize routine tasks, and increase boredom. Interdepartmental communication may break down and turf battles may ensue over new services offered. Working in a single department may leave an individual vulnerable when technology advances; that is, if a specialized expertise is no longer needed, the individuals who know just that one job may be out of work or require extensive retraining. Finally, department managers may become so protective of their own goals that the organizational goals may be compromised. These disadvantages can be minimized by supervisory awareness, however, and should not prevent management from opting for functional departmentalization.

Process and Equipment

Activities can also be grouped around the equipment, process, customer flow, and technology involved. This kind of departmentalization is often found in hospitals because hospitals usually operate sophisticated equipment and handle certain processes that require special installations, training, and expertise.

Every task involving the use of certain equipment and technology is then referred to the particular specialized department that is equipped to do the task. This type of organizational structure is similar to functional departmentalization, the major difference being the emphasis on person–machine relationships or a process that supports mass production. For instance, in imaging and nuclear medicine departments, specific equipment is used but only certain functions are performed. Another area in which organizing occurs around equipment is in large hospital laboratories, where the laboratory has discrete sections, each focusing on one high-volume type of testing. Here staff may be assigned to work with the microbiology equipment or the chemistry equipment and remain in this area for their entire career. Similarly, in radiology individuals with specialized training in nuclear medicine, tomography, ultrasound, and diagnostic radiology perform those tasks for other departments. Organizing by equipment, process, and technology results in the staff becoming very specialized in the defined area, but this is beneficial during disaster situations when patient care services are triaged in large numbers.

Departmentalization by function and by equipment frequently become closely allied. In fact, within a functional department, one may organize staff by process or equipment. However, departmentalization does create disadvantages for management and staff. Because employees are specialized, they may not be able to fill vacancies in other areas or positions because they lack the additional skills. Conversely, the employee is limited on positions into which she may advance because her skill set is technologically narrow.

Territory (Geographic Location)

An alternative way to departmentalize is according to location (see Exhibit 12.2). This means setting up departments based on defined geographic areas or sites. The extent of the area may range from the entire hemisphere to a number of cities, a few blocks of a large city, or different floors in the same building. This type of departmentalization is common in national and regional healthcare systems. For example, a hospital or nursing home in a large city may have several geographically dispersed units, such as St. Mary's East on one side of town and St. Mary's West on the other. If the same functions are performed in different locations and different buildings, geographic departmentalization is necessary. This type of departmentalization is also common for county health departments and home health agencies. As staff members join the agency, depending on their residence or client load, they are assigned to the agency's office that serves that region. The same considerations are applicable even if all activities are performed in one building but on different floors and wings, such as centralizing surgical services in the east tower with day surgery on the first floor, all operating rooms and recovery areas on the second floor,

EXHIBIT 12.2 Campus Departmental Structure

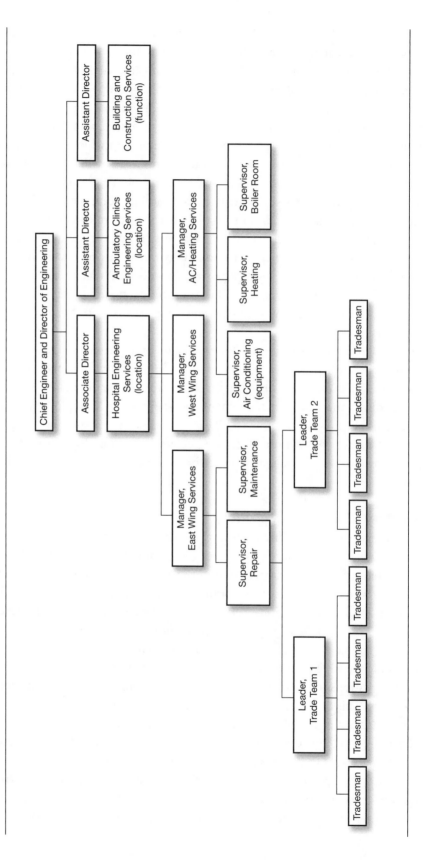

orthopedic surgery on the third floor, cardiothoracic surgery on the fourth floor, and so forth. In this example there is function, customer, and even equipment departmentalization in a territorial location.

One of the advantages of territorial departmentalization is placing decision making close to where the work is done; managers develop expertise solving problems unique to the location, and managers are familiar with their customers and their problems. Possible disadvantages of territorial departmentalization include duplication of effort and resources, focus on a given location's goals rather than the organization's, and the necessity of extensive rules or procedures to enable managers to coordinate and ensure uniformity of quality of care between locations. Consider the surgical tower mentioned above. One service that would likely be housed in this tower is central supply (instrument sterilization). However, this service also is required for the clinics, where some office-based procedures are performed, and for the emergency department. To support the needs of these departments, another instrument supply and sterilization unit may need to be established, staffed, and equipped in a location closer to these areas. On the positive side, this duplication of service provides opportunities for the development of more managerial talent.

Customer (Patient)

At times, management may group activities based on customer (patient) needs and characteristics, hence the term customer (or customer-focused) departmentalization. Two examples of organizations that have departmentalized along customer lines are universities and hospitals. In some universities, night programs and day programs comply with the requests and special needs of the "customers"—namely, part-time and full-time students. For example, in a hospital certain services and activities may be grouped for outpatients and inpatients, such as outpatient surgery. Some healthcare organizations have built entire facilities to specifically serve a patient type, such as women's centers and children's hospitals. In so doing, the healthcare center's services are less diverse and allow the staff to specialize in treating a certain customer or patient type. Healthcare services delivered by this approach are on the rise. Often, the distinction between customer and product structures is difficult to make because the product describes the customer. This is true of **centers of excellence** for cancer, cardiology, orthopedics, etc. The centers are product lines that treat patients with a common condition.

The customer departmentalization approach offers several advantages, including facilitating the attention to patient (customer) needs by centralizing specialists' focus on a specific patient or condition type and developing managers to become customer advocates. It may also have disadvantages, such as conflicts over resource allocation, the restriction of problem-solving skills to a single patient type, coordination problems between specialties or departments,

center of excellence
A department, such as cardiology or oncology, chosen by the healthcare organization to receive special attention and resources. Centers of excellence are sometimes called "institutes."

duplication of resources, and possibly decision making that pleases the customer but hurts the company.

Time

Some organizations find it helpful to group activities according to the period during which they are performed. An enterprise such as a hospital, which operates around the clock, must departmentalize activities on the basis of time, at least to a certain extent. The institution must set up different time shifts—usually day, afternoon, and night or only day and night. Activities typically are grouped first on some other basis, such as by function, and then are organized into shifts. Since the activities performed on each shift are largely the same, such groupings often create organizational questions of how self-contained each shift should be and what relationships should exist between the regular day-shift supervisors and the off-shift supervisors.

Product

This departmentalization approach is similar to customer departmentalization and is often seen in the establishment of centers of excellence. To departmentalize on a product basis in industry means that a division is responsible for a single product or group of closely related products; the emphasis is shifted from the function to the output or product. For example, a hospital supply company may have a separate department for furniture, another for surgical supplies, and a third for uniforms.

Product departmentalization in a healthcare facility involves the division into departments based on the "product" turned out—for example, maternity, surgery, oncology, cardiology, or psychiatry. Hospitals that have adopted this departmentalization approach often call it a product-line organization. Each such department has its own nursing, dietary, housekeeping, and maintenance staffs, and each such product department has its own boss—the director of oncology services, the director of maternity, and so on. These directors are in charge of all functions within their product departments, including nursing activities, therapy, food services, laundry, and maintenance. Often decision making is faster in this structure. While this compartmentalization approach may be seen within an existing organization, it is often seen when a parent organization establishes satellite locations. For example, a medical center may establish outpatient facilities throughout the community. One facility may be an urgent care center situated in an industrial area, and another may be a satellite laboratory adjacent to a medical office complex. Each community satellite is overseen by a director who must arrange for all services needed by the satellite location. Having total control over all or most factors allows economic and outcome performance of these individual products to be assessed.

As you can see, such product departmentalization can result in duplication of effort within the organization. Instead of a single director of nursing, there are as many as the number of existing departments. Moreover, coordinating all nursing services and ensuring that the same level of care is rendered throughout the entire organization are difficult because each supervisor reports to a different boss. Another potential disadvantage of this system is that the individual department managers may be "out of sight" of the overall leadership, especially if they are also geographically dispersed. This limits career opportunities.

There are advantages to the system, however. This system can be manipulated to gain economies of scale and the ability to leverage staff. For example, environmental services will be required for each of the different departments. A single department or outpatient center would not be able to command the pricing discounts on supplies that the medical center and its multiple satellites could. In the case of staffing, if one of the centers needs a nurse, she can more easily be assigned from the larger pool of nurses working at the medical center.

As hospitals have had to compete for market share, they have had to enhance, and to some extent exploit, those areas that are in demand by the population served. Some hospitals have created geographically separate facilities dedicated to one product, such as women's services or mental health services. Furthermore, the increased technology and advances in medicine in some product areas have forced healthcare enterprises to organize by product to permit the manager or product leader to focus on the product, the technology serving it, and the impact of medical advances on its future. Thus, product departmentalization, as practiced in healthcare institutions, also has encouraged specialization, can easily be aligned with customer departmentalization, and presents the same advantages and disadvantages.

Mixed Departmentalization (Composite, Hybrid Structure)

Departmentalization is not an end in itself. In grouping activities, management should not attempt to merely draw a balanced organizational chart. Its prime concern should be to set up departments that help bring about the institution's objectives and coordinate its functions. There are advantages and disadvantages to each method of departmentalization. Choosing a method is a question of balance and deciding which works most effectively. In so doing, often management uses multiple departmentalization options and creates a hybrid structure—that is, a mixed departmentalization; for example, a nursing supervisor (functional) on the surgical unit (subfunction), west wing, third floor (location), during the night (time), and in the women's center (customer). In practice, almost all hospitals have this composite type of departmental structure, combining function, location, time, and many other considerations (see Exhibit 12.2). Any mixture is acceptable, as long as it works and is consistent with the overall objectives of the institution.

Organizing at the Supervisory Level

Thus far, we have discussed the organizing process from an overall institutional point of view. We have explored how the chief executive establishes the formal organizational structure and makes it come alive by selecting the right supervisors to whom organizational authority is delegated.

Most department heads and supervisors are not likely to be involved in the major decisions concerning the overall organizational structure of their healthcare institution. However, they are likely to be concerned with the structure of their own department, including departmental goals and objectives, daily operations and activities, and existing personnel and resources.

The organizing process is basically the same regardless of whether it is performed by the CEO, COO, or first-line supervisor. Organizing involves grouping activities for purposes of departmentalization or subdepartmentalization on the supervisory level; assigning specific tasks and duties; and, most important, delegating authority. In essence, this means that the basic organizational principles must be understood and applied by supervisors when they are setting up their own departments, just as they were by the chief administrator when the overall institution was structured. How might a supervisor apply these principles daily, so that they are not just abstractions but parts of a healthy departmental body?

Ideal Organization of the Department

Most supervisors are placed in charge of an existing department; only a few have the opportunity to design a structure for a completely new department. When designing or rearranging the organizational structure of the department, the supervisor should conceptualize and plan for the ideal organization. The word "ideal" in this instance is not intended to mean perfect; rather, it is used to mean the most desirable organization for achieving stated objectives. It is the supervisor's job to design an organizational setup that is best for his or her particular department. In so doing, the principles and guidelines of organizing must be observed.

The manager must bear in mind that certain organizational concepts and arrangements that work well in a large organization may not be applicable to a smaller organization. In other words, supervisors must not blindly follow the idea that what is good for one enterprise is also good for another. Moreover, it is not essential that the manager's organizational plans for the department look pretty on paper or that the organizational chart appear symmetrical and well balanced. Rather, this ideal design should be uniquely tailored to suit the conditions under which the manager works, instead of some abstract image of what a "perfect" department should look like.

In planning this ideal, but realistic, organization, the supervisor must consider it as something of a standard with which the present organizational setup can be compared. The ideal structure should be looked on as a guide to the short- and long-range plans of the department. Although the supervisor should carefully plan for the ideal structure when becoming the department's manager, this does not mean that the existing organization should be forced to conform to the ideal immediately. Each change in the prevailing organization, however, should bring the existing structure closer to the ideal. In other words, the ideal organization of the department represents the direction in which the supervisor moves as time passes.

Internal Departmental Structure

When supervisors design the ideal departmental structure, they usually are being asked to subdepartmentalize. In other words, they establish subdivisions or subunits within their department—just as the chief administrator established the overall divisions or units for the whole organization. Several examples of how a director might subdepartmentalize are shown in the organizational charts throughout this chapter.

Supervisors consider the groupings of activities in the department, the various existing positions, and the assignment of tasks and duties to these positions. Is this the best possible arrangement for achieving departmental and institutional objectives? Are all the present positions necessary, or could some be eliminated or combined with others? Does each position have a fair assignment of tasks and duties, commensurate with its status and salary? Are the positions related so that there is no duplication of effort and that coordination and cooperation are facilitated? Are there any changes at all that the supervisor would like to see in the internal organizational structure of the department?

Such changes become the basis for the ideal organization of the department. They become the organizational goals toward which the department head strives when structuring the department.

Departmental Organizational Structure

A department can be organized by function, process and equipment, territory, and so on. A department may have sections, divisions, teams, or areas. Each subunit may have a lead employee, team leader, supervisor, or manager, or several subunits may report to one of these titled individuals. Regardless, the objective of the manager in creating the organizational structure is to ensure that the department's goals are achieved through the proper organization of staff and coordination of duties or work flow. Examples of different departmental structures are given in the following section.

Exhibit 12.2 displays a departmental structure where the engineering services are centralized under one executive, the chief engineer. He has responsibility for services across a healthcare campus that includes a hospital and several ambulatory clinics. This structure depicts an organizational structure that includes location, equipment, and function models and uses the relatively common titles of director, associate director, assistant director, manager, supervisor, and team leader.

Exhibit 12.3 depicts a health information management department that has chosen the self-directed team model. Self-directed teams may be found in tall or flat organizations. Some flat organizations, also known as horizontal organizations, may have customer-oriented processes performed by multidisciplinary teams (Dessler 1998; Dessler and Stark 2004; Osland et al. 2006) or microsystems, as discussed in Chapter 11. These teams are groups of people committed to a common purpose, with a set of performance goals, and an approach for which they hold themselves mutually accountable (Dessler 1998, 476). When a team approach is used, the manager establishes the objectives but has delegated authority to the teams to achieve the objectives. The team may use an authority template as explained in Chapter 11, or the manager may have met with each team one-on-one and discussed his expectations. To have fully decentralized authority, this manager may even allow each team to select its leader or to choose not to have a leader.

Earlier we discussed a product-line organization for surgical services. This example is displayed in Exhibit 12.4. All staff involved in the delivery of surgical services are aligned under the corporate director for these services. Note that practitioners with expertise in nutrition, financial management, pharmacy, and so forth are included in this product-line organization.

EXHIBIT 12.3
Single-
Department
Structure: Self-
Directed Teams

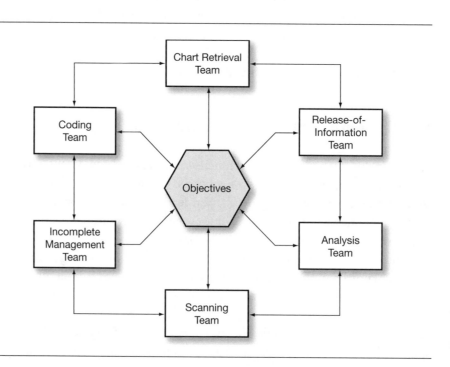

EXHIBIT 12.4
Product-Line
Organization

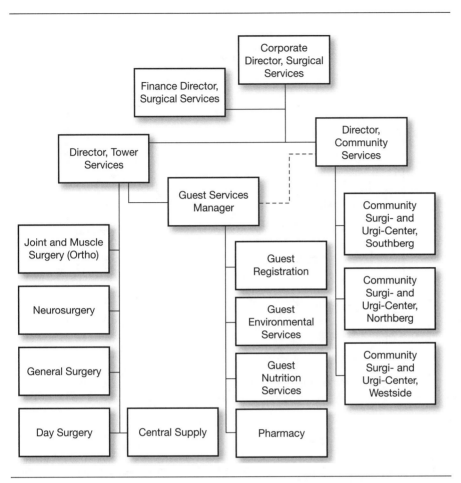

If a supervisor is setting up a new department or working in a newly established institution, much of the ideal structure can probably be implemented in the beginning. This is the most desirable situation, but it is not usually the case. In fact, often the structure that is established at the beginning of a new organization is rapidly changed.

Example of a New Department in a New Organization

Consider the case of a new 80-bed hospital in southwest Florida. The hospital expected to have 25 beds in operation on Day 1 and to be at the 80-bed level within six months. Clearly, the staffing level required for 25 beds was not the same as that required for 80 beds. Furthermore, it was inappropriate to hire staff for 80 beds only to have them be idle for up to six months until the census increased. To manage these staffing challenges, the activities of access, patient financial services, and health information were initially combined; these hybrid positions were titled personal account managers (PAMs) (see Exhibit 12.5). The PAMs were cross-trained to perform the duties of all three

Exhibit 12.5

New
Department
Organization
Chart

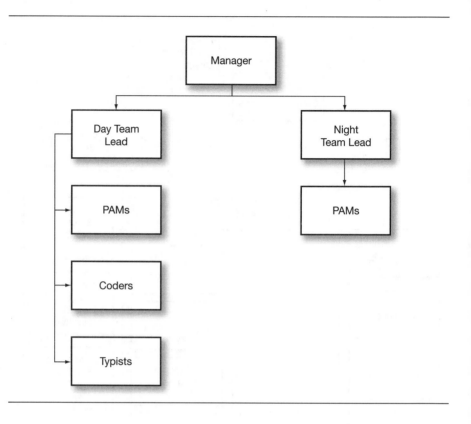

functions with the exception of coding and transcription. In fact, the PAMs even obtained the first meal selection from the patients and escorted the patients to the patient care area.

The PAMs worked 12-hour shifts three days per week and a four-hour shift on any day of their choosing. During peak registration hours they performed access functions; during slow periods or between patient registrations they obtained precertifications or certifications from insurers. Also during slower hours, the PAMs processed discharged patient records and completed the various billing functions for the day. In the early evening, these same individuals followed up on patient balances for collection purposes. Because they met the patients at the time of admission, PAMs developed rapport with patients and could check on their at-home recovery progress and report that information to performance improvement.

Generally, the supervisor implements organizational goals gradually while working within the existing departmental structure and with personnel. In this instance, the goals were to ensure the functions were adequately staffed with well-cross-trained individuals who eventually migrated to one specialized function or another as the hospital grew in size and complexity.

Organization and Personnel

The supervisor should design the ideal organization based on sound organizational principles, regardless of the people with whom he works. The problems of organization should be handled in the right order; the sound structure comes first, then the people are asked to fulfill this structure.

If the department setup is planned first around existing personnel, existing shortcomings are perpetuated. Because of incumbent personalities, too much emphasis may be given to certain activities and not enough to others. Moreover, if a department is structured around personalities, it carries an inherent flaw, which is revealed if a particular employee is promoted or resigns. If, on the other hand, the departmental organization is structured impersonally on the general need for personnel rather than on the incumbent personalities, it should not be difficult to find an appropriate successor for a particular position. Therefore, an organization should be designed first to serve the objectives of the department, then the various employees should be selected and placed into departmental positions. This, however, is easier said than done.

In most instances, the supervisor has been put into a managerial position in an existing and fully staffed department without having had the chance to decide on the structure or personnel of the department. Frequently, some of the available employees do not fit well into the ideal structure, but they cannot be overlooked or simply dismissed. In such cases, the best the supervisor can do for the time being is to adjust the organization to use the capacities of the existing employees. This is an accommodation of the ideal plan to fit present personalities and should be regarded as temporary. Then, as time goes on and attrition naturally occurs or a significant change in workflow is introduced, the supervisor can strive to come closer and closer to the ideal departmental setup.

Organizational Design

With the exception of team structures, the discussion of organizational structure has centered around traditional structure concepts. **Traditional structure** is the most studied and researched form of organization and has a long history of successful performance. Traditional structure is not inflexible or rigid. This structure functions successfully under most prevailing conditions and is capable of producing and accommodating change and adapting to contingencies as they arise.

Of course, even the best-designed organization cannot be left without change forever. Changes in technology, care delivery systems, the environment, human and social processes, organizational size, the workforce, economic

traditional structure
The most common form of organizational design, in which hierarchical relationships develop vertically, and each employee reports to one superior.

trends, regulatory activities, and so forth have to be accommodated. The institution must design a structure that works best under these contingencies. The organization is an open system, which means that changes in one part of it affect the activity in another part. The organizational concepts discussed thus far are applicable even under those new contingencies.

Matrix Organization (Matrix Design)

An alternative organizational structure building on traditional concepts is the **matrix organization**. This is an organizational structure in which employees have two bosses—one in the department to which they are permanently assigned and one who is directing a special project that crosses departmental boundaries or a service or product that spans several geographic areas. Matrix organization, also known as project or grid organization, does not do away with the traditional organization; it simply builds on it and, under certain contingencies, improves on it. It is superimposed on functional organization, creating a grid, or a matrix. Thus, it provides horizontal dimensions to the traditional vertical orientation of the functional organization. It is an organizational design that typically combines technical expertise found in the departmentalization model and product models simultaneously.

Exhibit 12.6 is the organizational chart of a national managed care organization (MCO). This example shows a matrix organization for the utilization review function of the MCO. The structure violates unity of command; for this organization it is imperative that utilization review policies be consistently applied nationwide. The corporate vice president of utilization review is responsible for ensuring this occurs, and she must have some authority to impose standard rules and procedures on the regional operations. Day-to-day oversight and control of these functions rests with the regional vice president. This structure can be used in a healthcare provider as well. For example, consider The Joint Commission's expectation for consistent nursing practice throughout a healthcare organization that has multiple outlying clinics, an ambulatory surgery center, a home health agency, community urgent care centers, and a hospital. The chief nurse executive must have authority to mandate certain nursing practices to ensure compliance with The Joint Commission's standard. In this scenario, a matrix organization may best meet this objective.

Matrix Structure in Project Management

High-technology fields such as healthcare often need to create project organizations to focus resources and special talents for a given time on a specific project. For example, if an organization is emphasizing oncology (cancer) care, the oncology division brings in dietitians, radiation therapy technicians, pharmacists, nurses, pastors, lab technicians, and physicians who specialize in cancer care. These members define the services to offer to cancer patients. They develop the plans, recruit the staff, organize the functions needed to serve the patients, and deliver the care.

---

matrix organization
An organizational structure that adds cross-departmental connections to a traditional vertical organization. These connections may unite departments for special projects or products or services that span several geographic areas. In a matrix organization, employees often report to more than one superior.

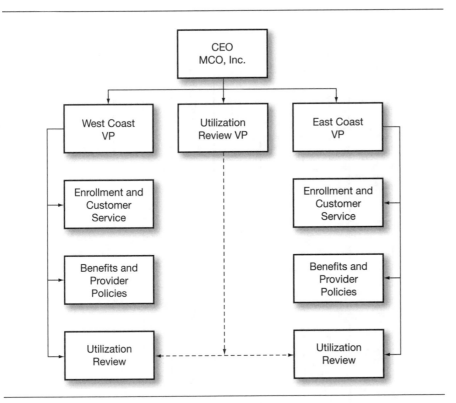

EXHIBIT 12.6
Utilization
Review Matrix

The essence of matrix management is a compromise between functional and product departmentalization in the same organizational structure. For example, Exhibit 12.4 demonstrates the matrix relationship for guest services between the tower and community directors. Exhibit 12.7 shows a more complex but not unusual matrix arrangement in a healthcare institution in which the functional managers are in charge of their professional function, with an overlay of two project managers (A and B) who are responsible for the end product—a specific project.

Some organizations are breaking down their functional organization structure and replacing it with project teams that focus on issues that cross many departments and tie to an organizational value such as clinical information or quality. The leaders of these endeavors often are certified as professional project managers (PMP®).[2]

Advantages and Disadvantages of Matrix Structures

A matrix organization gives an enterprise the potential to conduct several projects simultaneously. Say the president of a hospital sees the need for three projects to be phased into her institution within the next two years: a pharmaceutical barcoding system, an electronic record system, and preparation for the hospital's accreditation. The president could assign these projects to three different project managers, and matrix organizations could be established for each.

EXHIBIT 12.7 Matrix (Project) Organization

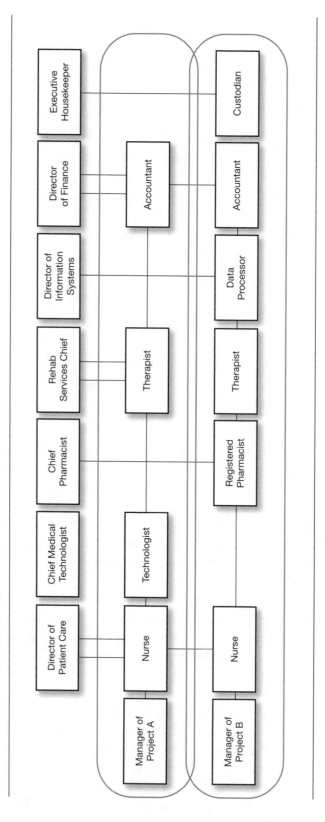

By establishing a matrix organization, better coordination can be achieved than would be possible in a traditional organizational structure because experts from throughout the organization are pooled together with a common charge and focus for a temporary period. The project is assigned to a project manager from the beginning to its completion, and people from the functional areas needed for the project are assigned either on a full- or part-time basis. The project matrix overlays the conventional structure; it draws on traditional structure for the various skills required for the project. When the project is finished, the project manager and specialized personnel return to their functional departments or are reassigned to a new project.

The advantages of matrix organization are that it

1. provides an effective way to focus on new products and customers and phase new projects in and out of operation;
2. improves coordination and establishes lateral relationships;
3. offers greater flexibility to consider and implement innovative ideas;
4. creates teams of experts quickly to cope with a sudden change or need;
5. dissolves teams without too much repercussion on the overall structure;
6. exposes members of a project to interaction with experts from other areas, thus offering an opportunity for personal development;
7 identifies individuals who may be selected to serve in future leadership positions; and
8. affords top-level management an additional way to delegate and decentralize.

Matrix design also creates a number of problems. The most common problem is that sometimes the roles of team members are not clearly defined. As noted earlier, the matrix organization is a system in which employees are supervised by two bosses, namely their functional director and the project manager. Recall Exhibit 12.4 and the dual-boss arrangement for the guest services manager. This structure clearly violates one of the major principles listed in Chapter 11—unity of command. The professional, when assigned to a project, may be faced with duality of command because conflicting directives may come from the two bosses. Additionally, when used in a project management context, the employees on the project may not be certain to whom they are supposed to report and whose assignments take priority; worse, there may be power struggles between the individual's two bosses. More confusion can arise when one person is assigned part-time to two or more projects.

Further sources of frustration for the project team members are that while assigned to the project, they may also feel isolated from the mainstream of their home departments and penalized because evaluations and possible promotion opportunities are usually vested in the functional department head and not in the project manager.

Most of these problems are caused by poor coordination, insufficient project preparation, and a lack of concise and clear statements of authority relationships. These symptoms introduce the concept of role theory. **Role theory** claims that when employees receive inconsistent expectations and little information, they experience role conflict, which leads to stress, dissatisfaction, and ineffective performance. Role theory supports the chain-of-command and unity-of-command principles (Roussel, Swansburg, and Swansburg 2006). Multiple lines-of-authority disrupt these principles, create stress, and reduce trust.

role theory
The concept that when employees receive inconsistent expectations and little information, they experience role conflict, which leads to stress, dissatisfaction, and ineffective performance.

If management creates an environment of support and communication, conflict can be avoided. Well-prepared projects have the following attributes:

- At the start of the project, the enterprise executive clarifies the relationships. He clarifies the authority and responsibility of the functional directors.
- The project manager has full authority and responsibility over the integrity of the design and over the budget. She is the decision maker and coordinator for the duration of the project.
- There are clear statements about the project manager's frequency of reporting and the scope of the project.
- The project manager makes schedules and works out priorities with the functional managers.
- The functional managers are responsible for the integrity of the service or products that their departments supply to the project.
- Statements concerning these decisions and responsibilities guide the project manager and the functional managers whose departments are involved in the project.

Despite the best preparations and clarifications, misunderstandings may still arise. Provisions to resolve such a dilemma should probably be made by referring the misunderstanding or dispute to higher management. Thorough preparation and clarifying authority and responsibility when the project is established minimize many of these problems. Some borderline cases involving problems of dual command may still arise. Remember that all organizational structures can create some problems occasionally. Matrix organization provides a system with a proven method of implementing a complex new task that has relatively short duration.

Additional Approaches to Organizational Structure

Two additional organizational approaches appear in the literature: mechanistic and organic (Burns and Stalker 1961). While classified as organizational structures, they speak more to the culture or atmosphere established within any of the other structures discussed in this chapter. Setting the tone for an organization starts at the top. Recognizing that labels have been created to define these tones is an important lesson for supervisors to learn, as these labels may affect recruitment and retention of talented staff.

A **mechanistic organization** is a structure that is characterized by high specialization, extensive departmentalization, narrow spans of control, many rigid rules and regulations, a limited information network, and authority vested in a few higher-level executives. In contrast, the **organic structure**, occasionally called the *thinking structure*, is one in which jobs tend to be general; few rules and regulations exist; communication is vertical, diagonal, and horizontal; and the organization is highly adaptive and flexible and encourages decentralized decision making by the employees.

Organizing defines the relationships between authority and activity and no one culture or structure works for every organization. Common sense helps the manager design the best one and create a culture that encourages productivity and employee satisfaction.

Organizational Charts

Many conflicts in organizations are caused by employees not understanding their assignments and those of their coworkers. Proper use of organizational charts, manuals, and job descriptions defining authority and informational relationships substantially reduces misunderstandings and clarifies doubts. The healthcare institution's structure is formalized graphically in charts and in words in the manual. To be helpful, these tools must be available all the time and be up to date, which means changes must be incorporated promptly.

Organizational charts are a means of illustrating the organizational structure at a given time—as a snapshot. The chart shows the skeleton of the structure, depicting the basic formal relationships and groupings of positions and functions; that is, it maps the lines of decision-making authority. Most of the time, the chart starts out with the individual position as the basic unit, which is shown as a rectangular box. Each box represents one function. The various boxes are interconnected horizontally to show the groupings of activities that make up a department, division, or whatever part of the organization is under consideration. They are connected vertically to show scalar relationships. Thus, one can readily determine who reports to whom merely by studying the position of the boxes in their scalar relationships.

Advantages of Organizational Charts
As the organizational chart is prepared, the organization must be carefully analyzed. Such analysis might uncover structural faults and duplications of effort, complexities, or other inconsistencies. Cases of dual-reporting relationships (one person reporting to two superiors) or overlapping positions

mechanistic organization
An organization whose structure is characterized by high specialization, extensive departmentalization, narrow spans of control, many rigid rules and regulations, a limited information network, and authority vested in a few higher-level executives.

organic structure
An organizational structure in which jobs tend to be general; few rules and regulations exist; communication is vertical, diagonal, and horizontal; and the organization is highly adaptive and flexible and encourages decentralized decision making by the employees.

might also be uncovered. Moreover, charts might indicate whether the span of supervision is too wide or too narrow, or if the organization is unbalanced.

Charts offer a simple way to acquaint new members with the organizational makeup and with their fit into the entire structure. Most employees have a keen interest in knowing where they stand, in what relation their supervisor stands to the higher echelons, and so on. Charts are also helpful in human resources administration; they can indicate possible routes of promotions for managers as well as for other employees.

Another advantage of charts is they assist in developing better communications and relations. Charts can also be valuable for future planning purposes. A supervisor may want to have two charts for his department, one showing the existing arrangements and the other depicting the ideal organization. The latter may be used so that all the gradual changes planned fall within the design of the ideal, representing the ultimate organizational goal of the department in the future. Charting shows what is changing and how that change affects the members of the organization.

Limitations of Organizational Charts

Charts also pose some limitations, especially if they are not kept up to date. It is imperative that organizational changes be recorded speedily, or they are of little practical use. Another shortcoming of charts is that the information they give is limited. A chart is a snapshot, not a CT scan; it shows only what is on the surface, not the inner workings of the structure. It shows only formal authority relationships, not the many informal relationships that exist (see Chapter 17). The chart also does not show the amount of authority and responsibility inherent in each position (sometimes even positions with similar titles have different levels of authority and responsibility).

Another problem with charts is that individuals confuse authority relationships with status. Sometimes people read into charts and come up with interpretations that are not intended. For example, a person may interpret an employee's degree of power and status by checking how distant that person's position is on the chart from the box of the CEO, or on which level it is shown.

Finally, some charts are so complex that they end up confusing the employees. To determine if your organization chart is too complex, supervisors should ask their employees to identify their position and then work their way up to the individual to whom the supervisor reports. If they cannot, the supervisor should reevaluate the chart.

vertical chart
An organizational chart that shows the different levels of the organization in a step arrangement in the form of a pyramid.

Types of Charts

Three main types of charts commonly used are vertical, horizontal, and circular. Of these, the vertical chart is used most often.

A **vertical chart** shows the different levels of the organization in a step arrangement in the form of a pyramid. The CEO is placed at the top of the chart, and the successive levels of administration are depicted vertically in the pyramid shape. One of the main advantages of the vertical chart is that it can be easily read and understood. It also shows clearly the downward flow of delegation of authority, chain of command, functional relationships, and the relationships between activities. Many of the general shortcomings of charts apply to vertical charts as well.

In addition to the vertical chart, some healthcare institutions prefer a **horizontal chart**, which reads from left to right (see Exhibit 12.8). The advantage of a horizontal chart is that it stresses functional relationships and minimizes hierarchical levels. The left-to-right chart of a matrix or project organization is a combination of these two arrangements. Horizontal relationships are superimposed on the vertical chart.

A **circular chart** can also be used. It depicts the various levels in concentric circles rotating around the top-level administrator, who is at the hub of the wheel (see Exhibit 12.9). Positions of equal importance are on the same concentric circle. This graphic portrayal eliminates the need to place positions at the bottom of the chart.

A few organizations might prefer an **inverted pyramid chart**, showing the chief administrator at the bottom and the associate administrators farther up. This type tries to express the idea of the "support" given to each manager by the "superior" (see Exhibit 12.10).

horizontal chart
An organizational chart that reads from left to right, stressing functional relationships more than hierarchical levels.

circular chart
An organizational chart that depicts the various levels in concentric circles rotating around the top-level administrator, who is at the hub of the wheel.

inverted pyramid chart
An organizational chart featuring the chief administrator on the bottom and others farther up. This chart expresses the idea that the superiors support those who report to them.

Summary

Management's overall organizing function is to design a formal structural framework that enables the institution to achieve its objectives. The CEO or COO establishes this framework initially, using the basic principles of formal organizational theory as guidelines. She begins with the principle that specialization is necessary for efficiency. This means grouping the various activities into distinct departments or divisions, assigning specific duties to each, which, in turn, assigns the tasks to multiple workers. The administrator can approach this departmentalizing effort in several ways. The most widely used concept of departmentalization is grouping activities according to functions—that is, placing all those who perform the same functions into the same department. Besides departmentalization by functions, it is possible to departmentalize by process and equipment, geographical (territorial) lines, customers (patients), time (shift), or product. However, a composite or hybrid structure made up of several of these alternatives is most often used.

Organizing on the departmental level involves the same general steps as organizing the overall institution—that is, grouping activities or subdepartmentalizing, assigning specific tasks and duties, and delegating authority. The supervisor should supplement these steps, however, by designing an ideal organizational structure specifically for his particular department. Such

EXHIBIT 12.8
Horizontal
Chart

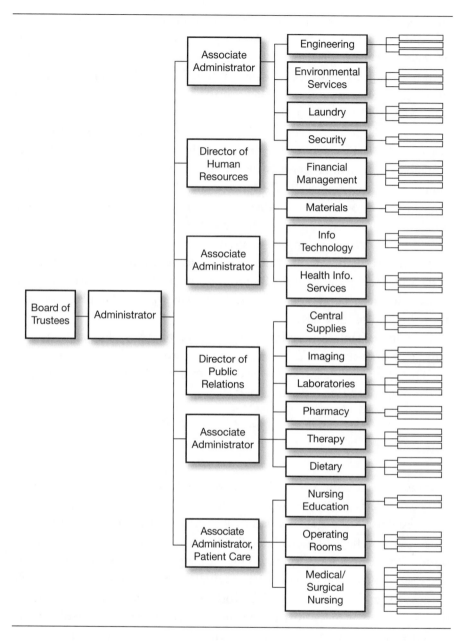

a structure represents the way the supervisor would organize the unit if starting from scratch and given ideal resources and personnel. In most cases, however, the supervisor comes into an existing department and cannot immediately implement an ideal organizational design. What must be done in that case is to plan changes or completely reorganize the department to make it come closer to the ideal. Such reorganization is a normal and important part of managerial life; however, it should not be done so frequently that it undermines the security and morale of employees. Organizational changes

EXHIBIT 12.9
Circular Chart

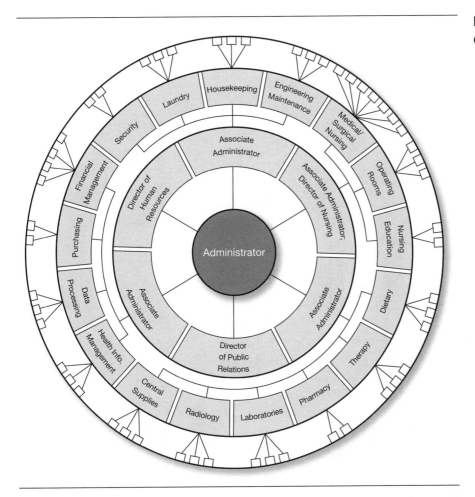

can be implemented either all at once or gradually, depending on the imminence of the need for them.

An approach that blends the functional and product organization structures is the matrix organization. This stresses horizontal relationships and combines functional and product departmentalization. Matrix design can be employed for achieving a special project with a definite result by superimposing a matrix over a traditional organizational structure. At the project's inception, the CEO or COO states the authority relationships to the project manager in charge, the functional personnel assigned to the project for the duration, and their functional department heads. This is necessary to minimize possible problems of dual command, dual allegiance, and other conflicts.

Two additional organizational approaches—mechanistic and organic—while classified as organizational structures, speak more to the culture or atmosphere established within any of the structures discussed in this chapter.

EXHIBIT 12.10 Inverted Pyramid Chart

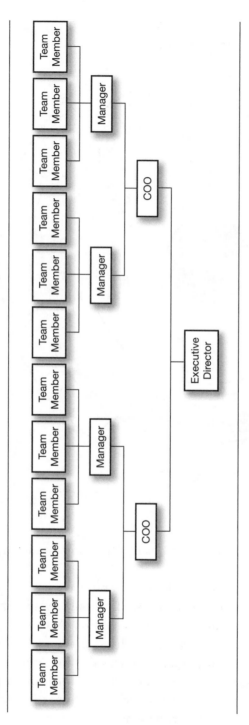

Notes

1. The term *function* in this context is used to connote organizational activities such as nursing, pharmacy, laboratories, dietetics, therapy, and environmental services rather than the basic managerial functions of planning, organizing, etc.
2. For more information on PMP certification visit www.pmi.org.

DELEGATION OF AUTHORITY

Chapter Objectives

After you have studied this chapter, you should be able to do the following:

1. Discuss authority as the lifeblood of the managerial position, and describe how the flow of authority throughout the organizational structure makes it operative.
2. Explain how delegating authority is key to creating an organization.
3. Define delegation of authority.
4. Describe the concepts of the scalar chain and unity of command.
5. Distinguish between authority and responsibility.
6. Describe the spectrum of delegation with centralization on one end and decentralization at the other end.
7. Identify some barriers to delegation.

The formal organizational structure, as stated in the previous chapter, is based on the division of labor and departmentalization. Once this has been accomplished, the second essential step for creating an organization is delegation of the organizational authority to qualified others. *Delegation* is the conferring or granting of authority from superior to subordinate to act as a representative of the superior. Authority is the lifeblood of the managerial position; without authority the manager's job is meaningless. In turn, the process of delegating authority breathes life into the organizational structure: the same process of delegation that brings authority to the manager is used to delegate it further down the line of command. As managerial responsibilities are divided, additional levels in the chain of command are created. The degree to which authority is delegated throughout the institution indicates the extent of decentralization.

The Meaning of Delegation

Delegation of authority makes the organization operative. Although the formal structure of an organization may have been meticulously designed by the administrator and carefully explained in manuals and charts, the organization

delegation of authority
The act of a superior granting authority on some level to a subordinate.

HOSPITAL LAND

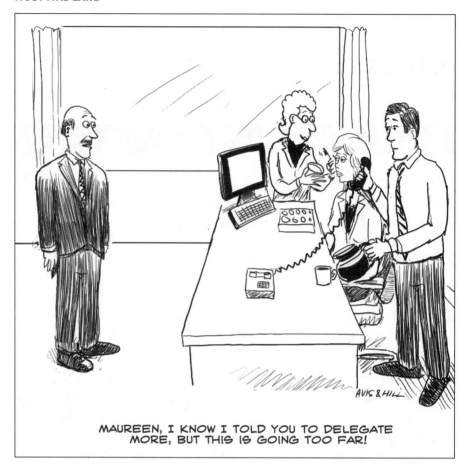

MAUREEN, I KNOW I TOLD YOU TO DELEGATE MORE, BUT THIS IS GOING TOO FAR!

still does not have life until authority is delegated throughout its entire structure. Through this process of delegation, the subordinate manager receives authority from the superior. In other words, if authority were not delegated, there would be no subordinate managers and thus no one to occupy the various levels, departments, and positions that make up the organizational structure. Only in delegating authority to subordinate managers is the organization actually created. Only with such delegation can the administration vest a subordinate with a portion of its own authority, thereby setting in motion the entire managerial process and life of the organization.

Delegation of authority, however, does not mean that the boss surrenders all of her authority. The delegating manager always retains the overall authority to perform her functions. If necessary, all or part of the authority granted to a subordinate manager can be revoked and reallocated. A good comparison can be made between delegating authority and imparting knowledge in an organization and using student teaching assistants (TAs) in college: The professor gives the TAs authority over a certain class period or lab, but ultimately the professor is still responsible for the class. If a TA fails to perform, the professor can revoke the authority.

The Scalar Chain (Chain of Command)

The line of vertical authority relationships from superior to subordinate is the **scalar chain**, or the chain of command. Through the process of delegation formal authority is distributed throughout the organization. It flows downward from the authority at the top, through the various levels of management, to the supervisor, and from there possibly to lower line supervisors. The broad authority necessary to run a private healthcare organization is usually delegated by the board of directors or trustees to the president (administrator or CEO), who in turn must delegate authority to subordinate managers (vice presidents), who then delegate authority to department directors, who then delegate to section managers, and so forth (see Exhibit 12.2).

scalar chain
The line of vertical authority relationships from superior to subordinate. Also called the *chain of command.*

An entity's organization chart should pictorially display the scalar chain so employees can see to whom each reports and from where their authority and assignments come. Solid lines typically represent line authority, while dashed or dotted lines represent staff or matrix authority (see Exhibit 12.4). Line and staff authority relationships are discussed in Chapter 14.

The chain of command must be clearly understood by every subordinate and must be closely adhered to, or the authority may be undermined. By the time the flow of authority reaches the supervisory level, it probably has narrowed considerably, thus focusing the supervisor's range of authority on the function for which he is responsible (see Exhibit 11.1). Nevertheless, it can be traced directly upward to the top executive, where authority is at its broadest scope.

Consider the following example. Most organizations have a finance division headed by the chief financial officer (CFO). This individual may have authority to sign contracts and authorize expenditures up to $500,000. The division may have several departments, including accounting, patient billing, accounts payable, cashiering, and auditing. Each department leader (manager or director) also may have contract signing privileges and expenditure authorization limits, generally at a substantially lower level, perhaps to $50,000. Amounts above $50,000 to $500,000 must be approved by the CFO, and amounts above $500,000 must be approved by her superior, the CEO. Further down the chain of command, the accounts payable clerk has no contract signing privileges nor expenditure authorization rights. Everything he processes has been authorized by someone superior in rank.

These scalar relationships are based on positional authority, as discussed in Chapter 11. They are also based on another important managerial principle—unity of command.

Unity of Command

Delegation of authority flows from a single superior to a single subordinate. Each subordinate reports and is accountable to only one superior—namely, that person from whom she receives authority. This is known as *unity of command*. A superior manager can have a number of subordinates reporting to him (span of control), but for each of these subordinates, the one-to-one relationship (unity of command) prevails.

The scalar chain provides the major route along which the process of delegation moves. Unity of command is a critical organizational concept; it enables the administration to coordinate activities, pinpoint responsibility and accountability, and define and clarify superior–subordinate relationships. Whenever the principle of unity of command is violated or compromised, management must anticipate complications; we discussed some of these in the matrix model in Chapter 12. Some potential complications include employee frustration because of conflicting directives, staff turnover, and poor employee morale.

The Process of Delegation

Every manager must be thoroughly familiar with the process of delegation.[1] It consists of three components, all of which must be present. These three components are inseparably related; a change in one of them requires an adjustment to the other two. The three essential parts of the delegating process are as follows:

1. the assignment of duties and the defining of the results expected by a manager to the immediate subordinates;
2. the granting of permission (authority) to the subordinates to make decisions and commitments, use resources, and take the actions normally necessary to perform their assigned duties; and
3. the creation of an obligation (responsibility) on the part of each subordinate to the delegating superior to perform the assigned duties satisfactorily (accountability).

Unless all three of these steps are taken, the success of the delegating process cannot be ensured. This is true no matter which level of management is doing the delegating. The chief executive officer does the initial delegation when he groups activities, sets up departments, and assigns staff their duties. All managers, from the chief executive officer down to the line supervisors, must do their part in delegating authority throughout the entire organization. The managers of each department or division must subdivide and reassign these duties within their own section, and delegate the appropriate amount of

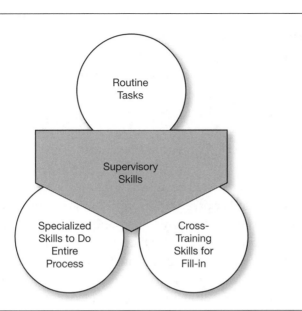

Exhibit 13.1
Delegation
Options

authority and responsibility to carry them out. Whether it is the chief executive officer who delegates authority to the vice presidents or associate administrators and directors, or the line supervisor who delegates authority to a team of non-managerial subordinates, the steps in the process of delegation are the same.

Delegation of Authority on the Supervisory Level

Once a supervisor has organized or reorganized the department's structure, or at least planned the changes that are needed and recorded them in an ideal organizational design or position description, she is ready to delegate or re-delegate authority in accordance with the organizational structure. We assume that the supervisor has been given sufficient authority and that she is in charge of all the activities within her section. Just as other managers, supervisors must delegate some of their authority. If this is not done, an organization has not been created. Specifically, the supervisor must assign tasks, grant authority to those assigned to perform the tasks, and create responsibility within each of the subunits and for each of the positions in the department.

In assigning duties, the supervisor determines how the work in the department is to be divided among the subordinates and the supervisor. All the tasks that must be accomplished in the department are considered; the supervisor decides which ones he can assign or delegate to a subordinate and which he must do (see Exhibit 13.1).

    First, the supervisor should assign routine duties that can be done by any subordinate. Second, he should assign duties that require special knowledge to those subordinates who are particularly qualified for the tasks.

Assigning Duties

Third, the supervisor must decide which functions only he should perform. Hence, delegation is the process by which managers assign a portion of their duties and resources to perform these duties to others.

Assignments should be made on the basis of logical guidelines, rather than on personal likes and dislikes or hunch and intuition. Ensman (1999) suggests delegating by task (e.g., picking up reports), by process (e.g., reconciling inventory), and by absence (i.e., tasks individuals can do in your absence). Assigning duties logically is important because the supervisor needs to explain his delegations.

The supervisor should be able to assign work so that everybody gets a fair share and can do her part satisfactorily. To achieve this fair distribution of work, the supervisor must clearly understand the nature and the content of the work to be accomplished. Furthermore, one must be thoroughly acquainted with the capabilities of the employees. The supervisor is often inclined to assign challenging work to employees who do that work best. In the long run, however, it is advantageous to train less-capable employees so that they also can perform the more difficult jobs. By building up the strength and experience (cross training) of all the employees, the supervisor's problems of assigning various duties become simpler.

The manner and extent to which the supervisor assigns duties to the employees significantly affect the degree to which the employees respect and accept the supervisor's authority (see acceptance authority theory in Chapter 11). Recall Barnard's communication recommendation from Chapter 2, which includes four conditions that must be met for an individual to accept a directive as authoritative. First, the person must understand the communication. Second, that person must believe that what is to be done is consistent with the organization's purpose. Third, the work must be something that the person has a personal interest in. Fourth, the person must be mentally and physically able to comply with the communication. However, the first step in delegating authority is to assign certain tasks or duties to each subordinate, recognizing that some duties may be retained by the supervisor.

Granting Authority

The second essential part in the process of delegation is granting authority—that is, granting permission to make decisions and commitments, use resources, and take the actions necessary to get the job done. As pointed out earlier, duties are assigned and authority is delegated to positions within the institution rather than to people. Because these positions are staffed by people, however, one typically refers to delegating authority to subordinates instead of to subordinate positions.

To be more specific, granting authority means that a supervisor confers on the subordinates the right and power to act and make decisions within a predetermined and limited area. The manager always must determine in advance the scope of authority that is to be delegated. The range of delegated authority is usually specific when a task is routine and more general when the task is less formalized. For example, the lab transporter has been assigned the job of picking up specimens from each of the physician offices in the medical office building. This is a routine task, and his authority is specific: He has authority over his own schedule and route, as long as he gets the specimens to the lab within two hours of collection. In contrast, the office manager's task is to run the office. This is a general task, and she has broad authority to make decisions regarding the operation of the office.

How much authority can be delegated depends on the amount of authority that the delegating manager possesses and on the type of job to be done. Generally, enough authority must be granted to the subordinate to perform the task adequately and successfully. There is no need for the degree of authority to be greater than necessary, but it must be sufficient to get the job done. If employees are expected to fulfill the tasks assigned to them and make reasonable decisions for themselves within this area, they must have enough authority to perform.

The degree of authority delegated is intrinsically related not only to the duties assigned but also to the results expected. Whenever management delegates authority, it is necessary to inform the subordinate of the expected results. For example, the employee should know what the superior expects, when he expects it, how much is expected, in what condition or format, and what resources may be available for her to complete the project. Good managers do not expect perfection on the first project. Subordinates learn from mistakes. Delegation is a process that facilitates grooming. **Grooming** is the process of preparing another individual to take on more authority and responsibility. Grooming also takes time.

grooming
The process of preparing another individual to take on more authority and responsibility.

If a supervisor is taking over an existing department consisting of a large number of employees, broad delegation of authority probably is in effect. It still is necessary, however, to check carefully whether the level of authority latitude is consistent with the ideal organizational plans. The supervisor should check the amount and type of authority delegated to each position and whether the three essential steps in the process of delegation were followed.

The supervisor must be specific in telling each employee what authority she has and what results are expected while exercising that authority. If this is not stated clearly, the subordinate has to guess how far the authority extends, probably by trial and error. Assignments are opportunities for supervisors to groom subordinates into members of the management team. As time goes on and the subordinates demonstrate that they are appropriately utilizing their authority to make appropriate decisions, less explanation will be necessary.

On the other hand, consider the situation in which the number of employees in the supervisor's department is rather small. Such a department consists merely of a supervisor and a few (three to six) employees. The supervisor may wonder if in these circumstances it is necessary to delegate authority. The answer is yes. Even in a small department, the supervisor needs someone who can be depended on to take over if the supervisor should have to leave either temporarily or for any length of time. Even in the smallest department, there should be someone who can work as the supervisor's backup.

It is a sign of poor supervision when no one in a department can take over when the supervisor is sick or has to be away from the job. The supervisor also may miss a promotion because there is nobody to take charge of the unit. Thus, sooner or later every supervisor needs one or more backups, understudies, next-in-command, or assistants. The supervisor needs to identify potential candidates and train them. As with any other new initiative, the department manager should always discuss this intention with his immediate boss to assure her that he is planning for the future of the department. In addition, because of compensation and job description changes that may be necessary down the road, it is beneficial to involve a human resources staff person for guidance on how to incorporate expanded authority into the subordinates' position descriptions. The human resources staff experts may be able to provide guidance for the selection process and may have evaluation tools to assess subordinates' strengths for this important role.

Remember that when authority is delegated, the supervisor remains accountable for the outcome. Therefore, it is advisable for supervisors and helpful to subordinates to have checkpoints to see how an assignment or project is progressing and for them to recognize that you are holding them accountable for completing the assignment as agreed. Furthermore, the supervisor should remember that if she changes an employee's job assignment, she must check to see that the degree of authority she has given is still appropriate.

The Exception Principle

exception principle
The principle that some decisions faced by an individual are beyond his scope of authority and must be referred to his superior.

Sometimes a supervisor is confronted by a problem beyond his scope of authority. Then the **exception principle** comes into play. A problem outside a supervisor's scope of authority is an exception, and must be referred to the supervisor's delegating manager (superior). The superior must make certain that the given problem is truly an exception, because a danger exists that some subordinate managers may refer too many decisions upward that they themselves should be making. In those situations, the superior should refrain from deciding, refer the problem back to the subordinate manager, and if necessary, do some additional grooming. If the supervisor continues to avoid decisions within his scope of authority, the supervisor's authority may need to be reduced or he may need to be replaced. If it is truly an exception, however, the superior manager must make the decision.

Only One Boss

In granting authority, the principle of unity of command must be followed. Employees must be reassured that all orders and all positional authority can come only from the immediate supervisor, the only boss they have. This principle should be stressed, as situations do occur in which two superiors issue directives and delegate authority to one subordinate. Dual command is bound to lead to unsatisfactory performance by the employee, and it definitely results in confusion about lines of formal authority. The subordinate does not know which of the two "bosses" has the authority that can contribute most to her success and progress within the organization. Eventually, such a situation results in conflicts and organizational difficulties as humorously depicted in Exhibit 13.2.

As stated before, delegating authority does not mean that management has divested itself of its authority. The delegating manager still retains authority and the right to revoke whatever part of the authority he delegated to a subordinate. Occasionally, as activities change, a need arises to take a fresh look at the organization and to realign authority relationships. Managers frequently speak of reorganizing, realigning, rightsizing, and so forth. What is meant by these terms is the revoking of authority and reassignment of it elsewhere. Naturally, realignments of authority should not take place too often because frequent changes create uncertainty, which affects morale. However, periodic reviews of authority delegations are advisable and are necessary in any organization. This applies to top-level administration as well as to the lowest-level manager.

   If recentralization of authority is called for, authority must be revoked or realigned. This is a form of reorganization that presents a difficult task for

Revoking Delegated Authority

EXHIBIT 13.2
Unity of Command

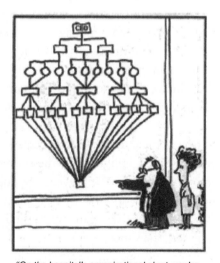

"On the hospital's organizational chart, you're right there, Mrs. Finkle. You report to everyone."

SOURCE: Reprinted with permission from *Hospitals & Health Networks*, Vol. 73, No. 10, October 1999. © 1999, by Health Forum, Inc.

the supervisor because subordinates are likely to feel suspicious, hurt, discouraged, or insecure. To mitigate these tensions, the supervisor must explain the reasons for this action. Such an unpleasant situation can be lessened by taking great care when choosing a subordinate to whom to delegate authority in the first place.

Because organizing is a dynamic process, it should be emphasized that regardless of the difficulties and unpleasant aspects involved, a supervisor must make organizational adjustments occasionally to keep the department as viable as possible.

Creating Responsibility

The third major aspect of delegating authority is creating an obligation on the part of the subordinate to perform the assigned duties satisfactorily. The *acceptance* of this obligation creates responsibility. Without responsibility, the process of delegation is not complete.

The terms *responsibility* and *authority* are closely related. Both terms are often misused and misunderstood. Although you may hear phrases such as "keeping subordinates responsible" and "delegating responsibility," these phrases do not describe the actual situation because they imply that responsibility is handed down from above, whereas it really is accepted from below.

Responsibility is the obligation accepted or agreed to by the subordinate to perform the duty as required by the superior. By accepting a job and accepting the obligation to perform the assigned tasks, an employee implies acceptance of responsibility. This responsibility cannot be arbitrarily imposed on a person; rather, it results from a mutual agreement in which the employee agrees to accomplish the duties in return for rewards. Thus, although the authority to perform duties flows from management to subordinate, the responsibility to accomplish these duties clearly flows in the opposite direction, from the subordinate to management. Once an assignment and resources are delegated to a subordinate, allow the employee to establish his or her own plan of action. This allows you to judge the employee's planning and decision-making skills.

It is essential to bear in mind, however, that responsibility, unlike authority, cannot be delegated. Responsibility cannot be shifted. Your subordinate accepts responsibility, but you still have it as well. The supervisor can assign a task and delegate the authority to perform a specific job to a subordinate. However, the supervisor does not delegate responsibility in the sense that once the duties are assigned, the supervisor is relieved of the responsibility for these tasks. A supervisor can delegate authority to a subordinate, but not responsibility. See the sidebar on the next page.

The healthcare facility administrator delegates a great deal of authority to the associate administrators for them to oversee the performance of various tasks and services. These associate administrators, in turn, delegate a large portion of their authority to the managers below them, but none of

---

Example of Delegation of Authority Versus Responsibility

The board approves funding for the renovation of an area of the hospital for a new medical staff lounge and library. The chief of the medical staff is notified of the approval. Additionally, the chairman of the board tells the CEO to proceed. The CEO accepts the authority to spend the funds authorized for this purpose.

The CEO asks the vice president of construction and design for the hospital to design the lounge and library. The vice president and CEO agree on a date when the preliminary drawing and cost estimates must be completed and presented to the medical staff.

The vice president needs the square footage and current layout of the vacated gift shop, which will be used for the new medical staff lounge and library. He asks his draftsman to measure and provide a perimeter drawing of the area. The draftsman agrees to do so, but with all the holiday activities going on around the hospital, he forgets to do it.

The vice president is unable to complete the drawings and cost estimates in time for the meeting with the medical staff. The chief of the medical staff complains to the chairman of the board.

In each step, authority has been granted and accepted. Ultimate responsibility for doing the project rests with the board, but one can be certain that others in the chain of command will be reminded of their failure to meet their obligations.

---

them delegates any responsibility. Each still accepts all the responsibility for the tasks originally assigned. Similarly, when a supervisor is called on by her boss to explain the performance within her department, she cannot plead as a defense that she delegated the responsibility for the activity to some employee. She may have delegated the authority, but she remains responsible and must answer to the boss.

Every supervisor should clearly understand this vital difference between authority and responsibility. When managers delegate the authority to do a specific job, they reduce the number of duties that they have to perform. They also conditionally divest themselves of a certain amount of authority, which can be taken back at any time if conditions are not fulfilled. In this process, however, managers do not reduce the overall amount of responsibility originally accepted. Although subordinates also accept a certain amount of responsibility for duties assigned to them, this does not in any way diminish the manager's responsibility. It does add another layer or level to the overall responsibility, thereby creating overlapping obligations. Such overlapping obligations provide double or triple insurance that a job gets done correctly and responsibly. The supervisor however is held responsible for what his subordinate fails to do.

Thus, even though responsibility is something you accept, you cannot rid yourself of it. This thought should not make you overly anxious. After all, delegations and redelegations are necessary to get the job done. Although a supervisor tries to follow the best managerial practices, she cannot be certain that each of her subordinates uses his best judgment all the time. Therefore, allowances must be made for mistakes. In evaluating her performance as a supervisor, her boss should notice how much she depends on her subordinates to get the work of the department accomplished. Although the responsibility has remained with her, her boss understands that she cannot do everything herself.

In appraising her skill as a manager, the boss considers how much care she has shown in the following areas: selecting the employees, training them, delegating appropriate levels of authority to the team members, providing constant supervision, and monitoring their activities. All these matters are taken into consideration in evaluating her ability as a supervisor.

Availability of Trained Subordinates

The process of delegation assumes that there is someone available who is willing to accept authority. Sometimes a supervisor wants to delegate more and more authority to subordinates, but no one in the department is willing or able to take on more authority. In such a case, authority, for the moment at least, cannot be delegated and must be withheld.

On the other hand, sometimes supervisors need to delegate authority even if they feel subordinates are not yet ready for it, because the subordinates will benefit from the experience. With additional experience and training, their judgment should improve and they become more capable subordinates. Although a lack of trained subordinates is often used by supervisors as an excuse for not delegating authority, they must always bear in mind that unless they begin to delegate authority and groom subordinates, no subordinate capable of being a backup and of taking over the department (if necessary) will ever be available.

It is the supervisor's duty to develop and train such a person, and in the process delegate more authority not only to the individual selected as a backup but to other employees as well. Moreover, this process of training for increased delegation gives the supervisor a much clearer view of his own duties, the workings of the department, and the various jobs to be performed. Bringing subordinates to the point at which they can be given considerable authority is a slow and tedious process, but it is worth the effort. In the early stages the degree of authority granted will be small, but as subordinates grow in their capacities, more and more authority can be delegated to them.

Selecting a Backup

The process of delegation of authority should include making one particular subordinate into an assistant for the supervisor. The role of this assistant or backup is to serve as a reserve person who is ready to support the supervisor and serve in the supervisor's absence. The first step is to select the right person for the job. The supervisor undoubtedly knows which employees are more competent and capable. These would be the employees to whom the other employees turn in case of questions and who are looked on as leaders.

Outstanding employees, moreover, know how to do their job well, are able to handle problems as they arise, and do not get into arguments. They should also have shown good judgment in the way they organize and go about their job, should be open minded, and should be interested in further development and moving into better positions. Outstanding employees must have shown a willingness to accept responsibility and must have proven dependability. Sometimes a worker may not have had the opportunity to show all these qualities. Whatever qualities have remained latent, however, show up rather quickly during the actual training process.

If the supervisor has two or three equally good employees in the department, training all of them for greater delegations of authority on an equal basis should begin. Sooner or later it becomes obvious which one has the superior ability, and this individual then becomes the major trainee for the backup position. Once the selection of a single person is made (in a large department there could be several), it is not necessary to announce this. Of course, the supervisor should discuss and explain the intentions fully to the employee chosen. More important, the supervisor must follow through by laying a thorough groundwork for good training so that chosen employee will work out as an understudy.

Training a Backup

Although the phrase *training a subordinate* is frequently used, the term *training* is really not appropriate. It would be more fitting to speak of developing, mentoring, or grooming the backup, or even self-development on the subordinate's part. Understudies must be eager to improve themselves and show the initiative to be self-starters.

The supervisor should gradually let understudies in on the workings of the department, explain some of the reports to them, and show them how needed information is obtained. The supervisor should tell them what is done with these reports and why it is done. The supervisor should also introduce an understudy to other supervisors and other people in the organization with whom they must associate; eventually the understudy should contact them herself. It is advisable to take the understudy along to some of the institution's meetings after this person has had a chance to learn the major aspects of the supervisor's job. On such occasions, the supervisor should show how the work of the department is related to that of the other departments in the healthcare facility.

As daily problems arise, the supervisor should let understudies participate in them and even try to solve some of them. By letting understudies come up with solutions to problems, the supervisor is given a chance to see how well they analyze and how much they know about making decisions. In time, the supervisor should give the understudy some areas of activity for which she will be entirely responsible. In other words, gradually more duties and authority should be assigned.

This whole process requires an atmosphere of confidence and trust. The boss must be looked on by the understudy as a coach and friend, not as a domineering superior and know-it-all. Supervisors should caution themselves that in their eagerness to develop their understudies as rapidly as possible they do not overload them or pass on problems that are beyond the understudies' capabilities. The supervisor must never lose sight of the fact that it takes time and experience to be able to handle problems of any magnitude.

All of this requires much effort and patience on the supervisor's part. With increased responsibilities, there should also be commensurate positive incentives for the backup. These may be in the form of pay increases, bonuses, a fancier title, recognized status within the organization, or other rewards of a tangible and intangible nature. Such rewards include the self-satisfaction that the subordinate feels when she is able to handle increased responsibility and is moving up in the organizational ranks. Conceivably, just about the time the understudy comes to the point of being truly helpful, she may transfer to another job outside of the supervisor's department. This may be discouraging for the moment, but the supervisor may rest assured that he has been recognized and given credit for developing a good new leader and for a training job well done.

Recognition

We have discussed how and why to delegate authority, who may be chosen to receive authority (an individual, a team, etc.), and the importance of clearly communicating expectations and periodically checking on the progress of the tasks assigned. The often forgotten step in delegation is recognizing individuals or the team for the job done and reviewing with them the work completed, including how it or the process might be improved the next time. Grooming subordinates to take on greater responsibility is a duty of every supervisor. The subordinate you assign a task to today may be your right hand tomorrow or may be able to cover for you during an emergency or a vacation. Employees want to improve. They want to feel appreciated for their efforts. A small amount of recognition goes a long way the next time an assignment is made. Personally recognizing the lab transporter discussed earlier for his ability to develop his route and schedule to get the specimens to the lab on time reinforces the transporter's decision making and the laboratory's emphasis on customer service and quality testing services.

Equality of the Three Essential Parts

Always bear in mind that the three components—duties, authority, and responsibility—must blend together to make delegation of authority a success. There must be enough authority (but not more than necessary) granted to subordinates to do the job, and the responsibility the supervisor expects them to accept cannot be greater than the area of authority she has delineated. Subordinates cannot be expected to accept responsibility for activities if they have not been handed any authority. In other words, do not try to keep your subordinates responsible for something that you have not actually delegated to them.

Inconsistencies between delegated authority, responsibility, and assigned tasks generally result in difficult and undesirable outcomes. In some organizations some of the managers have much authority delegated to them but have no particular jobs to perform; this creates misuses of authority and conflicts. Sometimes employees are put in positions in which responsibility is exacted from them when they did not have the authority to fulfill an obligation. When responsibility exceeds authority, it is nearly impossible to do the job. For example, assume you are the pharmacy director and have been granted authority to install a Pyxis system within three months. However, the chief nurse executive, chief information officer, and plant engineering director want nothing to do with the project because "their plates are full." You do not have the authority to order them to assist you because they are peers reporting to other administrators. This, too, is a most embarrassing and frustrating situation. Therefore, supervisors must make certain that the three essential elements for successful delegation are of equal magnitude and that whenever one is changed, the other two are changed simultaneously.

Some rare occasions occur when responsibility and authority are not equal and staff take action regardless. For example, in emergencies managers are often inclined and even forced to exceed their authority. One hopes this is the exception and not the normal state of affairs.

Centralization–Decentralization Continuum

As discussed earlier, delegation of authority is the key to the creation of an organization. If no authority has been delegated, one can hardly say an organization exists. Thus, from an organizational point of view, the problem is not whether to delegate or not delegate authority, but rather how much authority is delegated to middle- and lower-level managers. The question involves the degree of authority to be delegated or decentralized versus how much authority is centralized with a few individuals. Centralization and decentralization represent opposite ends of the delegation continuum.

This question about the degree of delegation is important because it determines the answer to another significant organizational question: to what extent is the organization decentralized? How much of what authority should be given to whom and for what purpose?

Variations in the extent of decentralization are innumerable, ranging from a highly centralized structure, in which the concept of an organization barely exists (such as the mechanistic model discussed in Chapter 11), to a completely decentralized organization, in which authority has been delegated to the lowest possible levels of management (as in the organic model). In the first instance, the chief executive is in close touch with all operations, makes all decisions, and gives almost all instructions. Hardly any authority has been delegated, and, strictly speaking, it cannot be said that an organization has been created. Many small enterprises regularly operate along these lines. Some small business owners or executives believe employees can never do anything as well as they can. They fear that something will go wrong or a customer will be lost if someone else takes over a job. Often, these same executives lack time for long-range planning because they are doing the work rather than delegating the work. Often such one-man shows collapse if the chief executive becomes incapacitated, dies, or for some other reason leaves the enterprise. Moreover, the same can be said for a large or physically dispersed department. A supervisor cannot single-handedly do all the work of a department, meet department goals, and focus on the objectives and action plans.

A less extreme situation is found in organizations in which authority has been delegated to a limited degree. In such organizations, the major policies and programs are decided by the top-level manager of the enterprise, and the task of applying these policies and programs to daily operations and daily planning is delegated to the first level of supervision. Few or no other levels exist between the top-level manager and the supervisors. This relatively flat organizational arrangement is often found in medium-sized enterprises. It is advantageous because it limits the number of unit managers or supervisors that the general manager must hire, thus keeping expenses down. Furthermore, the particular knowledge and good judgment the general manager possesses can be applied directly. A considerable number of enterprises have this type of organization.

At the other end of the centralization–decentralization continuum are those organizations in which authority is delegated as far down the chain of command as possible. To find out if an organization is this decentralized, one must determine the type of authority that has been delegated, how far down in the organization it has been delegated, and how consistent the delegations are. The more important the decisions made further down in the hierarchy are, the more decentralization is prevalent. The number of such decisions and the functions affected by them also serve as barometers of decentralization. Finally, the less checking that is done by upper-level management, the greater the degree of decentralization.

Most healthcare institutions probably find broad delegation of authority and decentralization advisable and necessary because of the nature of the activities involved and the skills, expertise, and expectations of the personnel. Today's better educated and more sophisticated healthcare workforce wants to use individual judgment and expects more authority and responsibility.

Achieving Delegation of Authority

Broader delegations of authority are not always easily put into practice. To be effective, a sincere desire and willingness to delegate must permeate the entire organization. Top-level management must set the mood by not only preaching but also by practicing broad delegation of authority. At times the desired degree of decentralization of authority may not be achieved. For instance, top management may find that authority has not been delegated as far down as it intended because somewhere along the line there is an "authority hoarder," a person who simply does not delegate authority any further. This person grasps all the authority delegated to him without redelegating any of it.

The Supervisor's Hesitancy to Delegate
Managers may resist further decentralization of authority for several reasons. To some, the delegation of authority may mean a loss of status (their subordinates "show them up") or a loss of power and control. Others may think that by having centralized power they are in closer contact with top-level administration. They think that they need to keep doing what got them promoted (Appold 2007). Still other managers may believe that their subordinates are already too busy to take on additional duties or are truly concerned with the expenses involved in delegating authority.

Occasionally, supervisors do not like the idea of developing an individual who could take their place, or they may be reluctant to delegate authority because they know that they cannot delegate responsibility. Because the responsibility remains with the supervisors, they may think it is best to make all decisions themselves. Thus, they overburden themselves. Their indecision and delay may often be costlier than the mistakes they hoped to avoid by retaining their authority. Always remember the likelihood exists that the supervisor may make mistakes as well. Moreover, if employees are permitted to learn from some of their own mistakes, they will be more willing to accept greater authority.

The supervisors' reluctance in delegating such authority is understandable in view of their continued accountability for the results. The traditional picture of a good supervisor was one who rolled up her sleeves and worked right alongside the employees, thus setting an example by her efforts. Such a description is particularly true of a supervisor who has come up through the ranks and for whom the supervisory position is a reward for hard work and professional or technical competence. This person has been placed in a managerial position without having been equipped to be a manager and is faced with difficult new problems. This person therefore retreats to a pattern in which she feels secure and works right alongside the employees. Occasionally such participation is needed, for example, when the job to be performed is particularly difficult or when an emergency has arisen. Under these conditions, the good supervisor is always right on the job to help. Aside from such emergencies and unusual situations, however, most of the supervisor's time should be spent carrying out the supervisory job, and the employees should be doing their assigned tasks. It is the supervisor's job not to do but to see that others get tasks done.

Frequently, however, supervisors do not trust their subordinates. They still think that if they want something done right, they have to do it themselves. Often they believe that it is easier to do the job than to correct a subordinate's mistakes. Even if the supervisor lets the subordinate do it, the supervisor may feel a strong temptation to correct any mistakes rather than explain to the subordinate what should have been done. It is frequently more difficult to teach than to do a job oneself. Moreover, supervisors often believe that they can do the job better than any of their subordinates, and they are probably right. Sooner or later, however, they have to get used to the idea that someone else can do the job almost as well as they can, and at that point they should delegate the necessary authority.

There are several ways to cope with this problem and to achieve the degree of decentralization that is desired by top-level administration. As stated before, the entire managerial group must be indoctrinated with the philosophy of decentralization of authority. They must understand that by carefully delegating authority they do not lose status, nor do they absolve themselves of their responsibilities. One way of putting this understanding into practice is to request that each manager have a fairly large number of subordinate managers reporting to him. By stretching the span of management, the subordinate manager has no choice but to delegate authority. By delegating, they can save their own time for more important managerial jobs, such as thinking and planning. If supervisors are willing to see to it that employees become more competent with each job, their own belief and confidence in their employees' work will also grow. This mutually advantageous relationship permits the supervisor to carry out the basic underlying policy of delegating more and more authority as the employees demonstrate their capability to handle it.

Another way to achieve broader delegation of authority is for the enterprise to adopt the policy of not promoting a manager until a subordinate manager has been developed who can take over the vacated position. By doing this, the manager is encouraged to delegate as much authority as possible at an early stage. Moreover, this process creates an ideal organizational climate in which the subordinates can find maximum satisfaction for many of their most important needs. Furthermore, by delegating, the supervisor captures time to do strategic planning and achieves management's purpose of accomplishing goals through others.

Despite the fact that a certain amount of authority must be delegated to create an organization, some supervisory duties cannot be delegated. The supervisor should always apply and interpret policies, give general directions for the department, take necessary disciplinary action, and appraise and promote employees. Aside from these duties, however, their subordinates should perform most tasks by themselves.

The Reluctant Subordinate

The delegation of authority and especially the development of an understudy are two-sided relationships. Although the supervisor may be ready and willing to turn over authority, the subordinates may sometimes be reluctant to accept it. Frequently subordinates feel unsure that they can handle the job assigned to them. They may be reluctant to leave the security of their job and their coworkers. They may have failed in the past or were excessively criticized about how they approached an assignment. Some may refuse because they see no reward for taking on the additional responsibility. Still others just prefer to avoid any additional workload, risk, or confrontation with peers. Merely telling them to have more self-confidence has little effect. When these situations arise, the supervisor should spend time with the subordinate to determine the reasons for the resistance. The supervisor, as we have said, must engender the subordinate's self-confidence by carefully coaching and training the subordinate to undertake more and more difficult assignments. Only then will the subordinate be able to accept the increased responsibility that goes along with harder tasks and greater authority.

Organizational Maturity

Timing also plays a role in solving the degree of delegation problem. Although centralized authority may be the most logical organizational form to use in the early stages of an enterprise, later stages usually require the CEO to face the problem of delegating more authority and decentralizing the organization to a greater extent. Such decentralization of authority becomes necessary when centralized management finds itself so burdened with decision making that the top executives do not have enough time to perform their planning function adequately or to maintain a long-range point of view. This situation usually occurs when an organization expands. The lack of time to plan should indicate to top-level management that they should delegate authority to lower echelons. In other words, there should be a gradual development toward decentralization of authority commensurate with the growth of the enterprise.

Delegation and General Supervision

Delegation ends, in the strict sense of the word, when the level of employees who are actually doing the work is reached. When no more authority can be delegated, the question arises as to how a supervisor can effectively reap the benefits of delegation—that is, how she can take advantage of the motivating factors of delegation in the daily working situation. The answer to this question can be found at the point in the philosophy of delegation that is commonly referred to as loose, or general, supervision. General supervision is closely tied to decentralization of authority.

general supervision
Supervision that provides orders in broad terms, with the expectation that the employees will decide how to reach those goals.

General supervision means merely giving orders in broad, general terms. The supervisor, instead of watching every detail of the employee's activities, is primarily interested in the results achieved. He sets the goals and expected results but permits the subordinates to decide how to achieve these results within accepted professional standards and organizational requirements. This is referred to as team management, and it gives each employee maximum freedom within the constraints of organizational and professional standards.

Employees' Reaction to General Supervision

Most employees accept work as a part of normal, healthy life. Accordingly, most managers display the underlying managerial attitude of McGregor's Theory Y (see Chapter 20) toward their employees. Such managers understand that in their daily jobs employees seek satisfaction that wages alone cannot provide. Most employees also enjoy being their own bosses. They like a degree of freedom that allows them to make their own decisions pertaining to their work. The question arises as to whether this is possible if one works for someone else, whether such a degree of freedom can be granted to employees if they are to contribute their share toward the achievement of the enterprise's objectives. This is where the ideas of delegation of authority and general supervision can help.

The desire for freedom, for being one's own boss, can be enhanced and fulfilled by delegation of authority, which in a working situation means general supervision. In the daily work environment, this broad, general type of supervision on the employee level has the same motivating results as the delegation of formal authority throughout the managerial hierarchy.

Advantages of General Supervision

Significant advantages result from this approach to supervision. These are similar to those cited in the discussion of the process of delegation. The supervisor who learns the art of general supervision benefits by having more time to be a manager and being less mentally and physically drained. The supervisor is freed from many of the details of the work and thus has time to think, plan, organize, and control. In so doing, the supervisor is positioned to receive and handle more authority and responsibility.

Moreover, the decisions made by employees under general supervision probably are superior to those made by a harried manager trying to practice detailed supervision. The employee on the job is closest to the problem and therefore is in the best position to solve it. Furthermore, opportunities to make decisions give the employees a chance to develop their own talents and abilities and become more competent. It is always difficult for a supervisor to instruct employees on how to make decisions without letting them make them.

This leads us to the third advantage of general supervision: it enables employees to take great pride in the results of their decisions. As stated before, employees enjoy being independent. Surveys reveal that the one quality employees most admire in a supervisor is the tendency to encourage independence by delegating authority. Employees want a boss who shows them how to do a job and then trusts them enough to let them do it on their own. In this way the supervisor provides on-the-job training for them as well as a chance for better positions.

The last advantage is that general supervision creates an environment for teamwork to thrive. When employees work together to achieve a goal, they learn that they achieve more working together than alone. Camaraderie also develops. In addition, individuals who may not have been recognized by their peers in the past may surface as knowledge leaders or display leadership skills that previously were not apparent to the department manager. Thus, general supervision allows for the progress not only of supervisors but of the employees, the department, and the enterprise as a whole.

Much more is said about general supervision in the discussion of the managerial function of influencing. Briefly, practicing the general approach to supervision (instead of an autocratic, dictatorial, and detailed approach) provides much of the satisfaction employees seek on the job, which money alone does not provide. Because this approach fulfills many of their needs, employees are motivated to put forth their best efforts in achieving the enterprise's objectives.

Advantages and Disadvantages of Delegation

Delegating and decentralizing authority provide numerous advantages, which become even more important as the enterprise grows. By delegating authority, the senior manager is relieved of much time-consuming detail work and subordinates can make decisions without waiting for approval. This increases flexibility and permits more prompt action. In addition, delegation of decision-making authority may actually produce better decisions because the team leader on the job usually knows more pertinent factors than the higher-up manager. Delegation to the lower levels also increases morale, interest, and enthusiasm for the work. It provides a good training ground and helps identify up-and-coming leaders. As Andrew Carnegie once said, "The secret of success is not in doing your own work but in recognizing the right man to do it" (Allen 2000). All these advantages serve to make the organization more democratic and more responsive to the needs and ideas of its employees, which ultimately results in delivery of better patient care.

Some disadvantages to extensive delegation also may arise. For example, the supervisor of a department may believe that she no longer needs the help of upper-level managers and can develop her own supporting services, known as "building an empire." This could easily lead to duplication of effort. Another disadvantage could be a possible loss of control, although the delegating manager can take steps to see that this does not happen. In most situations, however, the advantages of broad delegation far outweigh the disadvantages.

As stated before, the environment and contingencies of healthcare institutions are such that to deliver the best possible patient care, authority must be delegated broadly. Finding the proper degree of decentralization is important. Remember, no two departments are alike. Each has its own tradition, history, problems, challenges, workforce, and environment to integrate into an organizational structure. This is an ongoing process. One must constantly monitor and adjust the degrees of delegation and decentralization as the environment and the institution change.

Summary

In earlier chapters we defined authority as the power that makes the managerial job a reality. Authority is the lifeblood of the managerial position, and the process of delegation of authority breathes life into the organizational structure. Good managers must know how to use formal authority and how to delegate it to their subordinates. Through the process of delegating authority, management creates the organization. This process of delegation is made up of three essential parts: allocating or assigning a job or duty, granting authority, and creating responsibility. All three are inseparably related, and a change in one necessitates a change in the other two.

Managers can delegate authority, but they cannot delegate responsibility. Delegation does not relieve the manager from ensuring the work or task is being accomplished. Thus, the manager must clarify the expectations, define the subordinate's range of discretion, monitor its progress, hold the individual accountable for results, and recognize the subordinate for his performance. At all times, authority should equal responsibility. An imbalance may result in the task being left undone. When positions and position holders change, authority may need to be realigned or withdrawn. Finally, as mentioned in Chapter 12, supervisors should avoid making decisions for the subordinates to whom they have delegated authority. The subordinates need to plan and execute the assignments they accepted.

This process of delegation is the only way to create an operative organization. Thus, the question is not whether top-level management delegates authority, but rather how much or how little authority it delegates. An authority centralization–decentralization continuum exists in all organizations. If authority is delegated freely to the lowest levels of supervision, the organization is highly decentralized. If most authority is in the hands of higher-level managers, the organization is highly centralized. Although centralization might be appropriate when an enterprise is just getting started, far greater advantages arise from decentralization, or broad delegation of authority.

In a large- or medium-sized department, the process of delegation is similar to the one outlined in this chapter—assigning duties, granting the authority to carry them out, and encouraging employees to accept responsibility for them. In a small department, the delegation of authority takes the form of developing an understudy who can take over when the supervisor is not there. This is a long and tedious process because it involves careful development and progressively increasing delegations of authority. It is well worth the effort, as it contributes to high motivation and morale among employees. Moreover, unless the supervisor trains someone to be the backup and grants authority to that person, the department is bound to collapse if the supervisor is absent for any length of time or leaves the organization.

This decentralization of authority is not as easily achieved as it might seem. Management frequently runs into obstacles that must be overcome to achieve broad delegation. These obstacles may be caused by an authority hoarder somewhere down the line, a subordinate's reluctance to shoulder authority and responsibility, or the unavailability of suitable subordinates to whom authority can be delegated. Encouraging general supervision fosters an environment of decentralized authority.

At some point in the organization, further delegation of authority is not possible. This is at the interface between the supervisor and nonmanagerial employees as they go about performing their daily tasks. At this level, delegation of authority expresses itself in the practice of general supervision, which involves giving employees a great amount of freedom in making decisions and determining how to do their jobs. Such general supervision is probably the best way to motivate employees, whereas dependence on the sheer weight of authority normally brings about the least desirable results. Occasionally the manager must fall back on formal authority, but with the newer attitudes and expectations of our society, the general trend is toward more freedom and self-determination in management as well as in other aspects of life.

Note

1. A terminology change is occurring in the United States. Rather than using the term *delegation*, some organizations have adopted the term *empowerment*. The meaning is the same—you are empowering your subordinates to make decisions and to act.

Additional Readings

Chang, M. H. 2006. "Decentralization." Department of Economics, Cleveland State University. [Online information; retrieved 2/22/09.] http://academic.csuohio. edu/changm/main/research/papers/Decentralization_9.8.06.pdf.

Redding, W. 2008. "Big Vision, Local Focus." *Assisted Living Executive* 15 (8): 10–14.

PROCESS OF REORGANIZATION AND TOOLS TO IMPROVE THE PROCESS

Special thanks for their contributions to this chapter to Robert Sutter, RN, MBA, MHA, Six Sigma Master Black Belt, of Six Sigma Academy, Arizona, and Michael Troncone, MPH, FACHE, administrator, Calvary Hospital, New York, and principal, Michael T. Troncone & Associates, New Jersey.

Chapter Objectives

After you have studied this chapter, you should be able to do the following:

1. Discuss why organizations must reorganize.
2. Define reorganization and reengineering.
3. Review the various approaches available for organizing and reorganizing.
4. Distinguish between job design, job redesign, job rotation, job enrichment, and job enlargement.
5. Discuss approaches to quality and process improvement.

Previous chapters have discussed the fundamentals of organizing and how one departmentalizes within an entire healthcare organization as well as subdividing within a department. However, once organized, one should not assume that the structure will remain static. External and internal events may trigger the need to make modifications to the organization, a function known as *reorganization*. An example of an external event affecting an organization would be staff layoffs compelled by a decrease in hospital volume caused by the departure of a major employer near the hospital. Similarly, internal initiatives to improve processes and services may cause management to realign staff, positions, and authority. These internal initiatives often are driven by quality improvement activities, which will be discussed in this chapter.

Alfred Chandler (1962) did the original work on the strategy–structure relationship. His finding that *structure followed strategy* demonstrated that as organizations change their strategies, they must change their structure to support that strategy. Throughout Part IV of the book we discuss the executive's and the supervisor's roles in organizing staff, equipment, supplies, and other resources to achieve the goals of the entity. One must keep in mind that organizational structure is not static; its shape and needs change. For this reason, the manager's organizing function is constant; checking, questioning, and appraising the soundness and feasibility of the departmental structure are ongoing processes. The process improvement approaches discussed in this chapter will assist you in these endeavors. After all, organization is not an end in itself, but rather a means to an end—the accomplishment of the objectives of the department. A manager must be on the lookout for new developments, practices, and thinking in the field of organizing. The supervisor must be willing to reorganize the department if developments warrant it, if it is indicated that the existing structure does not permit effective and efficient functioning, or if it is apparent that the services or products being produced are defective.

The term reorganization has many connotations. In this discussion, the term refers to changes in the organizational structure, departmentalization, the assignment of activities, or authority relationships. From time to time, a manager makes such changes because of scientific and technological advances, the dynamic and changing nature of the department's activities, financial needs, or a change in supervisors. As noted previously, reorganization also may be necessary to overcome existing deficiencies. When supervisors study those deficiencies, they use a variety of tools to improve the processes of the department and organization. Often reorganization is closely aligned with reengineering and process improvement activities such as Six Sigma. Occasionally, it is confused with downsizing and rightsizing, driven by cost reduction.

In an effort to prepare for the future, improve patient care, meet regulatory demands, and reduce operating costs, healthcare organizations have concluded that they must replace labor-intensive manual efforts with technology-assisted alternatives such as implementing electronic health records (EHR) and computerized physician order entry (CPOE) applications. This trend toward more computerization will require a change in staff skills. With technology that permits clinical services to be performed, interpreted, documented, and monitored remotely, such as Picture Archiving and Communications System (PACS), robotics for diagnostic and surgical services, smart toilets,[1] and remote heart monitoring, there will be more healthcare workers and physicians working remotely or telecommuting, and using less space onsite at the healthcare entity. Healthcare organizations will need to reorganize or restructure to accommodate the advanced and modified services, establish opportunities for existing staff to gain new skills, and acclimate to the nontraditional staffing patterns that will result from having some staff that remain onsite at the bedside of the patient and some who serve the organization and patients from a distance. In addition, these technologies will affect the levels of staffing and skills required. EHRs will eliminate the need for clerical staff who now file or courier the record; laboratory staff who process samples may find their jobs changing as more technology, such as smart toilets and glucose monitoring units, are managed by the patient; and specialists will use robots to visit their patients so that they can "see" more patients in a given day. There are many tools available to organizations and their management teams to orchestrate the restructuring caused by these changes.

Reorganization Concepts and Tools

Two closely associated terms are **reengineering** and **Six Sigma**. Historically, reengineering has had a negative connotation as a harsh cost-cutting organizing approach. Yet when used properly, reengineering will reduce waste and improve services. Reengineering was introduced in the 1990s. According to Michael Hammer, "the simplest way to define reengineering is to say it means taking a 'clean sheet' approach to forget how you've done things in the past and to ask what's the very best way to get your work done. It's about rethinking how you do your work, working backwards from what customers need and then determining what's required to deliver it." Hammer contends that the concept has nothing to do with profit and loss, and it is not about buying and selling, merging, or divesting: "It's about serving customers' needs" (Deloitte & Touche 1996a).

With today's spotlight on implementing and expanding the use of EHRs to improve patient care, many healthcare organizations are to some degree performing reengineering endeavors. Using information technology to improve performance, cut costs, and deliver better patient care is a worthy project for any organization. EHRs will reinvent the way many processes in healthcare get done.

The increased focus on patient safety has caused healthcare organizations to examine their services, structure, and processes with a single goal in mind—to eliminate errors. Six Sigma is a combination of reengineering principles and quality improvement approaches that focus on delivering defect-free services and products. Six Sigma was developed by Motorola in the 1980s and subsequently has been used at many healthcare systems. "Six Sigma is a management method that addresses error prevention, problem solving, problem detection, and managed change. Six Sigma uses a collection of management practices to achieve its specified goal to achieve defect-free processes and decrease variation in services offered" (Barry, Murcko, and Brubaker 2002, 7; Woodard 2005).

Thus far we have identified the wave of transition to greater computerization of clinical documentation and processes, the need for different skills, and an approach to eliminate defects or reduce waste. These three initiatives are consistent with the Institute for Healthcare Improvement's charge to healthcare leaders to focus on the basics: "At the heart of sustaining better healthcare are three inextricably linked aims: a) reducing the burden of illness for individuals and populations; b) improving system quality, safety and value; and c) developing and maintaining a lifetime of professional competence,

reengineering
A reorganization process in which leadership determines the best way to accomplish its tasks, regardless of how those tasks were accomplished in the past.

Six Sigma
A combination of reengineering principles and quality improvement approaches that focuses on delivering defect-free services and products.

HOSPITAL LAND

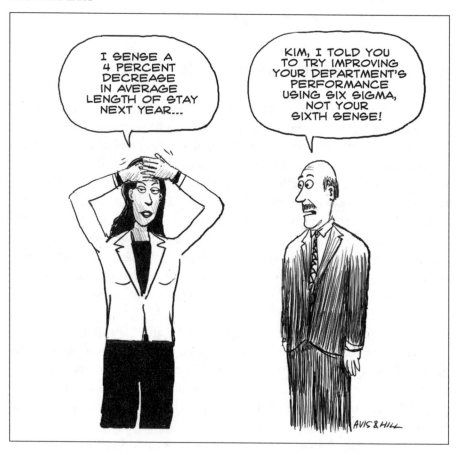

pride and joy in daily work" (Bataldan, Leach, and Ogrine 2009). Using these principles during troubling economic times and during times of dramatic change—such as that resulting from the pervasive and significant technology changes we have discussed—requires healthcare executives to think clearly and decisively to focus on the basics, reduce waste, add value in clinical care, and enable continual change (Bataldan, Leach, and Ogrine 2009). Doing so will result in reorganization.

In Chapter 2, we discussed the early theorists who focused on production improvement techniques during the scientific management era from 1890 through 1940. Additionally, we have said that supervisors should seek the input of their staffs for ideas to improve processes and the environment in which they work. Supervisors were encouraged to involve their staffs as early as the 1950s with the human resources school of management. Process or quality improvement approaches have attempted to merge the scientific management school with the human resources school.

Quality improvement programs are also known as total quality management, total quality control (Feigenbaum's term) (Nielsen et al. 2004), continuous quality improvement, companywide quality control (Ishikawa's term), Little Q and Big Q (Juran's terms), performance or process improvement, zero defects (Crosby's term) (Nielsen et al. 2004), quality circles, and multiple variations of these terms. Quality improvement is the practice of monitoring activities, identifying variations from expected outcomes, establishing corrective actions, and assessing whether the actions have corrected the variation. There is interdependence and overlap in the three reorganizing concepts of reengineering, Six Sigma, and quality improvement. Regardless of the trigger for reorganization, be it driven by the economy, regulation, technology, growth, or otherwise, the supervisor needs to understand the fundamentals for reorganizing the department or function. The quality and reengineering tools discussed above are instrumental to that task.

Reorganization Vocabulary

To help you through the reorganization effort, the following are some terms that describe activities and components of the reorganization process.

- *Job design* is the process managers complete to define the specific tasks, methods, and relationship of a given job or position to others in the organization. When a supervisor is first setting up a department or planning for a new function, job design is essential.
- *Job redesign* is the process by which the manager reviews the various tasks assigned to a job or position and alters the assignments to improve productivity, enhance quality, or enrich the employee's work experience. This is one reorganizing approach.
- *Job rotation* is an enlargement technique whereby employees periodically move from one job to another, thus expanding their skills and comprehension of the entire process.
- *Job enlargement* is a method used in redesigning the job by adding variety to it through more tasks of a similar nature.
- *Job enrichment* is similar to job enlargement in that it is a method used to redesign jobs. However, in the process of doing so, the employee is allowed more participation in decision making by increasing the depth of the employee's authority and adding a variety of tasks to the job.
- *Work redesign* focuses on the work itself—what is being done and how it is being done. The idea is to identify and eliminate duplication, waste, and process steps that do not add value. Organizations may be able to combine functions, merge units, redesign jobs, streamline processes, and/or eliminate organizational layers (bureaucracy) as a result of such efforts (Thomas 2002).

Each of the above tools evaluates jobs. Do not allow the redesign activity to become too complex or it will overwhelm you (Exhibit 14.1).

EXHIBIT 14.1

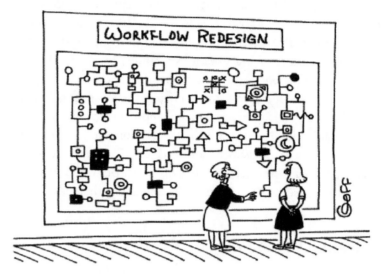

"And this is where our ED workflow redesign team went insane."

SOURCE: Reprinted with permission from *Hospitals & Health Networks*, September 2004, © 2004, by Health Forum, Inc.

However, recognize that every job does contribute to a process. For the reorganization process to effectively and efficiently use the resources (manpower, money, equipment, and materials) allocated, the supervisor must monitor the process changes to ensure that services and products being produced are at a quality level acceptable to the organization and the customer and, when necessary, to tweak the processes or organizational structure to achieve the goals of the organization. This tweaking may require reorganizing resources. When doing so, the supervisor reviews and possibly adjusts the authority he or she has granted to subordinates to ensure they have sufficient freedom to act to achieve the department's objectives.

The Supervisor's Role in Quality Management[2]

All managers are responsible for ensuring the quality of the product or service they oversee. The manager must continuously assess the performance of the operation within his span of control and maintain or improve its outcome. This is accomplished through others. The manager must monitor, motivate, and communicate with subordinates, peers, and superiors—team members who participate in the quality management process.

The customers, persons, or departments dependent on the manager's unit for their own satisfaction help the manager set the performance expectations necessary to achieve satisfactory results. Customers may be internal—other units of the organization—or external—the patients, families, and public the organization serves.

What Is Quality?

Many experts have attempted to define *quality*. While definitions vary, there are three standard levels of quality that are accepted today. At the most basic level is **conformance quality**. For the supervisor, this means ensuring that the outcomes of the work they oversee meet the minimum standard set by the organization. For instance, the new medical records supervisor may be responsible for ensuring that a given number of charts are coded each day or that the records are filed correctly. Conformance is the act of doing the right thing.

conformance quality
A level of work outcome that meets the minimum standard.

The second level of quality is often called **requirements quality**. At this level, the supervisor is responsible for meeting customer expectations. Every supervisor has a number of customers—their employees, the departments they interact with, and so forth. When a supervisor ensures requirements quality, she is perceived as running a good department.

requirements quality
A level of work outcome that meets customer expectations.

The highest level of quality is **quality of kind**. This means providing a service that exceeds customer expectations or that delights the customer. This is the quality that Deming (1986) alludes to when he defines quality as "pride of workmanship."

quality of kind
A level of work outcome that exceeds customer expectations.

Approaches to Quality

To achieve quality of kind, the supervisor must be familiar with and practice ongoing performance improvement techniques, both to motivate employees and to continuously improve the work product. Many of today's organizational approaches to quality are based on *DMAIR—Design, Measure, Assess, Improve, Redesign*. This process defines the continuous cycle of quality improvement. Its elements are as follows:

1. *Design*. The first step in improving any process is to understand its design. Questions to ask are
   - What is the purpose of the process? What is its objective?
   - Who is involved in the process?
   - What are the steps of the process? (These should be defined at the most basic level. Flowcharts are an excellent method to identify redundancies or inefficiencies in the process.)

2. *Measure.* "You can't manage what you don't measure" is an oft-quoted phrase. To obtain baseline measurement, questions to ask are
   - What parts of the process are being measured?
   - What parts of the process should be measured based on its design and the desired outcome?
   - Are the results satisfactory, or is there a need for improvement?
3. *Assess.* When the design of the process is understood and measurement results have been obtained, it is necessary to ask
   - Is the process efficient? Are there redundancies, extra or duplicate steps, inefficiencies, or unnecessary steps?
   - Can the results be improved?
4. *Improve.* Based on the assessment, changes to the process can be identified to improve the end result.
5. *Redesign.* As the improvements are implemented, two important steps must be taken:
   - Define the redesigned process and communicate it to all parties involved.
   - Establish measures to ensure that the improvements accomplish what was intended.

The Six Sigma approach to quality is quite similar to the DMAIR approach. Its steps are *DMAIC—Define, Measure, Analyze, Improve, and Control.* While the methodology calls for a rigorous, scientific approach to statistical analysis, the fundamental cycle of quality is quite similar. (Read more discussion of Six Sigma later in this chapter.)

However, an approach without a commitment from the workforce to achieve a quality-striving environment will not be successful. At Bronson Methodist Hospital in Kalamazoo, Michigan, employee understanding of and commitment to the strategic plan for clinical excellence, customer service excellence, and corporate effectiveness are the bases of individual and departmental goals (AHA-McKesson 2009).

Quality Improvement Teams

In the Word Web Online dictionary (2006), the primary definition of a *team* is a "cooperative unit." Each member of the quality improvement team (QIT) has a defined role in the performance improvement process. The manager may be called on to serve in any one of these roles:

- *Team leader.* The team leader is the owner of the performance improvement project under study and leads the team through the DMAIR or DMAIC process. The leader works closely with the facilitator to plan the work of the team. He must start meetings on time, assign roles and responsibilities, ensure that work is evenly distributed, ensure that everyone has an opportunity to participate, ensure accurate record keeping, and ensure that all tasks are accomplished.

- *Facilitator.* The facilitator is responsible for keeping the team on track by keeping time and ensuring that each topic is covered as laid out in the work plan.
- *Team member.* Team members are chosen because they are associated with the process under study, either as participants or customers, or because of their knowledge of the process. They must support the work of the team and support its recommendations throughout the organization.
- *Recorder.* The recorder is often a rotating role and is responsible for keeping an accurate record of the team's proceedings.
- *Consultant.* A consultant is an invited guest. She does not need to attend every meeting of the team but may be called on when her particular expertise is needed.
- *Team champion.* The team champion is a senior leader who has the authority to support the work of the team and ensure that the team receives resources and support needed.

In addition to utilizing the formally structured quality improvement team as suggested by the contributing author, Michael Troncone, there are other methods to gain employee participation at any level of the organization.

The *quality circle*, sometimes called the quality control circle (QCC) or do-it group (DIG) (see Exhibit 14.2), is a method of increasing employee participation in the daily work routine. The underlying ideas of this approach are derived from the work of McGregor, Maslow, Herzberg, Deming, Drucker, Sherman,[3] and others; the first practical applications of the quality circle were made in Japanese industries. The resulting Japanese management technique claims much credit for high levels of productivity, quality, and worker satisfaction. As performance and process improvement activities are part of the mainstream in healthcare institutions, both formal and informal process improvement techniques are being used to raise awareness at all levels of the organizations. Recognizing that healthcare delivery "takes a village," few healthcare professionals can do their jobs without relying on support from other individuals or teams (Scott 2009) to meet the organization's goals and maintain a safe environment for patients and staff.

In some settings, employees may recommend the establishment of a quality improvement task force. These members volunteer to meet regularly to discuss work, work processes, and quantity- and quality-related problems and to stimulate innovation. The task force is either assigned a project to assess or is asked to identify problems, isolate the causes, and develop practical solutions or more effective methods to ensure that the work is accomplished error free the first time. The supervisor may act as the facilitator of this group,

Exhibit 14.2

Do-It-Group
Establishment
Form

This DIG is __ intradepartmental (within 1 department) or __ interdepartmental (more than 1 department).

_____   _____   _____
Employee's Name   Department   Extension

We are looking for ways to improve what we do. We do that by offering suggestions and establishing DIGs to make our ideas work. A DIG idea may be started by anyone. If you have an idea or have identified a problem and would like to have a DIG created, complete this form. Discuss the idea or problem with your supervisor. Drop this completed form in the DIG Box next to the ATM machine.

Is this an idea? ____, or is this a problem ____?

(1) If this is an idea, please tell us more about it: _____

_____

_____

If this is a problem, tell us more: What is the problem? _____

_____

(2) Where is it located?_____

(3) When does it occur?_____

(4) Whom does it affect?_____

(5) How big is the problem? _____

(6) What do you think causes the problem?_____

Have you had DIG training? _____ Have you participated in a DIG before? _____ Have you ever been a DIG Chairman? _____ Will you join this DIG committee? _____ Will you chair this DIG? _____

If this problem is fixed or idea is implemented it will improve:
Customer satisfaction _____ Quality _____ Productivity _____ Organization _____
Finances _____ People skills _____ Other: _____

Supervisor's initials:_____ Date: _____

SOURCE: Adapted with permission from DIG Creation Form from Fayette Memorial Hospital, Connersville, IN.

but often a worker or individual from outside the work team serves in this capacity or in the role of team leader.

Usually the improvement team leader is first exposed to some basic training course in group dynamics, problem solving, and similar techniques.

The members are often given some training in problem-solving techniques, establishing priorities, brainstorming, and so forth. Because there are improvement opportunities or ideas to explore in any organization, the team may apply the Pareto Principle to determine which problems to solve and in what order (Spath 2001). The **Pareto Principle**, also known as the 80/20 rule, states that 80 percent of the results are caused by 20 percent of the causes. For example, the principle could be any of the following:

Pareto Principle
The principle that states that 80 percent of results are caused by 20 percent of causes.

- 80 percent of the ICU days are consumed by 20 percent of the patients treated in the hospital.
- 80 percent of the tardiness in a department is caused by 20 percent of the department employees.
- 80 percent of the needle sticks occur in 20 percent of the areas.

The thought underlying the use of an improvement team is to tap the minds of an organization's own workforce, realizing that the employees doing the job often know best why productivity may be hindered, why patient satisfaction is lower than desired, and why product quality is poor. Often they have excellent ideas and answers. These ideas may surface through the use of formal or informal team sessions coupled with an approach called brainstorming. Successful *brainstorming* sessions follow certain ground rules: (1) ignore the hierarchy (rank does not count); (2) suspend judgment (make it clear that ideas are being gathered); (3) encourage quantity, not quality (get as many ideas on the table as possible); (4) nurture a no-limits session (ask questions such as, "what would our competitor do in this case?"); and (5) don't rush (do not set a fixed time, serve refreshments, and so on) (*Journal of Accountancy* 2000). These brainstorming ideas and solutions are then presented to management or a performance improvement (PI) steering committee.

The QIT, QCC, or DIG fits into the existing organizational structures, following the existing channels of communication and authority. Because improvement teams are an application of participative management, the concept can be introduced with success into any organization in which administration's philosophy has been democratic, open, and participative. It is unlikely that these teams would produce results in an environment that practices autocratic and highly centralized management. The success of these teams is dependent on the recognition and support given by executive leadership. Winners of the prestigious Malcolm Baldrige Award and other similar awards attribute their success to an enveloping culture communicated and modeled by top management that stresses a belief that the organization can continuously improve the quality of its services through teamwork (NIST 2009).

The improvement team or task force may be empowered to implement their recommendations without a presentation to management (recall our discussion of decentralized authority in Chapter 13). In a quality-driven environment, much like that found in the culture of Japanese industries, total trust exists between management and employees. Employees are encouraged to make changes and test their hypotheses of improving processes and output without fear of management repercussion. The employees are empowered to make decisions about their work environments and are rewarded for taking the initiative. Management serves as coach and facilitator of the brainstorming effort. This type of managerial attitude develops over time and creates a culture of mutual trust and freedom of communication in a facility. This cultural style is more closely identified with the Theory Z philosophy. *Theory Z* is fairly new in healthcare, and the management culture it requires is different from that in most businesses in the United States; because of our litigious and rule-based environment, the likelihood that administrative oversight—even at the department level—will lessen to allow a Z-type environment to fully flourish in healthcare is unlikely in the near future.

One approach to help staff deal with redesigning a process is demonstrated in the chart developed by SSM HealthCare System (see Exhibit 14.3). This approach is used when a process or procedure for doing something, such as registering a patient for treatment, becomes so cumbersome or error prone that it needs streamlining.

Preparation of staff to participate in performance improvement teams may consume some productive time, but it must occur to make the process successful. All team members, whether they serve on the steering committee or the team assessing an opportunity to improve, must have a common vocabulary and use tools to transform data into meaningful information. Some of the tools used are shown in exhibits 14.4 and 14.5.

The success of any process that places subordinates and supervisors together requires communication. Duke University Hospital credits communication of priorities, tactics, and results as the basis for improving quality. At Duke, performance metrics, safety events, and examination of near-misses establish a culture of open communication in which all employees understand how their behavior affects quality and safety (AHA-McKesson 2009).

When individuals are initially convened to participate in a small quality improvement team there may be hesitance to openly share organizational concerns. To encourage communication without fear of reprisal, the **nominal group technique** is practiced. This technique tries to provide a way to give everyone in the group an equal voice in problem or process identification and is discussed in greater detail in Chapter 15.

nominal group technique
A method to allow all members of a group to have equal voice in discussions.

According to Witt (1996), the key questions that should guide the team or group are as follows:

- Who is the customer in the process?
- What is the desired outcome?
- What would the process look like under ideal conditions?
- What are key points where problems have been observed in the past?

EXHIBIT 14.3 Performance Improvement Model: Process (Re)Design Approach

Team Information	① Identify Opportunity
A PLACE TO:	OBJECTIVE:
	Identify an opportunity for improvement and the reason for working on it.
• Post Team Project Planning Work Sheet. • Display team meeting minutes. • Solicit comments using self-stick notes. • Recognize individuals who provided support to team.	KEY ACTIVITIES: • Research the opportunity: —Review indicators. —Survey patients and other customers and suppliers. —Interview individuals involved in the process. • Consider patient and other customers' and suppliers' needs to help select the opportunity. • Schedule the CQI Model activities.
	CHECKPOINTS: 1. The criteria for selection were customer oriented. 2. A schedule for completing the CQI Model steps was developed.
	OUTPUTS: • Mission Statement Form. • Team Project Planning Work Sheet.
② Conceptual Design	③ Analysis
OBJECTIVE: Develop ideal process flows.	OBJECTIVE: Design the control system for the process to prevent problems from occurring.
KEY ACTIVITIES: • Design the ideal process flows. • Perform customer needs analysis to define requirements at the hand-off and interfaces in the process. • Write a clear outcome statement. • Document mutually agreed upon requirements between customers and suppliers.	KEY ACTIVITIES: • Consider potential problems. • Consider potential causes. • Develop methods for preventing potential problems. • Design a measurement system.
CHECKPOINTS: 3. The sequence of activities in the new process was documented. 4. The potential benefits of the new process were clearly identified. 5. Customers' valid requirements were identified.	CHECKPOINTS: 6. Potential causes of problems were identified and prioritized. 7. Appropriate actions were taken on major potential causes. 8. The measurement and control system is specific enough to pinpoint future problems.
OUTPUTS: • Clear outcome statement of the process. • Flowchart of the ideal process. • Valid requirements of each customer/supplier relationship in the process.	OUTPUTS: • Control system with measurable indicators.

Continued

• How can we design quality into the process, rather than inspect for it after the fact?

For the healthcare supervisor, the most challenging part of any quality improvement process is the implementation of the improvement. Six Sigma has gained momentum as an approach that speaks to each of Witt's questions.

EXHIBIT 14.3 *Continued*

④ Implement New Process	⑤ Measure Results

④ Implement New Process

OBJECTIVE:
Put the new process in place.

KEY ACTIVITIES:
• Develop an action plan that:
—Identifies who, what, when, where, and how.
—Reflects the barriers and aids needed for success.
• Obtain cooperation and approvals.
• Implement the process.
• Develop performance targets for the process.

CHECKPOINTS:
9. Action plan addressed who, what, when, where, and how.
10. Action plan reflected the barriers and aids necessary for successful implementation.
11. Cooperation of relevant managers in impacted organizations was obtained.
12. Performance goals/targets were identified.

OUTPUTS:
• Action Plan.
• Targets for measurable indicators.
• Implementation of new process.

⑤ Measure Results

OBJECTIVE:
Confirm that the process is working well and that the performance targets for the process have been met.

KEY ACTIVITIES:
• Compare results obtained to the target.
• Change the process, as necessary, if results are not satisfactory.

CHECKPOINTS:
13. Data was collected to measure performance relative to targets.
14. Results met or exceeded targets. (If not, specific follow-up as planned.)

OUTPUTS:
• Compare the results obtained to the target.
• Change the process, as necessary, if results are not satisfactory.

⑥ Standardization

OBJECTIVE:
Ensure that the process is still working and is incorporated into daily work.

KEY ACTIVITIES:
• Ensure that solutions become part of daily work:
—Create/revise standards.
• Educate employees/medical staff on the process and/or standards and explain need.
• Establish periodic checks with assigned responsibilities to monitor the new process.

CHECKPOINTS:
15. Method to ensure process becomes part of daily work was developed.
16. All impacted personnel were trained (include explanation of need).
17. Periodic checks were put in place with assigned responsibility to monitor the proposed solutions.
18. Specific areas for replication were considered.

OUTPUTS:
• Education of people.
• Incorporation into standard operating procedures.
• Replication.

⑦ Future Plans

OBJECTIVE:
Plan what to do about any remaining problems and evaluate the team's effectiveness.

KEY ACTIVITIES:
• Analyze and evaluate any remaining problems.
• Plan further actions if necessary.
• Review lessons learned related to problem-solving skills and group dynamics:
—What was done well.
—What could be improved.
—What could be done differently.

CHECKPOINTS:
19. Plan for any remaining problems was developed.
20. Applied P-D-C-A to lessons learned.

OUTPUTS:
• Plan for the future of the team.
• Evaluation of the team and its work.

SOURCE: © SSM Health Care CQI Manual, St. Louis, MO, SSM Health Care System 1990 (pp. 279–80). Reprinted with permission.

CQI Data Tools	Purpose/Description of Tool
Brainstorming 	A discussion forum used to get a group of people to quickly generate, clarify, and evaluate a number of ideas that are listed regardless of their viability to support a solution to the problem.
Cause-and-Effect Diagram (also known as the "fishbone" and Ishikawa Diagram) 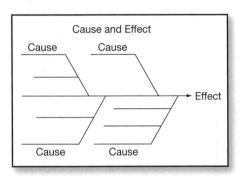	A diagram that depicts causes of a problem and attempts to narrow the problem down to the most likely, or root, cause. Contributing issues to the problem are grouped together, such as people, materials, machinery (equipment), and methods.
Flowchart or Process Diagram 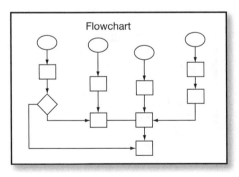	Pictorial description of the flow or steps in a process to allow visualization of the tasks. Flow charts are used to "document" a process or procedure.

Continued

Exhibit 14.4
Performance Improvement Model: Problem-Solving Approach

EXHIBIT 14.4

Continued

CQI DATA TOOLS	PURPOSE/DESCRIPTION OF TOOL

Pareto Chart (also known as 80/20 rule)

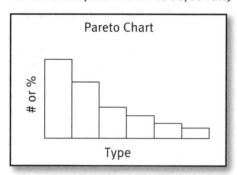

These charts are used to display data in the order of its relative importance or weight. It identifies the "few major causes" of variation from the "trivial" to many. It comes from the 80/20 theory that 80% of the results is directly related to 20% of the causes. For example, 80% of the delinquent medical records are for 20% of the physicians on the medical staff.

Run Chart (trend or line graph)

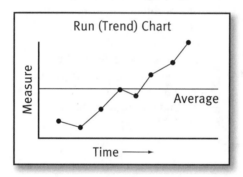

This graph shows with a single line data or results occurring at different times for a time period.

Histogram

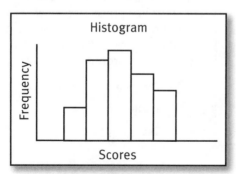

This graph, usually in bar format, displays the frequency with which something occurs. It shows a distribution that may or may not be bell shaped. It may illustrate the stability of a process.

EXHIBIT 14.4
Continued

CQI DATA TOOLS	**PURPOSE/DESCRIPTION OF TOOL**

Scatter Diagram

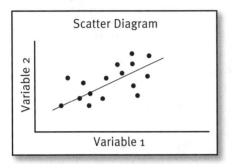

This diagram is used to demonstrate the relationship between two variables such as processing time and volume of specimens received.

Control Chart

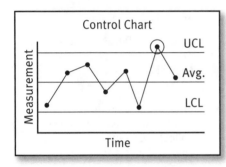

This chart reflects the tolerances of something happening within limits. Normal limits are established and concern should rise when the number of occurrences outside of the limits increases.
UCL — Upper Control Limit
LCL — Lower Control Limit

Affinity Diagram (also known as KJ Diagram and named for its founder, Kawakita Jiro)

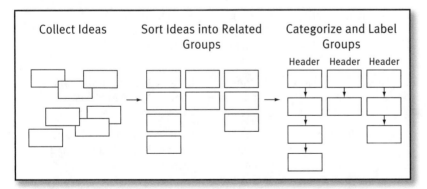

A tool used to sort large amounts of ideas or opinions gathered through brainstorming into groupings of similar ideas and then relationally into categories.

SOURCE: Adapted from *The Memory Jogger II*™ © 1994, GOAL/QPC, Methuen, MA. www.goal/qpc.com. Used with permission.

STEP	WHO	QI TOOL
1. List and Prioritize Opportunities	Steering Committee	Data Collection, Pareto Analysis, Brainstorming, Affinity Diagrams, Flowcharts, Graphs and Charts
2. Identify Customer(s) and Expectations	Steering Committee and Team	Brainstorming, Affinity Diagrams, Flowcharts, and Data Collection
3. Define Project and Team	Steering Committee	Flowcharts, Graphs and Charts
4. Formulate Theories	Steering Committee and Team	Brainstorming, Affinity Diagrams, Cause-and-Effect Diagrams, and Flowcharts
5. Test Theories	Team	Flowcharts, Data Collection, Graphs and Charts, Pareto Analysis, Histograms
6. Identify Root Cause	Team	Flowcharts, Data Collection, Graphs and Charts, Pareto Analysis, Histograms, Cause-and-Effect Diagrams
7. Identify Solutions and Control Systems	Team	Brainstorming, Affinity Diagrams, Flowcharts, Data Collection, Graphs and Charts, Cause-and-Effect Diagrams
8. Address Resistance to Change	Team	Brainstorming, Affinity Diagrams, Flowcharts, Cause-and-Effect Diagrams
9. Implement Solutions and Control Systems	Steering Committee, Team, and Others	Flowcharts, Graphs and Charts, Pareto Analysis, Histograms
10. Evaluate Performance	Steering Committee and Team	Data Collection, Graphs and Charts, Pareto Analysis, Histograms, Flowcharts
11. Standardize Process	Team, Steering Committee and Senior Management	Data Collection, Graphs and Charts, Pareto Analysis, and Histograms
12. Monitor Control Systems	Steering Committee and Senior Management	Data Collection, Graphs and Charts, Flowcharts, Pareto Analysis, Histograms

An Example of Six Sigma[4]

Six Sigma is permeating healthcare at an increasing rate. This is a favorable trend because it is a perfect fit for healthcare organizations: the methodology follows the medical model, and the healthcare industry is wrought with defects and process variation. Defects such as billing errors, postoperative infections, and unplanned readmissions are quite common in healthcare today. Also contributing to the adoption of Six Sigma is evidence that healthcare organizations have realized substantial improvements by deploying Six Sigma (Dlugacz 2004; Frankel et al. 2005; Lenaz 2004; Torres and Guo 2004; Young 2004).

Six Sigma is a systematic process improvement method that is focused on reducing process defects and variation. There are five phases associated with Six Sigma: define, measure, analyze, improve, control (DMAIC). These phases are collectively referred to as DMAIC, and as Exhibit 14.6 depicts, these five phases correspond to the medical model of diagnosis, treatment, and follow-up. In other words, dysfunctional processes are treated methodologically just like physicians treat sick patients.

Diagnosis: Define, Measure, Analyze
In the diagnosis phase, physicians conduct a history and physical as well as various diagnostic tests to determine the root cause of an illness. The define, measure, and analyze phases of Six Sigma are focused on diagnosing

MEDICAL MODEL	SIX SIGMA
• Diagnosis ⟶	• Define
— H&P	— Project Charter
— Laboratory	• Measure
— Imaging	— Process Maps
— Stress Testing	• Analyze
— Microbiology	— Regression
• Treatment ⟶	• Improve
— Medication	— Reengineer
— Surgery	— Design of Experiments
— Rehabilitation	
• Follow-Up ⟶	• Control
— Laboratory	— Control Plan
— Imaging	

EXHIBIT 14.6
Five Phases of Six Sigma
Imaging

SOURCE: Robert Sutter, RN, MBA, MHA, Six Sigma Master Black Belt.

the root cause of process defects and variation. The define phase establishes what process is to be treated and the process boundaries. Subsequently, the measure phase involves collecting data and establishing baseline performance measurements. The analyze phase identifies the root causes of dysfunctional processes through the use of various statistical methods. This rigorous use of data and statistical analysis is the hallmark of Six Sigma.

Treatment: Improve

Once a diagnosis of a patient's illness is confirmed, a physician prescribes a treatment to eradicate the cause of illness. During the improve phase of Six Sigma, methods such as reengineering and experimenting are employed to remove or fix the root causes identified in the analyze phase.

Follow Up: Control

Once a physician institutes treatment, a comparison of the patient's condition after treatment to before treatment is made to ensure that the treatment is effective and remains effective. The control phase of Six Sigma is designed to accomplish the same goal: to ensure that the process has improved and that the improvement is sustained. Six Sigma uses the control plan to achieve this objective. The control plan is a document that specifies what components of the process are measured, how they are measured, what constitutes acceptable measurements, and who is responsible for monitoring the measurements and taking action if the measurements are unacceptable.

The DMAIC methodology can be used to improve many processes in a healthcare organization just as the medical model—diagnose, treat, and followup—is used to treat virtually any illness.

Six Sigma Case Study: Thrombolytic Administration

The following is a brief description of a Six Sigma project to improve the timeliness of thrombolytic administration in patients with acute myocardial infarction in a community hospital. At the time of this project, the American College of Cardiology practice guidelines called for a thrombolytic to be administered within 30 minutes of a patient's arrival.

Define An initial meeting with the hospital's CEO, COO, and chief of the emergency department (ED) was held to garner the support of senior management and medical staff to the project. Subsequently, the problem was defined as excessive cycle time and variability associated with thrombolytic administration in the ED. The boundaries of the process were established as beginning with patient arrival to the ED and ending with thrombolytic administration in the ED. Project objectives and a multidisciplinary team of ED personnel were established.

Baseline data were collected to establish baseline performance measurements **Measure**
of door-to-needle time:

- Average (minutes): 44.3
- Standard deviation (minutes): 33.9
- Defect rate (proportion of patients with door-to-needle time = > 30 minutes): 68.75 percent

The data were then analyzed with a control chart, which revealed the process to be fairly stable. Subsequently, process mapping documented the process steps and flow as the current process is executed. Finally, a cause-and-effect diagram and a failure mode and effects analysis were conducted to identify factors that affected door-to-needle time.

The process map, cause-and-effect diagram, and failure mode and effects **Analyze**
analysis were reviewed to determine what data elements to include in the data collection plan. A data collection form and definitions were derived, and personnel from the medical records department were trained to collect the data. Variables, including age, EKG results, and the presence of chest pain, were analyzed using linear regression to ascertain which factors were statistically significant with respect to door-to-needle time.

The analysis revealed the time associated with acquiring the initial EKG was the only factor that affected door-to-needle time in a statistically significant manner. The quicker this occurred, the faster a thrombolytic was administered. None of the clinical characteristics—day of week or shift—statistically affected door-to-needle time.

Based on the results of the analyze phase, the team streamlined the process of **Improve**
acquiring the initial EKG, eliminated redundant and non-value-added process steps identified on the process map, and fixed problems ranked high on the failure modes and effects analysis. After the ED staff were trained on the new process and the process improvements were implemented, data were collected to ascertain if an improvement was realized. The results verified that the process changes were effective:

- Average (minutes): 24.8
- Standard deviation (minutes): 2.8
- Defect rate (proportion of patients with door-to-needle time = > 30 minutes): 5.0 percent

A control plan was formulated and implemented to ensure that the process **Control**
was continually monitored and that unacceptable performance was addressed immediately.

If implemented correctly, the Six Sigma methodology has repeatedly demonstrated its effectiveness in fixing myriad process problems in a variety of industries, including healthcare. However, Six Sigma is not a panacea for all of an organization's process-related problems. Instead, Six Sigma should be considered as one component of a comprehensive, integrated process management system. That is, Six Sigma should be incorporated with other process-management methods such as Malcolm Baldrige guidelines, root cause analysis, Lean manufacturing, and kaizen events. Just as a physician selects the best treatment for a patient's circumstances, an organization should choose the most appropriate process improvement method to achieve effective reorganization of its structure, processes, and services.

Six Sigma Versus Lean Versus Kaizen

Six Sigma, Lean, and kaizen are distinct process improvement tools, but they complement each other. Kaizen is a tool that works well for quick fixes, Lean often is used for simple work flows, and Six Sigma is used for more complex work flows. However, all may be used to address components of a problem.

Lean involves assessing value streams. *Value streams* are processing or work flows that deliver a service valued by a customer. An example of a value stream may be the admission of a patient. The various steps—including pre-registration data collection, pre-certification of the stay, collection of all laboratory data required for the admission, processing of the registration paperwork, and transporting the patient to the patient care area—would be studied; all should happen in a timely, accurate, and hassle-free fashion. If one of the steps is not perceived as having value, the step is considered wasteful and eligible for redesign or elimination. Assessing a wasteful step may involve kaizen or Lean tools and often requires more than a week to resolve. For Lean, or any of these process improvement tools to work, there must be a leadership mentality that supports improvement across turfs and through silos with a focus on improving the customer's experience.

kaizen (or kaizen blitz)
A Lean term for rapidly trying out improvements in processes.

Some problems can be addressed quickly by a process improvement team. These problems are sometimes called "low-lying fruit." Organizations may choose to use **kaizen** or a **kaizen blitz** to address these. Kaizen is Japanese for "improvement." During the blitz, teams test their solution or fix to a problem before agreeing upon a new process. But within a short time, usually less than a week, a new process commences. Anyone can kaizen. Employees at all levels are encouraged to identify problems that they individually or in a small team can fix, much like the DIG we discussed earlier in this chapter.

For example, on any given day a healthcare organization may receive many Fed Ex or overnight packages. Often these are shipped to the facility in this manner because the contents require expedited delivery. Let's assume that the receiving dock team is responsible for delivering these to the respective recipients but chooses to make a single delivery at 4 p.m. daily. In effect, packages that may have been delivered before 10 a.m. are now delivered six hours later. A possible quick fix would be to have the receiving dock personnel give these packages to the mailroom to place in the recipient mailboxes as soon as they arrive. Recipients would be advised to check their mailboxes at least twice a day. Problem solved. The issues addressed in a kaizen are often simple tactical problems, and empowering employees to solve these problems improves morale.

Business Knowledge Source (2010) defines the kaizen activity cycle:

- Standardize an operation.
- Measure the standardized operation.
- Gauge measurements against requirements.
- Innovate to meet requirements and increase productivity.
- Standardize the new, improved operations.
- Continue cycle *ad infinitum*.

This is also known as the Shewhart cycle (Business Knowledge Source 2010).

Toussaint (2009, 30) said "one thing is clear, after studying Lean journeys in many organizations, there is no one way to implement Lean. Lean is really about having the frontline workers design and improve the standard work. That should occur every day with real time measurement, not with control charts, but with simple hand-written performance measures done entirely by the frontline staff."

Reengineering

As the contributing author Robert Sutter noted in the section above, healthcare organizations attempt to demonstrate the results of their performance improvement efforts by pursuing such awards as the Malcolm Baldrige National Quality Award or the American Hospital Association's Quest for Quality Award or by seeking certification by demonstrating compliance with the ISO 9000-1 series of quality management system standards.[5]

Those who have implemented a reengineering process within their institution recognize the need to continuously improve. Reengineering requires you to focus on the customer's needs. By doing so, you are always looking to the customer (patient) for indicators of process modification. Once you begin reengineering, you really cannot stop. You continuously improve and inevitably reach a point when your patient requirements change. Then guess what? You will want to reengineer again, especially in healthcare, with its changing parameters and its constant reaching for better outcomes and measures (Deloitte & Touche 1996b).

Barry, Murcko, and Brubaker (2002, 8) describe the outcomes of reengineering as error-free provision of healthcare services that include:

- An organization that never makes errors has happy and loyal clientele.
- An organization that never makes errors is easy to manage.
- An organization that never makes errors has positive uses for resources.
- An organization that never makes errors attracts the best candidates for employment.
- An organization that never makes errors has peace of mind in the executive suite.

Reengineering has the potential to recreate organizations to improve quality and customer responsiveness, reduce costs, and streamline operations. It, too, relies heavily on employee teams coordinated by management to accomplish the change.

Technological, competitive, industry, and funding changes force department managers to rethink their organizational structure and work flow. When changes in the workplace occur, the administration, managers, and supervisors are called on to initiate programs that redefine the organizational structure, reporting relationships, chain of command, and processes throughout the organization.

Reorganization may take place to overcome existing deficiencies. For example, in the past, many nurses found themselves burdened with too much clerical work that kept them away from actual patient care and bedside nursing. This was an undesirable situation because the thrust of their education and purpose was the care of patients. Eventually, it became apparent that many of these functions could just as effectively be performed by someone without a nursing degree. This led to a job redesign and enlargement of jobs held by unit assistants. The care of non-patient-related things was assigned to these unit assistants, whereas the care of people reverted back to the nurses. As nursing shortages continued to threaten healthcare facility viability, job design and work redesign occurred again and patient care technicians evolved. These multiskilled individuals performed some of the patient care duties previously performed by nurses. By employing patient care technicians, the talents of nurses were used for those patient care activities requiring nursing education.

Once this or any other type of reorganization approach has been decided on, it can be implemented in various ways. A gradual, long-term plan provides for a period of adjustment as the organization changes. This approach is less disturbing than sudden, extensive changes, sometimes referred to as the "earthquake" or "shake-up" technique of organizational change.

Learning the techniques, putting them to use, and continuously seeking input from employees all take time. Moreover, encouraging employees to be open to and share constructive criticisms about processes established by their supervisors and encouraging supervisors to not react negatively to the criticisms have been major hurdles that only a few enterprises have successfully overcome. For healthcare organizations to flourish, this type of equal exchange between employees and their supervisors must occur.

Downsizing and Rightsizing

Reengineering is often confused with downsizing and reorganizing. Reengineering is initiated to cause dramatic improvements in services, while *downsizing*—also called *reduction in force* or *rightsizing*—is meant as a means for moderate to high cost reduction. Each is a top-down approach, in contrast to performance improvement that seeks changes from the bottom up. The focus of reegineering is strategic—that is, long term with a vision of sustained improvements. However, the focus of reorganizing through downsizing is to cut costs. These approaches can be painful to the staff involved. Not only are coworkers laid off, but layers of management can be collapsed, resulting in new management structures. For example, in 2008 the SSM HealthCare system in St. Louis initiated a reorganizing effort resulting in approximately 200 positions being eliminated from its six-hospital system. Four director positions of health information management were eliminated and replaced with two regional directors overseeing three of the hospitals' health information management departments (McClellan 2008).

Additional disadvantages to reorganization include hidden costs associated with poor morale, loss of knowledgeable and experienced employees and historians, and potential loss of customers who have established rapport with certain employees.

In reengineering, the employees become members of teams to determine how to do a job better. Because the team approach is employed, reengineering may take two to four years to implement, while downsizing and rightsizing are quickly initiated, usually with the assistance of external consultants and with little input, if any, from the employees.

Alternatives to Downsizing

Through employee input, a variety of alternatives have surfaced to address the fiscal crisis that often leads to downsizing. Some of these include **timesizing**, cross-training (job rotation), lowering wages, attrition, reassignment, leaves, and buyouts. Timesizing is popular in some organizations because it can be applied across the board to all levels of the organization. This technique requires all staff to take a designated number of hours off, with or without pay. No one loses her job, but everyone contributes to the fiscal situation by either using up accrued paid time off or taking time off at no cost to the company.

timesizing
A cost-cutting technique that involves employees taking unpaid time off, or using accrued vacation time.

attrition
The practice of not replacing employees who leave.

Attrition is another favored approach, whereby a position is not filled when an individual leaves. This approach requires the supervisor and his team to reassess the work of the department and reorganize to accomplish the efforts required with the remaining staff. Doing so may involve reassignments, job enlargement, job enrichment, and job rotation.

In any reengineering endeavor, circumstances often drive the approach that an organization must take. Changes are always disturbing to those who are affected by them, regardless of how well intended the changes are. A manager who frequently changes the department's organizational structure runs the risk of damaging the morale of the subordinates. To the supervisor suggesting the reorganization, it might seem trivial, but to the subordinates it probably appears frightening because it implies changes in their working environment, status, and security. The wise supervisor knows how to strike a balance with respect to organizational change. In most instances, the supervisor probably finds that most subordinates quickly adjust to change if it is properly explained, if the employees have input or even recommend it, and if the need for change is demonstrated. A more detailed discussion of the introduction of change appears in Chapter 20.

Recentralization of Authority

As you know, from time to time it is necessary to review the degree of authority that has been delegated. The supervisor may believe that she has lost control over certain activities and that it has become necessary to tighten up or to recentralize. Another reason to tighten or recentralize is the significant reorganization of an entity, such as might result from a merger. In a merger many site-specific services are no longer needed at each location. For example, human resources, materials management, accounting, patient financial services, and even telecommunication departments are frequently centralized at one location. This centralization effort streamlines the services, reduces staff, and requires the realignment of authority held by the remaining incumbents. Often reengineering tools are used to redesign critical systems and processes to accommodate the "new" organization. Clearly, involvement of some staff is necessary when such drastic organizational changes occur.

Summary

In this chapter, we considered the organizing process from the supervisor's point of view. Drastic reorganization is called reengineering. This reorganizing approach focuses on the customer (the patient in the healthcare setting). Reengineering endorses the involvement of employees in the restructuring efforts. It differs from reorganizing that uses downsizing, which primarily focuses on cutting costs and eliminating jobs.

A vast number of tools are available to assist management in assessing reorganization options for the structure of the entity, the department, a service, and even a procedure. Employee involvement is necessary to ensure that a broad range of ideas and opinions is collected about the change and to gain buy-in.

After a change in the organizational structure has been accomplished or at least planned, the supervisor can proceed to delegate or redelegate authority in accordance with the departmental structure or modified process.

Notes

1. For more information on smart toilets, see www.aahsa.org/pubs_resources/presidents_ messages/2003/cow_ chips_smarttoilets.asp.
2. This section is contributed by Michael T. Troncone.
3. V. Clayton Sherman has not been discussed in this book. However, Mr. Sherman authored *Creating the New American Hospital*. This book and his teachings have been embraced by many hospitals nationwide. He provides guidance for healthcare managers to balance the regulatory environment and monetary restrictions with the principal purpose of the organization—providing patient care. He encourages building an organization that is driven by customer satisfaction.
4. This section is contributed by Robert Sutter.
5. For more information on the ISO standards, see www.kvaliteta.net/N881R2_Sector_ Specific_Documentation_List_2007-12.pdf.

Additional Readings

Bandyopadhyay, J., and K. Coppens. 2005. "Six Sigma Approach to Healthcare Quality and Productivity Management." *International Journal of Quality and Productivity Management* 5 (1).

Chilgren, A. A. 2008. "Managers and the New Definition of Quality." *Journal of Healthcare Management* 53 (4).

Dreachslin, J. L., and P. D. Lee. 2007. "Applying Six Sigma and DMAIC to Diversity Initiatives." *Journal of Healthcare Management* 52 (6).

Frontiers of Health Services Management. 2009. "The Lean Advantage." *Frontiers of Health Services Management* 26 (1): (entire issue).

van den Heuvel, J. 2006. "The Effectiveness of ISO 9001 and Six Sigma in Healthcare." (thesis) [Online thesis; retrieved 12/06.] http://publishing.eur.nl/ir/repub/asset/8465/070126_Heuvel,%20Jaap%20van%20den.pdf.

van den Heuvel, J., A. J. Bogers, R. J. Does, S. L. van Dijk, and M. Berg. 2006. "Quality Management: Does it Pay Off?" *Quality Management in Healthcare* 15 (3).

Yap, C., E. Siu, G. R. Baker, and A. D. Brown. 2005. "A Comparison of Systemwide and Hospital-Specific Performance Measurement Tools." *Journal of Healthcare Management* 50 (4).

COMMITTEES AS AN ORGANIZATIONAL TOOL **15**

Chapter Objectives

After you have studied this chapter, you should be able to do the following:

1. Explain the need for committees in today's organizational setting.
2. Describe the purpose and authority of committees.
3. Discuss the various types of committees and their functions.
4. Describe the benefits and limitations of committees.
5. Discuss the major considerations about effective committee operation.
6. Discuss the importance of the chair's role.

A **committee** is a formal group with defined purposes and relationships within an organization. For example, the healthcare center's board of directors has a permanent position at the top of the management hierarchy and a defined structure and function. Although individual members may change, the purpose of the group is stable.

Committees, boards, task forces, commissions, and teams are everywhere—in business, government, schools, churches, and certainly in healthcare organizations. As an institution grows in size and specialization, administration and coordination become more difficult and, at the same time, more critical. One way to cope with this difficulty is to establish committees to assign and address specific issues.

Committees are an organizational tool that, if used properly, can help an enterprise function smoothly. A committee is a group of people who function collectively by working together, whether its purpose is to make a decision, submit a recommendation, solve a problem, conduct an investigation, or manage a government agency. Committees differ from other units of management in that members normally have other full-time duties in the organization and devote only part of their time to committee activities.

The amount of time management spends in committee activities is increasing. According to HealthGate Compass (2007), committee meetings account for approximately 120 days per year. The *Successful Manager's Handbook* projects that managers spend between 25 and 75 percent of their working hours in group meetings (Davis et al. 2000). The emphasis on committee meetings is growing for several reasons. First, because most enterprise activities have become more complex and specialized, organizations need to tap the specialized expertise of their staff. Complexity has created an urgent

committee
A formal group with defined purposes and relationships within an organization.

need for coordination and cooperation. Conferences and meetings answer these needs. Second, administrators now understand that people are more enthusiastic about carrying out directives and plans they have helped to devise than those handed down from above. Thus, committees are an additional means of effectively combining the formal (Chapter 1) and acceptance theories (Chapter 2) of authority, which gives employees more freedom, greater authority, and stronger motivation. You will recall that Chester Barnard is known for his acceptance theory. The *acceptance theory of authority* states that managers only have as much authority as employees allow them to have. In a committee context, the authority to make decisions and offer recommendations is *formally* given to the committee members, some of whom may be nonmanagers. Because the members include employees who are nonmanagers, the recommendations made by the committee are more likely to be accepted. HealthGate predicts that managers will spend even more hours in committee activities due to quality improvement activities.

Although we often hear people complain that too many meetings take up too much of their time, committees are still widely used, especially in healthcare organizations. They seem to have no substitute. Without committee meetings, it would be almost impossible for an organization of any size to operate efficiently and effectively. Of the many ways to collect ideas and opinions on how to handle certain problems, holding a meeting is the best. The real criticism is probably not that there are too many meetings, but that the results often do not justify the time and effort invested.

Everyone has experienced being tied up in a meeting in which the chair or another committee member rambled along in all directions with no purpose whatsoever. In the meantime, more important work accumulated on your desk. The lack of focus probably resulted from poor preparation by the chair, which did nothing to increase your respect for his managerial ability. Such an experience makes clear how important it is for supervisors to acquaint themselves with committee or conference leadership techniques. In other words, supervisors should learn how to run committees well and how to achieve effective participation. Meetings become interesting and stimulating when the participants know they are accomplishing something.

The Nature of Committees

A committee is a formal group with defined purposes and reporting relationships to whom certain matters have been committed. The committee meets to discuss matters that have been assigned to it. Committees have the following characteristics:

- Committees function collectively, and their members normally have other duties, making committee work a part-time assignment. Because committees function only in groups, they differ considerably from other managerial devices.

- Committees can be found at all organizational levels, and a committee likely exists or has existed for every organizational activity.
- Committees can have line or staff capacity. The committee works on the problem to which it is assigned. In a line capacity, the committee makes a decision when a solution is reached. In a staff capacity, the committee makes a recommendation after analyzing and debating the problem at hand.
- Committees can be classified as standing or temporary. A **standing committee** has a formal, permanent place in the organization. Typically, it deals with the same set of recurring issues on an ongoing basis. In a hospital, for instance, the performance improvement, surgical review, infection control, pharmacy and therapeutics, and safety and new products committees are considered standing committees. The nature and purpose of a permanent committee remain the same, although the individual members may change. A temporary committee, on the other hand, is one that is appointed for a particular short-term purpose and is dissolved as soon as it has accomplished its task. This type is also known as an **ad hoc committee**, and at times, it is called a task force or a team. The employee awards committee may be an ad hoc committee.

standing committee
A committee whose purpose is long term or permanent.

ad hoc committee
A committee with a temporary or short-term purpose.

Functions of Committees

Most committee meetings are either informational or discussional. In an **informational meeting**, the leader or chair does most of the talking to present certain information and facts. Assume, for example, that a supervisor wants to make an announcement about the new snow day policy. She calls a meeting instead of posting a notice or speaking to each employee separately. It may be expensive to take the entire workforce away from the job, but an informational meeting guarantees that everyone in the department receives the information at the same time. Such a meeting also gives everyone who is affected a chance to ask questions and discuss the implications of the announcement. The meeting leader should take care, however, that questions from participants are relevant and the meeting does not stray from its purpose.

informational meeting
A meeting in which the leader presents information and facts, usually with limited discussion from other members.

In a **discussional meeting**, the chair encourages members to participate more to secure their ideas and opinions. The chair could ask the individuals singly for suggestions, but it is probably better to call a meeting to allow them to make recommendations. While they may not have much control over the final decision, participants in such meetings nevertheless derive satisfaction from the knowledge that their ideas have been considered and may even be used. They are likely to offer valuable suggestions and may implement

discussional meeting
A meeting in which the leader encourages other members to participate.

HOSPITAL LAND

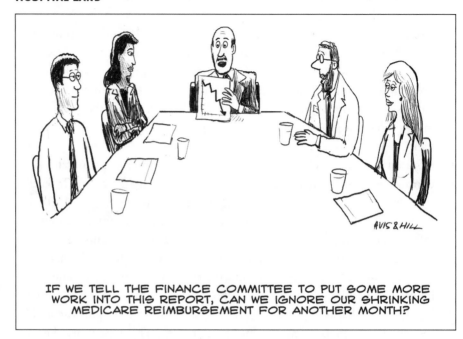

IF WE TELL THE FINANCE COMMITTEE TO PUT SOME MORE
WORK INTO THIS REPORT, CAN WE IGNORE OUR SHRINKING
MEDICARE REIMBURSEMENT FOR ANOTHER MONTH?

changes more enthusiastically if they participate in finalizing the decisions. In
a case such as this, the committee acts in a staff capacity.

Many questions in a healthcare organization affect so many departments that a committee representing several functions and specialties is better
able than an individual acting alone to make a decision. The same situation
can exist within a department. For example, employees may be dissatisfied
with the vacation schedule and weekend work, regardless of a supervisor's efforts to be fair. The supervisor can make a decision for the employees on these
matters, but it is better if staff can find a solution themselves. In such a case,
management is not concerned with the final decision so long as it falls within
the limits set—for example, that not all individuals who perform a single function are allowed to take vacation at the same time. If the group is allowed to
make this type of decision, it will come up with an acceptable solution. Even
if it is not the best in the supervisor's eyes, a solution that is implemented by
the group with great enthusiasm is better than a "perfect" decision that is met
with resistance.

Benefits of Committees

A group of individuals exchanging opinions and experiences often comes up
with a better answer than any one person thinking through the same problem.
This is perhaps the major benefit of group discussion. Various people bring to

a meeting a range of experience, backgrounds, information, perspectives, and ability far beyond what an individual can offer. As new members join the group, they bring new ideas and perceptions. This wider perspective would not be available if the problem were delegated to an individual decision maker. Indeed, many problems are so complicated that one person could not possibly have the knowledge to come up with a wise solution. Evaluating alternatives and ideas among several people stimulates and clarifies thinking.

Group deliberation can also promote coordination and cooperation. Committee members often become more knowledgeable and considerate of the problems of other employees, supervisors, and administration. They become more aware of the advantages of working together to seek solutions and the need to do so. Because they are involved in the analysis, logic, rationale, and solution of a problem, individual members are more likely to accept and implement the decision. It matters little how much a person actually contributed to the plan, as long as he was a member of the committee and sat in on the meeting. Probably the most significant benefit of committees in healthcare organizations is that they promote coordination and cooperation among the various units of the institution.

group deliberation
The practice of discussing issues among all members of a committee.

Committees have additional benefits. They produce continuity in the organization: Few committees replace all their members at the same time. Furthermore, they provide a good environment for junior managers and executives to learn how decisions are made, to absorb the philosophy and thinking of the hospital, and to see how the organization functions. As a result, committees provide a forum for identification of potential leaders. They also give representatives from various departments a chance to be heard and get involved in the affairs of the organization.

Disadvantages of Committees

Despite all these benefits, the committee function has often been abused. Sometimes committees are created to delay action, and many people have come to think of the committee as a debating society. Jokes about committees include calling them groups "that keep minutes but waste hours" and "where the unwilling appoint the unfit to do the unnecessary." Remarks that meetings go all day long and leave no time for anyone to get real work done are frequent.

Indeed, one of the most common complaints about committees is that they are exceedingly time consuming. Each member is entitled to have his or her say, and some individuals carry on too long about how valid their points are. According to Nelson and Economy (1996), meetings represent 25 percent of the average businessperson's working hours, 40 percent of the middle manager's, and 80 percent of the executive's. In addition to their cost in terms of time, committees also cost money. Time spent in committee meetings obviously is not spent on other productive activities. Thus, every hour taken up by a meeting costs the institution. Furthermore, expenses might be incurred for travel and preparation for meetings.

Another shortcoming of committees is that the sense of responsibility they evoke is limited. When a problem is submitted to a committee, it is submitted to a group and not to individuals. Responsibility does not weigh as heavily on the group's shoulders as it would on an individual's shoulders. The committee's problems become everybody's responsibility, which in reality means they are nobody's responsibility. It is difficult to criticize the committee as a whole, or any single member, if the solution proves to be wrong, because each person can say that the committee made the decision. Members are willing to settle for less-than-ideal solutions, and they blame the committee if the solution does not work. This dilution of responsibility is natural, and there is no way to avoid it.

Weak or compromise decisions and tyranny of the minority are other shortcomings of committees. Many organizations traditionally reach unanimous decisions based on politeness, cooperative spirit, mutual respect, and other considerations. Committees, in this instance, go with the lowest common denominator instead of the optimum solution. This often leads to weak, watered-down, undesirable compromises. Also, in their efforts for unanimous or nearly unanimous conclusions, committees may be tyrannized by a minority or a dominant individual who holds out as long as possible for the solution she advocates. The majority might allow itself to be dominated by such a minority or dominant personality because of a lack of time, interest, or sense of responsibility. This may even strain working relationships outside of the committee.

groupthink
The result of allowing group discussion to be dominated by a desire to find group concurrence on a conclusion, even if facts point to another conclusion.

Another danger is that committee members may become victims of the groupthink phenomenon. **Groupthink** is allowing one's deliberations to be dominated by a desire to concur with the group at any expense, even if the facts point to another conclusion. Pressure for unanimity may overwhelm some members, causing the group to overlook or negatively appraise alternative solutions. While consensus, in and of itself, is not bad, it has little value when it results from the belief that support means going with the flow or never challenging the judgment of the majority or the boss (Zarowin 2005). Under this influence, the group is likely to make decisions that are not in the best interest of the organization just to avoid conflict and dissent. Alfred Sloan, who ran General Motors from 1923 to 1956, once said at a director's meeting, "Gentlemen, I take it that we are all in complete agreement on the decision here. Then, I propose we postpone further discussion . . . to give ourselves time to develop disagreement and perhaps gain some understanding of what the decision is all about" (Zarowin 2005).

The Effective Operation of a Committee

Most healthcare facility administrations have established committees because they contribute to the smooth functioning of the organization. Some of these committees exist to fulfill the requirements of the healthcare facility's accreditation or licensing program. However, when considering establishing a committee, one should ask the following questions (Siegel 2004):

- Is it essential? An attempt to get more people involved in a decision is not in itself a bad thing, but as managers, we must be cautious to consider the productivity impact.
- Are the right people in attendance? For example, it is tough to decide on an infection surveillance program when the infection control nurse does not attend the meeting.
- What is the point? Those in attendance will not find the committee valuable if they do not know what its goals are.

Familiarity with the means for ensuring effective committee operation is essential. It is not easy to make committee meetings a success, because the goals may be numerous and members may have competing interests and demands on their time. As we have already indicated, the basic goals of committee meetings are (1) to develop the best suggestions or solutions for the problem under consideration, (2) to arrive at majority consensus—or, ideally, unanimity—on suggestions or solutions, and (3) to accomplish objectives in the shortest time. It is a challenge for any committee to fulfill these goals, but the following sections offer a guide for effective committee operation and conference leadership.

Scope, Functions, and Authority

The first thing a committee needs is a mandate. Members must know its scope, duties, and functions to operate effectively. The executive establishing the committee must define the subjects to be covered and the expectations to be fulfilled—the committee must have a job description. How the committee relates to other units within the organization must also be stated. This prevents the committee from floundering and enables the manager to check on whether it is meeting its expectations.

In addition to its functions and scope, the degree of authority conferred on the committee must be specified (see Exhibit 15.1). As we mentioned earlier, it must be clear whether the committee is to serve in an advisory (staff) or decision-making (line) capacity. For example, in many hospitals, the human research committee (sometimes referred to as the investigational review board) has line authority to decide whether to approve a proposed research project. On the other hand, in most hospitals the medical executive

Exhibit 15.1

Example of
Formalized
Scope of
Authority for
the Recovery
Audit
Contractor
(RAC)
Readiness
Committee

Purpose of Committee: To provide for a collaborative forum for those involved with ensuring the hospital's compliance with the national RAC initiatives.

Scope: The RAC Readiness Committee is charged with:

1. Understanding, keeping current with, and establishing a repository of the RAC regulations
2. Developing processes to address the regulations and respond to the RAC's requests in accordance with the timetable established by the RAC
3. Implementing corrective actions including system changes and updates, ensuring documentation education is provided and monitored, and modifying current procedures
4. Nurturing and maintaining collegial relationships with the federally assigned RAC for this region
5. Recommending policies to the medical staff and administration to ensure the hospital's compliance with the regulations and reducing the hospital's exposure to these external auditing initiatives
6. Implementing procedures to fulfill the policies approved
7. Identifying educational voids and offering educational programs for our staffs based on RAC regulations and findings

Composition: The following individuals shall participate on this committee:

1. Ambulatory care director
2. Case management director (vice-chair)
3. Chief financial officer
4. Clinical information data specialist
5. Compliance officer
6. Emergency department medical director
7. Health information management director (chair)
8. Operating room director
9. Patient care services director
10. Patient financial services director
11. Others on an ad hoc basis

Meetings and Reports: The committee will initially meet weekly until such time that it is determined that the Committee may meet less frequently, but no less often than monthly. At least monthly, the committee chair will issue a report to the administrative council that includes committee's initiatives, RAC findings, financial impact of RAC findings, and actions taken to reduce and/or eliminate repeated findings and recommendations. A summary report will be provided to the board of directors and executive committee of the medical staff at least quarterly by the chief financial officer and emergency department medical director, respectively.

committee acts in a staff capacity when it deals with a physician's or surgeon's application for hospital privileges. This committee makes a recommendation to the board of directors, and the board in turn decides. Committees may also have hybrid authority—that is, line authority for some actions and staff authority for others. The medical staff's executive committee may have line authority to remove an impaired surgeon from the operating room and staff authority to recommend to the board additional actions that should be taken relative to this surgeon.

For a formal, standing committee, all such information should be included in the organizational manual. Sometimes the function and scope of a committee may be defined by federal (e.g., compliance committee), state (e.g., information management committee), or local (e.g., disaster preparedness committee) regulations or accreditation or licensing (e.g., credentialing committee) rules. Scope, functions, and authority must also be explicitly stated for a temporary committee, but perhaps not so formally. An ad hoc committee should only be established for a subject worthy of group consideration. If a topic can be handled by one person or over the phone, there is no need to establish a committee.

Composition

Because the quality of a committee's work is only as good as its members, choose members carefully (see Exhibit 15.2). They should be able to express and defend their views, but they should also be willing to see the other party's point of view and able to integrate their thinking with that of the other members. They also should be honest with whomever appoints them. Every member's time is valuable, so if someone else on your team has more knowledge

EXHIBIT 15.2

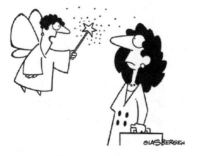

*"I'm your Corporate Fairy Godmother with three wishes!
I wish you'd get to meetings on time, I wish you'd stop
interrupting other people, and I wish you'd
contribute something besides cynicism!"*

SOURCE: Copyright 2001 by Randy Glasbergen, www.glasbergen.com. Used by permission.

about the committee's subject, recommend that person. This will save the time spent checking with that individual on specific items and reporting back to the committee. Depending on the purpose of the committee, members with certain expertise or knowledge may be needed. For example, a minister or priest would be a wise selection for a bioethics committee. If possible, choose members of approximately the same organizational rank to eliminate the complications of a direct superior–subordinate relationship. If committee members are chosen from different departments, the problems of rank are more easily overcome. Sometimes, however, the composition of a committee is dictated by outside regulations.

A committee provides a good opportunity to bring together specialists in different departments and activities in such a way that all concerned parties are properly represented. This results in balanced group integration and deliberation. The various representatives are assured that their interests have been heard and considered. Administration should make sure that concern with proper representation is not carried too far. It is more important to appoint capable members to a committee than representative members. The ideal solution is to appoint to the committee a capable member from each pertinent activity. Finally, asking others to participate on a committee carries with it an obligation; you want them to know that the time they invest will be put to good use.

Source of Talent   The committee chair and the administrative champion that appoints a committee should constantly assess the skills of the committee members to identify potential candidates for future leadership appointments. The ability to present one's position diplomatically and to identify unique and effective solutions is a desirable trait for managers and supervisors. Committees are an excellent place for administrators to identify potential leaders; committee chairs, especially, may be groomed for leadership opportunities in the organization.

Size   A committee should be large enough to allow thorough group deliberation and a broad range of information resources. It should not be so large, however, that it becomes unwieldy and unnecessarily time consuming. Usually, committees of four to ten members work best. If the subject under consideration requires a much larger committee, it might be wise to form subcommittees to consider various aspects of the problem. Then the entire committee can meet to hear subcommittee reports and decide on a final answer.

Effective Conference Leadership

Because the success of any meeting depends largely on the chair's ability to lead it, she must be familiar with effective conference or committee leadership techniques to guide the meeting to a satisfactory conclusion. The individual members undoubtedly bring to the meeting their individual patterns of behavior and points of view. The chair must know how to fuse the individual perspectives and attitudes so that the group can work together effectively. The chair needs considerable skill, time, and patience to bring together diverse members into the closely knit group needed to achieve integrated group solutions.

The chair is the most important member of the committee. This person is expected to (1) bring about the fulfillment of the task and (2) build and maintain successful group interaction. Because the committee is made up of individuals with different personalities, expertise, and demands on their time, the chair must help these individuals interact productively.

The Role of the Chair

Once the committee has convened, the first step is to ask for volunteers to serve as recorder and timekeeper. The chair may wish to design a standard format for capturing the discussion and decisions from each meeting (see Exhibit 15.3). Next, the chair should ensure that the members understand the issues. Too often, people think first of how a new proposition affects them and

EXHIBIT 15.3
Meeting Discussion and Decision Form

Meeting Date:
Recorder:
Committee Members Present (check if in attendance):

	Jane Jones (Chair)		Tim Thompson, CFO		Jim Johns, Compliance
	Alice Adams, RN		Betty Boop, PFS		Gayle Goodman, CM

(please submit summary within 10 working days of meeting)

Item #	Topic	Relevant Discussion Points	Decisions or Follow-up Actions (with due dates)
1.	Organizing Meeting/Call to Order		
2.			
3.			
4.			
5.			
6.	New Business		
7.	Adjournment	Next meeting— Scheduled Note Taker—	

their own working environments rather than how it affects the organization as a whole, which can create unnecessary friction in a committee setting. Also, people tend to see the same facts differently. The same words can mean different things to different people. Thus, the chair has to determine what the participants think the issues are. Committee members are reminded not to compete and to give others' ideas equal weight to their own.

Finding out how members interact takes work. A frequent comment about committees is that the issues on the conference table are easier to deal with than the people around the table. Individuals in a meeting often react to each other rather than to their ideas. For instance, just because Person A talks frequently, everything he suggests may be rejected; Person B may automatically reject whatever someone else suggests; and Person C may be that member of the committee who never speaks. If you are running the meeting, listen to everyone. Paraphrase what participants have said when appropriate, but do not judge the merits of their comments. Avoid putting anyone on the defensive. As the meeting leader, you must assume that everyone's ideas have value.

It is the chair's job to minimize personality differences using parliamentary procedure. Attempt to control dominant people without alienating them. The speaking time of each participant can be limited so that one person does not monopolize the entire meeting. Also, be careful to call on people who seldom speak. With the help of such leadership techniques, the committee will react to the meeting content and not the individuals around the table. For a meeting to be successful, participants need to forget their personalities and outside allegiances and work together toward a meaningful solution. In all this, the chair mediates.

The quality of the solution depends to some extent on the amount of time spent to reach it. Too much haste probably will not produce the most desirable solution. On the other hand, most meetings have a time limit. Ideally, each agenda topic has an assigned time period. If there are no time limits, members may monopolize a subject while others may become bored and frustrated.

The chair's levels of interest and alertness set an example for other committee members. It is the chair's job to give every member a chance to voice suggestions and opinions. This is especially important when the committee members are expected to execute the decisions they make. In such cases, the chair may need to persuade the minority to go along with the decision of the majority. On other occasions, the majority might have to make concessions to the minority. All this takes time and may result in a compromise that does not necessarily represent the best possible solution. If the committee has reached the solution democratically, however, the chair has demonstrated her leadership abilities and the committee has accomplished the major purpose of the meeting—finding a solution.

It is important to keep all participants informed about the committee's actions. The recorder keeps notes during the meeting on a flipchart or board that everyone can see. This helps members keep track of what they have discussed and decided. After each meeting, the recorder distributes copies of the minutes with a reminder of the next meeting, date, time, and location and any assignments made during the meeting. Some organizations prescribe the format of the minutes for all committees.

The function of a chair is to help the members of the group reach their own decisions and to bring out their ideas. If the chair expresses her own views, the members of the committee may hesitate to express their opinions, especially if they disagree. This is even more likely if the chair also happens to be their boss or holds a higher position. On the other hand, in many situations it would be unwise and unrealistic for the chair not to express her views. This individual may have some factual knowledge or a sound opinion regarding the subject at hand, and the value of the deliberations is lessened if these facts are left unknown to other members of the committee.

The Chair's Opinions

On the whole, it is best for the chair to express her opinions last and to let participants know that these opinions are subject to constructive criticism and suggestions. After all, silence on the leader's part may be interpreted as an inability to make a decision or a fear of assuming responsibility. On certain occasions, however, the chair must use sensitive judgment on whether or to what extent to express her opinions.

The Meeting Setup

At least initially, schedule meetings for a regular time slot when all members are available. Once the committee has met several times and a meeting schedule is established, members should take it upon themselves to reserve time in their schedules to attend future meetings. Always allow sufficient time between meetings to prepare for the next meeting and gather any required information.

Select a location that is convenient to all attendees. The room should be comfortable and stocked with the necessary supplies, such as a whiteboard, flipchart, and markers. Set up the room to maximize participation, either around a table or in a semicircle so that all participants can see each other and hear comments.

Today, many meetings are held via telephone, thus eliminating the need for a conference room. These audioconferences (with sound only) or videoconferences (with sound and view of other participants) serve committee members who are geographically dispersed. This format expedites the work of the committee and contains the costs of travel to a common location. However, it presents its own challenges, as the chair may not be able to assess member understanding of the issues or concerns without the visual advantage. Members may be distracted by other work on their desks or new e-mail; as a result, they may participate less in the discussion at hand.

Agenda and Task Control

Successful committee work requires thorough preparation. Before the meeting, the chair must carefully outline the strategy and establish an agenda. He should list the discussion topics in the proper sequence and decide how long the meeting will last. The chair may even want to establish an approximate time limit for each discussion item to ensure better control of the situation. (See Exhibit 15.4.) If possible, the agenda should be distributed to attendees before the meeting so they can prepare.

EXHIBIT 15.4

Meeting
Agenda

RAC's Readiness Committee
Meeting Agenda
Wednesday, February 25, 2009
1:00 pm–2:00 pm Central Time

Recorder: Tim Thompson

Item	Time	Topic	Who/Notes/Documents
1.	1:00 pm	Organizing Meeting/Call to Order: Jane Jones Action Items: Roll Call Review and approve Minutes	1. Meeting Summary from January 28, 2009 2. Recorder Rotation Schedule—see list at bottom of this page. 3. Meeting Summary Template:
2.	1:10 pm	Resource additions	1. Members to share copies of any new articles or information on RAC activities.
3.	1:30 pm	Monthly activity	Total requests—HIM Total denials (clinical)—Case Management Total Auto-takebacks—Patient Financial Services Overall financial impact (this month and YTD)—CFO Major findings—All
4.	1:45 pm	Nursing observation documentation procedure	Patient Care Director
5.	1:52 pm	Update on medical staff training	ED Medical Director
6.	1:57 pm	Announcements	
7.	2:00 pm	Adjourn—Next Meeting: March 25, 2009 Recorder: Betty Boop	

Summary Recorder Rotation:

Meeting Date:	Recorder:	Meeting Date:	Recorder:
January	Alice Adams	July	Tim Thompson
February	Tim Thompson	August	Betty Boop
March	Betty Boop	September	Jim Johns
April	Jim Johns	October	Gayle Goodman
May	Gayle Goodman	November	Alice Adams
June	Alice Adams	December	Tim Thompson

Chair's Contact Info: *JJones@ABCHealth.org*; 505-555-1212

A well-prepared agenda is the best way to keep members on task. Although the agenda sets the overall strategy and sequence, it must not be so rigid that there is no means to adjust it. If a particular subject requires more attention than originally anticipated, the agenda should allow for reduction of the time allotted to some other topic. In other words, the chair should not be too quick to rule people out of order. What seems irrelevant to him may be important to other committee members. Some irrelevancies can relax the atmosphere and relieve tension that has built up. Because it is the chair's job to keep the meeting moving toward its goal, he should occasionally pause to consult the agenda and remind the group of what has been accomplished and what still remains to be discussed. A good chair recognizes the opportune time for summarizing one point and moving on to the next.

The agenda should state the purpose of the meeting and any specific goals. It should also state the start and end times in consideration of employees' work hours. Occasionally, a meeting may not progress as planned. If it appears that the meeting will not end as scheduled, the chair should ask the group if they wish to extend this meeting or to table discussion of the remaining topics. If they choose the latter, the chair must make sure these topics appear on the next agenda.

Advance Preparation

The chair, the committee's own staff, or designated committee members should gather additional background information. The members should receive this information before the meeting. Meetings should be planned far enough in advance to give members adequate notice and time to review any materials that will be discussed. This preparation allows the committee members to minimize conflicting responsibilities.

Last, but not least, make specific arrangements for the room, setup, equipment, and food. Confirm the arrangements at least once before the meeting and again, in person, on the day before the meeting. Nothing is more frustrating than to arrive at a meeting only to find the room is not set up properly or, worse yet, is occupied by another committee.

The Committee Meeting

Now that you are familiar with some of the guidelines for effective committee operation, the next question to consider concerns how these guidelines can be applied in a typical committee meeting. How can a diverse group of people, with the help of an effective conference leader, hold a meaningful discussion and arrive at satisfactory answers to the problems under consideration?

Always start and end the meeting on time. After a few introductory remarks and social pleasantries, the chair should state the problem to be discussed. This provides an opportunity for all attendees to participate freely. Any member should be able to point out those aspects of the problem that seem important to him or her, regardless of how everyone else sees them. The chair should ensure that the discussion eventually gets to the relevant points.

There are always some meeting attendees who talk too much and others who do not talk enough. One of the chair's most difficult jobs is to encourage the latter to speak up and to keep the former from holding the floor for too long. There are various ways to do this. For example, after a long-winded speaker has expressed her opinions, it may be wise not to recognize that member again, instead giving others the chance to speak. It might also help to ask her to keep remarks brief or to arrange the seating at the conference table so that it is easy not to recognize her request to speak. Most of the time, however, the committee finds subtle ways to indicate that those members who monopolize the discussion are hindering others.

This does not mean that all members of the meeting must participate equally. Some people know more about a given subject than others, and some have stronger feelings about an issue than others. The chair must take such factors into consideration but still stimulate overall participation. The chair should accept everyone's contribution without judgment and encourage everyone to participate. He may need to ask controversial questions just to get the discussion going. Once members have started to participate, the chair should continue to throw out provocative, open-ended questions that ask why, who, what, where, and when. Simple yes-or-no questions should be avoided.

Alternatively, the chair can start at one side of the conference table and ask each member to express his or her thoughts on the problem. The major disadvantage of this technique is that instead of participating in the discussion spontaneously, members sit back and wait until called on. The skilled chair can also watch the facial expressions of the people in the group, which may indicate that someone has an idea but is afraid to speak up. Then, the chair can call on that person.

If a meeting involves many participants, the chair may want to break it up into small discussion groups, typically known as buzz sessions. Each subgroup holds its own discussion and reports back to the meeting after a specified period. In this way, people who hesitate to speak up in a larger group are more likely to participate. Buzz sessions are usually advisable when there are more than 20 participants.

While using these techniques to encourage participation, the chair should stick to the agenda and ensure that the discussion is basically relevant. Sometimes an inexperienced chair is so anxious for someone to speak that discussion occurs merely for discussion's sake. This confuses the issues and delays the decision-making phase of the meeting.

Group Decision Making

Once all committee members have a similar understanding of a problem, determine the facts as objectively as possible. Only after considering all the relevant facts will the group be able to suggest alternative solutions. The chair knows that the best solution is only as good as the best alternative considered. Therefore, meeting participants should contribute as many alternatives as possible so that no solution is overlooked.

Brainstorming is a popular and interactive group-discussion and decision-making technique. It encourages participants to be spontaneous and creative and gives them complete freedom of expression. Brainstorming helps a group create as many ideas as possible in as short a time as possible.

Brainstorming comes in two formats:

1. *Structured.* In this method, every person in a group must give an idea when his or her turn arises or pass until the next round. It forces even shy people to participate, but it can also create pressure to contribute.
2. *Unstructured.* In this method, group members simply give ideas as they come to mind. This creates a more relaxed atmosphere, but it is also open to domination by the most vocal members.

In both methods, the general rules are the same:

- Never criticize ideas.
- Write every idea on a flipchart or whiteboard. Having the words visible to everyone at the same time prevents misunderstandings and triggers new ideas.
- Once everyone agrees, write down the question or issue being brainstormed.
- Record the exact words of the speaker on the flipchart; do not interpret.
- Do it quickly; 5 to 15 minutes works well.

The next step is to determine which idea to work on. GOAL/QPC (1988, 70–71) describes a commonly used technique known as the *nominal group technique* (see Exhibit 15.5).

Next, evaluate the alternative solutions and discuss the advantages and disadvantages of each. In so doing, the committee can narrow the field down to two or three alternatives. These options must be discussed thoroughly to reach a solution. The chair should mediate as the committee works out a solution that is acceptable to all members.

Often the best procedure is to find a solution that synthesizes all the important points raised by the members. Throughout this process, the chair has the difficult job of helping the minority save face. It is easier to placate the minority if the final decision incorporates part of each person's idea. However, this can be a tedious process, and, as we have said, such a compromise is not always the strongest solution.

EXHIBIT 15.5

Nominal Group Technique

When selecting which problems to work on and in what order, it often happens that the problem selected is that of the person who speaks the loudest or who has the most authority. This often creates a feeling in the team that "their" problem will never be worked on. This feeling, in turn, can lead to a lack of commitment to work on the problem selected and the selection of the "wrong" problem in the first place. Nominal Group Technique tries to provide a way to give everyone in the group an equal voice in problem selection. The steps in the process are as follows:

1. Have everyone on the team write (or say) the problem that he or she feels is most important. If members of the team do not write the problems out, have someone write on a flipchart or whiteboard (or somewhere visible) the concerns as they are being communicated. If people do produce written problems, collect them when they are finished. Everyone may not feel comfortable writing, but it may make them feel safer by talking about sensitive problems at the beginning.

2. Write the problem statements where the team can see them.

3. Check with the team to make sure that the same problem is not written twice (slightly different words may be used for the same problem). If a problem is re-peated, combine the two listings into one item.

4. Ask the team members to write on a piece of paper the letters corresponding to the number of problem statements the team produced. For example, if you ended up with five problem statements, everyone would write the letters A through E on the paper.

5. Make sure that each problem statement has a letter in front of it. Then ask the team members to vote on which problem is most important by putting a "5" next to that problem's letter. For example:

The problem list would look like this:

A. Space
B. Safety
C. Housekeeping
D. Quality Going Down
E. No Preventive Maintenance

Each member's paper would look like this:

A. _____
B. _____
C. _____
D. _____
E. _____

So, if someone thought "quality is going down" was the #1 problem, it would look like this:

A. _____
B. _____
C. _____
D. ___5___
E. _____

Everyone then has to complete the list by voting the second most important, third most important, etc.

A. 2, 5, 2, 4, 1
B. 1, 4, 5, 5, 5
C. 4, 1, 3, 3, 4
D. 5, 2, 1, 1, 2
E. 3, 3, 4, 2, 3

EXHIBIT 15.5
Continued

An alternate ranking approach involves the "one-half plus one" rule. Especially when dealing with a large number of items, it may be necessary to limit the items to be considered. This rule suggests ranking only one-half of the items plus one. For example, if 20 items were generated, team members only rate 11 ideas.

6. Add up each line of numbers across. The item with the highest number is the most important one to the total team. In this case, B (Safety) is the most important item with a total of 20. Add up the numbers for each item, and put them in order.

7. You then work on Item B first, and then move through the list.

SOURCE: Reprinted from *The Memory Jogger.*™ © 1988, GOAL/QPC, Salem, NH. www.goalqpc.com. Used with permission.

Sometimes the group may not be able to reach a compromise or agree on a decision. This happens more often when the group is hostile. In such a situation, the chair should find out the source of the disagreement and discuss it. Committee participants may think first of a new idea's objectionable qualities rather than its desirable features. Discussing such objections may dispel unwarranted fears and may allow participants to see the positive aspects. On the other hand, the objections may be strong enough to void the proposition. In any case, the group must have a chance to voice negative feelings before a positive consensus can be reached.

Taking a Vote

The chair often must decide whether to take a vote or whether the committee should work until it reaches a final, unanimous agreement. Many people feel that voting is the democratic way to make decisions. Voting accentuates the differences among members, however, and once a person has made a public commitment to a position by voting, it is often difficult to change his or her mind without risking harm to the person's dignity. Also, members of the losing minority may not be able to carry out the majority decision with enthusiasm. Whenever possible, it is better not to take a formal vote but to work toward a roughly unanimous agreement, even though this may take more time.

However, the price of unanimity is often a solution that is not as ingenious and bold as it could have been. The situation and the magnitude of the problem involved dictate whether unanimity is worth this price.

A skilled chair can usually sense what the members are feeling, and all she needs to say is that a particular solution seems to be the consensus of the group. At this point, especially in a small meeting, the group can probably dispense with parliamentary procedure and a formal vote. In a large meeting, of course, unanimity may be impossible, and decisions should be based on majority rule.

Ending the Meeting

The chair should always end the meeting on time. She should alert the members when the meeting time is nearly over (approximately 10 minutes in advance of the meeting's scheduled end time) to move the discussion toward closure. Zarowin (2004) suggests that the chair plan a closing statement for each meeting. It should include specific agreements on who is to do what and when. Without such a close, you risk each attendee leaving with a different view of the meeting's results or his or her obligations. Restating conclusions reached, actions taken, deadlines imposed, and results expected should keep the committee's purpose and members on track.

Follow-Up of Committee Actions

Regardless of whether a committee is acting merely to make a recommendation or whether it has final decision-making authority, its results need a follow-up. After the chair has reported the committee's findings to the superior who originally assigned the problem to the committee, the superior should keep the chair or the committee posted about what action has been taken. It is common courtesy to give the committee some explanation; inadequate updates or no updates at all cause the committee to lose interest in its work. When the committee has had the authority to make a final decision, the chair generally keeps the committee members abreast of actions taken in response to the committee's decision. Depending on the extent of the line authority granted, the committee may be responsible for carrying out the decision, or the executive who normally deals with the matter at hand may execute the decision. In any event, the committee members must be kept informed of any developments.

Summary

Every supervisor has probably been involved in committees either as a member or as an organizer. Committees have become an important device for augmenting the organizational structure and the functioning of an enterprise. They allow the enterprise to adapt to increasing complexity without a complete reorganization. They permit a group of people to function collectively to solve problems an individual could not handle. Despite the disadvantages and other criticisms leveled against committees, they can be valuable if properly organized and led.

Committees meet either to disseminate information or to discuss a topic. If discussion is involved, the manager who appoints the committee should clarify whether the committee is to arrive at a final decision on the question under discussion and take action based on this decision, or whether it is to make recommendations. A committee can operate in a line or staff capacity.

Regardless of the committee's purpose, group deliberation will likely produce more satisfactory and acceptable conclusions than a decree formally handed down from above. When members of the organization have had a role in making decisions or recommendations, they carry out the work with more enthusiasm. To achieve high-quality group decisions and recommendations, however, committee members must be carefully selected. In composing a committee, one must ensure that as many interested parties as possible are represented. The people chosen as representatives should be capable of presenting their views and integrating their opinions with those of others. As to the size of a committee, there should be enough members to permit thorough deliberations, but not so many that meetings are cumbersome.

In addition to these factors, the success of committee deliberations depends largely on effective committee or conference leadership. The chair's familiarity with effective group work makes the difference between productive and wasteful committee meetings. The chair's job is to produce the best possible solution in the shortest amount of time, ideally with unanimity. While trying to achieve these goals, the chair must find the proper balance between running the meeting too tightly or too loosely.

The chair depends on his or her perception of the mood and climate of the meeting to know exactly how to lead it and bring it to a successful conclusion. Thus, the chair has to sense when there has been enough general participation in the discussion, when alternative solutions have been properly evaluated, and when a vote is necessary. In all these matters, the conference leadership abilities of the chair are of the utmost importance.

Additional Readings

Bosler, B. 2006. "The 15-Minute Meeting: Indicator of Organization Expectation?" *For the Record* 18 (20): 20–24.

Larson, L. 2009. "The Power of Committees." *Trustee* 62 (2): 8.

16

THE INFORMAL ORGANIZATION

Chapter Objectives

After you have studied this chapter, you should be able to do the following:

1. Discuss the origins of the informal organization.
2. Describe how informal small groups evolve.
3. Describe the structure, benefits, and costs of the informal organization for its members and the power it can exert on the functioning of the formal organization.
4. Suggest ways the supervisor can react to informal groups and their leaders to improve relationships, thereby achieving increased organizational effectiveness.

In almost all enterprises, informal structures arise from personal interactions, social activities, sentiments, friendship, common interests, and needs. This invisible, shadow organization produces intricate patterns of influence and communication beyond and between the lines of the formal organization. These informal structures are not written down, nor do they have manuals, charts, or titles. But they are influential on the functioning of the formal organization and can be supportive of or disruptive to managerial authority.

Whenever people work together, informal relationships exist and become a powerful source of influence on the formal organization. The formal task structure, goals, and functioning of the organization are affected by a social subsystem known as the *informal organization*. Early scholars maintained that an inherent conflict exists between the goals of the formal organization and informal relationships. Today we know that both formal and informal relationships are essential subsystems of a complex system and that the informal relationships help the functioning of the formal organization by providing individual satisfaction and aiding group morale, which otherwise might be lacking.

The Genesis of the Informal Group

The informal organization is closely related to the workings of groups and committees, but its origin is quite different. The informal organization is a powerful source of influence that interacts with and modifies the formal organization.

Although many managers conveniently overlook its existence, they readily admit that to understand the nature of organizational life fully, it is necessary to "learn the ropes" of the informal organization. In almost every institution, such an informal structure develops. It reflects the spontaneous efforts of individuals and groups to influence their working conditions. For example, two or three people who do not work in the same area may meet daily for lunch because they enjoy each other's company, or people may join together because they have similar ideas about how a task could be improved and they want to approach their supervisor to discuss changing it. Whenever people associate with each other, social relationships and groupings result. The informal organization can make a positive contribution to the smooth functioning of the enterprise or can be disruptive. It also serves as a source of information for the grapevine discussed in Chapter 5. Therefore, the manager must understand, respect, and even nurture the workings of the informal organization.

At the heart of informal organization are people and their relationships, whereas at the heart of formal organization are the organizational structure and the delegation of authority. Management can create or rescind a formal organizational structure that it has designed, but it cannot rescind the informal organization because management did not establish it.

At the base of all informal organization is the small group, consisting of a few people (five, for example) who share physical proximity and contact; this brings about an interplay of sentiments and interaction—sharing of ideas, feelings, and opinions. The group interacts regularly to accomplish a common goal or purpose (Homans 1950). The first question that comes to mind is why people join such groups. We may wonder what advantages they gain from groups, as they are already members of a department in which their duties are specifically assigned, channels of communication exist, and a line of authority has been established. The answer to this question is that employees have certain needs they would like to satisfy but that the formal organization apparently leaves unsatisfied. People have a basic need to associate with others in groups small enough to permit intimate, direct, and personal contact among individuals. The satisfaction derived from these types of relationships generally cannot be obtained from working within a large organization. Thus, the small group provides the individual with fulfillments that are different from those that can be obtained from any other source.

Benefits Derived from Groups

People join groups for various reasons, including interpersonal attraction, group goals, group activities, and social needs. Perhaps the most important reason people join groups is that doing so provides a sense of satisfaction. An individual in a group is usually surrounded by others who share similar values.

This reinforces his own value system and interests and gives him confidence because it is comfortable to be among people who think along the same lines. The group also fulfills the need for friendship and companionship. The employee needs and enjoys the social contact with fellow workers, with whom he shares experiences and jokes and in whom he finds sympathetic listeners. Similarly, being part of a small group may provide status for an individual, because many groups are more or less exclusive. The group thus fulfills the need for belonging.

Another need satisfied by belonging to a small group in many instances is the need for balance and protection. Social interaction may balance routine and tedious work, and a small group offers protection from what the members may consider overbearing or unsympathetic management. The small group is a source of security, support, and collective power—there is strength in numbers, as the saying goes. Often people who enter an organization for the first time are anxious; the surroundings are unfamiliar and uncertainty exists. When several people are in the same circumstance, they may form a small group on this basis alone, providing temporary support to each other in an unfamiliar environment. New employee orientation programs encourage the creation of these groups. Whenever people sense the need for protection, they form small groups.

Informal groups also provide access to the informal communications network known as the **grapevine**. The grapevine works effectively in small groups, providing speedy, although at times inaccurate, information. The network or pattern of communication often has no resemblance to the formal chain of command. Groups tend to form around an individual who seems to be the focal point in a communications network. An individual who has information is able to satisfy the communication needs of others, even though the information transmitted may be false or distorted.

grapevine
The informal communications network in an organization.

In addition to these emotional needs, the interaction, communication, and collaboration that informal groups engender sometimes help employees get more work done. Informal groups may help employees accomplish tasks that would be impossible to accomplish alone. They also serve to bring the goals of these tasks more into the realm of the employee. The objectives and goals of the formal organization may appear remote and meaningless to the average employee. It is much simpler to identify with the objectives and goals of one's immediate work group. Often employees readily forego some of their own goals and replace them with the goals of the group.

The informal organization influences the behavior of employees, regardless of the status they occupy within the informal group. This is important for a supervisor to remember because one cannot hope to understand individual behavior without understanding the behavior of the organizational forces that shape it.

By recognizing all these needs, the supervisor will understand the many reasons employees tend to join informal groups and can attempt to use these groups constructively.

The Informal Organization

Small informal groups, as mentioned, are the basis of the informal organization, and all such groups have the potential to become part of the overall informal organization that interacts with the formal structure of the institution. In every organization, unless it consists of only a few individuals, an informal or invisible organization exists. The informal organization probably differs from the lines of the formal organization, but it is a functioning entity (Exhibit 16.1).

The informal organization develops when small groups acquire a more or less distinct structure and a set of norms and standards, as well as ways to exert pressure for conformity and procedure and to invoke sanctions to ensure conformity to those norms. The informal organizational structure is determined largely by the different status positions that people within the small group hold. This is known as the "pecking order."

Status Positions

status position
One of four positions vis-à-vis the informal organization. These are the informal leader, members of the primary group, members on the fringe of the group, and those outside the fringe.

Generally, there are four **status positions**: the informal leader, members of the primary group, members who have only fringe status, and members who have out status. The informal leader of the small group is the person around whom the primary members of the group cluster; their association is close, and their interaction is intense. This is normally considered the small nucleus group of which newcomers would like to become members.

These newcomers are usually new employees of the department. They remain on the fringe of the group while they are being evaluated by the small nucleus for acceptance or rejection. Eventually these individuals either are gradually integrated into the primary or fringe groups, or move into the outer shell because they have been rejected.

People in the outer shell are still a part of the department, although they have not been accepted as members of the core group. Such rejection, however, can have serious behavioral effects, especially if a person strongly wishes to belong to the nucleus group. This happens because, in essence, the group causes members to modify their own behavior and to affect the behavior of those in the fringe shell or the outer shell. If the rejection is mutual, however, the person in the outer shell can survive very well on her own.

The person who plays the role of the informal leader is usually the dynamic force of the group. As with the committee chairperson, this individual engages in leadership activities, crystalizes opinions, and sets objectives. This

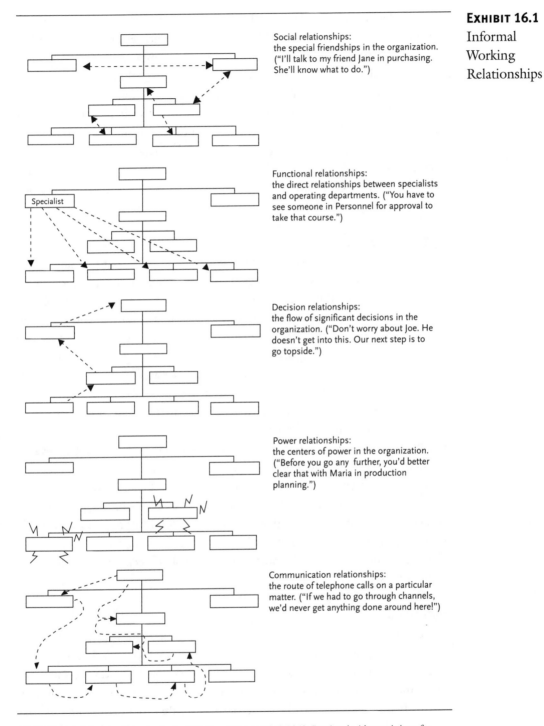

EXHIBIT 16.1

Informal
Working
Relationships

Social relationships:
the special friendships in the organization.
("I'll talk to my friend Jane in purchasing.
She'll know what to do.")

Functional relationships:
the direct relationships between specialists
and operating departments. ("You have to
see someone in Personnel for approval to
take that course.")

Specialist

Decision relationships:
the flow of significant decisions in the
organization. ("Don't worry about Joe. He
doesn't get into this. Our next step is to
go topside.")

Power relationships:
the centers of power in the organization.
("Before you go any further, you'd better
clear that with Maria in production
planning.")

Communication relationships:
the route of telephone calls on a particular
matter. ("If we had to go through channels,
we'd never get anything done around here!")

SOURCE: *Administrative Organization* by Pfiffner and Sherwood, © 1960. Reprinted with permission of
Pearson Education, Inc., Upper Saddle River, NJ.

group leader is generally democratically chosen by the group. The leadership role is created by consensus. This person usually possesses communication skills, sensitivity, and intelligence and helps the members achieve their tasks and emotional needs. The informal leader gains status, although without rank, and satisfies the group members' need for a leader to whom they can turn for support. Occasionally one might find small groups in which the leadership is shared and in which different leaders perform different functions, sometimes only for a brief time. For example, one leader may deal with administration, whereas another may deal with the union and another may try to maintain internal cohesiveness and morale. Most of the time, however, there is only one informal leader with whom the supervisor will have to deal.

Norms and Standards

Besides status positions, norms and standards are in place that regulate group behavior. Norms are expectations about how members of the group ought to behave. They define the boundaries between acceptable and unacceptable behavior (Feldman 1984). In addition to these standards for behavior between group members, norms relate to quality and quantity of work and to many other areas, such as honesty and loyalty. Norms promoting high performance, creativity, and an honest day's work are clearly desirable, whereas cheating, leaving work early, and limiting output are not beneficial. One should not assume that the norms of one group can be generalized to another group.

To be admitted to the group, an employee must be willing and eager to comply with such standards. Because groups are capable of granting or withholding the advantages of membership, individuals must modify their behavior so that it corresponds to that of the group. This is why the informal organization has such a significant influence over the behavior and work of employees who are primary group members. In addition, the interactions between primary group members also influence the behavior of those in the fringe shell and even possibly those in the outer shell because all are members of the total system.

Sanctions

Along with norms, there must be an effective procedure for invoking sanctions if a group member does not conform to the standards set. These sanctions can be elusive and evasive or overt. At first, sanctions can be mild; the group may try to bring the nonconformist back in line by friendly communication. If this does not produce the desired results, friendly comments may stop, and threats, ridicule, or possibly physical abuse may follow. The most powerful sanction is rejection. Employees who consistently do not comply with the group's norms are soon pushed to the outside shell. Their lives can then be made miserable, their work can be sabotaged, and eventually they may want to leave the institution completely. All these sanctions of the informal organization, whether subtle or strong, serve to ensure that group members adhere to the group's ideas of correct on-the-job behavior.

Resistance to Change

Another characteristic of the informal organization is inflexibility, especially resistance to change. It resists especially those changes that could be interpreted as a threat to the informal group. Over time, the small group develops satisfying social relationships, and any change that may challenge its equilibrium and stability is greeted with resistance. This resistance can take the form of complaints, work slowdown, excessive absenteeism, and reduction in the quality of the job performed. It is essential for a supervisor to understand the dynamics of these types of group behavior to introduce change successfully. This is discussed further in Chapter 22.

Interaction Between Informal and Formal Organizations

It might appear that the informal organization makes the job of the supervisor more difficult. Because of the interdependence between informal and formal organizations, the attitudes, goals, norms, and customs of one affect the other. Informal organizations do frequently give life and vitality to the formal organization, but this is not always the case. Informal organizations can have either a constructive or hindering influence on the formal organization and on the realization of departmental objectives. How the supervisor manages the informal structure has much to do with whether that influence is positive or negative.

The supervisor must respect the informal organization for the power it has; it cannot be ignored, and attempts to suppress it should not be made. It is important for the supervisor to be aware that these informal groups are strong, and they may often govern the behavior of employees to an extent that interferes with formal supervision. Sometimes it can even go so far that the pressure of the informal group frustrates the supervisor in carrying out objectives that the superior manager expects the supervisor to achieve. The wise supervisor, therefore, should work to gain the cooperation and goodwill of the informal organization and the informal leader and to use them to further the departmental objectives.

The Supervisor and the Informal Organization

One way the supervisor can put the informal organization to the best possible use is to let the employees know that its existence is accepted and understood. Such an understanding enables the supervisor to group employees so that those most likely to comprise a good team can work with each other on the same assignments. The supervisor's understanding of how the informal

HOSPITAL LAND

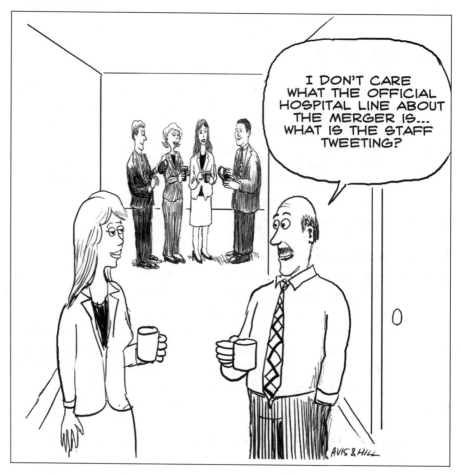

organization works also helps her avoid activities that would unnecessarily threaten or disrupt the informal group. The manager should do her utmost to integrate the interests of the informal organization with those of the formal organization.

The supervisor should exhibit this positive approach because she knows that there are positive attributes in a cohesive informal group. Morale is likely to be high, turnover and excessive absences tend to be low, and the members work smoothly as a team. This can make supervision much easier because the supervisor avoids hearing a lot of bickering; it can also ease the burden of communication because the group provides its own effective, although informal, channels.

Supervisors who encourage informal group leaders and informal relationships are likely to make their own jobs easier by gaining allies. Supervisors who suppress informal relationships risk creating enemies and fostering retaliation. By integrating formal and informal organizations, effectiveness is increased.

Group Decision Making

A supervisor can do even more to bring out the positive aspects of informal groups by sharing decision-making authority with them—that is, by practicing group decision making (Maier 1983). When problem solving demands a diversity of viewpoints and skills and when broad-based acceptance is needed, group decisions usually are superior. They enable the group to exercise control over its own activities and to make certain that all its interests are taken into account, with the result that no one comes out a loser. The advantages and disadvantages of group decision making are similar to those of committees discussed in Chapter 15.

The supervisor should establish ground rules for a group decision-making process; otherwise, the group decision process could bring about results that are opposite from those intended. First, the supervisor must sincerely believe in group decision making and want to use it. Second, the topic must be clearly set. For instance, if the group is to arrange its own vacation schedule, it should be stated how many employees with a special skill must always be present, what the time limits are, and so forth. Third, the group must be clearly told whether it is merely being asked for suggestions or whether the authority to find a solution and make a decision has been delegated. Finally, the supervisor should choose a problem in which the enthusiastic acceptance and execution are at least as important as, if not more important than, the specific elements of the decision itself. Under these conditions, group decision making can be an additional means of bringing out the positive aspects of the informal organization. These techniques can be equally beneficial in a task force or ad hoc committee in which group input and broad-based acceptance of a new process, policy, or the like are necessary.

The Supervisor and the Informal Group Leader

Informal leaders are powerful because of their status and power of authority; they can be a great help when they work in the best interest of the institution. When informal leaders are working toward achieving the same vision and goals as the formal leaders (and the organization itself), they can take a tremendous burden from the backs of managers and formal leaders. Some of the leadership functions and many management functions can be carried out informally by those without actual authority. This frees those with formal management responsibility to focus on what they themselves can uniquely do (Bacal 2009).

When informal leaders work against the goals of the organization, however, they can cause great difficulties. Therefore, supervisors should maintain a positive attitude toward the informal group leader. Instead of viewing this person as a "ringleader," supervisors should consider this individual as someone "in the know" and respect and work with him. Recall the discussion of personal authority and referent power. The informal leader has these traits and may be able to enlist followership from your staff to complete tasks and achieve goals. In an effort to build good relations with the informal leader, supervisors can pass information on to that person before giving it to anyone else. They can ask for advice on certain problems and, particularly if a rearrangement of duties is under consideration, may want to discuss the problems with the informal leader first to get some feedback and his support. Supervisors may also ask the informal leader to "break in" a new employee in the department, knowing that the leader would have done so anyway.

In taking this approach, the supervisor must be careful not to cause the informal leader to lose status within the group, because working with the supervisor means working with management. In other words, the supervisor should not extend too many favors to the informal leader, as this would ruin the latter's leadership position within the group. This discussion assumes that an informal group leader is easily visible in the department. Often it is difficult, however, for a supervisor, especially a new supervisor, to identify the informal leader of a group. Observation is probably the best means to find out. The supervisor should look for the person to whom the other employees turn when they need help, who sets the pace, and who seems to have influence over the other employees. The supervisor must continually and closely observe this because the informal group occasionally shifts from one leader to another, depending on the purposes to be pursued. Regardless of who the leader is, the supervisor should do all that she possibly can to work with the informal leader instead of against that person.

Summary

In addition to the formal organization, there exists in every enterprise an informal organization based on informal groups. These groups satisfy certain needs and desires of their members, which apparently are left unsatisfied by the formal organization. For example, an informal group can satisfy the members' social needs. It gives them recognition, status, and a sense of belonging. Informal information transmitted through the grapevine provides a channel of communication and fulfills the members' need and desire to know what is going on. The informal organization also influences the behavior of individuals within the group and compels them to conform to norms the group has established. Informal organization can be found on all levels of the enterprise—from the top to the bottom. It exists in every department, regardless of the quality of supervision.

The informal organization can have either a constructive or hindering influence on the formal organization. To make the best possible use of the informal organization, the supervisor must understand its workings and be able to identify its informal leaders. Then the supervisor can work with them in a way that helps accomplish the objectives of the department. Instead of dwelling on the informal organization as a source of conflict, the supervisor should remember that both the formal and the informal organizations are part of a complex system and interact with each other. The supervisor should approach the informal organization positively and emphasize its potential for the good of the enterprise. One way to emphasize the positive is to allow group decision making by the informal groups. The supervisor must not suppress the informal relationships. Formal and informal relationships should be integrated to increase organizational effectiveness.

Additional Reading

Bacal, R. 2009. "Benefiting from Informal Leaders in Your Organization—Communication Is the Key." [Online article; retrieved 3/2/09.] www.work911.com/leadership-development/articles/informalleadershipbenefits.htm.

STAFFING: HUMAN RESOURCES MANAGEMENT

THE STAFFING PROCESS

Chapter Objectives

After you have studied this chapter, you should be able to do the following:

1. Define the staffing function as the sum of activities required to attract, develop, and retain people who have the knowledge and skills needed to achieve departmental objectives.
2. Describe how equal opportunity laws and fair employment regulations affect the staffing function.
3. Describe the relationship between the human resources department and line management.
4. Describe the importance of job description and job qualifications based on job analysis.
5. Identify recruitment, staffing, and scheduling alternatives.

People are the most important and valuable asset of an organization. **Staffing** is the managerial function concerned with the procurement and maintenance of human resources to fulfill the institution's goals. It is the sum of activities needed to attract, develop, and retain people who have the necessary skills and knowledge to achieve departmental objectives. Once goals are determined, departments are set up, and duties and task relationships are established, people must be placed to give life to what would otherwise be an empty structure. It is the manager's responsibility to vitalize the department by staffing it properly.

      Human resources management begins with planning. Staffing begins with recruitment and selection. **Recruitment** is the process of locating qualified candidates, and **selection** is the process of choosing from the pool of applicants. Staffing also involves making sure the department's subordinates are properly oriented, placed, trained, developed, compensated, and given benefits. Some of these activities are handled by the human resources manager, while others are handled directly by the employee's supervisor or manager. The manager's staffing duties also include judging employees' work and evaluating their performance, promoting them according to effort and ability, rewarding them, transferring them, and, if necessary, disciplining or even discharging them. Only if a manager performs all these duties can one say that the managerial staffing function has been fulfilled.

staffing
The managerial function concerned with the procurement and maintenance of human resources.

human resources management
The management, including planning, of the staffing function.

recruitment
The process of locating qualified candidates.

selection
The process of choosing from the pool of applicants.

Staffing is a difficult task, and the importance of human resources management has expanded greatly in recent years. The oldest baby boomers started to retire in 2008. By 2015, baby boomers age 55 and older will compose only 20 percent of the workforce. This transition requires organizations to mitigate against the loss of organization memory and devise strategies to transfer knowledge from veteran employees to neophyte employees (Myers 2007). Good resource planning and maintenance have a major impact on the performance of the organization. Poor resource planning can result in shortages, and improper recruiting practices can lead to embarrassing situations. Many of these shortages or improper practices are caused by today's complex legal environment concerning human resources management. Thus, the supervisor depends heavily on the expertise of the human resources department, or an individual with human resources expertise. Nevertheless, good management considers human resources management the responsibility of all operating managers. The supervisor may be assisted by the human resources staff in performing these functions. For example, the human resources department does the recruiting and the initial screening, but the final hiring should be made by the supervisor of the department. The evaluation of the employees' performance should be made by the line supervisor, although the system, procedures, forms, and so forth are designed by the human resources staff.

The Staffing Function and the Human Resources Department

The human resources department is a staff department as defined in the Chapter 11 discussion of line and staff capacity. Its usefulness and effectiveness depend largely on its ability to develop a good working and sharing relationship with line supervisors. This relationship is governed in part by how clearly and specifically the CEO has outlined the activities and authority of the human resources department. In determining the human resources department's scope and relationship to the staffing function of line supervisors, line managers should understand the history of this department in organizations.

Historical Patterns

The predecessor of the human resources department was the personnel department. This function started primarily as a record-keeping department. It kept all employment records for the employees and managers, correspondence pertaining to hiring, applications, background information, various positions held within the enterprise, dates of promotions, salary changes, leaves of absence granted, disciplinary penalties imposed, and other information on the employee's relationship to the enterprise.

Proper maintenance of these clerical records is still of great importance today, especially with the growing emphasis on equal opportunity employment, pensions and benefits, insurance programs, unemployment claims, seniority provisions, and promotional and developmental programs. By assigning such clerical service activities to the staff in personnel, the administrator knows that the tasks will be handled competently and efficiently. If such a service were not provided by the personnel department, each supervisor would have to keep these records for his own department, jeopardizing consistency and spending the supervisor's time on noncore work.

In the 1920s, many managers in industry believed unionization might be thwarted if the industries gave employees such benefits as cafeterias, better recreational facilities, bowling teams, and company stores. The personnel department took responsibility for many of these programs.

During the 1930s, another shift in the emphasis of the personnel department took place. With the increase of union activities, the personnel department was expected to take direct charge of all employee and union relations. It often assumed full responsibility for hiring, firing, handling union grievances, and dealing with general labor problems. In other words, management believed that by having a personnel department, all personnel questions could be handled by the department, leaving the line supervisors with practically no staffing function.

This led to serious difficulties, however, because as the duties and power of the personnel department increased significantly, the standing of the supervisor as a manager decreased. The employees no longer regarded the supervisor as their boss. Because someone in the personnel department hired the employees; established their wages; and promoted, disciplined, and fired them, employees looked to someone in the personnel department as their leader. The demoralized supervisor justifiably complained that it was impossible to manage the department effectively without having the power to select, hire, discipline, and reward the employees. The evolution of the **unity of command** (see Chapter 11) concept forced management to clearly differentiate between the functions of the personnel department in a staff capacity and the supervisor's line role as the department's operating manager.

unity of command concept
Each person should take orders from and report to only one boss.

Current Patterns

During recent decades, most organizations have recognized the need for constant interaction and proper balance of influence and authority between the line managers and the human resources staff. Good management dictates that supervisors and human resources staff work together because their work is intertwined; however, their areas of authority and their roles must be clearly stated. Sound management principles advocate that the primary job of the human resources department is to provide the line supervisors with advice, suggestions, and counsel and support concerning fair and equitable employee practices and personnel problems. Going beyond this could lead to a fragmentation of the supervisor's job and make it difficult for the supervisor to be an effective manager. Of course, the supervisor must manage within the framework of the organization's human resources policies, procedures, and regulations. Line supervisors should take full advantage of the expertise and assistance that is available within the human resources department, but they must retain the basic responsibility for managing their department.

Exhibit 17.1 is an excerpt from *The Management of Human Resources* (Cherrington 1991). The passage emphasizes the distinction between management and human resources. Interestingly, this company continues to succeed, abiding by many of these same tenets while modeling corporate social responsibility within its community and for the customers it serves. You are encouraged to visit its website to learn more.

Because it is the supervisor's job to ensure the work is accomplished within the department, she must make managerial decisions that concern the department's employees. Generally, this means that the supervisor defines the specific qualifications expected from an employee who is to fill a specific position. It is the human resources department's function to develop sources of qualified applicants within the local labor market. This department must let the community know what jobs are available and, in general, create an image of the organization as an employer. These activities are known as recruiting. **Recruiting** is the process of attracting and seeking a pool of applicants from which to choose a qualified candidate. This can be accomplished by fostering good community relations and recruiting from high schools, training schools, colleges, and other sources of employees as well as using print advertisements in newspapers or professional journals or posting opportunities on various Web-based job boards. To promote the organization, the human resources department may tout the comprehensiveness of the benefits package in its open-position advertisements, mentioning benefits such as flextime or job sharing, telecommuting options, insurance coverage, and paid days off.

When individuals apply, the human resources department conducts screening interviews with the applicants to determine whether their qualifications match the minimum requirements of the job (e.g., education, certification, basic skills) as defined by the supervisor. The department also conducts testing (e.g., keyboarding speed and accuracy, spelling, math) if the position requires it, and sometimes administers personality assessments such as Myers-Briggs. Additionally, human resources personnel check references and verify

recruiting
The process of attracting and seeking a pool of applicants from which to choose a qualified candidate.

EXHIBIT 17.1 Management Versus Human Resources

We Don't Have an HR Department

An article in the *Personnel Administrator* described Nucor Corporation as the most productive steel mill in the world. When students in a human resource management class heard that a Nucor mill was located nearby, they thought it would provide an excellent field trip. One of the student leaders, Rebecca, called to arrange the visit. When she phoned she asked to speak with their human resource manager.

"I'm sorry, we don't have a human resource manager."

"Then could I speak with your personnel director?"

"We don't have a personnel director either."

"Then what do you call that position?"

"I'm sorry ma'am, but we simply don't have that position."

Assuming they had a special title for the position, Rebecca asked, "Who handles your compensation and benefits?"

"Our benefits are managed by our controller but our compensation is directed by a payroll clerk. Would you like to talk with her?"

"Is she also the one who manages the recruiting, hiring, and performance evaluation?"

"No, those activities are performed by our supervisors. Is there something I could help you with?"

Finally, Rebecca realized that they did not have a human resource manager or a personnel department. Eventually her call was directed to the general manager, who explained how the personnel functions were performed at that steel mill. Although Nucor Steel did not have a human resource manager at each mill, they had a manager of personnel services at the corporate headquarters who was responsible for creating personnel policies and programs for the mills.

The general manager explained that 335 employees worked at that location and all but 55 of them were directly involved in producing steel. These 55 included the supervisors, the clerical support staff, and six vice presidents. Although none of these people had the title human resource manager, they all performed various human resource functions. Wages, salaries, and benefits were distributed by the payroll clerk; health and accident insurance was supervised by an insurance clerk. The supervisors were responsible for most of the remaining personnel functions, including interviewing, hiring, discipline, safety, and training. Recruiting was not assigned to anyone since they had a long waiting list of job applicants and turnover was negligible.

Continued

EXHIBIT 17.1 *Continued*

The supervisors received a salary for 52 weeks per year, plus an annual bonus, while production workers received hourly pay plus generous productivity bonuses that were calculated daily and weekly. Everyone also participated in an annual profit-sharing plan. The productivity bonuses generally accounted for over two-thirds of the production workers' pay. Employees who came to work late forfeited their daily production bonus, and if they were absent they lost their weekly production bonus. Consequently, tardiness and absenteeism were not problems at this mill.

Rebecca asked if it would be possible to bring the student group on a field trip to visit the plant.

"I'm sorry, but we cannot accommodate you. It's not that we dislike visitors or want to be secretive, we simply don't have anyone to show you around. We are in the business of producing steel, not guided tours."

Nucor Steel is good at making steel. The top five steel mills in the United States average 347 tons of steel per employee per year, while the top five integrated steel mills in Japan average 480 tons of steel per employee per year. Nucor produces approximately 950 tons of steel per employee per year.

SOURCE: *The Management of Human Resources*, Third Edition, by Cherrington, © Reprinted by permission of Pearson Education, Inc., Upper Saddle River, NJ.

Note: For current information about Nucor's continued success, visit www.Nucor.com.

certifications and past records. Candidates who meet the stated requirements are referred to the supervisor.

Human resources personnel are guided by the organization's legal counsel as well as publications such as *Testing and Assessment: An Employer's Guide to Best Practices* published by the U.S. Department of Labor (2000). The human resources department works with departmental managers to ensure that skills testing remains current and that the hiring process does not discriminate against applicants.

It is up to the supervisor to interview, select, and hire from among the qualified available candidates. The supervisor assigns the new employee to a specific job and judges how the employee's skills can best be used and developed. While it is the human resources department's job to inform the new employee about the organization's benefits, general rules, shifts, and hours—typically during an employee orientation program—the supervisor explains the specifics of the position and department (i.e., wages, departmental rules, hours, and rest periods).

The department-specific orientation covers introductions to coworkers; a department tour; specifics about the assignment; and issues such as safety, security, computer passwords, and confidentiality. The supervisor either arranges to have another person, such as a department trainer or coworker, instruct and train the new employee on the job or does the training himself. The supervisor assesses the new employee's performance to determine whether she should be retained or retrained.

The supervisor also monitors compensation and decides whether the employee should eventually receive a pay adjustment or be promoted into a better job. If the need to take disciplinary measures should arise, it is clearly the supervisor's duty to do so. The supervisor should review planned disciplinary actions with the human resources department to make sure they are done properly. During the time an employee is with the organization, the complete employment record is maintained by the human resources department.

Throughout the entire staffing process, the supervisor is aided by the human resources department. As previously mentioned, this is particularly important because of the necessity of complying with nondiscriminatory employment, insurance, pension, promotion, and other practices and the standards of accreditation and regulatory agencies. The human resources department also provides expertise, advice, counsel, and guidance whenever personnel problems arise. In making decisions, the supervisor can follow, ignore, reject, or alter the personnel department's advice and counsel. In today's societal and legal environment regarding the staffing function, however, the input of the human resources liaison has become vital and has a strong impact on the practice of management.

Sometimes supervisors welcome the human resources department's willingness to help them out of a difficult situation. Frequently supervisors ask the human resources department to make a decision for them so that they do not become burdened with so-called personnel problems. These supervisors gladly accept the department's decision, believing that if the decision is wrong, they can always excuse it by saying the decision was made by human resources. As a supervisor, "passing the buck" is not an option. All supervisors must remember that it is their responsibility to execute the staffing functions.

Although it is understandable that the supervisor may be reluctant to question and disregard the advice of the human resources staff expert, she must bear in mind that the staff person sees only a small part of the entire picture and is not responsible for how the department performs. Many other factors that affect the department are involved in the overall picture—factors with which the human resources staff are not as familiar as the line supervisor. The supervisor cannot always separate her functions between personnel problems and performance problems. Every situation has certain personnel implications, and it is impossible to separate the various components of each problem within the department. Only the supervisor is likely to see the broad picture.

Staffing and Legal Implications

Employment law in the United States has traditionally been governed by the common law rule of "at-will employment," meaning that an employment relationship could be terminated by either party at any time for any reason or without a reason. This is still true today in most states. However, starting in 1941, a series of laws prohibited certain discriminatory firings. The federal government continues to address fair wages and immigrant employment practices and states have established state-specific employment-related legislation. In addition, local laws, executive orders and guidelines, and court decisions have made the staffing function more complex. Employment practices and policies must comply with these regulations, which in general prohibit discrimination against applicants and employees on the basis of race, sex, color, religion, or national origin. Also, employers cannot use age as a criterion of selection among applicants between 40 and 70 years old. Other laws request that an organization hire handicapped persons and veterans. Affirmative-action programs dictate that the institution give hiring preferences to minority members who are qualified or have the potential to fill available jobs.

A detailed discussion of labor laws is beyond the confines of this book; however, supervisors must be aware that information on these regulations is readily available from the human resources department or on the U.S. Department of Labor's website. Exhibit 17.2 is a partial listing of the major labor laws and their respective enforcement agencies effective at the time this edition of the text was prepared. Other legislative and regulatory issues are discussed in chapters 6 and 27.

It would be impossible for a line supervisor to keep abreast of all employment-related laws. This is where the expertise of the human resources department comes into play. The human resources department must make sure the organization complies with the multitude of laws and regulations. The human resources director should disseminate current information regarding fair employment practices to all first-line supervisors. For example, the department of human resources should familiarize the supervisors with recent issues and government provisions. Also, the various possibilities of conscious and unconscious discriminatory practices and sexual harassment should be brought to the attention of the supervisors, and supervisors should understand the meaning of affirmative action. Ideally this information is disseminated and discussed at a new supervisors' orientation program, either annually as a refresher or update course or regularly at management meetings.

EXHIBIT 17.2 Labor Legislation

LEGISLATION	CONCERN OR CONTENT	ADMINISTRATIVE OR ENFORCEMENT AGENCY
Fair Labor Standards Act of 1938	Minimum wage, overtime pay, and record keeping	U.S. Department of Labor
Fair Employment Act of 1941	Prohibits discrimination[‡]	Committee on Fair Employment Practices
Equal Pay Act of 1963	Compensation relative to the sex of a worker	Equal Employment Opportunity Commission
Title VII of the Civil Rights Act of 1964[†]	Sex, color, race, religion, and national origin	Equal Employment Opportunity Commission
Age Discrimination in Employment Act of 1967 (amended 1978)	Age (protection for those 40 to 70 years old)	Equal Employment Opportunity Commission
Occupational Safety and Health Act of 1970	Workplace safety	Occupational Safety and Health Administration
Rehabilitation Act of 1973	People with disabilities	U.S. Department of Labor
Employee Retirement Income Security Act of 1974	Pension and healthcare plan rules	U.S. Department of Labor
Immigration Reform and Control Act of 1986	Employment eligibility verification	U.S. Department of Labor
Employee Polygraph Protection Act of 1988	Prohibits use of polygraphs by most private employers	Secretary of Labor
Americans with Disabilities Act of 1990	People with disabilities	Equal Employment Opportunity Commission
Family and Medical Leave Act of 1993	Permits unpaid leave for certain reasons	Employment Standards Administration
Health Insurance Portability and Accountability Act of 1996	Health insurance coverage	U.S. Department of Labor
Nursing Relief for Disadvantaged Areas Act of 1999	Permits temporary employment of alien/foreign RNs	U.S. Department of Labor

[†]As amended by the Equal Employment Opportunity Act of 1972, the Pregnancy Discrimination Act of 1978, and in 1991 when a cap on punitive damages was applied.

[‡]Applied to national defense industry.

Functional Authority and the Human Resources Department

The beginning of this chapter stated that the human resources department is attached to the organization in a staff position, which means that staff's job is to advise and assist line managers. During the last few years, however, many CEOs of healthcare institutions, industry, and businesses have decided to limit the supervisor's authority to terminate an employee. In these organizations, all dismissals have to be approved by the human resources director or designated liaison. In this instance functional staff authority, as discussed in chapters 12 and 13, has been conferred on the human resources department.

There must be solid reasoning behind such a decision because it clearly runs counter to the principle of unity of command and weakens the authority of the line manager's position. While the CEO may have other reasons for delegating final authority to the director of human resources, he may make such a decision based on the need to comply with all fair and nondiscriminatory employment practices and regulations. In addition to this move, administration should explain the importance of documentation, and line supervisors should be urged to keep meaningful personnel selection and performance notes to which they and the institution can refer if necessary. If supervisors are kept up to date on these issues, it is unlikely that, for example, they will contemplate discharging an employee until all possible ramifications have been considered. Under these circumstances the director of human resources would probably go along with a proposed dismissal because the supervisor would have a well-documented and substantiated case that could become a valid defense.

Finally, the human resources department often has sole responsibility for many other activities, such as maintaining personnel records, complying and keeping current with equal employment opportunity/affirmative action regulations, overseeing insurance benefits administration, conducting exit interviews, negotiating and complying with union contracts, setting wage ranges, handling outplacement service, initiating and maintaining employee assistance programs, developing safety programs, and conducting attitude surveys.

The Supervisor's Staffing Function

The staffing function is an ongoing activity for the supervisor, not something that is required only when the department is first established. More typically, the supervisor has to staff a department that already has an existing number of employees. In this case, although there is a nucleus of employees to start with, staffing is still needed because the composition of a department rarely stays the same for long. Because every supervisor depends on employees for the department's results, it is the supervisor's responsibility to make certain that there is a supply of well-trained employees to fill the various positions.

Determining the Need for Employees

To make certain that the department can perform the jobs required, the supervisor must determine both the number and type of employees who will be needed for the department. The supervisor considers what competencies staff must possess that are most significant to the department's success. Some behavior competencies may be achievement orientation, customer service orientation, flexibility, ability to work on a team, conceptual thinking, self-confidence, assertiveness, persuasive ability, professional aspirations, and the ability to develop others. Required skill competencies depend on the department. An employee in a pharmacy, for example, requires skills different from those of an employee in the laundry department. Once the competencies are known, the supervisor can design a competency-based interview approach (Exhibit 17.3) and query applicants in these areas.

If the supervisor structured the department, she presumably designed it in a fashion that the functions, competencies, and jobs are shown in their

EXHIBIT 17.3

COMPETENCY INTERVIEW	PRESENT	
Explain the steps to add a column of numbers in Excel.		
When would you use the task manager on your PC with Microsoft products?		
Can you add numbers in Word?		
How do you color a field in Word?		
When would you use Access?		
What is a mouse?		
To open a file, do you right click or left click on the mouse?		
If you wish to scan both sides of a document, which feature will you select on the scanning menu?		
If you intend to convert single-sided originals to double-sided copies, you will choose which of the following: 1→1, 2→1, 2→2 or 1→2?		
To use the online calculator and keypad on your keyboard, which lock key should you set on?		
Other technologies/equipment skills:		

proper relationships. If the supervisor takes over an existing department, it is necessary to become familiar with the organizational structure by drawing a chart of the existing jobs and functions and assessing the competencies of the incumbents. For example, the supervisor of the maintenance department may find that there are groups of painters, electricians, carpenters, and other tradesmen within the department. After taking this inventory of personnel, the supervisor should create a "staffing table" to determine how many skilled positions there are and should be within the department, what shifts need to be covered, and if the incumbents are able to support the department's needs. The working relationships between these positions should also be examined and defined by the supervisor.

After determining the needs of the department, the supervisor may have to adjust her ideal department design temporarily to fit within existing limitations. For example, several positions may have to be combined into one if there is not enough work to justify more than one position. Then the competencies of the employee placed in that combined position must be assessed to determine if he needs additional training to be able to perform successfully in the restructured position. Only by studying the organizational setup of the department can the supervisor determine what and how many employees are needed to perform the various jobs.

To fill the various positions with appropriate employees, the supervisor needs to match the available jobs in the department with the qualifications of prospective employees. The supervisor makes such a match with the help of **job descriptions** and **job specifications** (Exhibit 17.4). Often these documents are included in the departmental manual. The job description tells exactly what duties and responsibilities are contained within a particular job. It describes what the employees do, how they do it, and what the working conditions are. A job specification, also at times referred to as job qualification, identifies and describes the minimum acceptable qualifications required of a person holding a job; it typically contains general qualification requirements such as experience and training, education, and knowledge and skills. Often, human resources departments create a single document that includes both the job description and job specification components.

Job descriptions and job specifications are based on **job analysis**—a study of the jobs within the organization. This consists of analyzing the activities the employee performs; the equipment, tools, and work aids the employee uses; and the working conditions. The supervisor who is taking over an already established department often finds a set of job descriptions available. If none is available, the human resources director will help establish a set. However, no one is better equipped to describe the content of a job than the supervisor. She is responsible for the accomplishment of the department's tasks and knows (or should know) the content of each position. Although the final form of the job description may be prepared in the personnel office, the

job description
A document that describes the duties and responsibilities of a position.

job specification
A document that identifies the minimum acceptable qualifications of a person in that position.

job analysis
A study of the jobs within an organization to document the activities, tools used, and working conditions of each position.

EXHIBIT 17.4
Example
of a Job
Description/
Performance
Appraisal Form

Employee Name_____

Employee Number_____

Department/Unit_____

Job Title: Cook   **Job Number:** 24   **Salary Grade:** 7

Reports To: Immediate supervisor   **FLSA Status:** Non-exempt

Date Prepared/Revised: December 6, 2000   **Licensure/Certification:**

Job Summary: Reviews menus for upcoming meals, pulls meats for thawing and prepares and cooks meats; prepares and cooks baked goods and desserts, vegetables, and soups; and cleans up cook's area.

Education and/or Experience: At least one year experience as a cook and the ability to speak, read, and write English is required; high school diploma or G.E.D. is preferred.

Environmental Conditions: Work occurs inside; work involves frequent exposure to extreme cold conditions and hot and elevated surfaces; work involves occasional exposure to extreme hot and wet conditions, high dust and noise levels, low light levels, confined space, hazardous materials, and sharps.

Physical Requirements: Work requires frequent standing, walking, stooping/bending, lifting up to 25 pounds floor to waist (25 to 50 pounds with assistance), lifting up to 20 pounds waist to shoulder, and pushing/pulling up to 400 pounds (with wheels); work requires the ability to taste and perceive colors.

Drivers License Required? No   **CPR Required?** No

Continued

supervisor should determine its specific content. Even when job descriptions are available, it is the supervisor's duty to become familiar with them to make sure they are realistic, accurate, and up to date.

Only by closely analyzing the job requirements is it possible to ascertain the skills necessary to perform the job satisfactorily. Even if the position is already in operation, it is still advisable to determine the major duties and responsibilities. Several questions a supervisor asks as she analyzes a position appear in Exhibit 17.5. If the older job description no longer fits the current content of the job, the supervisor should update it. Even if the job in question is a new position, the supervisor should proceed along similar lines. The supervisor should determine the job's duties and responsibilities and, with the help of the personnel department, draw up a new job description. Once the content of the job has been listed, the supervisor should specify the

EXHIBIT 17.4
Continued

Ratings for first four sections:

5	4	3
Much more than acceptable—significantly exceeds criteria for successful job performance	More than acceptable—exceeds criteria for successful job performance	Acceptable—meets criteria for successful job performance

2	1
Less than acceptable—generally does not meet criteria for successful job performance	Much less than acceptable—significantly below criteria required for successful job performance

Core Dimensions	Key Actions	Rating	Comments
Adaptability	• Tries to understand changes in work tasks, situations, and environment • Approaches change or newness positively • Adjusts behavior		
Building loyalty customer	• Uses Key Principles • Acknowledges the person • Clarifies the current situation • Meets or exceeds needs • Confirms satisfaction • Takes the "heat"		
Teamwork/ Collaboration	• Builds relationships (using Key Principles) • Exchanges information freely • Volunteers ideas freely • Builds on others' ideas • Supports group decisions • Puts group goals ahead of individual/own goals		
	Average Rating		

Role Dimensions (Skilled Role)	Key Actions	Rating	Comments
Managing work (includes time management)	• Prioritizes • Makes preparations • Schedules effectively • Leverages resources • Stays focused		

Exhibit 17.4
Continued

Job-Specific Tasks		Standards	Rating	Comments
Tasks:	*% of time*			
Reviews menus for upcoming meal(s).		• Completely • In appropriate amount of time for meat to thaw		
Pulls meats for thawing.		• Accurately • In a timely manner • According to policies and procedures		
Prepares and cooks meats.		• Safely • According to written or verbal instructions based on type of meat • Consistently • By time required		
Prepares and cooks baked goods and desserts.		• Correctly, according to package directions or recipe • By time required		
Prepares and cooks vegetables.		• Correctly • Appropriately • By time required		
Prepares and cooks soups.		• Correctly • Completely • Thoroughly		
Cleans up cook's area.		• Thoroughly • Completely • Practicing "clean as you go"		
		Average Rating		

Other Job Objectives (Optional)	Accomplishment	Rating	Comments
	Average Rating		

Continued

EXHIBIT 17.4
Continued

	Average Rating	Multiplied by:	Weighted Average	
Dimensions (50%)				
1. Core Dimensions		× 0.25	=	
2. Role Dimensions		× 0.25	=	
Performance (50%)				
3. Job-Specific Tasks		×	=	If **no** Optional Job Objectives, multiply Average Rating by 50% (0.50).
4. (Optional) Job Objectives		×	=	If **has** Optional Job Objectives, assign a percentage value, at your discretion, to "multiply by" in rows 3 and 4 to equal 50% (0.50).
Average Rating of All Previous Sections		(This column needs to total 1.00)	(Add these averages to get the final rating)	

Ratings for this section only:

Expert—*can use the knowledge or skill independently and is also able to assess others and/or teach the knowledge or skill*

Competent—*can use the knowledge or skill independently*

Novice—*little or no experience with the knowledge or skill; needs training and/or assistance*

Knowledge and Skills (Job-Specific Technical/ Professional Dimension)	*Results*	*Rating* **E**-Expert **C**-Competent **N**-Novice	*Comments*
Knowledge of department policies and procedures.	Policies and procedures are followed.		

EXHIBIT 17.4
Continued

Ratings for this section only:

Expert—*can use the knowledge or skill independently and is also able to assess others and/or teach the knowledge or skill*

Competent—*can use the knowledge or skill independently*

Novice—*little or no experience with the knowledge or skill; needs training and/or assistance*

Knowledge and Skills (Job-Specific Technical/ Professional Dimension)	*Results*	*Rating* **E**-Expert **C**-Competent **N**-Novice	*Comments*
Knowledge of safe food handling practices	Safe food-handling practices are followed.		
Ability to use basic mathematics	Calculations are correctly made.		
Ability to operate cooking equipment	Equipment is operated correctly and safely.		

Total number of Expert ratings _____

Total number of Competent ratings _____

Total number of Novice ratings _____

List any Corrective Actions received during the past twelve months and discuss progress to date with employee:

Key development (knowledge or skill) needs, including for a future responsibility: (Ask the employee to complete an Individual Development Plan for a future discussion)

Key strengths:

Has employee completed annual requirements (m3 and PPD test) within the last twelve months? _____

Employee Signature _____

Reviewer's Signature _____

Date _____

SOURCE: Adapted with permission from Deaconess Hospital, Oklahoma City, OK.

Exhibit 17.5

Job Description
Worksheet

Main Job Tasks:

1. What is the main purpose?
2. What are the essential duties?
3. What are the main priorities?
4. With whom will this candidate interact?
5. What deadlines does this job have?
6. What equipment does this job use?

Must-Have Requirements:

1. What basic skills must the candidate have?
2. What special skills should the candidate have?
3. What kind of experience should the candidate have?
4. How much experience is needed? (One month? One year?)
5. What level of education is needed?

Preferred/Personal Skills:

1. How much stamina is required?
2. What work characteristics are important? (Ability to work unsupervised? Manual dexterity? Detail orientation?)
3. What level of communication skills is needed? (Written, public speaking, etc.)
4. How long would you like a person to remain in this position?
5. What additional requirements are preferred, but not mandatory?

SOURCE: McGill, A. *Hiring the Best.* 1993. Reprinted with permission of the McGraw-Hill Companies.

knowledge, education, degrees, experience, and skills required of the prospective employee. It is acceptable to state in the job description that the employee must be able to work well with coworkers. In that way the supervisor is clearly telling candidates the job cannot be done just his way; he must always consider the feelings of colleagues as well (AICPA 2004). Asking current staff to provide input (see Exhibit 17.6) may reveal not only content overlooked by the supervisor but also retraining and job redesign needs.

Equal employment opportunity laws and rulings require that job descriptions must not discriminate against certain classes (e.g., age greater than 40 [ADEA], disability [ADA], and national origin [Civil Rights]) and must be job related. The supervisor should consult the human resources department for guidance on these laws. To comply with these laws and regulations, many personnel departments have assumed responsibility for the final review of the draft of the job descriptions. If they are kept current, position descriptions prove invaluable to many people throughout the organization. They inform the incumbent (and whoever needs or wants to know) what he is supposed to do (this part of the description includes some statement of authority and infor-

EXHIBIT 17.6

Questions to
Ask Your Staff

1. What is the primary purpose of your job? How does it contribute to the facility?

2. What are the essential functions of your job, and how much time do you spend on those tasks?

3. What are the peripheral functions of your job or tasks that someone else could do?

4. What amount of education and experience do you believe is needed for your job?

5. What skills are needed to perform your job?

6. How much reasoning is needed in your job?

7. What are the physical demands of your job?

8. What are the visual requirements of the job?

9. Please describe the noise level you experience in your job.

SOURCE: Adapted from "Need Job Descriptions? Let Staff Start Them Off via a Questionnaire." May 2002, pp. 3–4. Reprinted with permission from *Law Office Administrator*, P.O. Box 11670, Atlanta, GA 30355. (404) 367–1991.

mational relationships). The job descriptions also serve as a basis to recruit applicants for open positions and help evaluate incumbents in the positions.

In every job, an employee must know certain facts before he can perform the job effectively. For example, a certain position may require the ability to read simple blueprints or perform basic or higher-level mathematics. If a knowledge of mathematics is needed, the specific type of mathematics required should be clearly defined. The word mathematics could imply knowledge far beyond a working knowledge of simple arithmetic, or a knowledge of simple arithmetic might be all that is required in the job. The more precisely the supervisor defines the required job knowledge, the easier it is for her to select from among available applicants.

When stipulating the skills needed for a particular job, the supervisor should not ask for a higher degree of skill than is absolutely necessary. One way to avoid this is to compare the requirements in the position description with the qualifications of employees who are doing the same or similar work. Such an investigation may quickly reveal the minimum level of education necessary for a certain job. There is no need, for instance, to specify a certain number of years of formal education and experience if all that is required is simply job know-how. The job specifications should not ask for less than what is needed but should specify the requirements realistically. If the requirements are set too high, the department may end up employing an overqualified person who may become unhappy and bored with the position. It is just as disastrous to ask for less than the necessary requirements.

The human resources department can guide the supervisor in developing or drawing up these job descriptions. Once these job descriptions have been drafted, the supervisor should consult with some of the people who are holding these jobs to compare the job descriptions with the actual positions in question. The human resources department should review the description again after this process. Once all discrepancies have been resolved, the job descriptions are reviewed one final time by human resources and possibly by the supervisor's superior.

The final, approved description is maintained in the human resources department and also in the supervisor's file. This is necessary because the job description is constantly referred to when the human resources department recruits candidates, when the supervisor hires new employees, when the employees' performance is appraised, and when establishing equitable wage patterns within the department or comparing wage scales with other organizations that have similar positions. As new employees are hired into the positions, they should receive a copy of the job descriptions.

If staffing decisions are to be valid, they must be based on comprehensive job descriptions that are systematically revised to reflect the current job situation as accurately as possible and be adjusted to comply with current requirements of equal employment opportunity and nondiscrimination laws. Often the job description serves as the basis for performance evaluations, so every incumbent in the position described by the job description should receive a copy of the most current version.

Position Titles

No standard agreement exists on the use and meaning of titles, especially in the upper echelons of healthcare organizations. The role of the most senior executive has evolved from superintendent to hospital administrator to executive director to CEO or president. (Throughout this book the terms *president, chief executive officer*, and *administrator* have been used interchangeably.) The CEO in larger hospitals is no longer concerned only with the internal operations of the hospital but also with external community relations. The CEO title communicates to patients, relatives, visitors, physicians, and the public that the president is the chief executive officer in the organization.

Following corporate usage of titles, where the president is the CEO, implies that an executive vice president is on the second level, several senior vice presidents (e.g., for patient care and for fiscal affairs) are on the third, and vice presidents are on the fourth level (e.g., vice president of professional services, of ambulatory services, of human resources, of environmental affairs). If an organization is tall, there may be associate and assistant vice presidents as well.

Supervisors should not assume that every healthcare organization uses the same titles. A nursing home may use "administrator," while a home health agency may use "executive director" for its top employed position. Physician groups often use "executive director" or "practice administrator" for their top employed position. Although the titles of the upper echelons vary from one healthcare institution to another, there must be internal consistency. Similarly, titles must be consistent across a healthcare system that may include a hospital, several ambulatory clinics, a home health agency, a durable medical equipment company, and a freestanding ambulatory surgery center. One way to do this is to use a basic title, such as director, and add adjectives to indicate the rank and area of activity (e.g., executive, associate, or assistant director, nursing, medical and surgical; or chief technologist, radiology, ambulatory services).

How Many to Hire

Normally, the supervisor is not confronted with the situation in which many employees have to be hired at the same time. However, such a situation could exist when a new department is created and the supervisor has to staff it completely, if a strike is anticipated, or if part-time armed services personnel are called from their peacetime jobs to serve in a military action. More typically, the question of hiring a single employee will occur.

A supervisor usually needs to hire a new worker when one of the employees leaves. Each vacancy should be considered an opportunity for the supervisor to revisit the department's or section's organization and reanalyze the job and related jobs for possible process improvements that may negate the need to replace the person or transition the department's structure closer to the ideal organization. This reassessment may be required during economic downturns, especially if the organization freezes hiring. This forces the supervisor to modify processes or reduce services so that the remaining staff can do the same work with fewer people. Occasionally changes in the technical nature of the work take place, and manual labor may be replaced by machinery, sophisticated instruments, or other new technology. In this case a replacement may not be needed, or a new employee with the different technical skills will be hired. The supervisor's study of the processes and organization may also reveal opportunities to use volunteers or to outsource the work, either of which may be more cost effective than hiring a new employee.

Other situations arise for which additional employees have to be added. For example, when new duties are to be undertaken and no one within the department possesses the required job knowledge and skill, the supervisor has to recruit employees. Sometimes a supervisor is inclined to ask for additional help if the workload is increased or if the supervisor feels added pressure. Before requesting additional employees under those conditions, the supervisor should make certain that the current staff are working up to capacity and that additional people are absolutely necessary.

In summary, the actual hiring decision is not to be made in the human resources office but rather by the supervisor of the department in which the employee is to work. It is up to the supervisor to hire the employee or identify an alternative approach to getting the work done. Because all applicants are screened by the human resources department, the supervisor knows that all those sent to him possess the minimum qualifications prescribed for the job. It is the supervisor's job to pick out the one who can best fill the job. This is not an easy task, but the supervisor gains more and more experience in selecting the "right" applicant over time. The selection process is discussed below and in Chapter 18.

Finding the Right Person

Depending on the economy, applicants have different motivations to seek employment. During prosperous times, skilled workers such as nurses may be reluctant to seek night or weekend shift positions. Unskilled workers also benefit from prosperity, as humorously depicted in Exhibit 17.7. However, during poor economic times, employers, including healthcare facilities, may constrict the number of positions they will fill, and there often are more applicants than jobs.

Finding individuals who have the basic skill competencies adds another dimension to the recruiting problem. Sixty percent of human resources executives surveyed in the late 1990s reported that workers lack basic math skills, 55 percent cite serious deficiencies in workers' basic writing and comprehension skills, and 63 percent feel employees lack positive work habits (i.e., arriving on time and staying at work all day) (Snelling Report 1998). In 2003 the National Assessment of Adult Literacy reported that one in seven U.S. adults is unable to read (National Center for Education Statistics 2009).

EXHIBIT 17.7
Car Perk

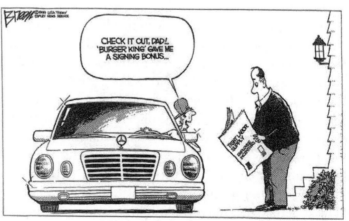

By Steve Breen, Asbury Park (N.J.) Press, for USA TODAY, Nov. 16 1999.

SOURCE: Courtesy of Steve Breen.

Of course, many employees of healthcare organizations require skills far beyond the basics, and there is a continuing shortage of highly trained healthcare workers. Thirty-seven percent of the respondents to a survey by the Healthcare Financial Management Association (2009) said they believe the nurse shortage will exceed 20 percent by 2019, and 91 percent of the respondents said they believe hospitals will be employing individuals with skill sets different from those required today. One suggestion offered by Jeffords, Scheidt, and Thibadoux (2000) for filling positions requiring college degrees is to develop work relationships with students. This may mean that supervisors need to tap local colleges and universities and offer to serve as training, internship, or cooperative work arrangement sites for undergraduates while the students progress through the curriculum. By participating in an ongoing program, the hospital has first choice of employees who are knowledgeable about the job and compatible with the department's culture. While these are successful tactics during up economies, they can help supervisors find the "best of the best" during down economies when there may be numerous applicants for a single opportunity.

The first step in establishing an internship program is to approach faculty of nearby technical schools, colleges, and universities that produce the graduates most in demand; examples may be nursing programs, physical therapy programs, heating and cooling technician programs, and radiology technician programs. Part-time employment arrangements could be developed to accommodate the students. Such arrangements test supervisors' skills as mentors, because they work one-on-one with the students, share the "tricks of the trade," and continually encourage the students to continue their education. At the end of the internship, you may even be required to complete a performance evaluation, including an assessment of the student's skill level, knowledge, and maturity.

Another arrangement similar to an internship or cooperative work arrangement is an externship. The externship is typically a short-term arrangement whereby the student spends from a few days up to a few weeks observing the work of others, working closely with one worker, or both. This option allows the student to determine if he truly wishes to pursue a healthcare career.

Internal initiatives also can assist with finding the right staff for your jobs. Some organizations have created their own internal "schools" to develop and educate needed staff. An example of this "growing-your-own" approach might be providing medical terminology, anatomy and physiology, and coding courses to groom coding technicians for filling health information, registration, clinic, and patient accounts positions. Cox Medical Center in Springfield, Missouri, established a state-certified school to train medical transcriptionists because the hospital had such difficulty hiring these specialized professionals.

Another alternative is to develop an in-house temporary agency that maintains a roster of individuals interested in part-time or temporary work on an as-needed basis. When a need arises, the agency coordinator starts down the list, calling those on the roster until one or more are able to fill the vacancy for the designated period of time or until a permanent replacement is found. Often these workers do not wish to have a permanent or full-time position but have the skills and are willing to fill in. Occasionally, these in-house agencies include staff who, because of health reasons, are on limited-duty restrictions or employees whose jobs were recently eliminated. Both of these groups of employees have knowledge of the organization, have contributed to the organization's goals, and wish to provide continued service to the facility.

Reevaluating the older-employee option is yet another alternative. Studies have found that older workers have better attendance records, are much less likely to file workers' compensation claims, use less healthcare benefits, and display a sincere willingness to learn new skills (Prenda and Stahl 2001; Allen and Wircenski 2005). More older Americans have remained in the labor force for several reasons, including the fact that many are staying healthier longer, some are feeling financial pressures, some desire more income for leisure activities, and many are able to find work that is less physically demanding. While some organizations thought it unwise to invest in retraining older workers, AARP revealed that employees in the 50 to 60 age bracket stay on the job an average of 15 years (Prenda and Stahl 2001).

Last but not least is a relatively popular approach for human resources recruiting efforts—offering perquisites such as sign-on bonuses, flexible work hours, and options for telecommuting. The most desirable candidates probably receive offers from competing healthcare organizations. Regardless of the condition of the economy, managers today must accept the reality that only 35 million people were born between the years of 1964 and 1978 (Generation Xers), considerably fewer than the baby boom generation, who competed for work with 85 million contemporaries early in their career (Jennings 2000). As these baby boomers retire, there are fewer Generation Xers and Millenials to replace them. Thus, there may be insufficient employees to fill openings in the years to come. The comic shown in Exhibit 17.7 depicts how desperate employers may be. You must discuss your staffing needs and difficulties with human resources and together create an innovative recruitment plan to meet the departmental objectives.

Transfers

transfer
A reassignment of an employee to another job of similar pay, status, and responsibility.

Transfers are another internal source of recruitment. A **transfer** is a reassignment of an employee to another job of similar pay, status, and responsibility. It is not a promotion because it is a horizontal move. Transfers take place either because the organization makes it necessary or because the employee requests it. Employees may want a transfer for various reasons—for example, to gain broader experience or to avoid some friction in a department. If an employee has problems that are causing friction, a transfer is not always the right solution unless it clearly resolves the problems. Sometimes technological changes in one department free a number of employees for transfer into a unit where needs for employees are expanding.

Transferring an employee from one position to another within the healthcare institution often results in greater job satisfaction. For example, a nurse's aide may consider a job as an aide in the operating room to be more prestigious than being an aide on the medical-surgical floor. The pay is the same and one cannot call it a promotion, but to the aide such a transfer means greater job satisfaction and constitutes an achievement. Transfers also provide employees with the opportunity to gain broader knowledge of the institution's activities. It is necessary, therefore, that a healthcare institution have sound transfer policies and procedures, always considering equal employment opportunity provisions, so that those who desire a lateral transfer are given the opportunity to do so. The director of human resources together with the various line managers should design these policies and procedures and ensure that employees are prepared to make successful transfers.

It is probably best for the human resources department to act as a clearance center for interdepartmental transfers. If the responsibility is given to supervisors, the employee may be reluctant to request an interdepartmental transfer for fear of alienating the boss. Some supervisors may be understanding in these matters, whereas others may be resentful and not give their consent. Whatever procedure is instituted must have provisions that the employee inform the immediate supervisor of the desire to transfer. It is only fair that the present supervisor should be aware of the employee's intent. In the event that the immediate supervisor does not recommend the transfer, the employee should be able to appeal this decision to a higher line officer or possibly to the personnel director.

Provisions must also be in place dictating whether transfers are to be made only within departments, only between departments, or both. The procedure must state whether the employee carries previous seniority credits with him, and it must make provisions for the situation when two or more persons want to transfer to the same job. For example, should length of service be the sole determinant, or should capacity to handle the job also be taken into consideration? Good transfer policies and procedures must cover many additional aspects, such as equal employment opportunities. In any event, the opportunity must exist for employees to be transferred, as this provides more job satisfaction and motivates employees in much the same way as a promotion.

Outsourcing

When traditional recruitment efforts are not successful in supplying a healthcare organization's labor needs, many consider **outsourcing**. Outsourcing means contracting out a part of or an entire function area to a third party who

outsourcing
Contracting with a third party to handle some aspect of an organization's work.

offshoring
Using an outsourcing contractor who uses labor from countries other than the United States.

supplies the appropriate staff. Some think of outsourcing as synonymous with offshoring. The term **offshoring** indicates that jobs performed by U.S. residents in the past are now being performed by residents of countries such as India, Switzerland, and Mexico. However, outsourcing means contracting out a part or an entire functional area to a third party who supplies the appropriate staff. The two may occur simultaneously if the outsource firm also uses residents of other countries to do the work.

Hospitals have recognized that they cannot provide every service to every patient. Thus, they are reengineering their structures and focusing on their core competencies. Those activities that are not in the patient care realm become ideal candidates for outsourcing. For example, food service, housekeeping, patient billing, laundry and linen, security, clinical equipment management, information systems, and other activities are now outsourced by many hospitals. In fact, some hospitals are outsourcing clinical areas as well, such as after-hours radiology readings.

Often-cited reasons for outsourcing given by *Controller Magazine* (1997) and *AHA News* (Boothby 1998) include the following:

1. The function is difficult to manage or is currently out of control
2. Resources (labor and expertise) are not available internally or externally
3. There is a need to reduce and control operating costs
4. The organization desires to improve its focus
5. The organization desires to improve patient satisfaction
6. The function will result in budget flexibility
7. The organization wants access to world-class capabilities or expertise
8. The organization will become more competitive
9. The organization wants to free resources for other purposes

Supervisors may find that evaluating outsourcing firms may be just one approach to filling jobs in the workplace. Supervisors who choose to investigate outsourcing possibilities and eventually recommend them must take into consideration the duties and roles the outsourcing firm may have in their departments and the parameters in which they are required to function. Some of these duties may include quality improvement, productivity and other reporting requirements, accreditation preparation, patient or customer satisfaction expectations, achieving expected savings, employee training, waste management, increasing staff morale, and smoothing interdepartmental relationships.

Outsourcing has its disadvantages as well. Quality control may be more difficult, especially if the outsourcing firm is doing its work off site. Some existing employees may lose their jobs when their work is outsourced, and other employees may fear for their own future employment. This fear could lead to increased turnover as employees leave for more secure positions elsewhere. The outsource firm may not be as cost-effective as initially thought, and costs may rise more quickly than anticipated. Careful consideration must be given before proceeding with this alternative, and a supervisor is wise to include her boss and human resources department in these deliberations before approaching any outsourcing firms.

The Organizing Side of Staffing

Thus far we have been speaking about the managerial function of staffing— that is, selecting individuals to perform designated duties for the organization. However, often we use the term "staffing" to mean to schedule. Scheduling is technically an organizing function because managers organize resources according to time of the day or day of the week that the duties must be accomplished to meet the department's objectives. Recognizing that the two functions are closely related, we will discuss some managerial tactics for scheduling and/or organizing one's staff to achieve the goals of the organization.

Traditional Work Schedules

Common work schedules are eight and one-half hour work shifts with a non-paid half-hour (or more) midway through the shift for a meal break. These shifts may be 7 a.m. to 3:30 p.m., 3 p.m. to 11:30 p.m., 11 p.m. to 7:30 a.m., 8 a.m. to 4:30 p.m., 4 p.m. to 12:30 a.m., midnight to 8:30 a.m., and so on. In a traditional structure, full-time staff work Monday through Friday or if working the third shift (11 p.m. to 7:30 a.m./midnight to 8:30 a.m.), Sunday through Thursday. Sometimes the third shift is a straight 8 hours (11 p.m. to 7 a.m., midnight to 8 a.m.) due to limited staff. Part-time staff are used to cover the weekend hours.

However, some supervisors find that these traditional shifts do not meet the needs of their department, or that their employees prefer other schedules. In some cases, alternative schedules are necessary.

Flexible Work Schedules and Other Alternatives

Work schedules for many employees have become more flexible. The idea behind this is that employees should have some autonomy to adjust their work schedules to fit their lifestyles and to choose the hours they would prefer to work while ensuring that a core workforce is available to attend to the department's operations. One such alternative is flextime. **Flextime** enables employees to choose a schedule that fits into their off-the-job activities. It enables working parents or others with responsibilities at home the opportunity to combine work with family life.

Another work-scheduling option that is popular is the 4–10 or 3–12 arrangement, which means employees work 10 hours, 4 days per week or 12 hours, 3 days per week. This is also called **compressed scheduling**. When

flextime
Scheduling that allows employees to modify their personal schedule to fit their off-the-job activities.

compressed scheduling
Special schedules—such as 10-hour days, 4 days per week—that squeeze more work into fewer days.

HOSPITAL LAND

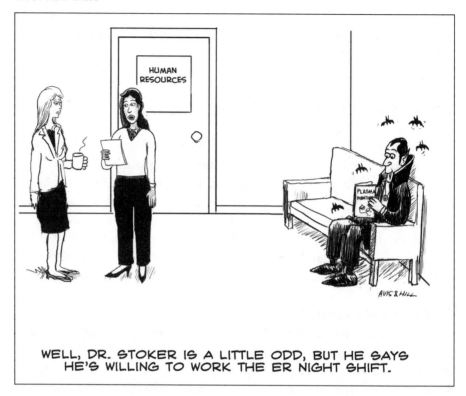

WELL, DR. STOKER IS A LITTLE ODD, BUT HE SAYS HE'S WILLING TO WORK THE ER NIGHT SHIFT.

gasoline prices rose, some employers offered compressed scheduling as a way to reduce consumption of gasoline and other out-of-pocket expenses for their staff. In addition, flexible work schedules tend to improve employee satisfaction and contribute positively to productivity and time utilization.

We usually think of staffing as assigning individuals to work *inside* our place of business, but today that is not necessarily so. Supervisors may consider establishing **virtual positions**, that is, positions manned by individuals who work at alternative workplaces, such as at home. This alternative work arrangement option, also called **telecommuting**, has gained popularity in many industries and is penetrating the healthcare industry for reasons other than employee convenience. Telecommuting reduces the amount of on-site workspace needed and allows employees to cope with the rising cost of gasoline. Some of the more common jobs using telecommuting include IT help desk support, coding, transcription, claims editing, collections, pre-registration, cancer registry abstracting, and order processing (materials management). Global Telematics offers a checklist that management can use to assess telecommuting options. This checklist appears in Exhibit 17.8.

Not all employees desire to work at home. Working at home requires self-discipline, telecommuting skills (e-mail, cell phones, faxes, repairing minor software/hardware problems, etc.), and communication skills (Jamison

virtual positions
Jobs that are held by employees who work off site.

telecommuting
Working from home or another off-site location.

EXHIBIT 17.8

TELEWORK SOLUTIONS CHECKLIST FROM GLOBAL TELEMATICS

Telework means using telecommunications and computers to let employees do their work in novel locations, such as new remote offices or their own homes.

Here are the main considerations in deciding to establish additional office work locations:

1. **Be on the lookout for business problems which telework helps solve.**
   - Difficulty filling jobs because appropriate workers do not live close to the office.
   - Employees who would be happier working closer to their homes.
   - Need for headquarters expansion or relocation.
   - Location- or facility-related operational problems.

2. **Consider all of the telework location options:**
   - In additional company facilities.
   - In employees' own homes.
   - In special work centers for employees from several organizations—"telework centers."

3. **Take a comprehensive approach to telework.**
   - Recognize that installing secure and reliable computer networking technology is critical, but only one piece of the telework solution.
   - New processes and procedures will be necessary also.
   - Involve business planning, personnel management, facilities planning, and operations management.
   - Don't count on telework as an easy "off-the-shelf" purchase.

4. **Encourage employees to submit proposals for new worksite locations.**
   - Let individual employees propose working at home (telecommuting).
   - See if any managers propose relocating their work groups.
   - Evaluate these proposals for energy and ideas to drive improvement.

5. **Look for opportunities to improve customer focus.**
   - Survey customer attitudes that reflect company locations.
   - Consider advantages of a second company location closer to the airport, a business center, an important customer, or a cluster of customers.
   - Examine if a second location would provide better facilities for meeting customers.

6. **Seek retention and recruitment improvements.**
   - Survey employee attitudes toward present and potential locations.
   - Map out where employees live to see a better location for certain offices.
   - Respond to individual employee needs by offering work-at-home opportunities.

7. **Evaluate the facility cost reductions from split operations.**
   - Back office operations—functions not requiring customer contact in the office—can be placed in lower cost space.
   - Mobile personnel who meet customers in the field instead of at the office can be placed in lower cost space.

Continued

EXHIBIT 17.8

Continued

8. Find potential operational improvements from telework.
- Moving a work group out of headquarters may support more creativity and single-minded focus.
- Logistical factors—moving people or materials in and out—may be eased for some work groups in a new site.

9. Use telework for additional flexibility to handle change.
- Work sites for temporary task forces, special projects, and seasonal hires.
- Multiply flexibility by using portable office equipment and modular furniture.

10. Check out the many telecommunications options for linking worksites.
- Define what you want in functionality and keep looking until you find it; technology is improving and costs are dropping.
- Seek long-term relationships with sources of expert technical support.
- Look at intranets (internal, private internets), document conferencing, remote access to the in-office local area network through a secure gateway, and enhanced voice messaging.

11. Address the teamwork and company culture issues arising from dispersed work sites.
- Make extra effort to maintain company teamwork and culture when employees formerly working together start to work apart.
- Schedule additional inter-facility meetings and social gatherings as telework replaces some of the daily face-to-face interaction.

12. Move forward on telework only on finding a "killer" advantage.
- Telework is complex and risky enough to be justified only when the advantages are projected to be very important and near certain.
- Start on the easy parts.
- Try telework confidently, but leave room for modifications as experience builds.

SOURCE: Prepared by Global Telematics, www.globaltelematics.com. Used with permission. © 2009, Global Telematics. All rights reserved.

and O'Connor 2002). And some employees prefer the socialization aspects that an office setting provides.

Alternative work schedules present challenges to managers. They must consider how to supervise staff working on different shifts, at home and on site, and how to coordinate activities with other departments. Managers should conduct periodic observations of the work being performed by all of their employees, regardless of their shift or location. This is more difficult for employees working late-night shifts and for employees working off-site, so often managers must focus on monitoring production instead of actually observing the work. However, as long as flexible working schedules and arrangements produce good results (e.g., easier staff recruitment, better staff retention, higher morale, fewer absences, less tardiness, less dissatisfaction, and better patient care), supervisors should make every effort to overcome these problems by better planning and supervision. More about flexible scheduling appears in Chapter 23.

Temporary Staffing to Fill Scheduling Gaps

Some departments must plan for variable workloads. When workloads fluctuate, especially at predictable times, the use of temporary staff, which may include **pro re nata** (PRN, which means "as needed") or part-time employees, is an ideal solution. For example, at year-end the central supply and materials management departments must take a physical inventory of all supplies both in stock and throughout the organization. This is no easy task. Accounting often has a fluctuation in its workload at year-end as well, because it needs to prepare statements, gather straggler expenditures to record in the proper year, and prepare for external auditors. Vacation months also frequently require the use of PRN or part-time employees to do the work of regular employees who are out. Using overtime may fill these needs, but overtime is costly. Hiring temporary or part-time employees may be the better solution. Baker (2005) reported that 70 percent of employers offer opportunities to work part time, and 66 percent offer flextime. The part-time staff can support workload peaks and scheduled absences of full-time staff members.

> **pro re nata (PRN)**
> Latin term that means "as needed." Used to identify healthcare workers who work only as needed, rather than on regular shifts.

The supervisor's plan should be one of ensuring that one or more of these part-time individuals are cross-trained to perform the seasonal duties and utilize them during those times. PRN or temporary employees often are used during vacation months to fill certain positions throughout an organization. Of course, some positions must be filled by coworkers during one's vacation or the individual who is taking vacation may be required to catch-up upon his or her return. This is often the case for management and supervisory employees. By recruiting staff who are willing to adjust their schedules at different times of the year, the supervisor is able to manage labor expenses and fulfill the work requirements.

Summary

Staffing is the managerial function of procuring and maintaining the department's human resources, a function every supervisor has to perform. Staffing means to attract, select, place, train, retain, evaluate, promote, discipline, and appropriately compensate the employees of the department. All this is the supervisor's line function. The human resources department aids the supervisor in fulfilling this duty. In most enterprises, this department is attached to the organization in a staff capacity, and its purpose is to counsel, inform, and service all other departments of the enterprise. Sometimes, to be of service to the line manager, the human resources department may be inclined to take over line functions such as hiring and disciplining. Supervisors must avoid turning over any of their line functions to the personnel department, although at times it might seem expedient to let them handle the problems.

Before a manager can undertake the staffing function, the number and types of employees and competencies needed in the department must be clarified. The organizational chart combined with job descriptions will help the supervisor decide what workers are needed to fill the various jobs. In addition, the supervisor must consider the amount of work to be performed and the positions allocated in the budget. In all these supervisory duties, the human resources department is available for assistance and service.

During the most recent decades, numerous federal, state, and local laws and regulations as well as executive orders have been enacted regarding equal employment opportunities, fair employment practices, and nondiscriminatory practices. All staffing practices and policies must comply with these requirements. Making sure the organization is complying with these regulations is best handled by specialists in the human resources department. Because of the vast impact this has made on the activities of managers and because of the importance of compliance, the influence of the human resources department within an organization has increased substantially. The CEO recognizes and deals with the need for a proper balance of influence and authority between the line managers and the human resources staff.

In a number of organizations, functional authority has been conferred on the human resources department, especially when the problem involves dismissals and fair employment practices. The average line supervisor could not possibly remain aware of new laws, court decisions, and so forth. Therefore, it makes good sense that the authority of the human resources department has been greatly increased, even if this means narrowing the supervisor's line authority.

Efforts to recruit employees vary by the type of employee and the state of the economy. To recruit qualified staff, various incentives may be offered. Sometimes managers consider outsourcing a function or part of a function to a third-party contract firm that has expertise in the function's duties and access to talented staff. Before proceeding with this option, however, management must consider the positive and negative aspects for the organization as a whole.

Flexible work schedules sometimes help healthcare organizations meet staffing needs. In cooperation with the human resources department, today's supervisor can find a variety of work schedules and technology-driven alternatives from which to choose.

18

THE SELECTION PROCESS

Chapter Objectives

After you have studied this chapter, you should be able to do the following:

1. Discuss the selection process.
2. Describe the purpose of the interview.
3. Discuss the difference between and purposes of directive (structured) and nondirective (unstructured, counseling) interviews.
4. Recognize that interview questions must be structured to avoid discrimination against applicants.
5. Understand the value of involving others in interviewing preferred candidates and supporting entity diversity missions.

So far we have defined staffing as the sum of the activities required to attract, develop, and retain people who have the knowledge and skills needed to achieve departmental objectives. We have learned how to successfully integrate the efforts of the human resources staff with supervisory efforts to identify viable candidates for open positions. In this chapter, we discuss the selection process. The goal of this process is to hire the best employees available for the organization. As Quicken Company (2000) says, "Hiring an employee is truly [about] making an investment in your organization. When you hire someone to work for you, you will invest time, money, training, and trust. If you do it right, your organization can move forward much faster than ever before; if you do it wrong, not only can you lose your investment, but you could be subject to lawsuits that might cause you to lose much more."

The selection process involves choosing the candidate who best meets the job demands, who is likely to perform well, and who will stay with the organization. Candidates for a position may come from within or outside the organization. Because selecting the right employee contributes significantly to the effectiveness of the department, the final decision should rest with the candidate's prospective superior. This way, the selector is completely responsible for the selected candidate's performance. Opinions of others, such as the selector's superior, those who will have working relationships with the selected candidate, and specialists from the human resources department, can help the supervisor make her decision. The final decision on selection, however, rests with the department supervisor.

HOSPITAL LAND

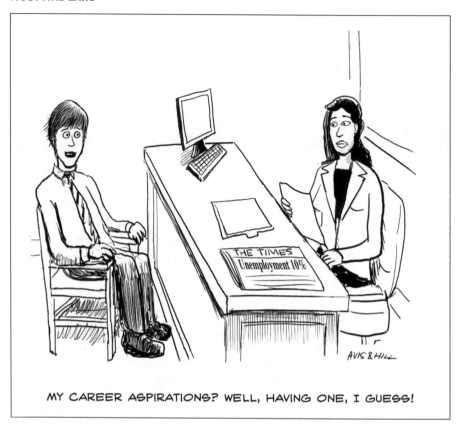

MY CAREER ASPIRATIONS? WELL, HAVING ONE, I GUESS!

After the human resources department performs all the preliminary work—such as recruitment, preliminary screening interviews, obtaining reference data, and relevant testing—the pool of applicants is reduced to three to five possible candidates. Line managers then interview these applicants and select the one who will best fill the vacant position. The personal interview between the supervisor and the applicant is essential to the selection process. This is the moment when the supervisor must match the applicant's personality and capabilities with the culture of the department, the demands of the job, the authority and responsibility inherent in the position, the working conditions, and the rewards and satisfaction the position offers.

Equally important is the applicant's decision to apply. The process may pose considerable risk to the candidate. The internal candidate may have to obtain his current supervisor's permission to interview, and the interviewer gains access to past performance evaluations. The external candidate probably needs to take time off from his current job to interview.

Although some people question the reliability of the interview as a means of selection and as a predictor of performance, it is an almost universally used selection device. The two-way communication enables the interviewer to learn more about the applicant's background, interests, and values and allows the applicant to ask questions about the institution and the job. The interview is not a precise technique, and it is difficult to interview skillfully. Because no fixed criteria exist for success or failure, prejudiced interviewers too easily evaluate an applicant's performance according to their own stereotypes. Job applicants may react differently to different interviewers. As a decision-making tool, however, interviews are probably more valid predictors of employee behavior than tests are.

Interviews

It is not easy to appropriately appraise someone's potential during a brief interview. Interviewing is an art that everyone can and should learn. There are several types of interviews, including pre-employment (or selection) interviews between the supervisor and prospective employees and counseling interviews or sessions during which the abilities and deficiencies of an employee are discussed. Other interviews occur when an employee is asked to leave the organization, when an employee voluntarily leaves the job, and when an employee wants to discuss complaints, grievances, and any other problems. In general, interviews can be grouped into two categories: directive (structured) and nondirective (unstructured or counseling). Some interviews have aspects of both categories. For example, the **appraisal interview** (see Chapter 19) is primarily a directive interview, but the discussion may take on some aspects of a nondirective counseling interview.

Directive Interviews

A **directive interview**, also known as a structured interview, is a discussion in which the interviewer knows beforehand the goals, objectives, and areas of discussion. A structured interview follows a predesigned format. The interviewer first encourages the interviewee to volunteer as much information as possible and then asks her additional direct questions. The interviewer frequently follows a standardized list of consistent, job-related, nondiscriminatory questions. The benefit of structured interviews is that they cover all pertinent topics and allow for direct comparison of the contents of all interviews.

Nondirective Interviews

Nondirective, or counseling, interviews use no checklist. The format develops as the interview unfolds. In this type of interview, the interviewer encourages the interviewee to express his thoughts freely.

Nondirective interviews are typically used in problematic situations in which the interviewer is eager to learn what the interviewee thinks and feels. A supervisor may conduct a nondirective interview when an employee has a

appraisal interview
An interview that may take on characteristics of both directive and nondirective interviews. Usually designed to discuss an employee's strengths and weaknesses.

directive interview
A structured interview between a supervisor and employee in which the interviewer knows beforehand the goals, objectives, and areas of discussion.

nondirective interview
An unstructured interview between a supervisor and an employee often used to discuss a problem or grievance. Also called a counseling interview.

grievance or an off-the-job problem. She may use this approach in an exit interview when the employee voluntarily leaves the job. Another reason for a nondirective interview is to collect opinions about the overall operation of the department or employee satisfaction with recent changes. The supervisor of the employees usually conducts such interviews; occasionally, however, a level of supervision is skipped and the manager at the next level may meet one-on-one with the interviewees. Affording subordinates the opportunity of counseling interviews is vital to good management.

Counseling interviews can be time consuming. Despite competing pressures, however, time for such interviews must be made. Listening improves a supervisor's relationships with his subordinates and decreases the likelihood of personnel problems.

Skillful listening is an art that can be learned through training and experience. It is better learned through practice than by reading books on the subject. Eventually one can develop a system of listening that is comfortable, fits one's personality, and puts the speaker at ease. A common purpose of directive and nondirective interviews is to promote mutual understanding and confidence. Neither is a cure for all human relations problems.

The Employment Interview

employment interview
An interview between a supervisor and a prospective employee designed to determine if the prospective employee is a good fit for the position, and vice versa. Also called a pre-employment interview.

The **employment interview**, also known as the pre-employment or selection interview, is an example of the directive, or structured, interview. The interviewer knows ahead of time what facts will be discussed, what the objectives will be, and what areas will be covered. The structured interview asks all applicants a set of standardized questions; this produces data that can be compared and provides a basis for evaluating the applicants. This does not mean that the structured interview must be rigid. The interviewer should prepare the questions in advance. The questions should be asked in a logical sequence, but the applicant should have ample opportunity to explain each answer. At times, the interviewer will need to probe until she fully understands the interviewee's response. The interviewer wants to learn as much as possible, first by letting the interviewee volunteer information and then by asking direct questions.

Preparing for the Employment Interview

Because the purpose of the directive employment interview is to collect facts and reach a decision, the interviewer should prepare for it as thoroughly as possible. First, he should examine the available background information. This allows the supervisor to sketch a general impression of the interviewee in advance.

Before conducting any employment interviews, the hiring manager should review the position description and identify the competencies the ideal candidate must have. For example, if the opening is for a lead radiology technician for the PACS (Picture Archiving and Communications System) and ultrasound section, some competencies may include the ability to develop and train others; technical expertise with PACS technology, duplicating digital images, and computers or other equipment used; good customer relations; a positive perspective; a history of high quality and productivity; and the desire to do things right the first time. Additionally, the manager may consider the diversity of the organization, the cultural backgrounds of the patients served, and the language skills required to communicate with coworkers, other departments, customers, and patients. The interviewer should structure her questions to encourage the applicants to discuss issues and experiences related to these competencies. This is also the time to clarify any questions that may concern results of skill and aptitude tests that human resources may have given before the interview.

The Application Form

The *application* is a form that seeks information about the applicant's background and present status (Exhibit 18.1). The completed application supplies facts such as the applicant's schooling and degrees; training; previous work experience, including nature of duties, length of employment, and salary; and other relevant data. The candidate completes the application on his first visit to the human resources department, and the data are evaluated to decide whether the applicant merits further consideration.

The information solicited by application is somewhat limited by laws, regulations, and court decisions regarding equal employment opportunities and discrimination. Generally, except under certain bona fide, job-related circumstances, federal regulations and guidelines prevent employers from requiring applicants to state their religion, sex, ancestry, marital status, age, birthplace, parents' birthplace, and other personal data.

Matters concerning the questions an interviewer is allowed to ask are discussed later in this chapter.

An application may provide the interviewer with a sample of the candidate's abilities to write, organize his thinking, and present facts clearly. The application indicates whether the applicant's education follows a logical pattern and whether he has consistently progressed to better jobs. It also gives the interviewer points of discussion for the interview and references to contact.

While studying the completed application before the interview, the interviewer should keep in mind the job for which the applicant is being considered. If questions arise while studying the application, the interviewer should write them down and ask them during the interview. For example, all previous jobs are stated in chronological sequence; however, these data might reveal a period of time during which the applicant did not work. Careful questions about this may reveal that the candidate spent the time unemployed,

EXHIBIT 18.1 Typical Employment Application Form

EMPLOYMENT APPLICATION - Anywhere Ambulatory Surgery

General Information

| NAME (LAST, FIRST, M.I.) | | | DATE | |

| PRESENT ADDRESS | CITY | | STATE | ZIP CODE |

| PERMANENT ADDRESS | CITY | | STATE | ZIP CODE |

| TELEPHONE NUMBER | SOCIAL SECURITY NUMBER |

Are you younger than 18 years of age? If yes, provide birth date | Available start date: | Salary requirement:
❏ Yes   ❏ No

Employment status desired: | Shift preference: | Can you work weekends/holidays?
❏ Full-time ❏ Part-time ❏ Temp ❏ Per-diem   ❏ Day ❏ Evening ❏ Night ❏ Rotation | ❏ Yes   ❏ No

POSITION DESIRED
1)_____   2)_____

Have you ever applied or worked for this facility before?   ❏ Yes ❏ No

If yes, facility_____   Date (s)_____   Position (s)_____
Supervisor (s)_____   Under what name (s)_____

Education

SCHOOL	NAME AND LOCATION	YEAR ATTENDED	DID YOU GRADUATE?	SUBJECTS STUDIED
High School				
Vocational/Technical				
College/University				
Graduate/Other				

Special courses, training, military service or experience acquired.

Skills

OFFICE SKILLS	SOFTWARE PROGRAMS	EQUIPMENT
❏ Typing _____ wmp ❏ Transcriber ❏ Shorthand _____ wmp ❏ PEX ❏ Ten key by touch ❏ Scanner ❏ Medical Terminology ❏ Personal computer		

Licenses

LICENSES, CERTIFICATIONS, OR OTHER	STATE	ID NUMBER	EXPIRE DATE

We are an equal opportunity employer and do not discriminate on the basis of race, color, religion, sex, national origin, age, disability, or veteran status as provided by law.

EXHIBIT 18.1 *Continued*

EMPLOYMENT INFORMATION					
(List below your employment history beginning with the most recent employer.)					

Employment History

Employer	Address: City:			Telephone Number	
Your Position title	Dates employed From: To:	Starting Salary	Ending Salary	Supervisor's name and title	
Describe your duties				Reason for leaving	

Employer	Address: City:			Telephone Number	
Your Position title	Dates employed From: To:	Starting Salary	Ending Salary	Supervisor's name and title	
Describe your duties				Reason for leaving	

Employer	Address: City:			Telephone Number	
Your Position title	Dates employed From: To:	Starting Salary	Ending Salary	Supervisor's name and title	
Describe your duties				Reason for leaving	

References

Please give two references (not relatives or persons previously listed) who are acquainted with your training or activities during the past five years. If recent college graduate, professors and faculty advisors in your field of concentration are particularly helpful.

Name	Address:	Telephone Number	Occupation	Years Known

Other

Have you ever been convicted of a misdemeanor or felony (other than a parking citation)?   ☐ Yes   ☐ No

If yes, explain_____

The type and seriousness of the crime, along with your entire work history, education history, and the position for which you are applying will be considered. A "Yes" response to the above question will not automatically disqualify you from consideration for employment.

Comments

Make any comments that you feel are important in regards to your application.

I certify that the responses given above are true and correct to my knowledge. I have not withheld any fact which might adversely affect my application, and understand that any omissions of fact or any false or misleading statements will be considered just cause for immediate dismissal, no matter when discovered. I further understand that I may be required to pass a physical examination including drug testing prior to final acceptance of employment

_____   _____
Applicant's signature   Date

We are an equal opportunity employer and do not discriminate on the basis of race, color, religion, sex, national origin, age disability or veteran status as provided by law.

recovering from an illness or assisting a family member with an illness, traveling abroad, or attending a specialized course of study.

Scheduling Employment Interviews

Not all interviews must be conducted in person. You may find, after careful review of a batch of applications and the accompanying human resources research, that six or seven candidates meet your requirements. You may choose to do a brief telephone interview with these candidates. Be careful not to call them at work. If you call them at home and connect to an answering machine, you may wish to be somewhat vague about your call—for example, "Hello, this is Mr. Smith calling from Littletown Ambulatory Surgery Center. This message is for Suzanne McKnight. We received the information you sent us and would like to speak with you further about the materials. You may reach me at (555) 444–1212. I look forward to speaking with you." The applicant may not have shared the fact that she was looking for a new job with her family or roommate.

To avoid interrupting candidates at work, try to arrange telephone interviews for when they are at home or at a private location. Furthermore, schedule the interviews ahead of time. It is only fair that they have time to prepare as you have. Based on the telephone interviews, you may select two or three people to interview in person. You may wish to send these candidates a copy of the job description in advance. If they do not like what they see, they may decide not to come in, which will prevent you from wasting an hour or more of your time and the time of others who participate in interviews.

Because the purpose of the employment interview is to gather enough information to make a hiring decision, the interviewer should prepare a schedule or plan for the interview. She should note any areas that need further clarification, keeping in mind that interview questions should focus on job knowledge, job situations, work requirements, and ability to handle various situations. Developing the questions in advance allows the interviewer to devote much of her attention to listening and observing the applicant, and writing the questions down helps to ensure that all the interview covers all key points. A well-prepared plan for the employment interview is worth the time spent on it.

Finally, the interviewer should be concerned with the proper setting for the interview. Privacy and some degree of comfort are normal requirements for a good conversation. If a private room is not available, the supervisor should create an aura of privacy by speaking to the applicant in a place where other employees are not within hearing distance. If possible, the interviewer should take precautions to avoid any interruptions during the interview that could distract her attention from the applicant. Placing the telephone line on "do not disturb" or "busy" and posting a sign on the door that reads "interview in progress" give the interviewee additional assurance of the importance the supervisor places on this interview.

Conducting the Employment Interview

The interviewer should create a comfortable atmosphere that puts the applicant at ease. A good interviewer thinks back to when he applied for a job and recalls the stress and tension of the experience. After all, the applicant is meeting strangers who ask probing questions and is probably under considerable strain. It is the interviewer's duty to relieve this tension. Opening the interview with brief general conversation, possibly about the weather, traffic, or some other topic of broad interest, might help put the applicant at ease. One question that helps ease the way through the warm-up period is, "Why did you choose to apply to this healthcare facility?" The interviewer may also offer water or coffee or may employ another social gesture, such as walking the applicant through the work area. A good starting question is, "How did you learn about this job opening?"

This informal warmup should be brief, and the interviewer should move the discussion quickly to job-related matters. Studies have shown that interviewers sometimes make selection decisions in the first minutes of the interview, and it would be inappropriate to do this before discussing job-related matters.

In addition to obtaining information from the applicant, the interviewer should ensure that the job seeker learns enough about the job to help him decide whether the position is a good fit. The interviewer should discuss the working conditions, wages, hours, benefits, the position's immediate supervisor (if he or she is not present and participating in the interview), and the job's relationship with other jobs in the department. The interviewer must describe the situation completely and honestly. In her eagerness to make the job look as attractive as possible, especially to professionals who are in short supply, the interviewer may make it sound better than it actually is. The interviewer must avoid overselling the job by telling the applicant the benefits or advantages that are available only to exceptional employees. If the applicant turns out to be an average worker, this may lead to disappointment.

After outlining the job's details, the interviewer might ask the applicant, "What experience from your prior positions will help you perform this job?" After this discussion, the supervisor should ask the applicant what else she would like to know about the job. If the interviewee has no further questions, the supervisor should proceed with questioning to find out how well-qualified the applicant is. The supervisor will have some knowledge about the applicant's background from the application, and there is no need to ask her to restate this information. However, the interviewer will need to know exactly how qualified the interviewee is for the job. Most of this information is obtained through direct questions. The interviewer should be careful to phrase these questions clearly for the applicant. In other words, he should only use terms that conform with the applicant's language, background, and experience. The interviewer should phrase questions in a slow and deliberate form, one at a time, to avoid confusing the applicant.

The interviewer should be careful not to ask questions that could be considered discriminatory or illegal. The human resources department can assist with designing questions to avoid pitfalls. Examples of appropriate and inappropriate questions appear in Exhibit 18.2. Finally, the best predictor of future behavior is past behavior. Typically, asking a wide variety of questions can help gain information that targets the specific job's skill requirements. The interviewer should probe until the question has been answered to his satisfaction.

EXHIBIT 18.2 Examples of Appropriate and Inappropriate Questions

---

Appropriate Interview Questions

1. What do (did) you like best about your present (most recent) job? Why? What do (did) you like least?
2. What special assignments have you taken on in the past (or in your current job) that will make you successful here?
3. Have you ever been convicted of any crime or misdemeanor other than parking violations?
4. Is there anything that would preclude you from traveling out of town overnight or working overtime?
5. Considering your previous bosses and without giving me any names, which one did you like the least and why?
6. If a physician yelled at you because you failed to chart something for her, what would you do? How would you respond?
7. Have you had to change the way you did your work in the past because a new procedure or policy was implemented? What would you do if you didn't agree with the change?
8. Give me an example of a new process or system change you proposed and tell me how you convinced your supervisor that it was the right thing to do.
9. If you found a copy of a patient's bill on the floor in the hallway, what would you do with it?

Inappropriate Interview Questions

1. Were you born in Cuba or the United States?
2. Will your husband (wife) have any problems with your working hours?
3. Have you ever been arrested for any crime?
4. Do you have babysitters arranged for your children?
5. Do you dislike your current job because you are reporting to a woman?

Peer Interviews

An organization that encourages employee participation may ask the coworkers to interview the one or two final candidates that the hiring manager prefers. To ensure that the coworkers ask legitimate questions, the human resources department may provide them with a structured interview form like the one shown in Exhibit 18.3.

One advantage of coworker interviewing is that the coworkers are more likely to support the individual hired because they had a say in the hiring. However, if the supervisor decides to select an individual other than the one the coworkers preferred, they may be reluctant to participate in future interviews or to help the new person overcome hurdles. Another advantage to coworker interviews is that candidates may feel more at ease being interviewed by peers and may disclose experiences that they did not reveal to the hiring manager. When this happens, the interview may take longer, since the peers and candidate will be engaged in sharing their common experiences and may veer off the structured interview path. Peers may judge candidates on appearance or find an applicant appealing if they live in the same neighborhood, have children in the same school as theirs, or if they attend the same church. While these attributes may encourage rapport between the peers and the potential incumbent, they do not tell the peer whether the individual will be able to do the job. Overall, the benefits of peer evaluations usually outweigh the disadvantages.

Before making the final selection, the supervisor should consider asking the applicant to return for a second interview. This return visit provides another opportunity for the hiring manager and applicant to converse. When an applicant returns for a second interview, the manager may notice other attributes or attitudes that were not apparent during the first interview.

Some employers publish guidance for their managers in policy manuals or on websites. The University of Maryland Eastern Shore (2001) advises its managers, "A structured interview may include four different types of questions concerning job knowledge, job samples/situations, work requirements, and handling various situations." Your organization may provide you with sample interview questions similar to those shown in Exhibit 18.2. Many sample questions are available on the Internet for you to incorporate in your screening process.

Tips for the Employment Interview

The employment interview is a forum for open dialogue and for determining whether the organization and the candidate are a good match. The interviewer should take care not to ask leading questions such as, "Do you have difficulty adjusting to authority?" or "Do you daydream frequently?" This form of questioning may lead to antagonism and does not encourage dialogue between the interviewer and the candidate. Open-ended questions are better—for example,

EXHIBIT 18.3

PEER INTERVIEW—CANDIDATE ASSESSMENT

Candidate Name: _____   Position: _____

Each member of team will select questions to ask the candidate in a uniform manner. Generally, two questions from each category; however, areas marked as "key" may require a question emphasis. The team will use their "best" judgment in determining the most applicable questions based on the position. If at any time it appears the candidate is having difficulty answering a question, the team member will put the candidate at ease by reminding him/her to take their time and think about the question prior to answering.

KEY AREA CHECK THOSE THAT APPLY	CATEGORY	TEAM MEMBER TO ASK QUESTIONS	QUESTIONS	WT 1-3	1=VERY POOR 2=POOR 3=FAIR 4=GOOD 5=VERY GOOD	TOTAL:	INTERVIEWER'S COMMENTS
	General		What are your strengths and weaknesses? Why did or why do you desire to leave your last/present job? What is most important to you in a job? What previous job was the most satisfying to you and why?		1 2 3 4 5 1 2 3 4 5		
	Motivation		How do you feel about the statement "Attitude is willingly helping out whenever and wherever necessary—even if it is not my job"? What career objectives have been met? How do you measure success? What motivates you most on the job? Give an example when you went beyond your employer's normal job expectations in order to get a job done. Tell me about a time when you felt like giving up on a certain job. What did you do? Tell me about an important goal that you set in the past and what you did to accomplish it.		1 2 3 4 5 1 2 3 4 5		

Beyond the total score, my general impression of this candidate was: _____ a great fit, _____ a good fit, _____ just "ok" fit, _____ not a fit for the position interviewed.
Interviewer: _____   Date: _____

SOURCE: Reprinted with permission from Knoxville Hospital and Clinics, Knoxville, IA.

"Could you describe how you handled the flooding disaster last fall?" "How do you view the nurse's right to not participate in a surgical abortion?" "Which responsibilities of this position most concern you?" "Why did you leave your prior position?"

The interviewer may take notes during or, preferably, immediately after the interview. This is especially helpful if several candidates are being interviewed. It is difficult to remember what each applicant said and to avoid confusing their statements. There is no need to take notes on everything, but the key points should be jotted down.

Every question the interviewer asks should be pertinent and job related. This brings up the area of questioning that, although not directly related to the job itself, can become relevant to the work situation. Problems of a personal nature, while only indirectly connected with the job, may be relevant. An interviewer must use judgment and tact in this respect, as the applicant may be sensitive about some personal topics. By no means should the interviewer pry into personal affairs that are irrelevant to the work situation merely to satisfy her own curiosity.

Reference checks can provide additional information about candidates. These are obtained from previous employers and are best handled by the human resources department; special care is advisable because of privacy regulations and potential exposure to damage claims. The information requested from references should be job related. All reference checks should be done with the knowledge and permission of the applicant. Exhibit 18.4 is a typical mail-out reference check form often used by human resources departments. However, a hiring manager may wish to contact the applicant's former supervisor(s) for more specific, job-related information. Exhibit 18.5 presents some tips to consider and suggests questions to ask when performing a telephone reference check.

Some applicants are skilled at designing—or inflating—their resumes. The hiring manager should warn candidates that their references will be carefully checked. Even if a colleague recommends a candidate, the hiring manager is wise to check other references the candidate provides. Further, if human resources has not checked education credentials and the Office of Inspector General's website for disbarred individuals, the hiring manager should.

Equal Employment Opportunity Laws

Before the 1960s, interviewers could ask almost any question that was job related in some way. The many laws, executive orders, and court decisions that now affect equal employment opportunities, discrimination, and affirmative action have made interviewing far more complicated. Obviously, many questions are still perfectly lawful. For example, the interviewer can ask for the applicant's first and last names, current address, employment history, and

EXHIBIT 18.4
Sample
Authorization
for Reference
Check

Deaconess Hospital

Authorized Release of Personal Data: Deaconess Hospital may request information regarding an applicant's education and work history from previous employers and educational facilities. Therefore, I, the undersigned, hereby authorize and request any present or former employer, educational institution, law enforcement agency, financial institution or other persons having personal knowledge about me to furnish Deaconess Hospital and/or its agents with any and all information in their possession regarding me, in connection with any application for or retention of employment. Further, I hereby release from liability and hold harmless all persons and corporations supplying this information to Deaconess Hospital and/or its agents. A photocopy of this authorization is as effective as the original.

Signature: _____ Date: _____

Release Authorization: I authorize the company and/or its agents, including consumer reporting bureaus, to verify any of this information including, but not limited to, criminal history and motor vehicle driving records. I hereby release without reservation all persons, schools, companies and law enforcement authorities from any liability for any damage whatsoever for issuing this information.

Today's Date: _____ Signature: _____

The following must be filled out completely for your application to be considered. PLEASE PRINT.

Last Name: _____ First: _____ MI: _____

Home Address: _____

City: _____ State: _____ Zip: _____

Social Security No.: _____ Date of Birth: _____

Driver's License No.: _____ Driver's License State: _____

If you have ever attended school or been employed under any name other than the one listed above, please indicate the name(s) used: _____

SOURCE: Adapted and excerpted from the Deaconess Hospital Application for Employment and related materials. Courtesy of Deaconess Hospital, Oklahoma City, OK.

educational background. Unlawful questions include those about the applicant's race or color, sex, religion, birthplace, and arrest record. Some questions toe the line between lawful and unlawful. For instance, it is certainly lawful to ask the applicant what languages he speaks, because bilingual ability is desirable, sometimes even necessary, in many healthcare positions.

EXHIBIT 18.5
Telephone
Reference
Check
Checklist

1. Identify yourself immediately, explain your position with the organization, and tell the reference party why you are calling about the applicant.

2. Ask if this is a good time to discuss the candidate. If not, arrange a time to discuss the applicant.

3. Assure the reference that any discussion you have will be held in confidence.

4. Offer to have the reference call you back collect or toll-free if you sense that the person doubts the legitimacy of your call.

5. Try to establish rapport with the reference you are calling to encourage freer exchange of information.

6. Tell the reference about the position for which the applicant is being considered. Ask the reference, "How do you think the candidate would fit into our vacancy?"

7. Ask questions about the candidate's relationship with the reference:
   • How is it that you know the applicant?
   • What are his or her strengths? Weaknesses?

8. How did he or she get along with peers? Supervisors? Physicians?

9. Did the applicant meet commitments? Deadlines?

10. Did you observe the applicant in any stressful situations? How did she/he handle her/himself?

11. What type of support will we need to provide him/her to ensure he/she will be successful in this position?

12. Why do you think the applicant is interested in this position?

13. Does the applicant work best alone or with a team?

14. How was the applicant's attendance?

15. Did you find him or her to be honest and trustworthy?

16. Compared to others, how would you assess this person's professional/clinical knowledge and skill?

17. How would you describe the individual's communication skills?

18. Did you observe this individual working with subordinates? If so, could you describe that interaction?

19. Would you rehire the applicant?

20. Is there anything else you think I should know about the applicant?

However, this question should not lead to asking about the applicant's native language or the language he uses at home.

It would be presumptuous to provide a comprehensive list of appropriate and inappropriate questions in this book because each situation could involve specific legal restraints and should be judged individually. The laws and regulations change frequently, and in some cases they are state specific. The courts and administrative agencies make new decisions almost daily, so it is a full-time job to stay abreast of them. The human resources staff are usually familiar with the most recent developments and proper current practices. The interviewer should consult with them to learn which questions are appropriate, which are lawful if properly worded, and which are unlawful. The interviewer may also seek advice on obtaining information that is necessary but that she cannot ask for directly. For example, rather than asking, "How would your spouse feel about you traveling a lot or working long hours?," the supervisor may try to get the same information from questions such as, "Can you be away from home overnight if the job requires it?," or "Will your home responsibilities permit you to work around the clock?"

Closing the Interview

Candidates no doubt have questions they wish to have answered so that they, too, may make an informed decision. Some may ask questions throughout the interview, while others may wait until the interviewer has finished asking hers. Regardless, the interviewer should ask the applicant if he has any questions. This provides both parties with an opportunity to clarify anything that was discussed during the interview. It also indicates how interested the candidate may be in the position. Did he prepare questions? Does he ask questions that popped into his head during the interview? Are the questions well structured? Do the questions seek specific information?

This closing period of the interview also permits the interviewer to inform the applicant of the next steps in the process. This is discussed in the next section; suffice it to mention here that the interviewer should give the applicant an idea of when he may expect a decision about his candidacy for the position.

Evaluating the Applicant

The chief problem in employment interviews is how to interpret the candidate's employment and personal history and other pertinent information. It is impossible for interviewers to completely eliminate personal preferences and prejudices. Interviewers should recognize their personal biases and make efforts to control them. They should be able to clearly write down their reasons for selecting one applicant over another. Also, a supervisor may overlook something on an application or a resume that another set of eyes may catch.

For these reasons, it may be beneficial to ask another peer supervisor or a coworker team to participate in the interviewing process. Having multiple interviewers helps the supervisor avoid some common pitfalls.

The first of these pitfalls is making snap judgments. While many rely on intuition when making hiring decisions, it is best to support feelings with facts. It is difficult to keep from forming an early impression and looking for evidence to substantiate this first impression during the rest of the interview. The interviewer should collect all the information on the applicant before making a judgment. This prevents the **halo effect**, which occurs when an interviewer bases an applicant's potential for job performance on one or two characteristics and allows this impression to color all the other factors. This may work favorably or unfavorably for the job seeker. In any event, it is wrong for the interviewer to base an overall opinion on a single factor, such as the applicant's ability to express herself fluently. If an applicant is articulate, there is no reason to automatically assume the rest of her qualifications are top notch. A glance at current employees in the department will remind the interviewer that some very successful employees have rather poor verbal communications skills.

halo effect
A circumstance in which an interviewer bases an applicant's potential for job performance on one or two characteristics and allows this impression to color all the other factors.

Another common pitfall is overgeneralization. The interviewer must not assume that because an applicant behaves in a certain manner in one situation he will automatically behave the same way in all other situations. There may be a special reason why the applicant may answer a certain question evasively. It is wrong to conclude from this evasiveness that the applicant is underhanded and probably not trustworthy. Remember that people tend to generalize quickly. Conducting a second interview of two preferred candidates allows the interviewer to assess whether the candidates' mannerisms change or whether they contradict information they provided earlier.

Comparing the applicant with current employees in the department is another common mistake. The interviewer may wonder how this applicant will get along with the other employees, the manager of the department, or other supervisors and how the candidate will fit into the corporate culture. The interviewer may believe that an applicant who is considerably different from current employees is undesirable. This thinking may harm the organization because it only leads to uniformity, conformity, and mediocrity. This does not mean that the interviewer should make it a point to look for "oddballs" who obviously do not fit in the department. But a job applicant's failure to resemble the other employees is no reason to conclude that the person will not make a suitable employee.

If a team interview is conducted, the team members may see attributes in this candidate that you as the supervisor would have never discovered. Team members can delve into the specific expectations of doing a job and find weaknesses or strengths in a candidate that the supervisor may not. The benefit of team interviews, however, is after the hiring. If the team was in favor of selecting the candidate, the team will support the candidate when he or she starts work. The contrary may be true as well: if the team is not favorably inclined toward this candidate, it may provide less enthusiastic support when he or she starts to work. The latter scenario is a disadvantage of team interviews.

As the principal interviewer, the supervisor must be wary of a candidate who has all the right answers. The interviewer should recognize when an applicant gives responses that are socially acceptable but not very revealing. The job seeker knows that the answer should be what the interviewer wants to hear. For example, if the interviewer asks a nurse what his aspirations are, the reply probably will be to be a head nurse one day. He settles for aspiring to be a head nurse rather than the director of nursing because the applicant knows that only a certain amount of ambition is socially acceptable. Asking a candidate how his former boss would describe him may yield a reply that describes him as hard working, motivated, willing to do what it takes, and a good team player. Each of these attributes is what every supervisor desires in an employee. They are also the answers that are written in every guide on how to interview.

To avoid receiving "canned" or rote answers, the interviewer should pose questions that require the applicant to explain how he handled a difficult situation such as an observed theft of patient cash, a loss of electricity to the operating rooms, an unexpected visit from an accrediting or licensing agency, or registration of a blind or deaf patient. The interviewer also may consider giving the candidate a copy of the job description and asking, "Which of these duties can you perform?" and "Is there anything here that you cannot do?" (*Medical Office Manager* 2001).

Another hazard for the interviewer to avoid is giving undue merit to excessive qualifications. While the applicant should be qualified, there is no need to look for qualifications in excess of those required to perform the job. An overqualified applicant may make a poor and frustrated employee who becomes bored with the job.

Testing the Applicant

The hiring manager may wish to have human resources test applicants for certain skills before considering their applications. Skills tested may include spelling, alphabetization, math, or typing. Several products are available for this type of basic testing. Beyond that, what if you want to test someone on a specific job, such as performing a screening mammogram or writing a specialized diet? Exhibit 18.6 includes information from the American Health Information Management Association (AHIMA 1999) on this type of pre-employment testing.

Prescreening tests can provide additional information about a candidate's ability to perform the job, but the organization must use caution to

EXHIBIT 18.6 Pre-Employment Testing

The Equal Employment Opportunity Commission (EEOC) enforces myriad federal equal employment opportunity laws. The EEOC does not provide guidelines for validating pre-employment tests. In fact, the EEOC does not take action unless a discrimination charge is filed. Once a discrimination charge is filed, an EEOC investigator and an industrial psychologist analyze the test in question by measuring it against accepted industry standards. However, there are guidelines published by the U.S. Department of Labor with which your human resources liaison should be familiar.

There is no formal organization or service that validates pre-employment tests. Any organization that needs assistance in developing pre-employment tests should seek the advice of a human resources consultant or an industrial psychologist. A number of published resources are also available.

There are five basic steps to creating a valid test:

1. *Job analysis*: The test writer must develop a "core competency model" for the open position, which identifies the knowledge, skills, and abilities needed to perform the actual job. For example, someone interviewing for a coder position should never be tested on codes for conditions that are not treated at the facility.

2. *Test blueprint*: The test writer should develop a test plan (or outline) that accurately reflects the competencies identified as essential to performing the open position. The test plan should be grouped by categories of performance. Each performance category should be weighted based on its importance to performing the job.

3. *Item writing*: The test writer should eliminate any question that carries an ethnic, gender, socioeconomic, or geographic bias. Questions should only reflect the actual tasks that are performed as part of the job.

4. *Field testing*: The completed pre-employment test should be field tested before it is given to any potential job applicants. Your current employees may be a good test group. The field testing process is an excellent opportunity to fine-tune the test questions so that they accurately reflect the job being offered.

5. *Item analysis*: Once the test is administered to job applicants, it is vital to refine and validate it as test data are collected and evaluated. Issues that the test writer should consider during evaluation include: Are any questions too difficult? Do any questions show a pattern of discrimination? Does the test correlate to the overall knowledge, skills, and abilities needed to perform the job?

SOURCE: Courtesy of the *Journal of AHIMA*, Vol. 70, No. 4 (April 1999). © AHIMA.

avoid discrimination charges. Putting in the effort to develop a sound and justified test may save turnover and recruitment expenses in the long term.

Diversity

Another issue that may factor into the decision is the organization's mission to have a diversified workforce. Diversity issues relate to race, gender, age, disabilities, religion, job title, physical appearance, sexual orientation, nationality, cultural identity, competency, training, experience, and personal habits. Kaiser Permanente's workforce of 181,000 employees and physicians is 74 percent female and 56 percent people of color, officials said, "mirroring and exceeding the racial, ethnic and gender composition of its health plan membership and the communities it serves." Kaiser has been recognized for its leadership on diversity by a host of publications and organizations in recent years (Rauber 2009). Employing individuals from a variety of backgrounds helps the organization understand the patients it serves and brings different perspectives to the workplace. When an organization makes diversity a goal, the leadership team must embrace it in daily management activities, including staffing.

Making the Decision

The final step in the selection process is choosing an individual for the job. It can be difficult to make a judgment based on the information gathered. However, if the hiring manager has followed the suggestions made in this chapter, the chances of making a successful decision improve. The assumption here is that it is within the hiring manager's sole authority to decide and that the organization's policies and procedures do not require authorization from the line superior or someone in the human resources department. However, in many organizations, the immediate supervisor may not actually extend the offer of employment or establish the starting wage. Today, more and more human resources departments have this functional responsibility. This ensures consistency in hiring practices and equity in pay and avoids favoritism and discrimination claims.

At the conclusion of the employment interview, the hiring manager will likely choose one of three possible actions: recommend hiring the applicant, defer the decision, or reject the applicant. The applicant will be eager to know which of these actions the supervisor chooses and is entitled to an answer within a reasonable period of time.

If the hiring manager decides to recommend hiring a particular applicant, he or she must recognize that the human resources department may require additional tests, such as a pre-employment physical that may include a drug screen. Additionally, human resources staff may conduct criminal checks once the recommendation has been submitted. It is not until after the candidate has successfully passed these additional screens that the human resources department establishes, with the hiring manager's cooperation, the start date and initial orientation for the candidate.

The hiring manager may instead decide to defer a decision until he has interviewed several other applicants. In this case, it is necessary and appropriate for the supervisor to inform the first candidate of when she will be notified. Such situations occur frequently, but it is unethical to use this tactic to avoid the unpleasant task of telling the applicant that she is not right for the job. While waiting for an answer, the applicant may let other opportunities slip by. It is unpleasant to tell an applicant that she is not suitable, but if the supervisor has decided that an applicant will not be hired, it is best to tell her so in a clear but tactful way.

It is better not to state the specific reasons for rejection. Giving reasons for not hiring someone may encourage arguments and comparisons and can lead to other problems, especially because the chances of being misquoted and misunderstood are great. It is best to turn the applicant down by stating, in a general way, that the match between the applicant's qualifications and the needs of the job is not sufficient. It is unfair to tell the applicant that she will be called if something suitable opens up if the interviewer knows that no hope exists.

Hiring managers should avoid rejecting candidates too quickly. It is best to wait until the chosen candidate has accepted the job—and in some cases you may wish to wait until after the new hire has started the job—before sending a rejection letter to your second-best candidate. However, you should promptly notify those applicants you would never consider hiring, those whose salary expectations are above the rate range permitted at your organization, or those who definitely lack the skill set you are seeking.

The hiring manager should always bear in mind that the employment interview is an excellent opportunity to build a good reputation for the institution. The applicant knows that he is one of several candidates and that only one person can be selected. The way applicants are turned down, however, can affect their impression of the institution. Often, the only contact the applicant has with the organization is the employment interview. It is necessary, therefore, that an applicant leaves the interview, regardless of its outcome, feeling that he has been treated courteously and fairly. It is a managerial duty to build as much goodwill for the organization as possible, and the employment interview presents one opportunity to do so.

Documentation

In recent years, the need for documentation has become evident, as supervisors' hiring decisions are increasingly challenged. The interviewer must write down the reasons for not hiring a certain applicant and why one was hired in preference to the others. This documentation is essential because the supervisor could not possibly remember all the various reasons, and she may be asked to justify the decision months later.

Generally speaking, the department of human resources informs line managers how to document the selection process. In some cases, supervisors might feel pressure from the human resources department, peer supervisors, or higher management to give preferential hiring considerations to minorities or women. Supervisors should realize that the organization might need to meet certain affirmative action goals. Again, only through careful documentation can supervisors justify hiring decisions. Notes recorded on a separate piece of paper and attached to the application serve this purpose.

Temporary Placement

Sometimes, although the applicant is not the right person for a particular job, he may be suitable for another position for which no current opening exists. The supervisor might be tempted to hold this desirable employee by offering temporary placement in any job that is available. The supervisor should inform the applicant of this prospect. At times, however, temporary placement in an unsuitable job causes misunderstanding and disturbance within the department. It is usually strenuous for an employee to mark time on a job that he does not care to perform while hoping for the proper job to open up. Normally such strain leads to dissatisfaction, which is usually communicated to other employees within the work group. Also, the expected suitable job may not open up. Therefore, interim placements should be approached with great care.

Summary

Available job openings may be filled in two ways: hire someone from the outside or promote someone from within the organization. In hiring from outside, the human resources department recruits and preselects the most likely applicants. For internal candidates, the human resources department screens for minimum job requirements but usually encourages employment from within and may, in effect, be less stringent on the referral of internal candidates. It is the supervisor's function and duty, however, to interview candidates appropriately and to hire those who promise to be the best fit for the job available. To accomplish this, the supervisor must acquire the skills needed to conduct an effective interview. The employment interview is primarily a directive (or structured) interview, in contrast to the nondirective interview often encountered in the supervisor's daily work.

During the employment interview, the supervisor tries to determine whether the applicant's capability matches the demands of the job and the organizational culture. To carry out a successful interview, the supervisor should become familiar with the candidate's background information, list points to be covered and questions to be asked, prepare in advance, and secure a proper setting. In addition to obtaining information from the applicant, the interviewer should discuss with the interviewee as many aspects of the job as possible. There will be a number of additional questions and answers before the interviewer is ready to conclude the employment interview, evaluate the candidate, and make a decision. All this must be accomplished while giving proper attention to the many aspects of equal and fair employment practices and other legal considerations.

One person will not see everything that may be known about an applicant. Supervisors are encouraged to ask peer supervisors to interview the candidate and to identify desirable and undesirable traits. A coworker peer or team interview can supplement the supervisor's interview and can yield benefits such as obtaining additional information about the candidate and providing after-hire support of the selected candidate. The human resources department can provide tools that will prevent interviewers from asking inappropriate questions. When an organization chooses to include diversity as a goal for the organization, the leadership team must embrace this concept in daily management activities, including staffing.

In addition to conducting directive interviews, the supervisor is often called on to carry out nondirective interviews. This form of interview usually covers problematic situations and gives the employees the opportunity to freely express their feelings and sentiments. Giving subordinates the opportunity for a counseling interview is another vital duty of the supervisory position.

Additional Reading

Goldsmith, J. 2007. "Baby Boomers and the Health System: It's the Workforce, Stupid!" In *FutureScan: Healthcare Trends and Implications 2007–2012*, 10–12. Chicago: Health Administration Press and the Society for Healthcare Strategy and Market Development.

PERFORMANCE APPRAISALS AND POSITION CHANGES

Chapter Objectives

After you have studied this chapter, you should be able to do the following:

1. Describe the purpose of periodic performance appraisals.
2. Discuss the role of the supervisor in performing the appraisal.
3. Understand the advantages to succession planning and mentoring.
4. Review the relationship between wage and salary structure and employee retention and recruitment.
5. Describe the purpose and methods of promotion.

The performance appraisal system is the ongoing process of gathering, analyzing, evaluating, and disseminating information about the performance of employees. These appraisals not only guide management in selecting certain individuals for promotion and salary increases but also are useful for coaching employees to improve their performance. Appraisals are an important part of long-range personnel planning and the supervisor's staffing function. In addition, well-identified and well-described appraisal methods and procedures contribute to a healthy organizational environment of mutual trust and understanding. This type of atmosphere is necessary for the healthcare organization to bring about increased productivity and better patient care. A performance appraisal system helps identify work requirements and performance standards, analyzes and appraises job-related behaviors, and recognizes those behaviors.

Performance appraisals are central to organizational and management development. Their purpose is to provide a measure of the employee's job performance that leads to counseling (motivation) and further development (training and succession planning). Because a **performance appraisal** is a formal system of measuring, evaluating, and influencing an employee's job-related activities, it identifies the types of training experiences that may enhance the employee's performance. As discussed in Chapter 17, today's economy presents an ample supply of applicants but limited funds to hire. Managers must be selective in their hiring choices to find individuals with specific skills upon which the supervisor can build and broaden his subordinates' expertise and scope of responsibility.

performance appraisal
A formal system of measuring, evaluating, and influencing an employee's job-related activities.

The performance appraisal process is a control system that serves as an audit of the effectiveness of on-the-job training programs, of supervisory coaching, and of each employee. Decisions regarding an employee's continued employment, promotion, demotion, transfer, salary increase, or possible termination are made on the basis of the performance appraisal. Performance appraisals are important to maximize employee motivation and productivity (Exhibit 19.1) and to minimize the chances of litigation. In the typical organization, every employee is subject to a periodic performance appraisal; every organization needs valid information that enhances management's effectiveness in directing human resources.

The Performance Appraisal System

The appraisal of an employee's performance is central to the supervisor's staffing function. It points to the need for further development, shows how effectively various subordinates contribute to departmental goals, and helps management identify those employees who have the potential to be promoted. It is important for a supervisor to be in a position to assess objectively the quality of the employees' performance in the department. Therefore, most organizations request that supervisors carry out the provisions of the institution's formal appraisal system and periodically appraise and rate their employees (see Exhibit 19.3). This formal appraisal system is also known as employee evaluation, employee rating, annual review, or merit rating. For the purposes of this book, assume that the system has been designed so that it is legally defensible and not discriminatory in any way.

According to Michael Holzschu (2001), preparing the performance review can be stressful and nonproductive: "sometimes the fault lies with the

EXHIBIT 19.1

How Am I Doing?

More than 600 employees responded to the survey question: "How valuable is the feedback you receive during performance reviews?"

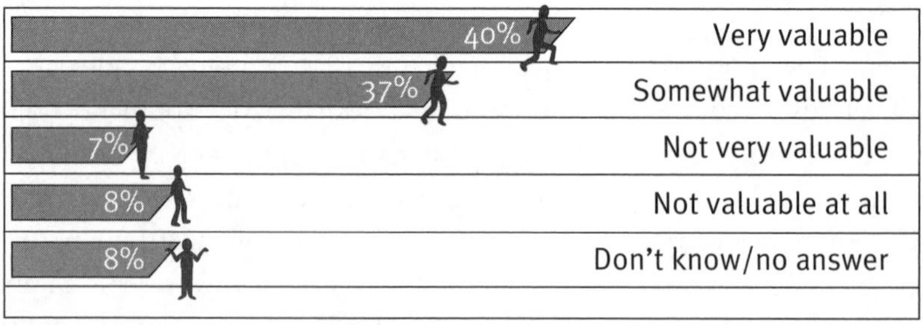

%	Response
40%	Very valuable
37%	Somewhat valuable
7%	Not very valuable
8%	Not valuable at all
8%	Don't know/no answer

SOURCE: Data from Office Team, Menlo Park, CA, 2004.

format of the appraisal instrument. A review should give an accurate appraisal of how well a staff member has done then show the person where and how to improve." Proper advance planning can prepare a supervisor for this important management responsibility. This chapter discusses appraisal methods, data collection, and the entire appraisal cycle.

Performance Appraisal Methods[1]

Performance appraisals take many forms. The written essay, the simplest appraisal method, is a written narrative assessing an employee's strengths, weaknesses, past performance, and potential and provides recommendations for improvement. Other types of performance appraisal methods include comparative standards (e.g., simple ranking, paired comparison, forced distribution) and absolute standards (e.g., critical incidents, BARS, 360-degree feedback).

Comparative standards, or multiperson comparison, is a relative assessment method that compares one employee's performance with that of one or more coworkers. In group rank ordering the supervisor places employees into a particular classification such as top one-fifth and second one-fifth. If a supervisor has ten employees, only two could be in the top fifth, and two must be assigned to the bottom fifth. In individual ranking the supervisor lists employees from highest to lowest. The difference between the top two employees is assumed to be equivalent to the difference between the bottom two employees. In paired comparison, the supervisor compares each employee with every other employee and rates each as either the superior or weaker of the pair. After all comparisons are made, each employee is assigned a summary or ranking based on the number of superior scores received.

Other performance appraisal methods include **critical incidents**, **graphic rating scale**, and **behaviorally anchored rating scales (BARS)**. For critical incidents assessment, the supervisor's attention is focused on specific or critical behaviors that separate effective from ineffective performance. The graphic rating scale lists a set of performance factors such as job knowledge, work quality, and cooperation that the supervisor uses to rate employee performance on an incremental scale. BARS combine elements from critical incidents and graphic rating scale approaches. The supervisor rates employees according to items on a numerical scale.

Another method is **360-degree feedback** or *multisource* or *multirater method*. The multisource feedback method provides a comprehensive perspective of employee performance by using feedback from the full circle of people with whom the employee interacts, including supervisors, subordinates, and coworkers. It is effective for career coaching and identifying strengths and weaknesses. However, there has been criticism of this tool indicating that performance may decline with its use and that it is less valuable to the appraisee

comparative standards
An assessment method that compares employees to other employees in the department.

critical incidents assessment
An assessment method in which the supervisor focuses on specific behaviors that separate effective from ineffective performance.

graphic rating scale
An assessment method that uses a list of performance factors that the supervisor uses to rate employee performance.

behaviorally anchored rating scales (BARS)
An assessment method that combines elements from the critical incidents and graphic rating scale assessments.

360-degree feedback
An assessment method that incorporates feedback from all of an employee's coworkers, including superiors, peers, and subordinates. Also called multisource or multirater feedback.

if coaching does not accompany the feedback to assist the appraisee in understanding the data and how to use it to improve one's performance (Nowack 2007). Widespread adoption of multisource feedback in healthcare has been impaired because many of the feedback instruments were developed in non-healthcare industry sectors. These often lack some of the unique challenges present in healthcare such as physician–manager relations and the frequency and gravity of ethical dilemmas (Garman and Tyler 2004).

Many other methods can be used for performance appraisals. Regardless of the method(s) a supervisor chooses, his goal is to ensure a comprehensive and factual evaluation with meaningful feedback to the employee.

Performance Appraisal Purposes

The performance appraisal system serves many purposes. It can provide a guide for possible promotion, further development, and a basis for merit increases. Garman and Tyler address this purpose by identifying 25 critical competencies for healthcare professionals based on one's career ladder progression (Exhibit 19.2). It also can translate the performance, experience, and qualities of an employee into objective terms and allow comparison with the requirements of the job. The formal appraisal system is designed to consider such criteria as job knowledge, ability to follow through on assignments, judgment, attitude, cooperation, dependability, output, housekeeping, and safety. Such a system of evaluations helps the supervisor take many factors into account when considering merit increases or a promotion. It also provides a rational basis for decision making, as it reduces the chances for personal bias.

Such a formal appraisal system forces the supervisor to observe and scrutinize a subordinate's work not only from the standpoint of how well the employee is performing the job but also from the standpoint of what can be done to improve the employee's performance. Such judgments are difficult to make in most healthcare settings because one is not dealing with concrete performance measures, such as units produced, but with concepts of leadership, teamwork, and cooperation. Because an employee's poor performance and failure to improve may result from inadequate supervision, a formal appraisal system is also likely to uncover supervisory issues.

A formal evaluation system also serves another purpose. Employees have always expected security from their work. In addition to that, they seek satisfying and interesting work that enables them to grow. Often employees are provided copies of their job descriptions but may not know exactly what is expected of them. A well-designed appraisal system reduces ambiguity concerning job requirements and uncertainty by providing employees with information about what is expected from them (Exhibit 17.4) and feedback on how they have performed.

EXHIBIT 19.2 Recommended Competency List, Based on Career Objectives

OBJECTIVES	FIRST PROFESSIONAL POSITION	PREPARATION FOR MID-LEVEL MANAGEMENT	PREPARATION FOR SENIOR MANAGEMENT	MEAN IMPORTANCE RATINGS		
				E	M	S
1. Charting the Course						
Strategic vision		X	X	2.77	4.23	4.61
Innovativeness		X	X	3.38	4.23	4.06
Systems thinking		X	X	3.15	4.46	4.22
Flexibility/adaptability	X	X	X	4.00	4.42	4.06
2. Developing Work Relationships						
Individual understanding	X	X		3.85	3.92	3.47
Mentoring	X	X		3.77	4.31	3.94
Physician/clinician relations	X	X	X	3.92	4.54	4.59
3. Broad Influence						
Consensus building		X		3.15	4.00	3.89
Persuasiveness	X	X	X	3.69	4.54	4.22
Political skills		X	X	3.38	4.15	4.29
Collaboration/team building	X	X	X	3.46	4.15	4.33
4. Structuring the Work Environment						
Work design and coordination	X	X	X	3.69	4.46	4.33
Feedback giving/performance management		X	X	4.00	4.54	4.33
Use of meetings		X		3.15	4.08	3.67
Decision making	X	X	X	3.62	4.62	4.39
5. Inspiring Commitment						
Building trust	X	X	X	4.54	4.69	4.61
Listening/feedback receiving	X	X	X	4.31	4.62	4.35
Tenacity		X	X	3.31	4.08	4.22
Self-presentation	X	X	X	3.92	4.46	4.12
6. Communication						
Energizing	X	X	X	3.46	4.00	3.94
Crafting messages	X	X	X	3.69	4.46	4.38
Writing	X	X		4.08	4.38	3.94
Speaking	X	X	X	3.38	4.31	4.06
7. Self-management						
Managing limits	X	X	X	3.92	4.31	3.72
Balance		X	X	3.85	4.00	4.12
Resilience/self-restraint[a]	X	X	X			

[a]Resilience was added after the CVI survey; thus, no mean ratings were available. Informal inquiries regarding this competency suggest it would be relevant to all levels, and thus its representation as such.

SOURCE: Reprinted with permission from *Journal of Healthcare Management* 49 (5): 312.

Every employee has the right to know how well he is doing and what can be done to improve his work performance. One can assume that most employees are eager to know what their supervisors think of their work. In some instances, the employee's desire to know how he stands with the boss can be interpreted as asking for reassurance about his future in the organization. In other instances this expressed desire may be interpreted differently. For example, a subordinate may realize that she is doing a relatively poor job but hopes to find that the boss is not aware of it. On the other hand, another subordinate who knows that she is doing an outstanding job may wish to make certain that the boss is aware of it. This employee will want to receive more recognition.

Regular appraisals are important incentives to the employees of an organization. In a large, complex organization, employees can easily feel that they and their contributions are forgotten and considered insignificant. Regular appraisals assure employees that the potential exists for improving oneself in the position and that one is not lost within the enterprise; they assure employees that supervisors and the entire organization care about them.

Some organizations employ team models that are empowered to take certain actions. Empowerment permits individuals within a work team to make certain decisions about their work assignments, schedules, and other related items. When teams were discussed earlier in the book, this decision-making freedom was explored in the context of delegation and authority. If a supervisor and his subordinates are working in an environment that supports empowerment and team structures, it may be appropriate to allow team members to prepare or contribute to the performance appraisal of a member of the team. Team members often know the strengths and weaknesses of a fellow team member better than the supervisor. Caution must be exercised against overly criticizing or praising an individual without adequate substantiation of the facts.

The performance appraisal is a critical tool at the disposal of the supervisor, as it influences all personnel functions. It is a determinant in the planning, developing, and recognition of the organization's human resources. Performance appraisals motivate employees, which benefits the organization. Because the appraisal interview is a directive or structured interview, the supervisor needs to prepare in advance the guidance she intends to give the employee to consider. The guidance should help him improve his performance, meet the supervisor's expectations, and improve his position in the department or the organization. This process is a component of the supervisor's mentoring duties. Furthermore, this constructive dialogue, held privately between the supervisor and the employee, helps build trust.

In addition to creating a healthy organizational climate of trust, performance appraisals help management:

- make decisions about compensation and employees' developmental and training needs,

- provide an inventory of employees suitable for promotions,
- facilitate succession planning,
- aid the supervisor by showing whether an employee is in the right job,
- identify for the boss those employees who are moving ahead and those who are not progressing satisfactorily, and
- show whether the supervisor is succeeding in the job as a coach and teacher.

As mentioned, an appraisal program also has many advantages for employees. It reflects the quality of their work and gives them a sense of being treated fairly and not being overlooked. It tells the employee what she can do to be promoted to a better job. Appraisals give the subordinate an opportunity to express concerns, personal goals, and ambitions. In this respect, appraisals are motivational because they create a learning experience for subordinates that inspires them to improve.

Mentoring, Skill Building, and Succession Planning

We have referenced the term **succession planning** several times already in this chapter, but what is it? Succession planning is how a manager ensures that individuals are prepared to take on new assignments within and outside of the department. When a subordinate is given that new assignment, most supervisors are proud to have a member of their team selected. Furthermore, this indicates that the supervisor (1) selected the right talent for the organization, (2) groomed and exposed the individual to others to allow them to gain an opinion about the individual's skill level, and (3) are a respected mentor of "new blood" for the organization. Now, how did the supervisor do it? Several factors tie into succession planning. These include recognizing the additional talents candidates may have when selecting new hires, inventorying the skills of existing staff to identify talents that can be applied to future projects, and being willing to allow staff to tag along to meetings as appropriate or volunteer to serve on interdisciplinary and interdepartmental committees.

Succession planning is particularly important in today's environment, with a generation of baby boomers nearing retirement. HCA has established a COO development program to address this reality (Commins 2009). The program pairs talented individuals with a CEO, who serves as a mentor and boss. Such leadership programs improve the pools of potential leadership in healthcare organizations and can be deployed for identifying leaders for any level of management within an organization.

A **skills inventory** is a list of skills that an individual possesses, regardless of whether the skill is applicable to the person's job. For example, John may be a payroll specialist processing the payroll for the medical residents and interns, but he also has a degree in journalism. Let's assume that the healthcare

succession planning
Preparing employees to take on new assignments within or outside of the employee's current department.

skills inventory
A list of skills an individual possesses, regardless of whether the skill is applicable to the person's job.

organization is celebrating its 50th anniversary and wishes to create a souvenir booklet that includes quotes from former and present staff about their memories of the organization. John may be asked to volunteer to that effort.

A skills inventory, also called a *talent review*, may result from the development section of performance appraisals or be conducted independent of the annual review. In the development section, the employee and supervisor discuss the individual's skill strengths and weaknesses; skills used on the job and off the job are noted. In this way the strengths of all staff are captured in the inventory. Strengths may include "Internet skills," "bilingual," "public speaking experience at the Chamber of Commerce," "pilot in training," "prior business owner," and "database experience." Ideally, these strengths and skills are entered into a centralized computerized repository. The benefit of a computerized skills inventory for the organization is obvious: it allows the organization to search within the organization for individuals with new or unusual skills before filling a position with an external applicant.

mentor
An individual who helps a subordinate establish goals and a path to achieve them.

Mentoring goes hand-in-hand with the appraisal process and skills inventory discussion. When mentoring, the supervisor (the **mentor**) has a good opportunity to dialogue with her subordinates about their future aspirations and help them establish a path to achieve them. This may include shadowing opportunities, whereby a subordinate works with the supervisor on higher-level projects, such as preparing capital expenditure requests, or joins the supervisor in meetings with others outside of the department. Another mentoring activity is assisting the subordinate with educational choices such as career choices or college selection. Using such competency guides as that in Exhibit 19.2, the mentor steers the young professional down various paths to sharpen his skills in these areas. Finally, the supervisor may recommend her subordinates to work on projects; for example, preparing and giving a presentation to the IT steering committee on the subject of "meaningful use" as initially introduced in the 2009 American Recovery and Reinvestment Act (Stimulus Package). Mentoring requires the supervisor to guide the protege and serve as a confidant. It may require some of the supervisor's personal time, but the rewards can be tremendous.

Timing of Appraisals

Appraisals must be conducted regularly to be significant to the employee and the organization. A one-time performance measure is of little use; the supervisor should formally appraise all the employees within the department at regular intervals at least once a year. If an employee has just started in a new or more responsible position, it is advisable to schedule an initial appraisal within three to six months.

Ideally, employees should be evaluated several times throughout the year to ensure that they receive timely feedback on their performance and to separate the performance review from the timing of a wage adjustment; this separation helps the supervisor focus on performance improvement and not the economic situation of the employee. However, often supervisors do not have the luxury of the time it takes to conduct this amount of structured counseling. Therefore, they must take advantage of opportunities to give immediate feedback when they observe appropriate and inappropriate actions. An advantage of doing these on-the-spot counseling sessions throughout the year with team members is that there should be no surprises at evaluation time.

Periodic appraisals assure the employee that whatever improvement was made will be noticed and that he will be recognized for this progress. As time goes on, periodic ratings and reviews become an important determinant of an employee's morale. It reaffirms the supervisor's interest in the employees and in their continued development and improvement.

Annual formal appraisals and the review of these appraisals do not replace the feedback on performance that is part of the day-to-day coaching responsibilities of the supervisor. Employees should receive feedback daily; it is well known that performance feedback is most effective when it occurs immediately after the event to which it relates. This applies equally to feedback on below-par performance and to recognition of above-par performance. Without this ongoing daily feedback, formal, once-a-year appraisals do not suffice.

Who Is the Appraiser?

A major difficulty in effective performance appraisal is that we as human beings can only make subjective appraisals. This creates intellectual and perceptual problems, leading to the rater's own interpretation of reality and not necessarily absolute reality. To minimize these shortcomings, some organizations devise an appraisal system in which the employee is evaluated by various appraisers. This may include self-appraisals and peer appraisals; in some systems, the appraisals are subject to reviews by those higher up in the administrative hierarchy. A few organizations have assessment centers for evaluating employees for their future potential as managers. (This concept is discussed more fully toward the end of this chapter.)

With the exception of team-cultured organizations, the appraisal is usually conducted by the individual's immediate supervisor. Formal authority inherent in the managerial hierarchy means, among many other aspects, that the supervisor has the right to make decisions in reference to the subordinate's performance. Among all other appraisers, the immediate supervisor is the person who should best know the duties of the jobs within the department. The immediate supervisor has the best opportunity to observe the appraisee on the job and provide feedback. Furthermore, most subordinates want to receive performance-related feedback from their immediate superior and feel more comfortable in discussing the appraisal with him.

Sometimes it may be necessary for the first-line boss to call on the next higher supervisor for assistance in making appraisals. To assist the new supervisor, the organization or the supervisor's superior should provide some training on performance evaluations, including discussing their preparation, evaluation methods, techniques for identifying obstacles to success and recommendations for ways to remove these obstacles, methods for creating goals, and relevant legal issues.

In some institutions the appraisal is made by a committee composed of the first-line supervisor, her boss, and possibly one or two other supervisors who have adequate knowledge of the performance of the person being rated. This approach has the advantage of reducing some of the immediate supervisor's personal prejudices or biases. These alternative approaches to the immediate supervisor appraisal are necessary in situations in which the superior has little opportunity to observe the employee on the job; for example, where an enterprise has employees who work around the clock, in a matrix organization, in project management roles, in remote facilities, or as telecommuters.

self-appraisal
A self-rating by an employee, which provides a supplemental source of appraisal input.

Self-appraisal, or self-rating, is a supplemental source of appraisal input. There are several advantages to self-ratings: they (1) often contain less "halo" error (employee self-ratings tend to be more critical than those done by supervisors), (2) show the supervisor how the employee perceives the responsibilities and problems of the position, (3) help identify differences of opinion, and (4) are particularly useful when employees work in isolation. However, self-appraisal can often lead to conflict if the supervisor's appraisal differs significantly from an inflated self-rating by the employee. When this occurs, the supervisor should prepare for an in-depth discussion with the employee. By asking the employee to explain her rationale for the self-ratings, the supervisor may learn about achievements of which he was previously unaware. Once the employee shares her opinions and justifications, the supervisor must show the employee the data collected since the time of the last evaluation and how these data compare to the expectations set forth. That is why the appraisal system often combines self-appraisals and supervisory appraisals into one comprehensive performance appraisal.

At times, in team settings or when more than one individual shares the same duties, peers are used as appraisers. They can often provide valuable information about their colleagues because of their daily interactions. They can observe how an employee interacts with peers, subordinates, and the boss.

Peer appraisals offer independent judgment, may provide the appraisee with "better" methods to improve his performance based on peer experience, and have often proved to be good predictors of performance when used as a basis for promotion.

However, some powerful influences in organizational life may distort or cloud a peer's perception. Most employees have a strong need for security and work for present and future rewards from the employer. If someone else receives additional rewards, the chances for additional rewards become smaller for everyone else. This competition for current or future employer rewards, whether apparent or not, could distort a peer's perception of a colleague's performance and potential. In addition, friendships and stereotyping may bias the rating. Friendship relates not only to individuals but also to groups. For instance, the appraiser may evaluate a peer in a group of which she is a member. The appraiser may be tempted to rate members of that particular group higher than individuals in another group. Also, at times peers are not willing to evaluate each other, considering it to be an inducement to snitching on one another. Some union contracts forbid peer participation in the evaluation process.

For all practical purposes, appraisal done by the immediate supervisor should suffice, and in most organizations the immediate supervisor is the primary, if not the only, appraiser of employee performance. However, the use of multiple sources of appraisals is likely to obtain a more comprehensive evaluation.

Performance Rating

To minimize and overcome the difficulties in appraising an employee, most enterprises find it advisable to use some type of appraisal form (see Exhibit 19.3). Appraisal forms are prepared by the human resources department in collaboration with the unit supervisor and possibly in conjunction with outside consultants. Often the appraisal form will include space for comments from both the appraiser and the appraisee. As mentioned, great care must be exercised to make certain that the system used is legally defensible.

Although many types of appraisal forms are available, most of them specify job-related and other important criteria for measuring job performance, intelligence, and personality traits. In addition to determining criteria, standards must be clarified to determine how well employees are performing. Ideally, criteria will tie directly to a clearly written and up-to-date position description that the employee has had for at least the same period of time as the period being addressed in the performance interview. The instruments most used in the appraisal process are based on both behavior and traits. Some are objective, whereas others are subjective.

Exhibit 19.3

Sample
Performance
Appraisal

PERFORMANCE APPRAISAL　　　　　　　Date: _____

Employee Name: _____　Title: _____

Department: _____　CC: _____　Emp. No. _____　DOH: __/__/__

Appraisal Period: _____　to: _____

Instructions: Carefully evaluate employee's work performance in relation to current job requirements. Check rating box to indicate the employee's performance. Indicate N/A if not applicable.

DEFINITION OF APPRAISAL RATINGS:

Outstanding (O): Performance is exceptional in all areas and is recognizable as being far superior to others.

Very Good (VG): Results clearly exceed most position requirements. Performance is of high quality and is achieved on a consistent basis.

Good (G): Competent and dependable level of performance. Meets performance expectations of the job.

Improvement Needed (IN): Performance is deficient in several areas. Improvement is necessary.

Unsatisfactory (U): Results are generally unacceptable and require immediate improvement.

N/A: Not applicable to this person's job.

APPRAISAL FACTOR	RATING
Applies past experiences to new problems?	
Retains information? Does not repeatedly ask the same questions or make the same mistakes?	
Follows instructions and takes notes when necessary?	
Has gained the skills necessary to navigate the computer system for the functions for which he/she is responsible?	
Takes care of equipment?	
Uses supplies wisely?	
Follows department procedures?	
Completes assigned work when expected?	
Completes assigned work accurately?	
Completes volume required?	

Continued

EXHIBIT 19.3
Continued

APPRAISAL FACTOR	RATING
Makes efficient use of time?	
Meets accuracy requirements?	
Completes assigned work with little or no dependence upon others?	
Handwriting legible?	
Does not transpose numbers?	
Willing to work overtime?	
Requires minimum supervision?	
Improved in all areas that were marked "improvement needed" or "unsatisfactory" in last evaluation?	
Achieved goals outlined in last evaluation?	
Maintained strengths in same areas as last evaluation?	
Days of absence?	
Tardies?	

Area(s) for Improvement:

Strengths:

Goals:
1.

Target Date: _____ Employee's Initials: _____
2.

Target Date: _____ Employee's Initials: _____

Employee Comments:

Employee's Initials: _____

Employee's Signature: _____ Date: _____

Supervisor's Signature: _____ Date: _____

Manager's Signature: _____ Date: _____

The following are qualities and characteristics that are most frequently rated. For nonsupervisory personnel, typical qualities include the following:

- quantity and quality of work produced,
- job knowledge,
- dependability,
- attitude,
- amount of supervision required,
- maintenance of work area and equipment,
- unauthorized absenteeism and tardiness,
- safety, and
- personal appearance.

For managerial and professional employees, typical factors include the following:

- analytical ability,
- judgment,
- initiative,
- leadership,
- quality and quantity of work produced,
- knowledge of work,
- attitude,
- dependability,
- emotional stability, and
- teamwork.

For each of these factors the supervisor is charged with selecting the degree of achievement attained by the employee. In some instances, a point system is provided to arrive at a numerical score.

Despite the outward simplicity of some rating forms, the supervisor will probably run into a number of difficulties. First, not all supervisors agree on what is meant by a simple adjective rating scale such as unsatisfactory, marginal, satisfactory, and above average. It is advisable, therefore, that the form contain a descriptive sentence such as shown in Exhibit 19.3, in addition to each of these adjectives:

- For unsatisfactory, "performance clearly fails to meet minimum requirements"
- For marginal, "performance occasionally fails to meet minimum requirements"
- For satisfactory, "performance meets or exceeds minimum requirements"
- For above average, "performance consistently exceeds minimum requirements"
- For superior, "performance clearly exceeds all job requirements"

Some performance appraisals may include a combination of points and adjective categories, where the adjective method is used for less objective conditions.

For example, in rating a nurse's degree of emotional stability, the appraiser may select among the following choices the phrase that is most descriptive:

1. "Unreliable in crises; goes to pieces easily; cannot take criticism"
2. "Unrealistic; emotions and moodiness periodically handicap his or her dealings; he or she personalizes issues"
3. "Usually on an even keel; has mature approach to most situations"
4. "Is realistic; generally maintains good behavioral balance in handling situations"
5. "Self-assured to a high degree; has outstanding ability to adjust to circumstances, no matter how difficult"

When weaknesses are identified during the performance period and noted in the performance appraisal, a **performance development plan** to facilitate correction should be established. This plan should include specific and objective measures or expectations to be achieved. For example, "Sue has not been able to complete the sorting of incoming mail by noon daily. I will review the mailroom's mailbox layout for her again. It is expected that she will be able to receive and sort the mail delivered by 10 a.m. into the mailboxes by noon each day." Make sure employees understand the performance expectations. To check whether an employee understands, one technique is to simply ask her to summarize the expectations (Spath 2006).

performance development plan
A plan to facilitate correction of weaknesses identified during a performance appraisal.

When encountering performance shortfalls, the supervisor may find Robert Mager's Performance Analysis Checklist (Exhibit 19.4) and the Performance Problem–Solution Checklist (Exhibit 19.5) beneficial. These tools help the supervisor analyze the cause(s) of the employee's performance gap and the actions that should be taken to close the gap.

The performance development plan should guide the appraisee in how to improve his performance. This may include remedial training, such as visiting the PC lab at the healthcare facility to become more comfortable with how to use a certain application or refreshing one's knowledge of anatomy and physiology by taking an online course.

In summary, the performance development plan should discuss what is expected and how one might successfully achieve the expectation. Supervisors should strive to objectively evaluate employee performance in such a way that employees will welcome the perceptions shared and seek to improve themselves. The goal of performance appraisals is multifaceted: to help retain good performers, to facilitate retraining or counseling when necessary to help people become better employees, and to make sure employees have the skills and resources they need to effectively perform their jobs and meet management's expectations.

Exhibit 19.4 Performance Analysis Checklist

1. Whose performance is at issue?
2. What is the performance discrepancy? What is actually happening? What should be happening?
3. Is the problem worth solving? What would happen if you ignored it?
4. Can we apply fast fixes? Are expectations clear? Are resources available and adequate? Is quality of performance easily observed?
5. Are the consequences appropriate? Is desired performance punishing to the performer? Is poor performance rewarding to the performer? Are consequences arranged effectively?
6. Do they already know how? Could they do it if their lives depended on it? Could they do it in the past? Are the tasks performed often?
7. Are there more clues? Can the task(s) be simplified? Can obstacles to performing be removed? Can the performer(s) learn to perform?
8. Describe solutions.
9. Calculate the cost of each solution.
10. Select the most practical of the cost-effective solutions.
11. Implement the solution(s).

SOURCE: Robert Mager, © 1999, The Center for Effective Performance, Inc., 1100 Johnson Ferry Road, Suite 150, Atlanta, GA 30342. www.cepworldwide.com 1-800-558-4237. Reprinted with permission. All rights reserved. No portion of these materials may be reproduced in any manner without express written consent from The Center for Effective Performance, Inc.

Problems in Performance Rating

Performance rating systems can have weaknesses, often because rating employees is largely a subjective process. The supervisor should be aware of these pitfalls and try to minimize errors in processing, storing, and recalling observed behavior.

Some supervisors have a tendency to be overly lenient in their ratings, rating appraisees higher than they deserve. They are afraid they might antagonize those being evaluated if they rate them low.

Other supervisors are overly harsh in rating their employees and appraise them lower than they should. To give consistently low ratings is as damaging as being too lenient.

For example, if the operating room personnel on day shift are consistently appraised higher than those on the evening shift, it is difficult to determine whether this is because of the evening supervisor's strictness or the day shift supervisor's leniency or whether this reflects real differences in the employees' abilities and performance.

EXHIBIT 19.5
Performance
Problem
Solution
Checklist

PROBLEM	SOLUTIONS
They can't do it, and... the skill is used often:	Provide feedback Simplify the task
the skill is used rarely:	Provide job aids to promote desired performance Simplify the job Provide periodic practice

Training will be required if the above remedies are inadequate.

They can do it, but... doing it right leads to punishment:	Remove the sources of punishment
doing it wrong is more satisfying:	Remove the rewards for incorrect performance
nobody notices when they do it right:	Apply rewards to the performer for doing it right
there are obstacles to performing as desired:	Remove the obstacles (or help people work around them)

central tendency
The tendency to appraise all employees as roughly average.

halo effect
The tendency to give high or low marks on an entire appraisal because of high or low marks on one aspect of the appraisal, even if other aspects of the appraisal do not deserve the high or low marks.

Another common error is **central tendency**, in which the appraiser rates the employees consistently as average or around the midpoint in the range, although some employees' performance warrants higher or lower ratings. Such a tendency shows that the supervisor may be unprepared for the formal appraisal and avoids being decisive. Another subjective error of the appraiser is to be influenced by the **halo effect** (discussed in Chapter 18), which is the tendency to let the rating they assign to one characteristic influence their rating on all subsequent characteristics. This works in two directions. Rating the appraisee as excellent on one factor influences the rater to give the employee undeserved high ratings on other factors. On the other hand, rating the employee as unsatisfactory on one factor influences the appraiser to give the appraisee another low or lower-than-deserved rating on other factors—again possibly undeserved.

One way to minimize the halo effect is to rate all employees on a single factor or trait before going on to the next factor. In other words, the supervisor only rates one factor of each employee at a time and then goes on to the next employee for the same factor, and so on. This enables the supervisor to standardize the ratings; however, the supervisor should not feel compelled to strive for or expect that the distribution of ratings resemble a normal, or bell-shaped, curve.

similar-to-me appraisal tendency
The tendency of a supervisor to rate employees whose attitudes resemble their own higher than otherwise deserved.

Some raters are tempted to judge more favorably those employees whose attitudes resemble their own; this is the **similar-to-me appraisal tendency**. A further distortion can be caused by interpersonal relations and bias. The ratings may be influenced by the supervisor's likes and dislikes about each individual working in the department. This is especially apparent when objective standards of performance are not available.

Organizational influences, or the way administration uses the ratings, may give rise to another source of difficulty. Often raters are lenient when they know that pay raises and promotions depend on the appraisals. Conversely, if the organizational emphasis is on further employee development, appraisers may be inclined to be harsh and emphasize weaknesses.

The supervisor's judgment must be based on the total performance of the employee. It is unfair to appraise a subordinate based on only one assignment on which she did particularly well or poorly. The evaluation should be based on the employee's performance during the entire appraisal period, not just on the appraisee's most recent behavior. If periodic appraisals are performed at intervals throughout the evaluation period, a supervisor is less likely to judge an individual on the most recent experience. Employees know when their appraisal is due and will act accordingly by increasing their productivity, curbing their tardiness, and so on. The supervisor may notice this other aspect of the halo effect—sudden improvement in performance—just prior to an evaluation period.

Compiling the information needed for an appraisal is no simple task. Because memory tends not to go beyond about two months, it is to the supervisor's advantage to keep dated notes throughout the year of observations of and conversations with staff members. These notes can simply be dropped into a folder for each employee. Another source for recall may be e-mail messages the supervisor has sent to employees acknowledging their accomplishments throughout the year. Additionally, the supervisor should review the employee's prior evaluation or evaluations to assess whether the employee is progressing as anticipated. This approach provides the supervisor with a year-long basis from which to develop the appraisal, which shows the staff that the supervisor took care in preparing their evaluations.

Some managers seek the subordinate's opinion of their performance in advance of conducting the evaluation discussion. In these cases, the subordinates appraise themselves first. This gives the appraisees the opportunity to state their side of the story first. It is easier for many subordinates to criticize themselves than to take criticism from the supervisor. After reviewing the employee's self-rating, the supervisor offers his comments on the subordinate's strengths and weaknesses and proceeds with preparing the evaluation for the discussion.

Supervisors must take care not to let random or first impressions of an employee influence their judgment. The evaluation should be based on the employee's total record of performance, reliability, initiative, skills, resourcefulness, and capability. Obtaining input from peers and customers served by the employee and combining these observations with the supervisor's impressions result in a fairer assessment of the individual's performance.

Supervisors also should not allow past performance appraisal ratings to influence current ratings unjustly either way. An aid to minimize these errors and biases is to document employee behavior as soon as possible after each occurrence. When the formal appraisal takes place, supervisors can refer back to the documentation to assess whether the employee's performance has improved as a result of the immediate feedback at the time of the occurrence. If so, then the need to address past poor performance is minimized. However, if even after several counseling sessions performance has not changed, this pattern should be addressed. The goal of the performance review is to provide a balanced assessment that is not biased by some event that is no longer pertinent.

Observing all these problems in rating helps supervisors overcome subjectivity in processing, storing, and recalling observed behavior when evaluations are made. Training for those who do appraisals also helps. Such training is necessary because appraisals that are biased, inaccurate, or distorted do not increase an employee's motivation. These errors also may lead to poor promotion and retention decisions and even possibly to charges of discrimination. Training supervisors on how to observe behavior is an ongoing process. The success of the performance appraisal largely depends on the supervisor's ability to obtain accurate information and then to discuss it with the appraisee in a nonthreatening and constructive manner.

Preparing for the Interview

Everything regarding general techniques of interviewing (see Chapter 18) is applicable to the appraisal interview. Additional skills are necessary as well because the direction of evaluation interviews cannot be predicted. At times it may be difficult for the supervisor to carry on this interview, especially if the subordinate shows hostility when the supervisor discusses a negative evaluation. Of course, employees need to know if and where their performance is inadequate. Positive judgment can be communicated effectively, but it is difficult to communicate criticism without generating resentment and defensiveness. It takes much practice and insight to acquire skills for handling the evaluation interview.

Some supervisors do not believe they need to conduct an evaluation interview because they are in daily contact with their employees. These supervisors claim that their door is open at all times. However, this approach is not enough. Many employees want a formal, written appraisal in which they receive a substantiated report on their performance that others can see should the employees apply for advanced positions. Also, employees may have some things on their mind that they do not want to discuss in the everyday contacts with the supervisor in the open office. To ensure a productive appraisal interview, it is appropriate that the employee be provided sufficient notice of the date to gather his thoughts and facilitate a two-way discussion. The supervisor may wish to provide the employee with a written notice and agenda such as that shown in Exhibit 19.6. Regardless, the objectives displayed should be the objectives the supervisor seeks to achieve when conducting the appraisal interview.

The supervisor must be well prepared for this review session. The appraiser must know what should be covered and achieved in the meeting and gather all the information relevant to the discussion and re-review the information to refresh her memory about the reasons behind the opinions expressed in the appraisal. The various events that occurred during the evaluation period must be clear in the interviewer's mind. The supervisor may want to prepare an outline for this meeting. Thorough preparation enables the appraiser to be ready for any direction the discussion takes.

Predicting what will happen in this review session is difficult. It may be an uneventful meeting, and the appraisee's responses may be minimal—an occasional yes or no, or a nod of the head. Another meeting, however, may end up as a bitter confrontation. Because of the importance and sensitivity of the performance review, the appraiser must also be skilled in interviewing and counseling. The reviewer must ask the right question at the right time and be a constructive listener. In the review session, information must be shared. The appraisee must feel that his concerns are important. Success of this review session can be improved if the appraiser has empathy, listens constructively, asks the right questions at the proper time, and observes keenly. Lastly, the appraiser must allow enough time to conduct the interview and ensure that no distractions or interruptions are allowed to occur during the session.

PERFORMANCE APPRAISAL MEETING FOR: JANE SMITH **11 A.M., 5/30/2010**	**EXHIBIT 19.6** Notice of Appraisal Meeting

Objectives:

- Communicate my evaluation of your performance
- Resolve any concerns
- Accept ratings
- Identify areas for improvement and/or advancement
- Discuss your personal career goals
- Commit to future goals and expectations

The Appraisal Interview

Although experienced supervisors probably do not need to follow a formalized system, administration often suggests that all supervisors follow a standardized agenda similar to the one noted above.

The appraisal interview should be conducted in a private place that is not in earshot of coworkers and is free of interruptions. An atmosphere that is relaxed and as informal as possible will likely make the employee feel comfortable and encouraged to voice his opinions on performance-related matters.

At the outset of the appraisal, the supervisor should state the purpose of the evaluation procedure and the interview; state that the interview is to be a constructive and positive experience for both the person being appraised and the appraiser; and indicate that it is being conducted for the benefit of the employee, the supervisor, and the institution. As part of this warmup, the supervisor may wish to comment on the progress the worker has made since the preceding counseling interview and compliment him on his achievements. The discussion then gradually moves to areas that need improvement. One should use as many examples as possible when discussing both strengths and weaknesses. Be aware that the formula of starting with praise, following it up with criticism, and ending the interview with another compliment is not necessarily the best method. Good and bad may cancel each other out, and the worker may forget the criticism. A mature employee is able to take deserved criticism when it is appropriate. By the same token, when praise is merited, it should be expressed. It is not always possible to mix praise and criticism effectively. Finally, focus on performance, not on the employee's personality. If personality conflicts do exist, discuss how these conflicts affect performance rather than how one should adjust his personality.

Some supervisors prefer not to have to tell their subordinates how they stand in the department and what they should do to improve. They are reluctant because, unless it is done with great sensitivity, this type of interview can lead to hostility and even greater misunderstanding. However, every employee is entitled to an honest, accurate, comprehensive, and fact-based performance evaluation. Many employees distrust anything that relates to their review, starting with the validity of the measuring instrument used and the appraiser's ability to observe. Employees may be reluctant to discuss their workplace behavior. However, this discussion is absolutely essential to ensure effective appraisals.

Because the idea of being rated imposes some extra tension and strain, the institution should provide supervisors with learning opportunities to conduct appraisals effectively. Many facilities provide training such as practice sessions, behavior modeling training programs, role-playing experiences, in-basket exercises,[2] and assessment centers. All this is done to increase the supervisors' effectiveness in dealing with those being evaluated, to improve their observer accuracy, and to aid them in carrying out appraisal interviews effectively. The four major formats for this interview are (1) the tell-and-listen/listen-and-tell format, (2) the tell-and-sell approach, (3) the problem-solving approach, and (4) a mixed interview combining all these formats.

Effectively utilizing these interview approaches and providing for a friendly, collaborative atmosphere in a private area for the review are most important. As personal feelings and opinions most likely will be brought out in the discussion, the appraisee must be assured of privacy and confidentiality. The supervisor should not discuss specifics of the interview with the appraisee's coworkers even though some issues may arise in the session that will require further action or investigation. The employee should be assured that the content of this counseling session will be held in confidence.

The supervisor should next proceed to a discussion of the evaluation itself. The subordinate's strong points and then weak points are stated, followed by a general discussion that allows the employee an opportunity to state her opinions and feelings. This is the tell-and-listen format. The supervisor should stress that everyone in the same job in the department is rated according to the same standards and that the employee has not been singled out for special scrutiny. The supervisor should be in a position to support the rating by citing specific, documented instances of good and poor performance. The supervisor should be careful to relate the measured factors to the actual demands of the job. The rating must be geared to the present qualities of the employee's performance.

This last point is particularly important if some employees are already doing good work and the supervisor is tempted to leave well enough alone; these are probably the very employees who are likely to make further progress, and to tell them simply to keep up the good work is not sufficient. These employees may not have major problems; nevertheless, they deserve thoughtful counseling with a focus on their future. Such employees are likely to continue to develop, and the supervisor should specify future development plans. The appraiser must be familiar, therefore, with the opportunities available to the employee, requirements of the job, and the employee's qualifications. Whenever he is discussing a subordinate's future, the supervisor should not make promises for promotion that may not be possible to keep.

The interview should end with a discussion of what the subordinate can and wants to do about any deficiencies and what the supervisor will do for the employee in this regard. In contrast to the tell-and-listen format of the discussion of the evaluation, this is a listen-and-tell format. Comments and conclusions pertaining to the appraisee's responsibilities should be specific, unambiguous, and in writing. If applicable any commitments by the appraiser, such as providing training or other resources, should be noted.

The tell-and-sell format requires the supervisor to do much of the communicating. Often, it is used when a subordinate believes she did nothing wrong and the supervisor is placed in a position of "selling" her evaluation and performance improvement plan to the employee. This approach does not have to have a negative result, however. The format may be acceptable to subordinates when a supervisor is trusted and is known for her expertise and her insight is valued by subordinates.

The problem-solving approach is most often used when a single issue concerns the supervisor, such as a subordinate's excessive tardiness. Both the supervisor and subordinate discuss how this problem will be solved.

When using any of these approaches, supervisors should remember to avoid using the word "I" in the interview. This is a time to discuss your employee's performance—what he has done, not how you feel about it or how you performed that job in the past.

One of the pitfalls of appraisals is the lack of objectivity. This flaw may surface during the interview and create an impasse when trying to deal with the employee's weaknesses. If practical, the supervisor may wish to use a **management by objectives (MBO)** approach. The underlying concept of MBO is that identified, measurable, and workable objectives are agreed on by the supervisor and the employee, which leads to improved performance and a motivating environment. MBO creates a participative climate because the subordinates help decide what their goals are. Although MBO is primarily a planning tool and a process that goes beyond performance appraisals, it can be logically and conveniently linked with performance evaluations and appraisal interviews. The review lends itself well to measuring the quality of an employee's on-the-job performance and achievements, and is a good time for the employee to help set new objectives. These new objectives are to be achieved during the next period, and should be regularly monitored with the use of monthly or quarterly report cards. The regular monitoring makes sure

management by objectives (MBO)
A management tool developed by Peter Drucker that uses measurable objectives to motivate and evaluate performance.

there are no surprises at evaluation time. Since the subordinates are judged on objectives they helped determine, they are more likely to achieve them.

Closing the Evaluation Interview

The interview should also give the employee an opportunity to ask questions. Any misunderstanding cleared up at this time may avoid future difficulty. The appraiser should also clarify that further performance ratings and interviews will occur regularly. The supervisor should always remember that the purpose of the appraisal interview is to help employees see their shortcomings and to aid them in finding solutions. The real success of the interview lies in the employees' ability to see the need for their own improvement, stimulating in them a desire to change.

At the end of the appraisal interview, the supervisor should make certain that the employee is clear on his performance expectations and the ways in which he can improve. He also should come away with a desire to improve. It is hoped that employees will establish goals that are mutually satisfying to themselves and the supervisor. An employee's commitment provides some measurable goals against which future performance can be judged. Furthermore, the supervisor must agree to set aside time to retrain the individual on processes that are not being performed well or coach the individual on ways to enhance performance. At the end of the next appraisal period, both supervisor and subordinate will meet to evaluate how well the goals have been achieved and what the next objectives will be. This gives the subordinate a custom-made standard for evaluation. It provides him or her with a specified goal within a specified period. The employee will be that much more motivated because the goal was a commitment on his or her part.

Custom requires that the person being appraised sign the evaluation form on completion of the review. Usually a statement appears above the signature line saying that the employee's signature merely confirms that the interview occurred and that the appraisee in no way approves or disapproves of the statements contained in the evaluation.

With this understanding, the subordinate will probably sign. If, however, the appraisee would like to state personal views, no harm is done in letting her do so. Many employees will not verbalize their disagreement with the rating, and signing the forms with such feelings can create resentment against the organization. The real purpose of the signature is to document for the supervisor's boss that the evaluation interview took place. As stated, many supervisors have mixed reactions about the appraisal interview. Because it provides essential feedback on the entire evaluation procedure, administration must make certain that it occurs, and the signature is the simplest way to confirm this.

As a reminder, the appraiser should note any important issues that were raised during the evaluation and any personal commitments he made to the employee, and note dates for follow-up and feedback to the employee.

Proper Wages, Salaries, and Benefits

Some experts strongly advocate that the annual performance appraisal review be separate from salary review. They suggest that the discussion of the employee's past performance, future potential, and further education and development, as well as the coaching and counseling taking place, should not be tainted by discussing pay and compensation. Whether a salary adjustment will be made does not depend only on the performance but also on the financial condition of the enterprise, wages paid elsewhere, the economic conditions, and many other factors. Most likely if both reviews are done together, the appraisee will interpret everything that is said in relation to future reward opportunities and possible promotions. A proposed solution is to have two separate review sessions. The first may be concerned with the review and employee development, and the second session (four to eight weeks later) may cover the compensation issue.

Although people want more from their jobs than just a wage or salary, the latter are basic necessities. Pay provides more than the means of satisfying physical needs; it provides a sense of accomplishment and recognition. Most people at work consider relative pay as important, and real or imagined wage and salary inequities are frequent causes of dissatisfaction, friction, and low morale. It is top-level management's duty to pursue a sound policy of wage and salary administration throughout the entire organization; the goal is to have a nondiscriminatory compensation structure. By setting wages high enough, the healthcare organization is able to recruit satisfactory employees and motivate their present employees to work toward pay increases and promotions. Reducing inequities among employees' earnings raises morale and reduces friction.

Wage rates and schedules are usually set by top-level administration. The supervisor's authority in this respect is quite limited. Nevertheless, it is a part of the supervisor's staffing function to make certain that the employees of the department are properly and equitably compensated. It is every manager's job to offer the amount of compensation that will retain competent employees in the department and, if necessary, attract good workers from the outside. Monetary rewards are an exceedingly important factor for all employees. However, many employees are much more concerned about how their salaries compare to the earnings of others than they are about their absolute earnings. No doubt many wage rates and schedules follow historical patterns, whereas others are often accidental or due to exceptions. For example, certain wage rates can be distorted when positions are difficult to fill, when individuals are retained because of certain knowledge or skill, or when the administration prefers different wage-scale philosophies. In the long run such situations cannot be tolerated.

internal alignment
Aligning salaries of positions within a department, relative to the monetary value of the positions. That is, paying people who are equally valuable approximately equal pay.

It is the supervisor's duty to see that the wages paid within the department are properly aligned internally and externally. **Internal alignment** means that the jobs within the department and institution are paid according to what they are worth. Internal consistency based on equity provides a system of compensation that is acceptable to the employees involved, resulting in satisfaction and a desire to be promoted and to remain with the present employer. External alignment means that the wages offered for the work to be performed in the department compare favorably with the going rate in the community and area. External competitiveness refers to the pay relationships among organizations and the competitive positions reflected in these relationships. If wages do not compare favorably, the supervisor knows that some of the most experienced workers will leave and that attracting new ones from the outside will be difficult. All of this applies also to an appropriate benefits program, often called "fringe benefits."

Internal Alignment

job evaluation
A method of determining the relationships between pay rates and the relative monetary value of jobs within a department.

To pay the various jobs within the department according to what they are worth, the supervisor should ask the human resources department to conduct a **job evaluation**. Sometimes an outside consultant is used. Job evaluation is a method of determining the relationships between pay rates and the relative monetary value of jobs within a department. In such a procedure, a committee guided by the human resources staff evaluates the jobs according to various factors, such as competence, problem solving, and accountability, then devises an appropriate wage rate based on the worth of each job and institutes an appropriate wage schedule. Of course, some questions will arise about what to do with exceptional cases—that is, those employees who are receiving either excessively high or exceedingly low salaries in relation to others. Once a plan has been designed, it is necessary to maintain it properly so that no new inequities arise.

There are several methods of job evaluation. Although they are systematic, they are not totally precise because they involve questions of human judgment. In addition to the most widely used point system, other methods, such as ranking, factor comparison, and job classification, are typically used.

External Alignment

wage survey
A survey that collects data on wages paid in the community for similar key jobs in similar or related enterprises.

If the wage and salary policy of the institution is to be externally competitive, pay rates must be approximately the same as those prevailing in the community. Thus, accurate wage and salary data must be collected through surveys. Job evaluations establish differentials between jobs based on different job content; **wage surveys** provide management with information on whether the organization's wage level is competitive externally and aligned. A wage survey involves collecting data on wages paid in the community for similar key jobs in similar or related enterprises. The jobs that are similar in every healthcare organization are called **benchmark jobs**. Examples of benchmark jobs are dietitian, housekeeper or custodian, registered nurse, health information director, and patient billing clerk (Exhibit 19.7). The benchmark positions in your organization are adjusted based on data from these surveys. Then the job evaluations of the other positions can be adjusted accordingly, causing what some term the "ripple effect." These routine adjustments are important. Without proper **external alignment**, the supervisor cannot recruit competent employees or prevent present employees from leaving for better-paying jobs.

To conduct such a survey is a rather costly and sophisticated procedure; performing one's own survey probably produces the most meaningful results. Alternately, one can use a survey published by a reputable external source. Reputable sources of wage surveys are government agencies such as the Bureau of Labor Statistics, professional associations, industry newsletters (see Exhibit 19.7), and hospital associations. The area usually considered in the survey is the geographic region within which workers seek employment and employers recruit workers.

Depending on the focus of a survey, benefit information may be included in a wage survey. Most enterprises provide benefits for employees, such as pensions, insurance, education reimbursement, healthcare, dental plans, maternity leave, daycare, vacation time, and pay for time not worked. These are often called fringe benefits, although these benefits often account for 25 to 35 percent of the cash payroll. Most of these additional benefits are established by top-level administration as institutionwide measures. The supervisor has little to do with such benefits other than to make sure that the individual who has been evaluated understands how benefits operate and that each receives her fair share. However, supervisors may be able to implement other types of "benefits" in the department that will appeal to the employees and make up for shortfalls in the compensation program. Flexible schedules, remote working environments or telecommuting, and educational opportunities are all examples of perks that can satisfy and retain employees.

To determine whether the rates offered by the department are competitive, the supervisor *may* request that the human resources department undertake a wage and salary survey unless recent reliable information is available. By comparing this information with outside wage patterns, the supervisor can determine if his staff's wages are properly aligned externally. A sound wage and salary pattern should always be of great concern to the CEO. Although the supervisor has little direct authority in this area, pointing out inadequacies and inconsistencies may cause the administrator to launch an evaluation. Supervisors should definitely plead their case to upper management when multiple vacancies occur because of employees leaving to assume similar positions at other hospitals for higher wages and different benefits, or when the type of person required to fill a position is in short supply. To make

benchmark job
Jobs that are similar in every healthcare organization, such as dietitian and housekeeper.

external alignment
Aligning salaries within an organization with salaries of similar positions outside the organization but within the surrounding community.

EXHIBIT 19.7 Examples of Salary Survey Information

Table 5. Median hourly earnings of the largest occupations in health care, May 2006

Occupation	Ambulatory health care services	Hospitals	Nursing and residential care services	All industries
Registered nurses	$26.25	$20.12	$25.03	$27.54
Licensed practical and licensed vocational nurses	16.78	16.89	18.35	17.57
Dental assistants	14.50	14.76	–	14.53
Medical secretaries	13.62	13.30	12.66	13.51
Medical assistants	12.58	13.14	11.60	12.64
Receptionists and information clerks	11.55	11.74	10.07	11.01
Office clerks, general	11.47	12.55	11.12	11.40
Nursing aides, orderlies, and attendants	10.76	11.06	10.30	10.67
Home health aides	9.15	10.64	9.23	9.34
Personal and home care aides	7.23	9.17	9.36	8.54

2008 Hospital Compensation Report   **HayGroup**

Manager of Admitting - 7708

	Nbr. of Cos.	Nbr. of Incs.	Salary Range Midpoint ($000)						Annual Base Salary ($000)						Annual Total Cash ($000)					
			P90	P75	P50	P25	P10	Avg	P90	P75	P50	P25	P10	Avg	P90	P75	P50	P25	P10	Avg
Referenced by Job Title																				
All Hospitals	166	288	81.7	74.0	74.0	58.6	50.0	68.4	92.6	79.6	70.0	59.7	50.4	70.5	96.2	82.4	71.5	61.0	50.4	72.8
Independent Hospitals	38	53	82.4	71.1	59.6	57.1	48.9	65.3	86.8	75.7	62.9	53.8	47.6	66.7	89.1	76.7	64.0	54.0	47.6	68.3
System-Affiliated Hospitals	128	235	81.7	74.0	74.0	61.6	50.2	69.2	92.8	80.1	70.7	61.6	50.5	71.4	97.7	82.9	73.0	63.1	50.5	73.8
Referenced by Hospital Ownership																				
For-Profit	1	1	*	*	*	*	*	*	*	*	*	*	*	*	*	*	*	*	*	*
Religiously Sponsored	62	81	81.7	72.3	61.5	56.4	50.2	63.8	93.6	81.4	67.5	56.4	48.7	69.9	100.1	84.9	70.0	57.0	48.7	72.4
Not-For Profit Secular	93	192	83.7	74.0	74.0	67.3	56.6	70.7	89.6	79.6	71.4	62.6	52.2	71.9	94.7	82.4	73.4	64.8	52.2	74.2
Government	10	14	73.6	67.1	67.1	51.9	43.6	61.0	74.4	62.9	57.0	54.0	43.2	58.9	74.4	65.9	58.3	54.1	43.2	59.4
Referenced by Hospital Bed Size																				
500+ Beds	32	47	99.0	83.7	69.9	62.3	50.2	74.1	104.4	85.8	73.8	61.2	52.3	76.1	113.0	85.8	76.5	61.2	52.3	78.3
350-499 Beds	30	50	81.7	75.7	65.0	57.0	50.1	65.6	93.3	80.2	67.5	58.0	51.1	70.4	98.3	84.8	69.8	58.0	51.1	72.4
200-349 Beds	49	88	76.1	74.0	74.0	58.2	46.5	66.1	92.1	81.3	70.0	58.6	47.2	69.9	95.7	83.6	71.5	59.9	47.2	72.2
100-199 Beds	29	40	74.0	74.0	74.0	65.0	58.8	69.7	79.6	74.2	68.4	60.8	58.5	69.1	83.0	77.0	70.6	62.3	58.9	71.6
Less than 100 Beds	17	17	74.0	67.5	56.4	48.6	36.3	56.8	78.5	67.0	56.2	47.8	42.9	58.4	81.1	68.4	59.3	47.8	43.1	60.0
Referenced by Hospital Revenue Size																				
$500 Million +	40	70	84.2	77.8	67.1	56.9	55.2	69.3	95.6	80.6	71.6	57.3	52.3	71.8	99.3	82.9	73.1	57.3	52.3	73.8
$250 to $499 Million	53	67	87.2	81.7	64.2	50.2	47.7	66.2	96.0	87.0	70.0	52.7	48.5	71.4	103.0	88.5	71.3	52.7	48.5	73.5
$100 to $249 Million	34	49	74.0	71.1	64.7	60.1	50.5	63.8	90.9	75.0	66.7	60.1	48.3	68.9	95.5	76.2	67.4	62.0	48.7	71.5
$50 to $99 Million	12	35	74.0	74.0	74.0	74.0	74.0	72.0	84.8	78.1	71.1	63.2	59.2	71.5	88.5	79.7	73.6	68.2	59.5	74.1
$0 to $49 Million	19	35	74.0	74.0	74.0	74.0	52.4	69.0	78.9	75.7	68.6	60.8	49.4	67.4	82.3	78.9	71.3	61.7	49.4	69.7
Referenced by Geographic Location																				
Northeast	5	6	*	78.9	66.7	63.0	*	74.4	*	78.8	66.5	61.9	*	72.9	*	78.8	66.5	61.9	*	73.7
Mid-Atlantic	13	17	91.4	77.9	69.5	48.8	47.7	68.5	104.4	85.6	66.9	58.1	48.5	72.5	112.4	88.3	66.9	58.1	48.5	74.9
Southeast	19	29	70.5	66.0	57.1	56.6	43.8	58.8	77.6	69.7	59.7	52.4	44.0	60.7	80.1	69.9	60.1	52.4	44.0	61.5
Florida	4	7	*	*	*	*	*	*	*	*	*	*	*	*	*	*	*	*	*	*
East Central	17	23	79.1	73.1	64.6	50.2	48.9	63.2	92.3	81.7	72.5	52.2	50.5	69.3	96.0	81.7	72.5	52.2	50.5	69.8
West Central	15	17	102.6	73.9	55.0	43.0	41.9	63.9	80.7	79.5	64.4	43.5	42.7	64.0	86.3	81.4	65.9	43.5	42.7	66.3
North Central	8	8	*	76.9	72.0	67.2	*	70.8	*	82.9	78.7	69.5	*	75.7	*	82.9	78.7	70.5	*	78.5
South Central	20	26	66.8	60.8	56.4	56.4	52.1	59.4	75.4	66.3	58.1	54.1	48.9	61.1	76.4	66.3	58.1	54.1	48.9	61.7
Inter-Mountain	8	12	*	*	*	*	*	*	78.5	76.1	63.7	60.1	56.7	67.8	84.1	76.4	68.7	60.4	56.7	70.7
Pacific Northwest	5	7	*	*	*	*	*	*	*	72.4	68.7	66.0	*	67.4	*	73.8	71.1	68.3	*	69.6
California	45	125	74.0	74.0	74.0	74.0	74.0	75.0	91.2	80.5	73.7	67.3	62.6	75.3	96.8	83.8	76.8	70.2	64.9	78.9

SOURCES: (*Top*) U.S. Department of Labor, Bureau of Labor Statistics. (*Bottom*) Reprinted with permission from HayGroup. 2008. *2008 HayGroup Hospital Compensation Report*. HayGroup Reward Information Services.

an intelligent presentation, the supervisor must know the value of the various jobs within the department and also the going rate within the community. As every supervisor knows, proper compensation of employees is a significant aspect of the employee's continuing satisfaction and motivation. Without a sound wage and salary pattern, it is almost impossible for a supervisor to recruit competent employees or keep the subordinates motivated.

Promotion

Promotions provide an internal source of potential applicants. A promotion is the reassignment of an individual to a position higher in rank. This higher-level job entails more demands on the individual but results in higher pay, more authority and responsibility, more privileges, increased benefits, and greater potential for advancement. A promotion may also carry symbols of higher status, such as a more important job title, a larger cubicle or office, a bigger desk, or a secretary. Although some people do not want to advance, promotions are sought by most people who have a high level of aspiration. It is part of our culture for one to start at the bottom of the ladder and rise in status and income as one grows older. Because most people in our society look on promotions in this way, it is essential that organizations develop and pursue sound promotion policies.

Promotion from Within

Organizations depend heavily on promoting their own employees into better and more promising positions. The policy of promoting from within the organization is one of the most widely practiced personnel policies today. It helps achieve the organizational objective of being a good employer and a good place to work. The latter is undoubtedly one of the many goals of all healthcare centers.

Establishing and maintaining a policy of promotion from within versus external recruitment is important to the enterprise and the individual employee. For the enterprise, it ensures a constant source of trained people for the better positions; for the employees, it provides a powerful incentive to perform better. After an employee has worked for an enterprise, much more is known about that person than is known about even the best potential candidate from outside the organization.

Internal promotion often is less expensive to the institution in time and money than luring applicants from the outside. Additional job satisfaction results when employees know that with proper efforts they can work up to more interesting and more challenging work, higher pay, and more desirable working conditions. Most employees like to know that they can get ahead in the enterprise in which they are working and feel more secure in a setting that provides future job opportunities. All this provides strong motivation. On the other hand, little motivation exists for employees to do a better job if they know that the better and higher-paying jobs are always reserved for outsiders.

The internal promotion policy should be applied whenever possible and feasible. Most organizations are aware that under special circumstances outside people must be hired; sometimes strict adherence to internal promotion does harm to the organization. For example, if no qualified candidates are available or appropriate for the job, the internal promotion policy cannot be followed. Also, an organization may be forced to look outside because employees with inadequate potential for promotion have been hired in the past.

At times the injection of "new blood" into an organization may be necessary because it keeps the members of the enterprise from becoming too complacent. Bringing in new people is important primarily in high-level managerial jobs and for highly trained professionals. It is less important in hourly paid jobs.

Another reason the enterprise may have to recruit employees from the outside is that the organization cannot afford the expense of training and educating current employees. A particular position may require a long period of expensive and sophisticated schooling, and the institution simply may not be able to afford this type of upgrading program. Only large organizations can usually afford such expenses.

Another problem with promotion from within is that the organization must continue to live amicably with those who were bypassed. Such a problem, however, does not exist with an applicant from the outside who was rejected. In all this, as mentioned throughout this discussion, considerations of equal employment opportunity and possibly affirmative action must be included.

On the other hand, the supervisor should remember that not every employee wants advancement; many people know their limitations. Some employees are quite content with what they are doing and where they are within the enterprise. They prefer to remain with employees whom they know and responsibilities with which they are familiar. These employees should not be pressured by the supervisor into taking or seeking better positions. The supervisor should also bear in mind that what he may consider a promotion may not seem like a promotion to the employee. An ultrasound technician may believe that a promotion to an administrative position is a hardship, not an advancement. She may find the administrative activities less interesting than direct patient care duties and may be concerned about her loss of skills over time. The supervisor has to provide promotional opportunities that do not entail compromising professional aspirations.

Sometimes a supervisor sees an employee as indispensable and does not want to release him to take a better job in another department. As mentioned earlier, often the opportunity for an employee's advancement is a reflection of the supervisor being extremely good at developing subordinates. For exam-

HOSPITAL LAND

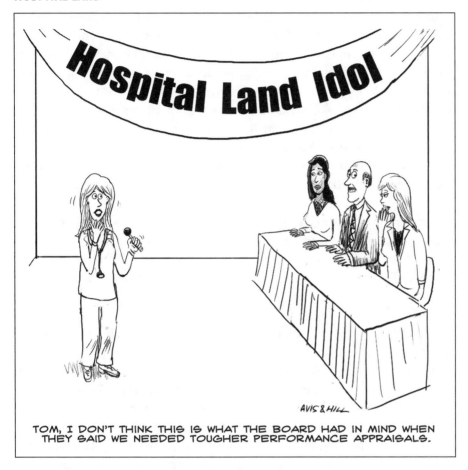

TOM, I DON'T THINK THIS IS WHAT THE BOARD HAD IN MIND WHEN THEY SAID WE NEEDED TOUGHER PERFORMANCE APPRAISALS.

ple, as a patient accounts manager develops outstanding billers and collectors, they are generally promoted out of that department to become assistant physician practice managers. The patient accounts manager may believe that the department suffers because of the loss of these outstanding professionals. In such a situation, administration should give credit to this manager for consistently developing promotable employees and should assure her that good employees will continue to enter the department from other hospital areas.

At times, the supervisor may be inclined to bypass someone for promotion within his department to avoid the extra work of replacing the promoted employee and training a new one. The supervisor may fear that the productivity of the department will suffer. This is shortsighted, as promotion from within is a prime motivator for employees to excel. Supervisors who are tempted to think this way should ask themselves where they would be today if their former superiors had had this attitude.

Basis of Promotion

Usually more employees apply for promotions than there are openings within an organization. Because of this, it is important for the organization and supervisors to formulate a sound basis on which employees are chosen for promotion. Because promotions are considered an incentive for employees to do a better job, it follows that the employee who has the best record of quality, productivity, and skill should be promoted. In many situations, however, it is difficult to objectively measure some employees' productivity, even though the supervisor has attempted to do so through merit ratings and performance appraisals. The most important criteria for choice are merit (current performance), ability (potential future performance), and seniority (experience).

Merit   Because promotion is an incentive for good performance, the best-performing employees should be promoted. Our discussion of performance appraisals emphasized the difficulty in measuring performance. The differences in merit among different employees in a healthcare job are also often difficult to measure precisely.

Ability   Ability and potential to assume the responsibilities of a higher-level position are additional criteria to consider. Perhaps an employee has extensive public speaking experience outside of the organization in his volunteer role as chairperson of the local Chamber of Commerce. This may be a skill that was captured during the skills inventory or development section of the performance appraisal. The supervisor should consider whether this person or another without public speaking skills is better suited for a promotion into a public relations position. Perhaps an individual has a baccalaureate degree in science and a master's degree in gerontology. The person's education adds depth to her set of core competencies. If the organization decides to open a skilled nursing facility or swing bed unit, this individual may have the competency to fill a top position in this endeavor, even though her current position does not utilize these competencies.

The performance appraisal process is a major source of information. While performance appraisals are used as a means of measuring performance, they are just as important as an appraisal of an employee's potential. A person's potential is based on the processes and personal resources the employee uses to achieve results—that is, intellect, maturity, and the ability to lead. In appraising potential and future performance, the supervisor should evaluate the employee's oral and written communication skills, flexibility, and his decision-making, leadership, and planning abilities.

Use of the Assessment Center

Some of the shortcomings of traditional methods used for selecting candidates for a position have been discussed above. In response to these shortcomings, thousands of industries and some healthcare organizations have adopted an **assessment center approach** for evaluating and selecting managers (Sullivan, Decker, and Hailstone 1985). An assessment center uses a process in which current employees seeking promotions to managerial jobs are administered individual and group exercises. The exercises and activities include job-related simulations such as interviews, in-basket exercises, tests, questionnaires, videotape exercises, and group problems. These exercises are designed to bring forth skills the organization considers critical to success. As the candidates go through these exercises, they are observed by a group of specially trained observers (assessors, evaluators) who are members of the institution's management group. After the session, the candidates are evaluated by this panel of assessors to make selection recommendations or placement decisions or to determine a candidate's future promotability. Generally, the composite performance evaluation is communicated to the candidate. Additional guidance about the use of assessments and assessment centers may be obtained from the U.S. Department of Labor in its guide to testing and assessments.

assessment center approach
A method of evaluating in-house candidates for promotion to management. Assessment centers include a battery of exercises and activities that allow observers to evaluate the management prospects of those seeking promotion.

Seniority

The exclusive use of merit and ability, which are to a great degree subjective criteria, and assessment centers, which may be considered burdensome, often gives employees the feeling that promotions are not made fairly. Frequent charges of favoritism, bias, and possible discrimination have caused managers to search for more objective decision criteria that would not create morale problems. However, it is difficult to find objective criteria that completely eliminate favoritism and possible discrimination; the only objective criterion is length of service. Supervisors generally believe that their relations with their employees will be easier if they promote on the basis of seniority. For unionized entities, promotion may be restricted to seniority in the labor contract. However, this factor is used even by those enterprises that do not deal with unions and may be applied to those jobs not covered by union agreements.

Basing promotion on the length of service assumes that the employee's ability increases with service. Although this may be questionable, with continued service the ability to perform and the knowledge about the organization probably do increase. If management is committed to promotion based on length of service, it is likely that the initial selection procedure of a new employee will be made carefully and that the employee will get as much training as possible in various positions. Most managers believe that an employee's loyalty is expressed by the length of service and that, consequently, this loyalty deserves the reward of promotion. On the other hand, some good employees may become discouraged and leave the organization, realizing that their chances for promotion are slim because many long-service employees may be ahead of them in line for such promotion.

Balancing the Criteria Good supervisory practice attempts to strike a "happy medium" between the criteria of merit and ability on the one hand and length of service on the other. When the supervisor selects from among almost equally capable subordinates, the one with the longest service will no doubt be chosen. If an employee with less seniority stands head and shoulders above one with longer service, the employee with more core competencies will probably be promoted. As much as this selection process seems to make sense, these decisions are difficult, and it is easy to see why some supervisors make length of service the sole determinant of selection for promotion. However, the ideal solution is to combine both factors. Rarely does a supervisor choose a person with the greatest merit and ability from all eligible candidates without giving any weight to length of service.

Selection for promotion also depends on the type of work involved, demands of the position to be filled, degree requirements prescribed by accrediting and professional associations, and many other factors. More emphasis is placed on merit and ability when the position to be filled is a demanding and sophisticated job on a higher level, whereas more weight can be given to seniority for promotion into a lower-level position. Every organization must decide on the relative weight of these factors in each case when deciding who is to be promoted.

Summary

Performance appraisals are central to organizational and management development. They are formal evaluations of employees' job-related activities. Such a system not only guides management in gathering and analyzing information, it also provides guidance for merit increases, promotions, and coaching of employees. The purpose of the appraisal system is to provide a measure of the employee's job performance that leads to counseling and further development. An evaluation system consists of rating the employee and the appraisal interview, which usually occurs later. Although the appraisal interview between the supervisor and the employee may be awkward or difficult, the entire performance appraisal system is of no use if this aspect is ignored and not carried out appropriately.

An important source of candidates for job openings is the reservoir of employees who are currently with the institution. Whenever possible, promotion from within is one of the most rewarding personnel policies any enterprise can practice. It is of great benefit to the enterprise and to the morale of the employees. Although it is difficult to specify clearly the various criteria for promotion, it is normally acknowledged that merit and ability factors should be balanced with length of service. To be able to assess the ability, merit, and future potential of the employee, supervisors must remain aware of the employee's performance. Therefore, the supervisor must regularly appraise the performance of the employees in the department. In addition to all these duties, the staffing function includes making certain that the employees of the department are properly compensated and have a benefits program. Although much of this is out of the supervisor's domain, it is a supervisory duty to make certain that good internal wage alignment exists, meaning that each job is paid in accordance with its worth and difficulties. The wages paid must be high enough to attract people from outside the organization, if necessary, and to prevent present employees from leaving for higher wages. To do this, the supervisor must be familiar with the rates being paid in similar occupations in the community. Such information can be obtained by wage and salary surveys conducted by the human resources department.

Notes

1. The Performance Appraisal Methods section is adapted from Allen (2000).
2. An "in-basket" exercise includes actual examples of items that may be on the supervisor's schedule for the day or in the supervisor's "in-basket" to do. An example of an in-basket exercise for a new supervisor relative to learning how to do appraisals effectively would be: "You arrive at your office this morning and your interoffice mail has arrived. Included in the mail are some advertisements for seminars, a catalog for PC gadgets, a request from your local professional association asking you to do a presentation on a new piece of technology you installed earlier this year, and a brochure about a new book. You receive an e-mail from the budget director with an attached budget worksheet for next year. It's due in 30 days. Also you get an e-mail from human resources with 15 attachments. The attachments are employee performance appraisals. Seven are due in 14 days; 8 are due 21–35 days from now. Which of these items will you work on first and what will you need to do to prepare to work on them?"

Additional Readings

Burt, T. 2005. "Leadership Development as Corporate Strategy: Using Talent Reviews to Improve Senior Management." *Healthcare Executive* 20 (6): 14–18.

Collard, D. 2008. "Hardwiring Accountability: Sustaining Results Through an Objective Leader Evaluation System." *HR Pulse* (Winter): 46–48.

Garman, A. and J. L. Tyler. 2004. "Development and Validation of a 360-Degree-Feedback Instrument for Healthcare Administrators." *Journal of Healthcare Management* 49 (5): 306–21.

U.S. Department of Labor. 2009. "Testing and Assessment: An Employer's Guide to Good Practices." [Online information] www.ipacweb.org/files/ONetasmtguide.pdf.

INFLUENCING

20

GIVING DIRECTIVES AND MANAGING CHANGE

Chapter Objectives

After you have studied this chapter, you should be able to do the following:

1. Define the managerial function of influencing.
2. Describe the essential characteristics of good directives.
3. Compare and contrast the major techniques and theories of directing.
4. Describe the role of teams as a motivational instrument to achieve the work of the organization.
5. Review tools for group decision making.
6. Relate the function of influencing to changing environments.

Influencing is the managerial function by which the supervisor motivates others to accomplish organizational objectives. It is vital to achieving goals and implementing change. In the context of human resources, the influencing function is particularly concerned with behavioral responses. William Drayton (n.d.) states, "Change starts when someone sees the next step," while Nathaniel Branden (n.d.) says, "The first step toward change is awareness. The second step is acceptance." The role of the supervisor is to draw the next step for the employees to see and motivate them to accept it.

The influencing function is also known as leading, motivating, directing, and actuating. Regardless of the terminology, it is the managerial function that the supervisor exercises to get the best and most out of the subordinates. At the same time, the supervisor strives to create a climate in which the subordinates find as much satisfaction of their needs as possible. We learned in Chapter 2 that until the mid-1900s, managers depended largely on negative persuasion, disciplinary action, and a few incentive programs to influence their employees. The notion of organizational hierarchy dominated managerial thinking until the behavioral sciences brought about new understanding of human motivation and taught us better methods of influencing. Today every manager must understand some of the psychology involved in interpersonal relations.

It is the role of every supervisor to influence employees to get the work done. Influencing is the managerial function that initiates action. In most work settings, little may be accomplished without influencing by the manager. Influencing includes issuing directives, instructions, assignments, and orders as well as guiding and overseeing employees. It also involves motivating employees.

Moreover, the manager should also consider the influencing function as a means of developing employees. The most effective way to develop employees is through diligent coaching and teaching by their immediate superior. Influencing means building an effective workforce and inspiring its members to perform their best.

Influencing is the job of every manager, from the CEO of a healthcare facility to the supervisor of one of its departments. The amount of time and effort a manager spends in this function varies, however, depending on the level, number of employees supervised, and other duties. The supervisor of a department spends more time influencing and supervising than the administrator of the institution does.

Influencing is a continuous function that connects the other managerial functions, including planning, organizing, staffing, and controlling. It plays a role in planning because the supervisor influences his staff to complete the plans. Obviously it affects organizing and staffing because the department's employees are whom the supervisor influences. The controlling function is likewise affected by influencing, inasmuch as control often involves identifying the causes of variances to plans, some of which may be human problems.

To get the job done, every supervisor spends much time and effort directing subordinates. Recall the principle of unity of command, which means that each employee has a single immediate supervisor, who is in turn responsible to her immediate superior, and so on up and down the chain of command. As discussed in Chapter 12, in healthcare organizations the unity-of-command principle may be violated by the presence of two sets of instructions: one from an immediate administrative supervisor and another from a patient's attending physician. Most times these instructions do not conflict, but if they do, the subordinate should refer the conflict to the supervisor. The supervisor or manager should confer with the physician and the administrator if necessary to resolve the issue. If time does not permit such deliberations, which is often the case in healthcare, the action that delivers the most appropriate clinical care to the patient should occur—that is, the instructions that benefit the patient should be followed.

Characteristics of Good Directives

Because issuing directives is such a basic and integral part of the supervisor's daily routine, it is often assumed that every supervisor knows how to give orders. This is, in fact, a skill that must be learned; some ways to issue directives are more effective than others. The experienced supervisor knows that faulty or bad order giving can easily upset even the best-laid plans and can create a general state of chaos, instead of coordination of efforts. Giving directives takes practice and proactive anticipation of the reaction(s) from the receiver. Since directives often involve changing something—one's assignment for the day, the way a procedure is done, when a process will occur, rules, etc.—the new supervisor may consider the common reactions to changes as displayed in Exhibit 20.1.

To the uninitiated outsider, it may seem that some supervisors get excellent results even though they appear to break every rule in the book. Other supervisors may use all the best techniques of order giving and phrase their requests in the most courteous ways and still get only grudging compliance. The question of the most appropriate method of order giving depends on the employees concerned, the work situation, the supervisors and how they view their job, their attitude toward people, and many other factors.

Because the supervisor's own success depends largely on how the subordinates carry out the orders, the manager must possess the knowledge and skill for good directing. In other words, because directing is the fundamental tool employed by supervisors to start, stop, or modify activities, it is necessary for every supervisor to become familiar with the basic characteristics that distinguish good and accomplishable directives from those that are not. These characteristics are fulfilled when directives are reasonable, intelligible, worded appropriately, compatible with the objectives, and posed within reasonable time limits.

Reasonableness

The first essential characteristic of a good directive is that it must be reasonable—that is, the supervisor can reasonably expect compliance. Unreasonable orders not only undermine morale but also make controlling impossible. The requirement of reasonableness immediately excludes orders pertaining to

Nature of Resistance	Common Staff Reactions	Reactions Caused By	Approaches to Reduce Resistance
Psychological	Anxiety Nervousness	Uncertainty	Communicate Educate staff
Perception	Anxiety Disinterest in organization activities Inattention to work	Loss of status Loss of control Loss of job satisfaction	Sell idea(s) Provide information Lead by example Facilitate change Upgrade skills
Economic	Sabotage Strike Leave job	Uncertainty Insecurity Instability	Involve staff Initiate change often

Exhibit 20.1
Resistance to Change

activities that physically cannot be done or are dangerous. In judging whether a directive can be reasonably accomplished, supervisors should not only appraise it from their own point of view but should also try to place themselves in the position of the employee. The supervisor should not issue a directive if the capacity or experience of the employee is not sufficient to comply with the order. This becomes particularly important in the case of recent graduates who may have had an excellent education in many areas but lack working experience and even some of the basic knowledge required. Supervisors should not forget the value of their own on-the-job training.

Sometimes supervisors indeed issue unreasonable instructions. For instance, to please the CEO, a supervisor may promise the completion of a job earlier than feasible. The supervisor tells an employee to complete the job in that time frame without considering whether she can actually do it. Bad plan. Instead, the supervisor should have placed himself in the position of the subordinate and asked if compliance reasonably could be expected. The decision will depend on many factors prevailing at the time. In some cases the directive may actually be intended to stretch the subordinate's capabilities a little beyond what had previously been requested. Then the question of reasonableness becomes a question of degree. Generally, however, a primary requirement of a good directive is that it can be accomplished by the employee to whom it is assigned without undue difficulty.

Intelligibility

Another requirement is that a good directive be intelligible to the employee—that is, the employee should be able to understand it. For example, a directive in a language not intelligible to the subordinate cannot be considered an order. The same also applies if both speak English but the supervisor uses words that the employee does not comprehend. This is a matter of communication (see Chapter 5).

Appropriate Wording

Every good supervisor knows that the tone and words used in issuing directives significantly affect the subordinates' acceptance and performance of them. A considerate tone is more likely to stimulate willing and enthusiastic acceptance. In the patient care field, the word *order* in connection with the attending physician's directives is normally used without unpleasant connotations. However, most supervisors should refrain from using the term *order* as much as possible and instead use such terms as *directive, assignment, instruction, suggestion,* and *request*. A directive followed by a sincere thank you is always appropriate. Tactfully delivering directives is a learned skill.

Requests   Phrasing orders as *requests* does not reduce their character as a directive, but a request usually gets a better response than a command. For example, "Mary, as time permits this morning, could you help Tina with her backlog of physician orders so that she is caught up by 10:00 a.m.? Thanks for your assistance." This style of directing works well and usually does not rub anyone the wrong way. It is a pleasant and easy way of asking an employee to get the job done.

In other instances it might be advisable to place the directive in the form of a **Suggestions** *suggestion*, which is an even milder form than a request. For example, the supervisor might say, "Mary, we are supposed to get all of this work done before noon and we seem to be a bit behind. Do you think we can make it?" Suggestions of this type accomplish a great deal because they are understood and accepted by responsible and ambitious employees. Such employees like the feeling of not being ordered around and of being on their own to get the job accomplished. Suggestions, however, are not advisable when dealing with new employees, who may not be familiar with the supervisor's expectations or the department's activities. Suggestions also do not work with employees who are less competent and less dependable.

Some subordinates must be told what to do simply because they do not re- **Commands** spond to less forceful orders. For example, "Mary, I need the status on those two patient bills I gave you last Friday by 10:00 a.m. Before you go on break today, stop by my office with your report. Thanks." The command or directive style leaves no room for questioning expectations.

Everyone remembers commands from parents and school teachers as part of growing up. Most people, however, think that once they are adults, commands are no longer necessary. Thus, the best rule for a supervisor is to avoid commands whenever possible but to use them when necessary.

Compatibility with Objectives

A good directive must be compatible with the purposes and objectives of the organization. If the instructions are not in accordance with these objectives, the subordinate may not execute them adequately or may not execute them at all. Thus, when issuing directives that appear to conflict with the organizational objectives, the supervisor must explain to the employee why such action is necessary, or the supervisor should explain that the directive merely appears to be but actually is not contrary to the institution's objectives. Instructions must also be consistent; they must not be in opposition to orders or directives previously given unless there is a good explanation for the discrepancy.

Ethics

Incompatible orders also may require an employee to do things that the employee finds inappropriate, unethical, or contrary to his values. Ethical theories offer a means to explain and justify actions and serve as guides for making moral decisions (Munson 1992) and, thus, influence behavior.

Some organizations have written codes of ethics (see Appendix 20.1 and Exhibit 6.1) to provide a road map for staff of ethical practices and expectations. These provide guidance on issues such as gifts from equipment manufacturers and exaggerations in publicity materials. Furthermore, many organizations have increased staff education in this topic. So when a supervisor issues a directive that appears contrary to the organization's published practices, staff should resist. In these situations, the supervisor must clearly explain her rationale to staff and possibly include her superior or the organization's compliance officer to ensure that staff recognize that the requirement being placed on them is not unethical.

Ethics has roots not only in published guidelines but also in cultures, religions, and families. Therefore, a supervisor in a culturally diverse environment may encounter resistance because of perceptions of those team members who grew up in a different culture or during a different period in time. Consider the younger generation of today. The mores under which they practice and how they conduct their day-to-day relationships differ substantially from those that predominated 40 years ago. Many factors affect healthcare today—including cost containment, genetic testing, discontinuation of life-saving measures, abortion, and privacy—that the supervisor must address in order to gain support from staff; many of these issues may cause ethical discomfort for some staff.

Time Limitations

An additional characteristic of a good directive is that it specifies the time within which the instructions should be carried out. The supervisor should allow a reasonable amount of time and, if this is not feasible, must realize that the quality of performance is only as good as can be produced under the time limit. In many directives, the time factor is not stated, although it is probably implied that the assignment should be carried out within a reasonable time.

Because the performance of the employee depends to a great extent on the format and content of directives given, the supervisor should make certain that the directive is in accordance with these most essential characteristics.

Directing Techniques

In previous chapters, various theories were discussed describing the supervisor's underlying managerial attitudes, such as Theories X and Y, autocratic and democratic styles, participation in decision making, and broad or narrow delegation of authority. The following is a more detailed discussion of how these managerial attitudes manifest themselves in the daily working environment.

Generally the supervisor adopts attributes from two basic supervisory techniques: autocratic (or close supervision) and consultative (participative) supervision. This discussion clearly distinguishes between these two extremes, but in practice the supervisor usually combines and blends the techniques. For example, the manager might use the autocratic technique for one situation and the democratic technique for another. Similarly, the supervisor might find one style more effective with some employees than others. No one form of supervision is equally good in all situations. Whether it is better to apply a more autocratic or a more democratic type of supervision depends on many factors, including the type of work; current situation; attitude of the employee toward the supervisor; personality and ability of the employee; and personality, experience, and ability of the supervisor. A good supervisor is sensitive to all these factors and to the needs of each situation, so the style of supervision should be adjusted accordingly.

Autocratic (Close) Supervision (Theory X)

Autocratic leadership usually reflects tight supervision with a high degree of centralization and a narrow span of management. The autocratic style is repressive, and this type of supervisor normally withholds communication except that which is absolutely necessary for doing the job. Autocratic management leaders make decisions unilaterally and do not consult with the members of the department. Therefore, the autocratic style of leadership minimizes the degree of involvement by subordinates.

In more specific terms, autocratic leadership is described by Douglas McGregor (1985) as **Theory X**. According to McGregor, a Theory X manager leans toward an organizational climate of close control, centralized authority, authoritarian practices, and minimal participation of the subordinates in the decision-making process. One may consider this the "big stick" approach. A Theory X manager makes certain assumptions about human behavior, including the following:

Theory X
A theory that employees perform best under supervision that involves close control, centralized authority, authoritarian practices, and minimal participation of the subordinates in the decision-making process.

1. The average person dislikes work and will avoid it to the extent she can.
2. Most people have to be forced or threatened by punishment to make the effort necessary to accomplish organizational goals.
3. The average individual is basically passive and therefore prefers to be directed rather than take any risk or responsibility. Above all else, he prefers security.

When the autocratic or close technique of directing is employed, the supervisor gives direct, clear, and precise orders to the subordinates with detailed instructions as to exactly how and in what sequence things are to be done. This allows little room for the initiative of the subordinate. The supervisor who normally uses the autocratic technique delegates as little authority as possible and believes that she probably can do the job better than any of the subordinates. The supervisor relies on command and detailed instructions, followed by close supervision. An autocratic supervisor believes that subordinates are "not paid to think"; they are expected to follow instructions. The boss alone is to do the planning and decision making. This type of supervisor does not necessarily distrust the subordinate but believes that without detailed instruction the subordinate could not properly carry out the directive. This person believes that only she can specify the best method and that there is only one way, the supervisor's way, to get the job done. In other words, Theory X management is practiced.

autocratic supervision
A management style based on Theory X, i.e., that involves little participation by subordinates in the decision-making process.

With most people, the consequences of **autocratic supervision** can be disastrous. Employees lose interest and initiative; they stop thinking for themselves because no need or occasion arises for independent thought. They are obedient but silent and lack initiative and ingenuity. It becomes difficult for the subordinates to remain loyal to the organization and to the supervisor, and they secretly rejoice when the boss makes a mistake. This form of supervision tends to make the employees somewhat like robots. Freedom is curtailed, and it is difficult for them to learn even by making mistakes. They justly conclude that they are not expected to do any thinking about their job, and, although they perfunctorily perform their duties, they find little involvement in the work. They are certainly not motivated.

Shortcomings of the autocratic technique of supervision are obvious. Generally, men and women who have been brought up in a democratic society resent autocratic order giving. It is contrary to the traditional democratic way of life in the United States. An ambitious employee will not remain in a position where the supervisor is not willing to delegate some degree of freedom and authority. Subordinates who are eager to learn and progress will resent being constantly given detailed instructions that leave no room for their own thinking and initiative. Frequently, this type of management is referred to as **micromanaging** because the supervisor directs every detail of the subordinate's action. The employee is stifled and eventually will leave the enterprise if possible. This method of supervision does not produce good employees and only chases away those who have potential.

micromanaging
The practice of directing every detail of a subordinate's action.

On the other hand, one must not forget that under certain circumstances and with certain people a degree of close supervision may be necessary. Suppose, for example, that the subordinate is the type of person who does not want to think for himself and prefers to receive clear orders. Firm guidance gives reassurance, whereas loose and general supervision may be frustrating. Some employees lack ambition and imagination and do not want to become involved in their daily job. Other employees have been brought up in an authoritarian manner and their previous work experience leads them to believe that general supervision is no supervision at all. Moreover, a work setting sometimes is so chaotic that only autocratic techniques can bring order. Aside from these rather unusual situations, however, it can generally be assumed that autocratic, or close, supervision is the least desirable and effective method.

Consultative (Participative, Democratic) Supervision (Theory Y)

The opposite of autocratic supervision is **consultative supervision**. Consultative supervision is also known as participative, democratic, or permissive supervision. It is similar to the concept of general supervision referred to earlier. Its basic assumption is that employees are eager to do a good job, have the motivation to perform their best, and are capable of doing so. The supervisor behaves toward them with this basic assumption in mind, and the employees in turn tend to react in a manner that justifies the expectations of their supervisors.

The democratic style emphasizes a looser type of supervision and greater individual participation in the decision-making process. Authority is delegated as far down as possible, and a wide span of management is advocated. A free flow of communication is encouraged among all members of the department so that a climate of trust and confidence can be established.

In McGregor's (1985) terms, the democratic style is represented by Theory Y. The Theory Y manager operates with a completely different set of assumptions regarding human motivation. She maintains that an effective organizational climate uses more general supervision, greater decentralization of authority, democratic techniques, consultation with subordinates on departmental decisions, and little reliance on coercion and control. The assumptions on which this type of organizational climate is based include the following:

1. Work is as natural to people as play or rest, and therefore it is not avoided.
2. Self-motivation and inherent satisfaction in work will be forthcoming when the individual is committed to organizational goals; thus, coercion is not the only form of influence that can be used to motivate.
3. Commitment is a crucial factor in motivation, and it is a function of the rewards coming from it.
4. The average individual learns to accept and even seek responsibility given the proper environment.
5. The ability to be creative and innovative in the solution of organizational problems is widely, not narrowly, distributed in the population.
6. In modern businesses and organizations, the intellectual potential of employees is only partially utilized.

McGregor underscores the notion that Theories X and Y are beliefs held by management about the nature of human beings. As such, they constitute the foundation on which the organizational climate is built. The supervisor who follows Theory X has a basically limited view of people and their capabilities. He believes that individuals must be controlled; closely supervised; and motivated by money, discipline, and authority. Thus, the autocratic

consultative supervision
A type of supervision based on the assumption that employees are eager to do a good job, have the motivation to perform their best, and are capable of doing so. Also called participative, democratic, and permissive supervision.

manager believes that the key to motivation is satisfying the lower-level needs of people.

The Theory Y supervisor, however, has a different opinion of the capabilities and potential of people. She believes that if the proper approach and conditions can be presented, people exercise self-direction and self-control toward the accomplishment of objectives. The Theory Y manager recognizes that the supervisor's activities must fit into the scheme of each employee's own needs. She also believes that the higher-level needs of people, such as personal growth and self-development, are more important than other needs.

This democratic approach to the directing function manifests itself in the way the supervisor makes routine assignments. He makes those assignments by consulting with his employees, and then assumes that they are more motivated if they are left to themselves as much as possible.

The essential characteristic of consultative supervision is that the supervisor consults with employees concerning the extent, nature, and alternative solution to a problem before the supervisor makes a decision and issues a directive. The supervisor who uses the consultative approach before issuing directives is earnestly seeking help and ideas from the employees and approaches the subject with an open mind. More important than the procedure is the attitude of the supervisor. A subordinate can easily sense superficiality and is quick to perceive whether the boss genuinely intends to consult her on the problem or only intends to give the impression of doing so.

Some supervisors use such pseudo-consultation merely to give employees the feeling that they have been included in the decision-making process. These supervisors often ask for participation only after they have already decided on the directive. In such cases the supervisor is using the consultative technique as a trick, a device for manipulating people to do what he wants them to do. The subordinates quickly realize that they are not being taken seriously and that this participation is not real. The results achieved will be worse than if the superior had used the most autocratic method. To practice actual consultative management, the supervisor must take it seriously and be willing to be swayed by the employees' opinions and suggestions. If the manager is not sincere, it is better not to apply this technique at all.

Most supervisors find that numerous occasions arise during a typical work week to employ consultative supervision; however, there should be some limits on its use. If this approach is used too frequently, subordinates may begin to doubt whether the supervisor has any opinions of his own or is able to make decisions. In short, they may wonder if the supervisor can manage.

Consultative direction does not lessen or weaken formal authority, as the right of decision making still remains with the supervisor. Although the supervisor seeks employee input, he may still express an opinion. It must be expressed in a manner that indicates to the employee that even the supervisor's opinions are subject to critical appraisal. Similarly, participative consultation does not mean that the suggestions of the employee cannot also be criticized or even rejected. True consultation implies a sharing of information between the supervisor and employee and a thorough and impartial discussion of alternate solutions, regardless of who originated them. Only then can it be said that the manager really consulted the subordinate.

For consultative supervision to succeed, the employees must prefer it. If the employees believe that "the boss knows best" and that making decisions and giving directives are not their concern, the opportunity to participate is not likely to motivate them or improve morale. The supervisor must also make sure that she is seeking employee input only in areas that are within the employees' scope of experience. Consulting them on areas that they are unfamiliar with may make them feel inadequate and frustrated instead of motivated.

When using the consultative method, the supervisor should summarize the conclusions so that everyone is clear on them. This is even more essential if several employees participated in the consultation.

The consultative approach is comparable to the **4 Es approach** developed at Humana, Inc. and described by LeTourneau (2004). While the approach was developed to help clinicians communicate better with patients, the concepts apply to communication between supervisors and staff about proposed changes. The first E is *engage*: "The goal of the engage stage is to introduce and generate interest in the change"; this step introduces the subject and encourages dialogue and awareness. The second E is *empathize*; during this step, the supervisor's role is to listen to and empathize with employee concerns and gather their questions and comments about the proposed change. The third E is *educate*, during which the supervisor explains how the change will be implemented, taking into consideration the comments and concerns that were raised and, ideally, responding to the various questions raised. LeTourneau states that "As change progresses, the teaching process should continue to include the skills and information needed for success." Finally, the fourth E is *enlist*: "Early involvement with engagement and empathy help to entice" employees to "become involved with the change. The process of explaining, listening, answering questions, and listing and addressing concerns is the start of enlisting them in the change process. When [employees] become drawn into planning and developing a change, it is much more likely to meet their needs" and influence their actions (LeTourneau 2004).

4 Es approach
A technique to engage subordinates in planning for changes that involves engagement, empathy, education, and enlistment.

One of the obvious advantages of the consultative or 4 Es approach is that the emerging directive does not appear to the employees as an order but rather as a solution in which they participated. This ensures the subordinates' cooperation and enthusiasm in carrying out the directive. It imparts a feeling of importance because their ideas evidently were desired and valued. Active participation also provides an outlet for reasoning power and imagination and an opportunity for employees to make worthwhile contributions to the organization. Employee ideas often prove to be valuable in improving the quality of directives. The approach may even bring the employee closer to the supervisor, which will make for better communication and understanding between them. Considering these advantages, it becomes apparent that consultation is by far the best method to use whenever the supervisor has to issue new assignments, directives, and instructions.

This democratic, participative approach to directing subordinates leads to what we have already referred to as general or loose supervision. General supervision means allowing the subordinate to work out the details of the job and make decisions on how best to do it. Through this process, workers gain satisfaction from being on their own and from having a chance to express themselves. Instead of having a specified, detailed list of orders to comply with, the supervisor generally indicates what the end result needs to be and makes a few suggestions as to how to go about it. In so doing, the supervisor assumes that given the proper opportunity, the average employee wants to do a good job. The supervisor is primarily interested in the results. Once the subordinate is told what is to be accomplished and goals are established and limits defined, the employee is left on his or her own. This form of thinking and supervision usually leads to higher motivation and morale and ultimately better job performance. It gives employees the opportunity to satisfy their needs for self-expression by being their own boss. In this atmosphere, team management thrives.

Theory Z Approach

Theory Z
A management approach that is based on lifetime employment, slow promotion paths, consensual decision making, collective responsibility, and informal controls. Theory Z assumes workers want to build strong relationships with their colleagues.

In addition to the autocratic and democratic management styles, there is the managerial approach that William Ouchi highlighted. The **Theory Z** approach, influenced by practices in Japanese industry, has been successful due to a managerial philosophy about people and organizations that is different from that generally accepted in the United States (Ouchi and Jaeger 1978; Ouchi 1981). The Japanese organizational climate is based on lifetime employment, slow evaluation and promotion paths, nonspecialized careers, consensual decision making, collective responsibility, informal controls, and a holistic concern toward the company. From this basis, Ouchi's Theory Z makes certain assumptions about workers, including the notion that workers tend to want to build cooperative and intimate working relationships with those that they work for and with as well as the people who work for them (Flinn 2001). In brief, this approach fosters a trust relationship between workers and supervisors that results in high-quality output because fear of reprisal is absent and emphasis on teamwork dominates the workplace. This is contrary to many current practices in the United States, such as short-run employment expectations, rapid evaluation and promotions, specialized careers, individual decision making and responsibility, severe disciplinary actions for errors, and explicit controls. Although some of the characteristics of this theory are being phased out in Japan, Theory Z is an approach that U.S. managers could use to increase productivity and job satisfaction.

Quality circles and total quality management, discussed in Chapter 14, are an outgrowth of the Japanese approach to management. Ironically, much of the Japanese management approach was taught to them by Americans W. Edwards Deming and Joseph M. Juran after World War II (Walton 1986). Today more healthcare CEOs are pursuing the Theory Z environment in their organizations, and those individuals exhibiting the related leadership traits are being sought.

Free-Rein Leadership

Finally, the **free-rein** style goes beyond Theories Y and Z. It is often called *laissez-faire leadership* because the climate of the organization is such that people are left almost entirely alone to do their jobs. On the assumption that individuals are self-motivated, a minimum amount of supervision is imposed. Although the manager is available as a consultant to help out if necessary, the individuals have enough authority to devise their own solutions. Sometimes this approach is used in settings in which an entire department is managed by self-directed teams that receive periodic guidance or direction from an administrator whose office is outside the department.

free-rein leadership
A leadership approach that assumes that individual employees are self-motivated and perform well with minimum supervision. Also called laissez-faire leadership.

Each of these four styles has a place in management. The free-rein approach is probably the most useful in an organization of professional people who desire and have shown the capacity for independent work. This would apply, for example, to research scientists and professors. The democratic style seems to be appropriate when a relatively unfettered environment is necessary, under which skilled and educated people seem to thrive. This probably includes most activities performed in a healthcare center. It is wrong to state, however, that a democratic leadership style is beneficial for all organizations, regardless of the nature of their activities and skill levels of their employees. In some situations even the autocratic leadership style produces good results, especially among unskilled subordinates who are poorly prepared to participate in decision making and who might be uncomfortable if urged to do so.

In conclusion, leadership style must be adapted to each specific situation. In general a more democratic, open style seems to achieve greater leader acceptance than an autocratic one. Such a style is more humanistic and more optimistic, which also makes it more acceptable to most employees. In addition, much of the research evidence indicates that the Theory Y democratic leadership approach is more likely to achieve better results.

Explaining Directives

The supervisor who practices general supervision creates an atmosphere of understanding and mutual confidence in which the employee feels free to call on the boss whenever the need arises without fearing that his call for help may indicate incompetence. Such a supervisor takes the necessary time to explain to the worker the reasons for general directives. Knowing the purpose behind the directives, the employee is able to understand the environment of the activities. This makes the employee better informed, and the better informed the subordinate is, the better he can perform the job.

In many enterprises, a common complaint is that subordinates are kept in the dark most of the time and that supervisors hoard knowledge and information that they ought to pass on. In most instances, it is difficult to issue directives so completely as to cover all factors and issues involved. If the person who receives the directive knows the purpose behind it, however, she is in a better position to carry it out than one who does not. This enables the worker to put the environment in total perspective and make sense out of it so that she can take firm and secure action. Without such knowledge, employees may feel anxious. Also, subordinates may run into unforeseen circumstances; if they know why the directive was given, many can use their own judgment and carry out the directive in a manner that brings about proper results. They could not possibly do this if they were not well informed.

Sometimes a supervisor can overdo a good thing, however, and instead of clarifying the situation, provide so much information that the subordinate is utterly confused. Explanations should include only enough information to get the job done. If the directive involves a minor activity and not much time is available, the explanation should be brief. Supervisors must use their own judgment in deciding how detailed their explanations are. They should take into consideration such factors as the capacity of the subordinates to understand, the training they have had, the content of the directive, the underlying managerial attitude, and the time available. After evaluating these factors, the supervisor is in a better position to decide what constitutes an adequate explanation.

General Supervision Compared with No Supervision

As mentioned, general supervision is not the same as no supervision at all. General supervision requires that the employee be given a definite assignment, but one that is definite only to the extent that the employee understands the results expected. It does not include specific instructions on how the results are to be achieved. General supervision does not mean that subordinates can set their own standards. Rather, the supervisor sets the standards and makes them realistic—high enough to be a challenge, but not higher than possibly can be achieved.

Although general supervision excludes direct pressure, employees know that their efforts are being measured against the standards, and this knowledge alone should lead them to work harder. By setting the standards reasonably high, the supervisor applies a degree of pressure, but it is quite different from that exerted by "breathing down someone's neck."

General supervision requires the supervisor to keep developing the potential of the employees. Everyone knows that active learning is more effective than passive learning. Employees learn more easily when they work out a solution for themselves than if they are given the solution. It is also known that employees learn best from their own mistakes. In general supervision, ongoing training of employees is an absolute necessity; the supervisor spends considerable time teaching employees how to solve problems and make decisions as problems arise at work. The better trained the employees become in basic problem-solving methods, the less supervision is needed. One way to judge the effectiveness of a supervisor is to see how the employees in the department function when the boss is away from the job.

General supervision, however, should be introduced slowly. The supervisor cannot expect instantaneous results if general supervision is introduced into a situation in which the employees have been accustomed to close supervision. It takes time before the results can be seen. The supervisor who uses a generalist approach is just as interested in results as any other supervisor, but he is also interested in the employees' individual development, which differentiates him from the autocratic supervisor.

Although the supervisor may be a firm believer in general supervision and practices it whenever possible, under certain conditions firmness, fortitude, and decisiveness must be shown. Certain employees simply may not thrive under loose supervision. Although general supervision is not a cure-all for every problem, most research studies indicate that it is more effective than close supervision in terms of productivity, morale, and achievements. General supervision permits the employee to take pride in the work and in the results achieved. It helps develop the employee's talent and capabilities and permits the supervisor to spend less time with the employees and more time on overall management of the department. General supervision provides the motivation for the employees to work on their jobs with enthusiasm and energy.

Team Management

Teams are mentioned throughout this book. They can play a major role in influencing the action of others in the department. Teams may be established to temporarily address an issue or as a formal structure within a department or organization. Temporary teams such as quality improvement or project teams are cross-functional and gather workers from various parts of an organization to focus on a process or project. Departments or organizations that have established self-directed teams as part of the formal structure have long-term purposes that are related to producing a product or delivering a service.

One advantage to establishing teams is that it places authority in the hands of those closest to the product or service to make decisions that will affect that product or service. Employees often appreciate being given this level of authority. It shows that management acknowledges their wisdom and trusts them to do the assignment. Another advantage is that it allows the supervisor's span of control to be enlarged because some of the decision-making efforts have been pushed down the ladder of the organization. By pushing some of the authority lower, supervisors can oversee more employees, or, conversely, fewer supervisors are required. Improvement in both the quality and cost of processes may result as well. Christian Hospital in St. Louis achieved a 50 percent reduction in turnaround time for transcribed reports after implementing a process improvement team. The team was given the freedom to address the situation and used that freedom to identify the causes of the problems and initiate solutions (Peckron and Herbst 2006).

However, the supervisor's role to provide clearly stated directives and goals is imperative for a team's success. All the members of the team must have a clear understanding of what the ongoing goals are and why they are important to the success of the organization (Colonna 2005). Colonna identifies other factors for team success, including clearly defined roles and responsibilities, good communication, productive disagreement, agreement to support decisions, strong external relationships, and routine self-assessment.

Teams fail as well. The most commonly cited reasons for failure are having unclear goals, changing objectives, lack of accountability, lack of management support, lack of role clarity, ineffective leadership, and no team-based pay (Neuborne 1997). One can see the need for communication and clarity in objectives as a recurring theme from both of these references. All employees need some degree of clear direction.

Even teams that do not fail have disadvantages. Conflict between team members is a disadvantage that could affect the morale of an entire department. Conflict within the team can also affect the product or service, especially if the team cannot come to agreement on the method to produce the product or deliver the service.

Staff sometimes need a decision maker. As the supervisor, you must take these advantages and disadvantages into consideration when you establish short- and long-term teams and recognize the symptoms of team breakdown that may lead to poor results.

Change and Influencing

All organized activities are under continuous pressure for change. There are various reasons for change, but the most common are economics, scientific and technological developments, disasters, people, competition, and regulatory issues. As this edition was being developed, the United States was in a recession, unemployment was hovering around 10 percent, the country was fighting wars in Afghanistan and Iraq, and many businesses had closed. That economic instability led to an increase in the uninsured and underinsured, causing bad debt and charity care to rise for healthcare organizations. As a result, many supervisors have been asked to reduce their workforce (also known as a reduction in force or RIF). Knowing that coworkers and team members may be struggling already at home, delivering this message may be the most difficult part of a supervisor's job. She may be asked to identify who goes and who stays. She needs to focus on objective criteria such as length of service; performance; disciplinary history; versatility (recall our discussion about skills inventory); and, if a labor union is involved, seniority (Coburn 2009, 47). The supervisor must document her rationale for each individual, and make certain that she takes into consideration anticipated changes. For example, she may write that she does not wish to trim the case management department at a time when external medical necessity audits are increasing trifold with Medicare, Medicaid, and third-party payers. Once the decision is made relative to who will be laid off, it should be done promptly but not until the supervisor personally plans what she will say to each employee. It is difficult for managers to face team members who they know will be terminated in a few weeks. Shortly after the layoff, the supervisor should meet with remaining staff to explain the layoff and the organization's plan. Typically, this will occur in collaboration with a human resources person or at an organization-wide meeting with the CEO. The effects of layoffs can hurt morale and linger for months. The supervisor's ability to encourage the team to move on will be reinforced by her communication and influencing skills.

Supervisors' effectiveness in the influencing function is extremely important whenever they are faced with change. Change is inevitable and is a part of everyday life. In fact, the growth of most undertakings depends largely on the concept of change and the ability to accommodate it. Communicating the reasons for change may reduce rejection and hostility. While changes are often the result of outside events that force the enterprise to alter its practices, sometimes changes must occur for the enterprise to stay alive.

Although all organized activities are subject to change, the degree and complexity of change vary considerably from one activity to another. This is particularly true in the healthcare field because of the changes in medical sciences and technologies and in the regulatory and economic environment. The supervisor's own department is a small social subsystem, interdependent on the larger system of the healthcare center. Any change imposed from outside is likely to shift the equilibrium of forces within each department as well as within the organization as a whole.

The departmental supervisor is at the forefront of change. He must sell the idea of change to the subordinates. Most often the supervisor has had little to do with the decision to make the change or with its timing; it originated higher up in the administration or outside the organization. However, the supervisor should understand and accept the change because his duty is to introduce it, explain it to the subordinates, and lead its implementation. The true beauty of leadership lies in the leader's and followers' ability to together create a new, different, and better future. The science behind change management is not complicated; it simply states that all human beings prefer to do things that have the most meaning for them (Atchison 2005). The supervisor who has not learned the art of communicating change effectively may encounter reactions from the employees that range from ready acceptance to outright rejection and hostility (these last should be reported to one's superior when they occur).

Resistance to Change

When it comes to jobs and interpersonal relations, many people resist change. This is important to realize because if a healthcare entity is to survive, it must be able to react to the prevailing forces. The main reasons for resistance to change are uncertainty, perception, loss, self-interest, and insecurity.

One of the important factors of internal inflexibilities is psychological. Supervisors and employees may develop patterns of thought and behavior that are resistant to change. Supervisors are often frustrated in instituting a change by the unwillingness or inability of people to accept it. To overcome these inflexibilities, the supervisor must patiently sell the idea, educate the staff, carefully disseminate information, provide good leadership, and develop a tradition of change among the department's members. An earlier chapter discusses the importance of humor. If some humor can be infused into the environment, change can be perceived as a time for fun. For example, consider the department that was converting over to a new information system. The facility chose to do it during a two-day period. To reduce anxiety and add a bit of levity to the atmosphere in the department, the director did two things: she hired a massage therapist who gave back massages to everyone throughout the day and had ice cream and cookies delivered by the catering department mid-afternoon. The supervisor must realize that even a small and seemingly insignificant change may cause strong reactions by some of the employees. "Fun" may reduce those reactions.

Another issue with change is the problem of erroneous perceptions. For example, employees may believe that a new organizational arrangement will reduce their influence or control. Even if the new structure will not reduce staff's influence or control, the fear that it may do so will increase staff resistance.

To a large degree these sources of resistance to change center around a major consideration—uncertainty about the effects of change. An impending change is likely to cause anxiety and nervousness. The employees may worry about being able to fulfill the new job demands.

Another reason for resisting change is that it disturbs the equilibrium of the current state of affairs. The change may threaten, prevent, or decrease

HOSPITAL LAND

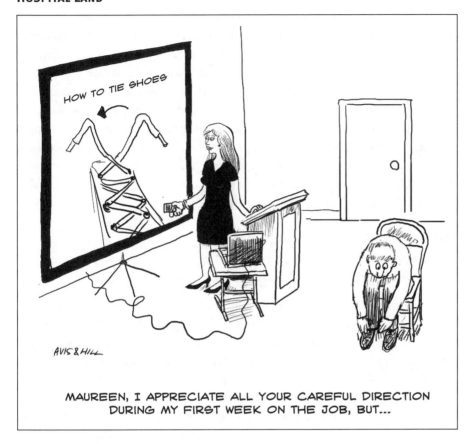

MAUREEN, I APPRECIATE ALL YOUR CAREFUL DIRECTION DURING MY FIRST WEEK ON THE JOB, BUT...

satisfaction with the environment. Therefore, it is natural for some employees to thwart the change. A further reason for resisting change is that any change is seen as a potential threat to the employee's security and self-interest. The subordinate must give up the known familiar routine for something new and unpredictable. For example, a new apparatus in the cardiopulmonary lab could make some of the technologists' previous skills unnecessary. The change may require the technologists to upgrade their skills, and they may not be sure they can master the new responsibilities.

Change may also threaten the employee's status within the organization and the existing social networks. The employee may fear that her status will be lowered and someone else's will be raised; such feelings of loss are common when mergers occur. A merger announcement can appear to be threatening and expected to produce changes in the reporting relationships and status of numerous employees.

Often threats of an economic nature provide another reason for resistance to change. The subordinate may fear that the change will affect his job economically. During the 18th and 19th centuries, Dutch hand-weavers in the

Low Countries of Europe (Belgium, The Netherlands, and Luxembourg) tried to destroy mechanical looms by throwing their wooden clogs (sabots) into the machinery (hence the word sabotage) because they feared that the machines would destroy their jobs and income. The same fears of loss prevail today.

In general, a change that causes great disturbance to one person may create little problem for another. The severity of the reaction that occurs in a particular situation depends on the nature of the change and the person concerned. The important factor for the supervisor to recognize is that changes do disturb the equilibrium of the employee and that when individuals become threatened, they develop behaviors that serve as barriers to the threat (see Exhibit 20.1). Therefore, it is the supervisor's duty to facilitate the inevitable process of adjustment when changes are necessary.

Overcoming Resistance to Change

In his book, *Resistance*, Pritchett (1996) offers the following analogy that serves as our starting point for ways to overcome this condition:

> Resistance is the most common side effect of change. If you don't encounter it, you have to wonder if you've really changed things much. Here's how it works. Change triggers the organization's immune system. People start to resist, trying to fight off the change. It's sort of like antibodies attacking some organism that invades a person's body. This just seems to be the natural order of things. Upset the status quo, and here comes the opposition. Look at it this way, and you see how resistance can be a valuable protective device. For example, strong resistance to change might cause a company to ditch some dangerous new plan or project, just like your body's white blood cells fight off an infection. Resistance can defend the health of organizations as well as individuals.

Kotter (1996) identified eight steps to create change that are categorized by their effect. Kotter's three stages are comparable to Kurt Lewin's three stages of change: "unfreezing, change, and refreezing." Kotter's eight steps appear in Exhibit 20.2.

The supervisor should always remember that employees seldom resist change just to be stubborn. There usually are valid reasons for resistance. Subordinates resist because the change affects their equilibrium socially, psychologically, and possibly economically. Understanding the reason for change is imperative for the employee. To facilitate this, the supervisor should allow the employee to "see" the problem and identify a solution that allows the employee to "feel" the change. Doing so permits the employee to "direct" the change, thus creating a feeling of control over the change and overcoming the negative feelings toward the change. When employees are motivated to accept and drive change, it will be something they feel in their hearts, not their heads, that will impel them to action (Campbell 2008, 24). One of the factors that is particularly important in gaining acceptance of change is the relationship

		EXHIBIT 20.2 Kotter's Eight Steps to Effect Change
CREATING A CLIMATE OF CHANGE	• Establishing a sense of urgency: What is forcing this change? • Building a guiding team: Assembling the players to lead the process change and define the "picture" of the organization after change. • Developing a vision and strategy: Where are we going and how will we get there? How will it affect: support staff, patient care staff, patients, the care we provide, competitors, and revenue? (Campbell 2008, 26–27)	
ENGAGING AND ENABLING CHANGE IN THE WHOLE ORGANIZATION	• Generating short-term wins: As changes occur and result in positive changes—promote them. • Empowering broad-based action: Encouraging others in the organization to proceed with process changes for the benefit of the organization. • Communicating the change vision: Repeating over and over again, the vision—where we're going and why. Campbell coins this "continuous dialogue."	
IMPLEMENTING AND SUSTAINING CHANGE	• Consolidating gains and producing more change: Publicizing successes and encouraging others to add to the list. • Anchoring new approaches in the culture: Continuous process improvement.	

that exists between the supervisor who is trying to introduce the change and the employee who is subject to the change. If a relationship of mutual confidence and trust exists between the two, the employee is much more likely to go along with the change. Mutual confidence and trust are emotional ties.

The supervisor should assume that a considerable amount of time is necessary to implement a change; a rigid timetable for change is unrealistic. Lewin (1947) conceived three stages of change as (1) an unfreezing or disruption of the current approach or process, (2) the change period during which various options may need to be implemented, and (3) a refreezing of environment during which the changed process continues and becomes routine. Given that changes and their resulting effects will take some time to be ironed out, the change must be planned far in advance, and its impact on each position and job should be anticipated. Even if the change is well thought out and carefully planned, some ramifications will probably be overlooked. With the proper attitude and the right techniques, the supervisor can facilitate the introduction of change. Involving subordinates in change discussions and decisions helps to overcome the various types of resistance.

Explanation and Communication

As noted earlier, the most important aspect in facilitating the introduction of change is the supervisor's duty to explain the change to the employees in advance. This should begin long before the change is to be initiated. It must be clear to the employees what the organization is trying to achieve with its change initiative and how it connects with the organization's goals. There should be ample time before the changeover to familiarize the employees with the idea and allow them to think through the implications and ask questions for more clarification.

In explaining the change, the supervisor should put herself into the subordinate's position and discuss its pros and cons from the subordinate's point of view. Referring to the earlier discussion on consultation or the 4 Es, this discussion should explain what will happen and why. It should clarify the way in which the change will affect the employee, what it means to that person, and, if applicable, how it will improve the present situation.

force-field analysis
An approach to overcoming resistance to change that involves openly discussing the pros and cons of a planned change.

In this process of communication, the manager might want to interject what is often referred to as the **force-field analysis**, an approach to overcoming resistance to change. In every change process forces act for and against the change. The supervisor should comment on the pluses and minuses connected with the change from the employee's point of view, then try to tip the balance toward acceptance so that the forces for the change outweigh the forces against the change. All this information should be communicated to the entire department, both to employees who are directly involved and to those who are indirectly involved. It is essential to be absolutely truthful. Pritchett (1996), in fact, says one should promise problems. Even the best planned change will encounter some unpredictable problems. Insinuating that there will be no problems is risky. The supervisor cannot afford a credibility gap.

The supervisor must also try to explain to the employees what they consciously and subconsciously want and need to know to resolve prevailing fears. Only then can employees assess and understand what the proposed change means in terms of their positions and activities. If the goals are easy to see and employees can identify an endpoint that is better for the team, department, or organization, staff will perceive the struggle to make the change as worthwhile. The subordinate who has been informed of the reasons for change, recognizes that the change is purposeful, and knows what to expect and why will be committed to the change. Instead of blind resistance, intelligent adaptation to the instructions will occur; instead of insecurity, a feeling of security will emerge. It is not the change itself that leads to so much misunderstanding as it is the manner in which the supervisor introduces the change. In other words, resistance to change that comes from fear of the unknown can be minimized by supplying an appropriate explanation.

Participation

Another effective way of reducing resistance to change is to permit participation in planning and implementing it. Playing a part in planning the change reduces uncertainty and removes some of the fears and threats to social relationships and self-interest. Furthermore, those who are affected by the change may have something to contribute, as they are close to the situation and may see some weaknesses in the change proposal that management might have overlooked. Last, if the plan for change is their plan, acceptance by the employees is greater.

This participation may be in the form of consultation, whereby criticism and suggestions are sincerely solicited from the employees. In face-to-face conversations, the supervisor discusses problems, asks questions, and tries to get the employees' ideas and reactions. Management can then incorporate as much of this into the change as possible, and the employees can consider themselves partners in the change.

A more advanced stage of participation occurs when the supervisor lets the employees make the decision about how to resolve a problem. The supervisor defines the problem and sets the limits but allows the subordinates to develop the alternatives and choose between them. Group decision making could also produce a better decision because pooled expertise is likely to identify and evaluate more alternatives than an individual could; those who are involved in this process are probably more deeply committed to the alternative selected. Therefore, group decision making is an effective means for overcoming resistance to change. Such an approach recognizes that if the employees who are threatened by a change have the opportunity to work through the new ideas and methods from the beginning and can be assured that their needs will be satisfied in the future, they will accept the new ideas and methods as something of their own making and will support the changes. Group decision making also makes it easier for each member to carry out the decision once it is agreed on, and the group will put strong pressure on those who have reservations or who do not want to go along.

Both types of participation should be encouraged because they help facilitate the introduction of change. Of course, in trying to implement change in the department, the supervisor makes use of all means available, including persuasion, discussion, participation, and group decision making. Participation is not always possible, however; in extreme situations, it may be necessary to make unpleasant changes unilaterally, impose them, and then help the subordinates understand and accept them.

Survival During Change

Even though the supervisor buys into the reasons for change, and even if he is successful in influencing his staff to accept the change, adjusting to new circumstances can drain him. The desire to successfully pull off a major change in his department can result in exhaustion, irritability, dissatisfaction, and insomnia. These are all symptoms of stress. They are the hormonal and mental reactions to internal and external pressures. Practicing stress management techniques and maintaining a sense of humor will help the supervisor get through this challenging time.

Summary

The influencing function of the manager forms the connecting link between planning, organizing, and staffing on one side and controlling on the other. Issuing directives is perhaps the most important part of the influencing function because without them, very little would be achieved. Certain prerequisites ensure that a directive is properly carried out. A good directive must indicate who, what, where, when, how, and why. It should be accomplishable, intelligible, properly phrased, and compatible with the objectives of the enterprise. In addition, a reasonable amount of time should be permitted for its completion.

In issuing directives, the supervisor may employ two major techniques: (1) the autocratic technique, which brings about close supervision, and (2) the consultative technique, which is characterized by general supervision. For certain occasions, employees, and conditions the autocratic technique is probably more effective, but for most situations it is better for a supervisor to apply consultative techniques to produce the highest motivation and morale among employees. This means that in the case of new assignments, the supervisor consults with the employees about how the job should best be done.

Managers use several supervisory styles, including autocratic (Theory X) and democratic (Theory Y), in their efforts to emerge as leaders. A manager who is appointed to a position of organizational authority is not generally perceived as a leader at the outset. It is hoped, however, that this person will emerge as a leader of the subordinates by effectively achieving results through them. This requires that the leader issue directives that are accepted by the staff members.

In directives primarily concerned with routine assignments and the daily performance of the job, the supervisor employs a form of general supervision instead of close supervision. In so doing, the supervisor gives the employees the freedom to make their own decisions on how the job is to be done, after she has set the goals and standards to be achieved. This also gives employees the freedom to use their own ingenuity and judgment; experiences of this type offer continuous room for further training and improvement. In addition, general supervision motivates employees to the extent that they find satisfaction in their jobs. General supervision normally produces better results than close supervision.

The general supervision environment provides an appropriate setting for teams to function. Team members influence themselves to achieve the organization's objectives. Teams can be long term or short term in nature. Long-term teams (such as self-directed work teams) are part of the formal organizational structure. Short-term teams often work on quality or process issues and as such require a cross-functional representation. These teams may be called quality improvement teams, do-it groups, quality circles, or any title that encourages a teamwork attitude. Teams have advantages, such as reducing cost for additional layers of management, improving processes that result in cost-effective and efficient ways of delivering services or products, and improving morale. They also have disadvantages in that team discontent can result in production delays, damaged morale, and conflicts with management. Clear communication of the team's purpose and authority is necessary to guard against these disadvantages.

Because the healthcare field is dynamic, necessitating constant and often substantial changes, the supervisor is confronted with the problem of how to introduce change. To cope successfully with average employees' normal resistance to change, the supervisor must realize that there are valid social, psychological, and possibly economic reasons for this resistance. By involving employees in change discussions and decisions, much of the resistance can be overcome. The supervisor is in the front line, and it is his responsibility to accommodate change and make it reality. If one endorses Lippitt's model (1987), a supervisor will be successful in managing change if he has a vision that is adequately communicated and understood; has the skills to communicate why the change is necessary; has individuals within the team who have the skills to implement the changes; establishes tangible and intangible incentives to achieve the vision; provides his staff with the resources (tangible resources, time, and support) needed to effect the change; and creates a flexible and dynamic action plan that strives to achieve continuous change for the betterment of the unit, department, or organization.

Additional Readings

Kotter, P., and D. S. Cohen. 2002. *The Heart of Change: Real Life Stories of How People Changed Their Organizations.* Cambridge, MA: Harvard Business School Press.

Kusmierek, K. N. 2001. "Understanding and Addressing Resistance to Organization Change." White paper prepared for the project on Managing Institutional Change and Transformation in Higher Education at the University of Michigan. [Online paper; retrieved 10/15/09.] www-personal.umich.edu/~marvp/facultynetwork/whitepapers/kusmierekresistance.html.

APPENDIX 20.1

Code of Ethics

Guide to Ethical Behavior for the Staff of Anytown Hospital

This guide for acceptable conduct was developed to give all employees, physicians, suppliers, lenders, customers and prospective customers, and the members of Anytown's general public an understanding of how Anytown Hospital's staff is expected to conduct the operations of this hospital and its affiliated services. For purposes of these guidelines, the use of Anytown Hospital means the hospital, its clinics, home health center, rehabilitation center, ambulatory surgery center, and physician practices.

All members of the Anytown Hospital staff (employee, board, auxiliary, medical, and volunteer staffs) are expected to carry out their activities responsibly; comply with all state, federal, and local rules and accrediting agency regulations; avoid any behavior that could reasonably appear to be improper or that could injure their own or Anytown Hospital's reputation for honesty and integrity in all its activities; and follow the policies listed below.

Failure by staff members to comply with these ethics guidelines; other codes provided upon employment, appointment or reappointment, or election; and acceptable standards of business conduct set forth by the hospital places it in a position of risk. When appropriate, the violator could be subject to disciplinary procedures, up to and including termination of the relationship the individual has with Anytown Hospital.

Alleged violation of or related dilemmas arising from these guidelines shall be referred to one or more of the following bodies for further action:

- Ethical issues related to patients or patient care shall be referred to the Bio-Ethics Committee;
- Ethical issues related to physicians or medical staff services are referred to the Executive Committee; and
- Ethical issues related to employees, suppliers, or any other not otherwise specified group or entity shall be referred to the Human Resources Director, unless Human Resources is at issue, then the referral shall be to the Administrator.

Employee Conflict of Interest
All employees are expected to exercise sound judgment that is not biased by individual interests or personal loyalties. Employees should refer to the Compliance Manual and the Code of Conduct received upon employment. One should have no personal, business, or financial interest that could compromise the objectivity, responsibility, and loyalty owed to Anytown Hospital. It is not possible to identify

every activity that might cause a conflict of interest or an appearance of such conflict. A conflict of interest exists if your circumstances would lead a reasonable person to question whether your motivations are aligned with the business' best interests (Duffy 2006, 62). Following are some examples of practices and circumstances in which conflicts might occur:

Our goal must always be to obtain goods and services and promote Anytown Hospital services on terms most favorable to the hospital when buying and selling. Neither you nor any of your immediate family members should (1) have or acquire by gift, inheritance, or other means, any interest in a supplier, customer, or its business (other than owning a small—five percent or less—percentage of the stock of a publicly held corporation); or (2) perform services for such a firm, unless properly disclosed. You should disclose any such holding or relationship to your immediate supervisor, department director, clinical service chief, or administrator, as such a relationship could appear to have the potential for biasing your judgment or activities.
Dealing with Suppliers and Customers

You must disclose to your immediate supervisor, department director, clinical service chief, or administrator if you or any of your immediate family members: (1) receive by gift, inheritance, or otherwise, an interest in a competitor or its business; or (2) are performing services for a competitor of Anytown Hospital other than serving as a member of the medical staff of a competitor hospital.
Dealing with Competitors

You or any of your immediate family members should not accept compensation or entertainment having more than nominal value, commissions, property or anything else of personal financial advantage from any outside parties in connection with any transactions involving the hospital. This does not apply to personal loans from a recognized financial institution made in the ordinary course of business on usual and customary terms. At no time shall staff accept cash or gifts of more than nominal value from patients or their families.
Compensation or Favors from Others

No gift (regardless of value) or other thing of value shall be given to or received from a supplier, lender, or customer representative with the intent to corrupt or bias that person's or the employee's conduct.
Giving or Receiving Gifts

No funds or assets of Anytown Hospital shall be used for, or in aid of, any candidate or nominee for local, state, or federal political office in the United States or for, or in aid of, any political parties or committees in connection therewith unless allowed by law and authorized by the Administrator of Anytown Hospital. These prohibitions cover direct contributions and indirect assistance such as the furnishing of goods, services, or equipment to candidates, political parties, or committees.
Political Payments

We encourage our employees and staff to participate in community activities and volunteer their time to bona fide charitable, educational, civic and trade organizations. Participation in these types of activities does not generally require prior approval, but you should guard against possible conflicts of interest, especially when the goals of the organization compete or conflict with those of Anytown Hospital.
Serving on Community, Civic, and Non-profit Boards (Duffy 2006, 62)

Accounting Systems: Books and Records

Anytown Hospital policy requires that its books and records shall accurately reflect transactions and disposition of assets. Books and records will be kept in accordance with Generally Accepted Accounting Principles (GAAP) in the United States. No false, artificial, or misleading statements or entries shall be made in Anytown Hospital's books or records including, but not limited to, time reports, accounts, and financial statements. No unrecorded "slush" funds or secret assets of any kind shall be maintained for any purpose whatsoever. Staff is expected to follow the hospital financial and information management policies regarding retaining documentation in their area of responsibility.

Patient Billings and Records

All initial patient billings shall be itemized. Patients are entitled to receive an itemized bill upon request. Patients are also permitted to receive a copy of their record in accordance with the Health Information Management Department policies and procedures.

At least annually, Patient Financial Services and Health Information Management will have an external agent audit a sample of accounts to ensure proper billing and coding practices have been followed and that adequate documentation exists to justify the billings.

From time to time, Administration will evaluate its charges against the prevailing charges in the region to ensure its charges are consistent with others providing similar services.

Privacy

At all times, employees, board, volunteers, and medical staff members will protect a patient's right to privacy by avoiding discussions of the patient's condition with those who are not involved in the patient's care, ensuring patient care documents are not in view of those not involved in the patient care, not accessing patient information that is not needed to perform one's job, and not disclosing patient information to unauthorized parties.

21

LEADERSHIP

After you have studied this chapter, you should be able to do the following:

1. Define leadership.
2. Discuss the various leadership theories.
3. Distinguish between emotive and task-oriented leadership roles.
4. Identify key management style factors.
5. Discuss the challenges that diversity in the workplace creates for leaders.

Leadership, one of the most popular and important topics in the field of management, is a key process in any organization, and an organization's success or failure is largely attributed to it. It is an essential component of the organizational climate. Ultimately, an organization's leadership is responsible for establishing an environment that facilitates the organization's successful performance and staff's motivation toward that end. Atchison (2004) describes a leader as one who has inspired others to be the best they can be, a definition that clearly defines the challenge for every healthcare manager.

The concept of leadership is of great importance because every organization is concerned with attracting and developing people who will be effective leaders. Leadership plays an important role in organizational life and ultimately makes the difference between an effective and an ineffective organization.

Leadership can further be defined as a process by which people are imaginatively directed, guided, and influenced to select and attain goals. It is helpful to look at leadership in an organizational setting as a behavior, as an action one person takes to influence others (Steers 1988). Kouzes and Posner (2003, 78–83) define leadership as a shared responsibility. For the purposes of this book, *leadership* is the process by which one person influences others to do something voluntarily rather than out of fear or as a result of coercion. This voluntary aspect is different from other processes such as influence by authority or power.

Much of this book uses the terms "leader" and "manager" interchangeably. In this context we distinguish between the terms. According to Kouzes and Posner (1987, 27), "managers ... get other people to do, but leaders get other people to *want* to do." Management is concerned with "doing," or executing. Managers execute plans, assign work, rearrange staffing to complete a project, and so forth. Leaders, on the other hand, provide an environment in which managers are able to execute. Leaders create the vision and point managers to the paths, and managers go down the paths. Leaders also encourage their managers to act responsibly by being socially responsible role models (see the "Social Responsibility" section later in this chapter). A good manager does not just act but also takes the right action.

Atchison and McDonagh (2007) further clarify the difference between managers and leaders. They state that leaders inspire, influence, establish strategies, and analyze relationships. Managers organize, control, establish tactics, and create plans. In other words, leaders lay the track, and managers make sure the trains run on time. This chapter provides information to help the new supervisor to become an efficient manager and to build the skills necessary to be an effective leader.

Leadership Theories

In any organized activity a leader mediates between organizational and individual goals to maximize the satisfaction of both. A manager also plays this mediating role, but not necessarily in the same manner as a leader. Although the terms *manager* and *leader* are often used interchangeably, they are not synonymous. A person who has formal positional authority may use formal legitimate authority and power to get things done; on the other hand, an individual who has no position of formal authority may use the leadership influence but is not the manager. From the view of organizational effectiveness, however, it is desirable for the manager to also be the leader. With that in mind, we consider those qualities an individual must display to function as a leader as well as a manager. The following theories posit what constitutes a good leader and what enables some people to be a leader and not others.

Early Genetic Theory
For hundreds of years observers recognized leadership as the ability to influence people in such a manner that they willingly strove toward an objective. It was believed that this ability was a quality separate from official position. This view holds that certain people are born to be leaders, having inherited a set of unique traits, characteristics, or attributes that cannot be acquired in any other way. This position, also known as the "great man" theory of leadership, concludes that leadership qualities are inherited simply because the leadership phenomenon emerged frequently within the same prominent families. In reality, however, strong class barriers made it difficult for anyone outside these families to acquire the skills and knowledge required to become a leader. In the beginning of the twentieth century, this belief in inherited leadership characteristics lost ground.

Trait, or Attribute, Theory

In the 1920s and 1930s, as social and economic class barriers were broken down and leaders began to emerge from the so-called lower classes of society, the early genetic theory was modified. Behavioral scientists began to contribute to the literature on leadership and determined that, rather than arising only from inherited characteristics, leadership could also be acquired through experience, education, and training. Efforts were made to identify all the traits—inherited and acquired—found in individuals regarded as leaders. These traits frequently included physical and nervous energy, above-average height, a sense of purpose and direction, willingness to accept the consequences of their actions, enthusiasm, friendliness and affection, integrity, technical mastery, decisiveness, verbal fluency, assertiveness, initiative, originality, intelligence, teaching skill, faith, ambition, and persistence.

The inadequacy of this approach soon became obvious. No satisfactory answer could be reached about which traits were most essential for leadership or whether a person could be a leader if certain traits were lacking. Also, how to isolate and identify all the specific traits common to leaders was not clear. A further weakness of the trait approach was that it did not distinguish between those characteristics needed for acquiring leadership and those necessary for maintaining it.

Although the trait approach is partially discredited today, a considerable body of research shows that leaders have in common certain general characteristics. Some of these are intelligence, communication ability, and sensitivity to group needs. Such traits are woven into the personality of the leader. These studies led researchers to question the validity of the trait approach as the predictor of leadership. Subsequent research determined that leadership style varies based on the managerial situation being confronted, the types of employees or skill levels they may have, or both.

The Contingency Approach

In their search for other variables, behavioral scientists discovered the importance of situational factors present in acquiring positions of leadership. This theory assumes that leadership behavior varies according to the situation (Fiedler 1967; Vroom and Yetton 1973). This approach, also known as the contingency model of leadership effectiveness, points out the interdependence between leadership style and the demands of the situation. Consider the role that Lee Iacocca played when he assumed leadership of the Chrysler Corporation in the late 1970s. Chrysler turned to him in its time of need, and he brought a "broad, popular, and galvanizing vision" to the organization that changed Chrysler's future (Peters 2001) for at least 25 years.

For nearly 40 years, Fred Fiedler (1967) studied the relationship between workplace situations and an individual's character and abilities (his values, vision, morals, initiative, and so on). His contingency theory states that there is no best way for managers to lead. Leadership in one group differs from leadership in another group; in one situation a certain person might evolve as the leader, whereas under different environmental conditions someone else would emerge as the leader. For example, in a political meeting an individual with good public speaking ability may rise to the top, and in a natural disaster someone with tactical skills may emerge as the leader. In other words, the leadership characteristics and behavior needed are a function of the specific situation.

In their desire to deemphasize the traits approach, however, some behavioral scientists may have ruled out the possibility that at least some characteristics predispose people to attain leadership positions or at least increase their chances of becoming leaders. It is clear today that both a person's characteristics and the situation in which she functions are involved in the concept of leadership.

The Follower Factor

A still better understanding of leadership incorporates the input contributed by followers. This theory maintains that the followers and the makeup of the group must be studied because essentially it is the follower who either accepts or rejects a leader, depending on whether his needs are satisfied. Proponents of this approach further maintain that followers' persistent motives, points of view, and frames of reference determine what they perceive in terms of leadership and how they react to it. The follower approach emphasizes the importance of the group at a particular point while it acknowledges that certain characteristics help one person emerge as the leader over another person. At times, a leader may become a follower if he perceives another will more effectively lead the charge and achieve the desired end. Therefore, satisfaction of the followers' needs is an important aspect.

More specifically, the follower factor stresses the idea that the leadership function must be analyzed and understood in terms of a dynamic relationship, a social exchange process between the leader and the followers. The followers bring to the situation their personalities, needs, motivations, and expectations. The leader appears to the followers as the best means available for the satisfaction of their needs, whether those needs are emotive or task oriented (see the discussion on need categories later in this chapter). A leader is essential for influencing a group to act as a unit to move toward task accomplishment. The members look to this individual as their leader not only because she possesses certain characteristics, such as intelligence, skill, drive, and ambition, but also because of her functional relationship to the members of the group.

Leadership Roles

Consider the different roles individuals play in groups. One person may organize the group to achieve goals, whereas another may serve as the "devil's advocate," raising a stream of objections; yet another is a "synthesizer," who pulls together the ideas of all group members. These roles and many others fulfill the needs of the group's members and are vital to the group's accomplishments. The group's leader is not necessarily expected to assume all these roles, but he is expected to fulfill some of them. Generally, leadership roles fall into two broad classifications of need: task oriented and emotive.

Task-oriented roles are those assumed by the leader to organize and influence the group to achieve specified objectives. Usually in an organized activity, these objectives are imposed on the group from above. In groups that arise spontaneously, however, tasks and objectives are generated from within the group itself. In both instances, the leader must facilitate the accomplishment of the group's goals.

Emotive leadership roles are employee centered and provide satisfaction for the individual needs of the group's members. George Bailey, the main character in *It's a Wonderful Life*, exemplifies this set of roles by treating customers and employees with generosity. The emotional needs of people are of a social and psychological nature. A leader in the emotive role helps members of the group to satisfy these needs; at the same time she prepares the way for task performance, an indication of how these roles may overlap.

Ideally, one leader plays both types of roles effectively. In some instances, however, group leadership can be shared without diminishing the group's performance or morale; one person plays the task role and another takes the emotive role. The formal organization of a healthcare institution, for example, often forces a supervisor to be primarily concerned with getting the job done. He must concentrate largely on task leadership. Under these conditions, the group may select another individual, the informal leader, who can function in the emotive role. The supervisor should not object to the informal leader's role. Rather, the supervisor should realize that it is a necessary part of the leadership process, one that fulfills important human needs and is an essential component of high employee morale.

Schein (1996) states that leaders of the future will be people who, paradoxically, "can lead and follow, be central and marginal, be hierarchically above and below, be individualistic and a team player, and, above all, be a perpetual learner." Deming (1994) says the primary responsibility of leaders is to manage the transformation of the organization. Another leadership role is to ensure that the organization works effectively with respect to the interactions between individuals, groups, and business units both within and outside the organization and that behaviors meet accepted standards for business ethics. Finally, Warren Bennis and Joan Goldsmith (2003) define the difference between managers and leaders as doing the right thing (leadership = effectiveness) versus doing things right (management = efficiency).

Leadership Style

Whatever leadership style is adopted by a supervisor influences her acceptance by her subordinates. According to Peters (2001), "The best leader is rarely the best pitcher or catcher. The best leader is just what's advertised: the best leader. Leaders get their kicks from orchestrating the work of others—not from doing it themselves." Bill Bradley (2005), retired U.S. senator from New Jersey and former professional basketball player, once said, "The business of leaders, of heroes, is tricky. Leadership is not something that is done to people, like fixing your teeth. Leadership is unlocking people's potential to become better." Thus, the supervisor's skills are used to enable employees to achieve at least partial satisfaction of their needs for esteem and self-actualization on the job.

The concept of leadership is closely tied to management style. We discussed several management styles in earlier chapters, including autocratic and democratic styles. Depending on the approach taken, a manager may be perceived as a leader, someone whom subordinates will follow to achieve a cause, or as a manager in title only, someone they may resent and for whom they will do only the minimum required. Tom Peters (2001), contemporary management theorist and author of *In Search of Excellence*, says that we should "think of pre-1990 as the Age of Sucking Up to the Hierarchy," while the "Age of the Promise 'Em Everything Pitch lasted from 1995 to 2000." He states further that the years 2001 through 2006 are the "Age of No-Bull Performance, which means that we're going to see leadership emerge as the most important element of business—the attribute that is highest in demand and shortest in supply." More than ever, leaders are expected to achieve results through people. No single leadership style is appropriate for all situations. A leader must be able to call on a whole range of responses. A good manager knows when to use one or another style of leadership to "involve the right people, at the right place and at the right time" (Peters 2001).

Healthcare leaders can strengthen their personal leadership skills by (1) gaining a deeper understanding of their personal convictions; (2) requesting regular feedback regarding their leadership approach; (3) defining the key competencies needed to help their organizations succeed; (4) reflecting on department-specific results from employee opinion surveys and conversations with staff and making behavioral changes, when appropriate, in response (Williams 2007, 51); and (5) studying the vision and mission of the organization and communicating it in such a way that people feel empowered and energized to help the organization succeed (Fontaine 2009, 2). The supervisor's goal should be to make herself a better leader and in doing so inspire others to effectively lead as well.

Underlying all management styles is interpersonal communications. Most people in healthcare management have perfected their technical skills—drawing blood, monitoring patient conditions, moving supplies, conducting specialized invasive studies, and so on. Often our technical duties do not require us to communicate with an audience beyond a colleague who has similar skills. A leader must be able to communicate with peers, superiors, subordinates, and customers in meaningful and sincere terms.

Leaders often exemplify professional and ethical conduct, aligning their personal conduct with ethical and professional standards that include a responsibility to the patient and community, a service orientation, and commitment to lifelong learning and improvement (Stefl 2008, 364). Williams (2007) indicates that one way for a leader to hone her skills is to read biographies of great leaders. Appold (2006) suggests going a step further and speaking with great leaders: Ask how they struggled with failures and how they overcame them; ask what they learned and why they were successful.

Another competency of leaders is the ability to demonstrate knowledge of the healthcare environment or, for the department manager, knowledge of department-specific healthcare specialty and expressing how it contributes to the quality and overall delivery of healthcare for the organization while galvanizing people to action and applying business principles to the efficient operation of the department (Stefl 2008, 364).

The leader must fine-tune these competencies or skills (see Exhibit 21.1) to draw individuals to follow him, encourage them to listen, and energize them to achieve organizational goals. In fact, developing and sustaining a high-energy workplace may be one of the most difficult tasks healthcare leaders are charged with; however, research shows that employees working in these climates outperform peers working in a less robust environment by as much as 30 percent (Fontaine 2009).

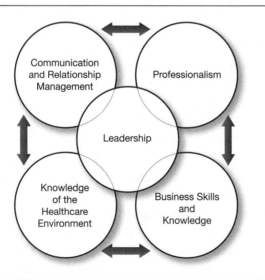

EXHIBIT 21.1
The Healthcare
Leadership
Alliance
Competency
Model

SOURCE: Reprinted with permission from Stefl (2008).

Another factor to consider is the healthcare industry's turnover rate. A number of factors affect an organization's ability to maintain its workforce. Job hopping is rampant in high demand–low supply positions. With many workers retiring, the numbers of younger people poised to take their place are fewer. Workers tend to leave a job in the first year to 18 months of employment, largely in response to poor leadership, inability to perform meaningful work, and a lack of opportunities to develop professionally. The cost of employee turnover is significant and may range from 70 percent to 200 percent of the replaced employee's salary. The cost of replacing a member of a healthcare team includes the time spent recruiting, interviewing, training, overseeing, and assimilating the newcomer. A workplace dominated by good leaders is conducive to productivity, efficiency, job satisfaction, and stability (Jackson 2004, 30–31). Success in this area often clearly differentiates the truly great leaders from the good leaders (Dye and Garman 2006).

Energizing Staff

To *energize staff* means to set a personal example of good work ethic and motivation; talk and act enthusiastically and optimistically about the future; enjoy rising to new challenges; take on the work with energy, passion, and drive to finish successfully; help others recognize the importance of their work; be enjoyable to work for; and have a goal-oriented, ambitious, and determined working style (Dye and Garman 2006). Setting this example draws staff and colleagues into a finely tuned follower–leader dynamic.

Effective leaders know which management style to use with each individual or group of individuals with which they work. We have discussed various management styles and know that individuals respond differently to each style, requiring the leader to blend styles to motivate certain individuals. To know which approach to take requires the leader to understand both the organization's and the individual's goals. This understanding is gained in interviewing and selecting staff; conducting annual appraisals; observing how individuals deal with coworkers and others inside and outside the department; and recognizing what "excites" them about their job, the department, or the organization.

Fontaine (2009, 1–2) recommends that a manager keep his team energized by creating clarity and buy-in while keeping people focused on the work at hand. Good leaders do this by being authoritative—creating the vision, providing the context, and gaining commitment—not leaving employees in the dark about the organization's strategy. When required, effective leaders reach out to others for help and expertise; take a more democratic approach to decision making; support employees, especially during economic downturns; and coach and develop people.

When the excitement increases, the team will be energized and some followers will seek to be more like the supportive, enthusiastic supervisor. When this occurs, the manager should guide or mentor these followers by developing their leadership competencies. Good mentors will listen rather than problem solve, make individuals think, and provide feedback (Mackenzie 2008, 52). Effective leaders know that only by developing other leaders will breakthroughs to success occur. They realize that people who do not assume greater responsibilities, creatively problem solve, or continuously learn will ultimately limit their own and the organization's possibilities (O'Leary 2009).

Diversity

The diversity challenges confronting leaders today are unlike those of just a decade ago. Today, leaders must understand the needs of a culturally and generationally diverse workforce.

Generational Diversity

Members of four generations of the U.S. population may be working together in the same department—the silenters, the baby boomers, generation Xers, and generation Yers. While stereotyping is not a reliable way to address issues related to generational differences, the following general descriptions may provide some insight on the needs of each generation and a leader's approach to each.

The silenters, or veterans, often have chosen a career, and possibly an employer, for life. If they decide to change employers, they typically seek a leader who directs their assignment. The boomers may be anxious to take on more assignments as they ascend the career ladder, focusing on personal growth. Gen Xers will seek a standard workweek that provides them with the flexibility to take care of family and attend to volunteer obligations. The gen Yers, or millennials, often expect flexibility and, because they are typically so technologically proficient, are usually highly productive. To members of this latest generation currently in the workforce, if they can do the job in 30 hours, why sit around for that extra 10? Don't think that means the gen Yers skip out on hard work, though; productivity is more important to them than the face time (Jusinski 2007). Gen Yers will ask questions, unlike boomers, who will dig and find answers. Gen Y workers spend a mere 1.6 years at one job (Jusinski 2007), and because they grew up in an era marked by school violence, natural disasters, and September 11 (Hartner 2007), they seek to live well-balanced lives rather than be bogged down with bureaucracy and a 9–5 job. Unless their supervisors catch and maintain their attention, gen Yers give their supervisors little time to develop them into leaders within the organization.

Not only will the healthcare workforce be populated with these four generational categories but our medical staffs will reflect the same diversity.

Coping with the newest generation in particular requires tact, patience, and restraint (Katz 2008), and building harmony among the generations will challenge the most talented leader.

Cultural Diversity

The healthcare workforce has also become global and culturally diverse. Understanding the unique experiences and personal and professional needs of individuals from different world regions who speak languages other than English, knowing how to best engage them to seek common goals, addressing and accepting ethnic differences and attitudes, and determining how best to encourage them to take on leadership roles will require study. Research findings thus far clearly establish that diversity tests leadership skills at a deeper and more personal level than does homogeneity because diverse groups are likely to encounter socioemotional conflict (Dreachslin 2007, 152).

When considering diversity issues, one should first understand the meaning of culture. Culture, in short, is the sum total of one's way of living. It includes values, beliefs, standards, language, thinking patterns, behavioral norms, communications styles, and other background and experience factors. Each person's culture, just as each organization's culture, guides decisions and actions of the groups in which he is involved through time (UCLA Health System n.d.). Recognizing the need to gain at least some understanding of each staff member's culture, it may be beneficial to do some advance research prior to the selection interview. It would be inappropriate to ignore differences in cultures and assume that each employee can be treated the same. Known as **cultural blindness**, this approach only serves the dominant groups of employees in your team.

cultural blindness
The practice of ignoring cultural differences among employees.

When a workplace or any other setting is represented by several cultures, it is considered multicultural. Multiculturalism is based on the idea that cultural identities should not be discarded or ignored but instead maintained and valued.

The importance of cultural diversity in the workplace has been, for the most part, accepted in American business (Leadership-Tools.com n.d.). As of the 2000 U.S. census, minorities have become the majority population in six of the eight largest metropolitan areas in the United States. Thus, living with and managing diversity has become a central theme of the twenty-first century. Many studies, in fact, have shown that diversity in human capital leads to increased creativity and efficiency in many cases. Studies have also shown that the failure to successfully integrate a diverse workforce has negative implications for organizational performance. This is most publicly expressed in legal actions, such as recent discrimination suits against multinational corporations such as the Coca-Cola Company, Wal-Mart Stores Inc., and Xerox Corporation (Sinha n.d.).

Brett, Behfar, and Kern (2006, 2–3) note four challenges that arise when managing and leading multicultural teams: (1) differing use of direct versus indirect communication, (2) trouble with accents and fluencies, (3) differing attitudes toward hierarchy and authority, and (4) conflicting norms for decision making. Western-style communications are typically direct, whereas non-Western communications are often delivered in an indirect manner. Furthermore, while a native of a non-Western culture will likely understand a directive, a supervisor from the West may not be able to determine whether that individual accepts it. A reply of "yes" from a non-Western staff member may simply mean, "I'm listening." In addition, frustrations can arise among team members and between you and a staff member when language is a barrier and one of you is not fluent in the other's language. Tone of voice and the volume at which one speaks may imply disrespect to someone from another country.

Just as U.S. employees respect the chain of command in organizations, so do managers in other cultures. However, in some cultures, the chain of command is not only followed but followed up through managers of the same culture rather than crossing over to a manager from another culture. For example, a Korean employee may express concerns to a Korean superior in the organization rather than to her direct supervisor, if that supervisor is non-Korean. Finally, decision making differs between the style typically practiced in the United States and that seen in other countries. While U.S. leaders often make decisions quickly and then move on, leaders from other countries may prefer to discuss decisions at length.

How can a manager prepare to deal with multiculturalism and rise to a leadership role when so many mores and values must be considered? In a study of Sodexo (formerly Sodexho), Dreachslin (2007, 152) suggests that one must buy into the other culture, perhaps by mentoring someone from a culture different from his.

Nevertheless, it is a sign of a good manager and a good leader to be able to recognize that a barrier may be present, diplomatically address it, and use a mixture of techniques to maintain team collaboration whenever the occasion arises. Employing the appropriate style largely determines the degree to which the leader can influence others in performing tasks and addressing situations.

Social Responsibility

Social responsibility (or corporate social responsibility) dictates that companies contribute to the welfare of society and not be solely devoted to maximizing profits. According to Walonick (n.d.), the accountability concept states that organizations receive their charter from society as a whole, and therefore their ultimate responsibility is to society.

Providing care to those community residents unable to pay, offering training and apprenticeship opportunities, ensuring employees are compensated at an acceptable level, thoroughly evaluating the competency of medical and other patient care staff, continuously improving the quality of services and facilities, offering health screenings and education, and other actions all represent socially responsible actions. McDonalds Corporation's funding of its Ronald McDonald Houses is an example of corporate social responsibility. Healthcare organizations such as Catholic Healthcare West (n.d.) publicize activities aimed at fulfilling their social responsibility, including efforts to conserve energy, use water-saving devices, and build mercury-free hospitals.

The proliferation of regulations governing reporting, protecting employees, maintaining physical plant and equipment, and protecting consumers demonstrates that profits cannot compromise the welfare of staff and patients. The moral organization will have an infrastructure that has implemented processes to comply with these regulations not just because it is mandated to do so but because it believes making moral choices on behalf of its employees, staff, and consumers will return greater profits than those lost by not doing so. In fact, Orlitzky, Schmidt, and Rynes (2003) found a positive correlation between social and environmental performance and financial performance. The ethical corporation places social responsibility at its center and bases its existence on ethics.

Summary

Leadership is a process by which one person tries to influence others in the performance of a task. Through effective leadership, subordinates are imaginatively directed, guided, and influenced in choosing and attaining goals. The concepts of leadership and management are not interchangeable; a person does not have to be a leader to be an adequate manager, but the supervisor of the department who is also the leader is ideal.

Much research has been conducted on leadership. The early genetic theory maintained that leadership was a function of specific characteristics with which a leader was born. Later the genetic approach was altered to state that leadership was a function of numerous personal traits that could be acquired as well as inherited. More recent studies point out that the situation in which a group is placed has significant bearing on who emerges as a leader. Furthermore, the follower factor adds to the concept of leadership the importance of the followers' perception and the group they constitute.

Many variables play a role in the leadership process. The leader is an individual perceived to be in harmony with the needs of the group and responsive to the group situation. However, because leaders must always be recognized as such by group consensus and because managers who are appointed do not necessarily reflect subordinate group choice, they are not generally regarded as leaders, at least at the outset of their assignment. It is desirable from an influencing standpoint that subordinates accept the manager as a leader and not merely as the head of the department. Thus, each manager must adopt a leadership style that facilitates such acceptance.

In the leadership process, it is necessary to fulfill both the task role (influencing the group to achieve its goals) and the emotive role (satisfying the emotional needs of group members). If it is impossible for the leader to fulfill the emotive role, an effective leader will not object to the group choosing an informal leader to fulfill this role. Although much about leadership remains to be studied, the research into this concept has given us a better understanding of the types of behavior needed in different settings and the importance of leadership for organizational effectiveness.

Today, leaders are challenged by a work environment that includes a multigenerational and culturally diverse workforce and a demand for a morally responsible organization. Understanding the needs of this workforce and blending management styles to energize staff to achieve goals and serve the community in a socially responsible manner will be paramount in the years to come.

Additional Readings

Exceptional Leadership. Dye, C. F., and A. N. Garman. 2006. Chicago: Health Administration Press.

Stefl, M. E. 2008. "Common Competencies for All Healthcare Managers: The Healthcare Leadership Alliance Model." *Journal of Healthcare Management*, 53 (6).

22

MOTIVATION

Chapter Objectives

After you have studied this chapter, you should be able to do the following:

1. Outline the major theories of motivation.
2. Describe the motivational processes.
3. Define perceptions, values, attitudes, and the factors that affect each of these.
4. Discuss the supervisor's duty in minimizing frustration and conflict.

Motivating employees is important to managers because motivation affects performance. Motivation is closely related to the crucial managerial function of influencing because it deals most intimately with the individual. Thus, we must understand what motivates a person and, more basically, what underlies a person's motivations. Peter Drucker maintains that people motivate themselves. He says you cannot motivate them; you can only thwart their motivation. To be an effective leader you must recognize that the business you are really in is the obstacle identification and removal business (Golden Business Idea 2005).

Motivation is the process affecting the inner needs or drives that arouse, move, energize, direct, channel, and sustain human behavior. Generally, the motivational process begins the drive that impels individuals to work toward certain goals they believe will satisfy their inner needs. Once these goals are attained, we judge whether these efforts were worthwhile. If deemed worthwhile, the result is reinforcement, and we continue to pursue these and other needs and drives. Understanding motivation will enable managers to help their employees achieve higher levels of job satisfaction and job performance.

motivation
The process affecting the inner needs or drives that arouse, move, energize, direct, channel, and sustain human behavior.

Theories of Motivation

Managers have long been aware of the importance of motivation, and many theories have attempted to explain how people are motivated. There are several ways to interpret the concept of motivation; two of the major categories of contemporary motivational theories are the content theory and the process theory. We do not discuss all of the motivational theories in this chapter, but we touch on several in both the content and process arenas.

content theory
The theory that individuals are motivated by needs. Also called *need theory*.

Content theory focuses on determining what factor or set of factors moves, energizes, and starts the behavior of an individual. This theory discusses the concept of needs or motives that drive people and the incentives that cause people to behave in a particular manner. Some authors call this school of theory *need theory*. A need is anything that is required, desired, or considered useful to obtain an item, feeling, or status. Four of the most publicized content theories of motivation are (1) Maslow's hierarchy of needs; (2) Alderfer's existence, relatedness, and growth (ERG) theory; (3) Herzberg's two-factor approach of satisfiers and dissatisfiers; and (4) McClelland's needs for achievement, affiliation, and power. Each content theory tries to explain individual behavior from a slightly different perspective.

process theory
The theory that individuals are motivated by equity and expectancy, i.e., that they expect equal compensation and treatment (equity) and that they will be rewarded for their effort (expectancy).

On the other hand, **process theory** examines how and why people choose a particular behavior to accomplish a goal and how they evaluate their satisfaction after reaching the goal. Equity and expectancy are the two major process perspectives on motivation. The first approach stresses the equity of effort in relation to the results; that is, there should be a balance in the amount of effort one must put forth for the resulting rewards—compensation, benefits, and so forth. The other approach emphasizes that one will exercise a certain level of effort if she expects to receive some reward, promotion, or recognition. If there is inequity or imbalance, staff will not be motivated. We discuss two process theorists: Victor Vroom (expectancy model) and B. F. Skinner (reinforcement model).

Model of Motivational Processes

Although the complete set of processes is complex, a generalized model of basic motivational processes is presented in Exhibit 22.1. This model shows five basic parts of the process: (1) needs and desires; (2) expectations, perceptions, motives, values, and attitudes; (3) tactical behavior action plan; (4) goal; and (5) results or feedback. At any point, individuals are likely to have a mixture of needs, desires, and expectations. For instance, one subordinate may have a strong need to achieve and a desire to earn more money; this person expects that doing the job well will lead to the desired rewards. This expectation is likely to cause behavior that is directed toward specific goals. Achieving the goals serves as feedback on the impact of this behavior and reassures this individual that the behavior is correct to satisfy the needs and expectations. On the other hand, if the action plan fails, it may tell the person that the present course of action is incorrect and should be altered.

This model of motivation is oversimplified because it does not take into account all influences on motivation; however, it shows the basic cyclical nature of the process. People strive to satisfy a variety of needs and expectations, and the success of one effort triggers the pursuit of another need and desire.

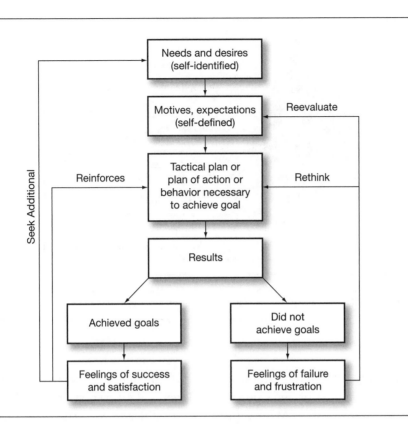

EXHIBIT 22.1
Model of the
Motivational
Process

Once a need has been met, another need or desire emerges and stimulates further action.

Maslow's Hierarchy of Human Needs (1954)

One approach to employee motivation is based on individual human needs. Every action is motivated by unsatisfied needs. These unsatisfied needs cause human beings to behave in a certain manner and to try to achieve certain goals in hopes of reducing the tensions that arise from unmet needs. A person eats because hunger creates the need for food. Similarly, an individual may have a strong need to achieve and strives to advance in his field of work. In other words, there is a reason for everything that people do. It is often observed that human beings never seem satisfied; we are continuously fulfilling needs. After the successful fulfillment of one need, we start on another round of pursuits.

Probably the most widely known and accepted theory of needs and motivation is the model designed by Abraham H. Maslow consisting of deficiency needs and growth needs. Deficiency needs must be satisfied if the individual is to be healthy and secure. They are the physiological needs for food, water, clothing, and shelter; needs for safety; and needs to feel a sense of

Maslow's Hierarchy of Needs
A motivation model that involves levels of needs, from basic physiological needs to the need for self-actualization.

Exhibit 22.2

Maslow's
Hierarchy
of Needs

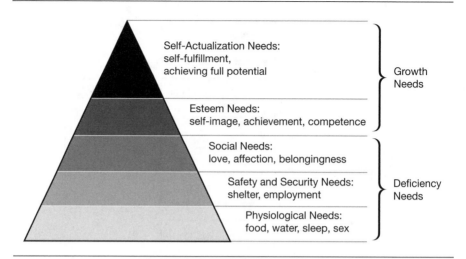

SOURCE: Maslow, Abraham; Frager, Robert (editor), Fadman, James (editor), *Motivation and Personality*, 3rd edition, © 1987. Adapted by permission of Pearson Education, Inc., Upper Saddle River, NJ.

belonging, love, and respect from others. Growth needs refer to development and achievement of one's potential. All needs, however, are not of the same order of importance. Many different kinds of needs exist, and some produce stronger motivation or demand more immediate satisfaction than others. Maslow suggests that these needs are arranged in a hierarchy (Huitt 1998) (see Exhibit 22.2).

Maslow's model contains five levels of needs that can be visualized as forming a pyramid. The most basic needs are physiological needs. Normally, in organizational settings, adequate wages and the work environment itself enable an individual to obtain the necessities and comforts of life that are vital to fulfilling these physiological needs.

When the physiological needs are reasonably satisfied, needs at the next higher level begin to dominate. These are usually called safety needs, such as those that create safe physical and emotional environments. They are the needs that, when fulfilled, protect against danger and threat. Such needs are natural reactions to insecurity. We all desire more control over and protection from the uncertainties of life. In a work environment, these uncertainties would produce security needs caused by, for example, an unstable economic climate (e.g., recession), fear of seemingly arbitrary management action (e.g., decision to close a clinic), loss of job, favoritism, discrimination, or unpredictable administration of policy. Most enterprises today offer various programs designed to satisfy and fulfill these safety or security needs. For example, most enterprises have grievance systems, adequate medical and other insurance plans, provisions for retirement benefits, provisions for unemployment compensation, and seniority benefits. Especially during times of economic instability, this set of needs tends to dominate employees' concerns. Therefore, the manager must attempt to respond to security needs when they arise.

Once the physiological and safety needs are satisfied, social needs become important motivators. Social needs consist of belonging, association, acceptance by one's peers, and giving and receiving friendship and love. These needs are often identical to the needs people have for a feeling of group identity—that is, being part of a group or team and being accepted and respected by their peers. A supervisor must be aware of the existence of these needs, which can be fulfilled in organizational settings by informal groups. As we know, tightly knit, cohesive work groups generally enable employees to gain greater on-the-job satisfaction and produce a better climate for motivation. This is why the supervisor should look at the positive aspects and strengths of informal groups. Often supervisors go to great trouble to control and interfere with the natural grouping tendency of human beings. This is ill advised. When a person's social needs are thwarted and frustrated, he will behave in ways that are likely to hurt organizational objectives. The manager should always realize that social needs are fulfilled largely by informal groups and informal organization, as discussed in Chapter 18.

Once the first three needs, also known as deficiency needs, have been satisfied, people generally attempt to satisfy growth needs. These are the needs for esteem and self-actualization. Esteem needs focus on one's desire to have a worthy self-image and receive recognition from others. Self-esteem includes the need for self-confidence, a positive self-image, self-respect, independence, achievement, competence, and knowledge. These needs are often fulfilled by mastery over part of the environment—for example, by knowing that you can accomplish a certain task.

However, a person also needs the esteem and recognition of others for her accomplishments. These needs relate to reputation, status, recognition, appreciation, and the deserved respect of colleagues. Many jobs in industrial settings offer little opportunity for satisfaction of such needs. However, many positions in the healthcare field are conducive to achieving these needs because of their challenging nature. The manager can satisfy those needs by providing external symbols of esteem such as appropriate titles and offices. Of course, it is desirable that both aspects of the need for esteem are fulfilled. Frequently, however, the esteem of self comes before esteem from others.

The highest level of needs is the need for **self-actualization**, self-fulfillment, or self-realization. These are the needs for realizing one's own potential, for continuing one's self-development, and for being creative in the broadest sense of the term. It has often been said that this is the need to become what one is capable of becoming. Unlike the other four needs, which typically are satisfied, self-actualization is seldom fully achieved. It is a process of becoming, and as one gradually approaches self-fulfillment, this process is intensified

self-actualization
Realizing one's potential.

and sustained. Because this need can be met only from within, there is little the manager can do to facilitate the achievement of this need except to provide an organizational climate conducive to self-actualization. The focus of contemporary American lifestyles leaves little time to fulfill this need. Most employees are continuously struggling to satisfy the lower needs and must divert most of their energy to satisfy them.

There seems to be a relationship between the hierarchy of needs and age. Physiological and safety needs are paramount in the life of an infant. As a child grows up, love needs become more important. When the adolescent reaches young adulthood, needs for esteem seem to take precedence. If the person is successful in meeting the lower-level needs in life, the move to self-actualization later in life is likely. Such a step does not necessarily follow because pressing circumstances may arrest the route of progress at the esteem level or at lower levels. As seen in the following discussion, this situation is often the basis of conflict between organizational and individual goals.

Maslow's hierarchy of needs is popular among managers. Because it is the supervisor's job to create a climate in which employees can satisfy the multitude of needs, this theory makes clear recommendations to management (see Exhibit 22.3). Some of the specific dynamics of Maslow's theory may still be in question, however, and have been challenged. Nevertheless, Maslow's hierarchy was the first clear theory urging managers to recognize the importance of higher-order needs. It caused a shift from the traditional lower-order motivators to higher motivators. While most healthy and normal employees are not hungry, feel reasonably secure, and have sufficient social relationships, others may yet have to fulfill such needs. Consider a dietary worker who is the sole supporter of her extended family, including her husband, three children, a grandchild, and her mother. Thefts of food items, such as whole chickens or boxed items, may require management to investigate this employee's lower-order needs.

Supervisors also must emphasize a working climate conducive to satisfying the higher-order growth needs by offering some variety of duties, delegation of authority, autonomy, and responsibility so that employees can more fully realize their potential and their growth needs.

Alderfer's ERG Model (1972)

Content or need theorist Clayton Alderfer did not totally agree with Maslow. He identified three categories of needs: existence, relatedness, and growth (ERG). These needs may surface when frustration occurs. His frustration–regression hypothesis states that when individuals are frustrated in meeting or achieving higher-need levels, they regress and seek to fulfill lower-level needs again. Furthermore, more than one level of need can cause motivation simultaneously.

Existence needs are those that are material or psychological desires. These are satisfied by basic support resources such as food, water, shelter,

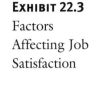

EXHIBIT 22.3

Factors
Affecting Job
Satisfaction

% who rate as very important:

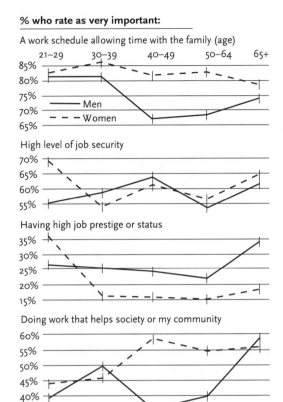

A work schedule allowing time with the family (age)

High level of job security

Having high job prestige or status

Doing work that helps society or my community

SOURCE: Adapted with permission from *Business & Health*, Vol. 18, No. 8. Medical Economics Co., Montvale, NJ.

working conditions, and pay. They are items that are divided among people, and one person's gain is another's loss.

Relatedness needs involve relationships. These are satisfied by having friends, family, and coworkers. These friendships allow for sharing feelings and thoughts, being accepted and having one's worth confirmed by others, and understanding.

The last category of need is that of growth. Growth needs encourage a person to be productive or creative. This need is satisfied by contributing in a problem-solving environment or having opportunities for personal development.

Alderfer's ERG model can be placed on a dimensional plane across Maslow's hierarchical pyramid, revealing a distinction between the degrees of introversion and extroversion. For example, an introvert at the level of relatedness might be more concerned with her own perceptions of being included in a group, whereas an extrovert at that same level may pay more attention to

Alderfer's ERG model
A motivation model based on three levels—existence, relatedness, and growth.

how others value that membership (Huitt 1998). More apparent is the correlation between Maslow's and Alderfer's need categories. Maslow's physiological and safety needs tie to Alderfer's existence needs. The social needs described by Maslow compare to Alderfer's relatedness needs. Finally, Maslow's remaining two tiers are consistent with Alderfer's growth needs.

Herzberg's Two-Factor Motivation–Hygiene Theory
The theory that workplace factors can be divided into two categories, those that do not motivate (hygiene factors) and those that do (motivators).

Herzberg's Two-Factor Motivation–Hygiene Theory (1959)

Another approach to the content theory of motivation as a need classification system was Frederick Herzberg's Two-Factor Motivation–Hygiene Theory. As a psychologist, Herzberg has done much research on job satisfaction and has developed a number of conditions on which satisfaction is based. He distinguishes between those factors at the workplace that are unlikely to motivate employees (hygiene factors) and those that tend to motivate employees (motivators). In essence, he states that the hygiene rewards satisfy what are commonly known as lower-order needs, whereas the motivators satisfy higher-order needs. Herzberg identifies the groups listed in Exhibit 22.4 as hygiene factors and as motivators.

Herzberg (1966)[1] measures satisfiers and dissatisfiers by how frequently they appear and how long they produce either a significant improvement or reduction in job satisfaction (see Exhibit 22.5). The five hygiene factors are environmental. When they are at an unacceptable level, that is, they are negative or lacking, they are noticed, and dissatisfaction occurs. When they are at an acceptable level, they are unnoticed, and satisfaction results. The factors most frequently involved in events causing job dissatisfaction (dissatisfiers) are company policy and administration, supervision, interpersonal relations, working conditions, and salary. Even when they are positive and appropriate, these factors do not tend to motivate people; they are expected. At this level, they are satisfiers.

This, however, does not mean that the hygiene factors are unimportant. They are essential because whether they exist or not is either satisfying or dissatisfying. Therefore, the manager must make certain that administra-

EXHIBIT 22.4
Herzberg's Two-Factor Motivation–Hygiene Theory

HYGIENE FACTORS	MOTIVATION FACTORS
The organization's policy and administration	Achievement
Technical supervision	Recognition
Interpersonal relations	The work itself
Working conditions	Responsibility
Salary	Advancement

EXHIBIT 22.5

Factors
Affecting Job
Attitudes

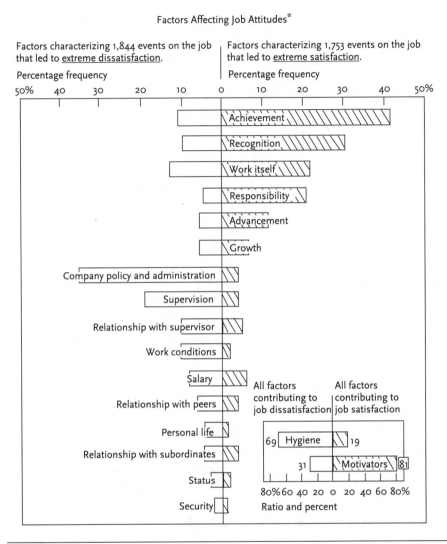

Factors Affecting Job Attitudes*

Factors characterizing 1,844 events on the job that led to extreme dissatisfaction.

Factors characterizing 1,753 events on the job that led to extreme satisfaction.

*As reported in 12 investigations. Exhibit does not include duration data.

SOURCE: Herzberg (1966). Used with permission.

tion and policies are fair and suitable, that pay and benefits are appropriate, that technical supervision is acceptable, that working conditions are safe and healthy, and so forth. By providing these factors at the proper level, the manager does not give the employees the opportunity to feel motivated, but these factors do keep them from being dissatisfied.

If managers really want motivated employees, they should use motivators. Herzberg's study indicates that the most frequently mentioned factors in improved job satisfaction are achievement, recognition, the work itself, responsibility, and advancement. It is the opportunity for advancement; greater responsibility; and promotion, growth, achievement, and interesting work that make a job challenging, meaningful, and really motivating to subordinates. A Watson Wyatt (2000) survey found that the top three nonmonetary rewards for employees under the age of 30 were (1) advancement opportunities (76 percent), (2) flexible work schedules (73 percent), and (3) the opportunity to learn new skills (68 percent). Interestingly, the factors that affect job satisfaction differ somewhat for people of different ages and genders (see Exhibit 22.3). The manager, therefore, should give the employees an opportunity to experience these motivational factors in an environment conducive to growth. Such motivational factors are obviously associated with the higher-order needs of people: They are related to the work content, whereas the hygiene factors relate to the work environment.

Herzberg's findings have important implications for the supervisor. Although management strives for good organizational hygiene through sound wage administration, enlightened supervision, pleasant working conditions, appropriate fringe benefits, and so forth, these factors alone normally do not produce a motivational climate. If properly fulfilled, they merely minimize dissatisfaction. What is actually required to achieve motivation is a two-way effort that is directed first at the hygiene factors and then at the development of motivation. In addition to the need to avoid unpleasantness that comes from largely dissatisfying conditions, the supervisor must produce positive motivation through a more sophisticated set of factors, which is closely related to the concept of self-actualization. Although it is difficult to apply these motivators in some situations, most positions in the healthcare setting provide ample opportunity for a manager to emphasize them. More information on Herzberg's theory appears in Appendix 22.1.

McClelland's Achievement Theory
The theory that individuals are motivated by their needs for affiliation, achievement, and power.

McClelland's Achievement Theory (1961)

Another approach to the content view of motivation concerns other important needs, as defined by David McClelland's Achievement Theory. McClelland and colleagues' (1953) research in organizational behavior led to what he has termed *learned needs* and is now commonly known as need for achievement (*n Ach*), need for affiliation (*n Aff*), and need for power (*n Pow*). The need for achievement is a need for personal challenge and accomplishment. It involves the desire to assume personal responsibility and pursue reasonably difficult goals, a preoccupation with the task, and specific and quick feedback as to accomplishment. This *n Ach* is obviously essential for a successful manager; it is critical for development in early childhood and can be used by adults as well. McClelland defines it as behavior toward competition with a standard of excellence.

The need for affiliation is the need for human companionship, support, and reassurance. People with a strong *n Aff* look for approval and reassurance from others, are willing to conform to the norms and wishes of others, and are sincerely interested in the feelings of others. They are likely to do well in situations that include a lot of social interaction. On the other hand, this trait can be distracting and have a negative impact on work performance.

The third need is the need for power, or need for dominance. The *n Pow* is a need to influence others and to lead and control them. Today we call this type of individual a driver. Those with strong *n Pow* are willing to make decisions. One of McClelland's studies concluded that all managers tend to have a stronger power motive than the general population and that successful managers tend to have stronger power motives than do less successful managers (McClelland and Burnham 1976).

Human behavior is controlled by these three needs. The intensity of desire for each may vary from situation to situation. For example, some people are drivers at work and become followers when at home (Exhibit 22.6).

Levels of Aspiration

A person's level of aspiration is closely related to the order of needs. Shifts in level of aspiration cause an individual to adjust his goals upward as various needs are satisfied. For example, suppose an individual is highly motivated by the need to achieve, and attitudes and personality cause him to look for such satisfaction by working as a laboratory technician in a healthcare center.

This person will not be satisfied for long by being a phlebotomist. Once the phlebotomist position has been attained, he is likely to strive for the next higher position, such as laboratory technician, then laboratory scientist, then laboratory director, and so on. The objectives that present possibilities for the satisfaction of the achievement needs also may shift to something outside the hospital, such as governmental activities, perhaps serving as deputy director of the Centers for Disease Control and Prevention.

This endless search for alternatives to satisfy increasing aspirations is an important aspect of human motivation. If an organization can provide an individual with a wider range of need satisfactions, this person will have a greater commitment to the organization.

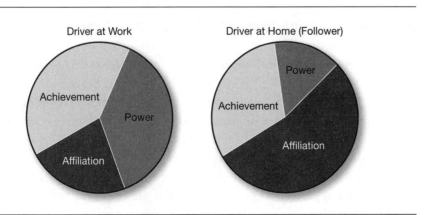

Driver at Work

Driver at Home (Follower)

Exhibit 22.6
McClelland's Achievement Theory of Influence, by Situation

Vroom's Expectancy Model
The theory that people act in a certain way because they anticipate that the behavior will achieve the outcome or goal desired.

Vroom's Expectancy Model (1964)

Process theorists speculated that motivation was driven by external influences. Theorists Victor Vroom and B. F. Skinner assess why and how people choose certain behaviors to meet their needs. **Vroom's Expectancy Model** suggests that people tend to act in a particular manner because they anticipate that the behavior will achieve the outcome or goal desired; that is, the amount of effort put forth by a person is directly related to the reward expected and the person's perceived ability to reach the goal. For example, if I pursue this certification program, I expect to be promoted to shift supervisor. Expectancy is the belief that if one puts forth effort X, the direct result will be Y. There must be a willingness on the individual's part to exert a high level of effort to reach an objective and satisfy an individual need.

The degree of effort is based on the individual's belief that the probability of achieving the goal will be reached and a reward will be received. This is the equity consideration each employee gives when completing an assignment. *Equity* is the perception of fairness in rewards or compensation given. Individuals perceive rewards differently and consequently exert more or less effort to obtain them. If rewards are given out inconsistently, employees may perceive the distribution as inequitable and hold back their contribution of effort. This theory has a significant bearing on facts we must consider when conducting performance evaluations (see Chapter 19) and may identify why some individuals with ability do not demonstrate merit.

Thus, for one to proceed through Vroom's expectancy model, three steps must occur. First, the individual must assess the probability that she can complete the assignment or do the job. If that probability is high, she will take the second step—evaluate the probability of getting a reward for doing the job. In this step she must determine how well the job or assignment must be performed to get a reward and try to accurately speculate what the reward will be. If the desire still exists to pursue the assignment and now the reward, she will take step three—do the job and hope that she will get what is expected.

Skinner's Reinforcement Model
The theory that behavior can be controlled through the use of rewards.

B. F. Skinner's Reinforcement Model (1938 and 1953)

Another process theory is that of reinforcement. B. F. **Skinner's Reinforcement Model** ties nicely to Vroom's theory because it is the reward that reinforces certain behavior on the part of the employee. However, reinforcement can also be negative. Punishment, such as counseling for excessive absenteeism or suspension for using inappropriate language, discourages an employee's behavior.

Skinner, a psychologist, determined that behaviors can be controlled through the use of rewards. He believed that employees who receive rewards for exceptional performance on one assignment are willing to take on other assignments and perform them well as long as the employee knows he will be rewarded. Under Skinner's approach, to get people to behave in a certain way, the supervisor must reward them every time. Rewards can be symbolic, monetary, or related to prestige or public recognition. This may explain why programs modeled after the **Pike Place Fish Market** in Seattle are popular and successful in organizations today: individuals strive to accumulate a large number of certificates or fish charms to demonstrate their exceptional performance. The important point is that a reward is offered that is desired by the employee, it is given as soon as possible after the employee has accomplished the task, and the employee perceives the reward worthy of his efforts. Failure to perform in a way that was expected results in no reward.

Pike Place Fish Market model
A motivational model based on the practices at a popular fish market in Seattle where employees perform for customers to show how much they enjoy their work.

Who Is Right?

If we follow Vroom's and Skinner's notions, motivation simply is one of the rewards for good work and deprivation of rewards or punishment for bad work. Clearly, motivation starts with personal recognition and appreciation (*Medical Office Manager* 2000). However, the employee will also apply probability to his decision—that is, his risk in performing or not performing the assignment or the degree of effort he will put forth. The calculating effort is directly related to the realistic level of the work assigned. Just because an employee was able to unpack 40 cases of canned goods in central supply today does not mean that giving him a reward will encourage him to unpack 80 cases tomorrow. Remember that as supervisors you have different needs than your staff. You need higher productivity from your team, but your team desires shorter shifts.

Lastly, supervisors should be motivators, but they can be motivation destroyers, too. Remember that rewards do not need to be monetary to be considered rewards by an employee. The simple pat on the back or thank you can motivate an employee to exhibit a certain behavior. Moreover, rewards that show an extra effort by the supervisor, such as issuing a certificate or writing a thank you note, can significantly increase motivation levels. Failing to distribute those rewards in a timely and sincere fashion is sure to kill motivation in the workplace.

Delnor Hospital in Geneva, Illinois, used simple rewards as motivators that paid back the hospital handsomely. The organization took the position "that satisfied employees provide better patient care. In a time of national shortage of healthcare workers, the best way to fill vacancies may be by preventing them" (Solovy 2001). The hospital's recognition program was publicized, praise was given publicly in mini-celebrations at the rewarded employee's worksite, and coworkers were given the means to reward each other with $5 gift certificates. Departments rated each other, and the ratings were published. When the organization achieved its financial, patient satisfaction, and turnover goals, everyone received a bonus (Solovy 2001).

HOSPITAL LAND

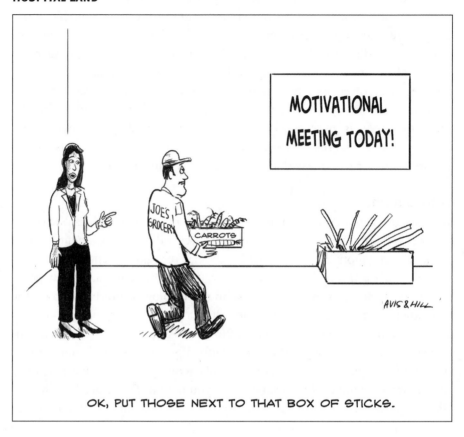

No one motivational technique works all the time. An approach that encourages one employee to perform a task well may not be the best technique to encourage another employee to execute the same task. Much has been written on motivational techniques, and this chapter has not discussed all the theorists. Additional research may yield information on a theorist who may have the right solution for your situation.

Perceptions, Values, and Attitudes

As we have said, all human behavior is motivated by unsatisfied needs. These needs spring from causes that are deep within the person and, together with other motives, attitudes, and behaviors, form the configuration usually called the personality. From this point of view, the motivation that contributes to personality can be defined as the potential to act to satisfy those needs that are not met. The phrase "potential to act" implies that some motives are stronger than others and thus more likely to produce action. The strength of motivation is determined by the strength of a particular need and the probability that the act required to satisfy that need will be successful and the rewards forth-coming. An individual is more likely to act if her motive is stronger, the probability for success is high, and the reward is perceived by her to be significant.

Other factors are also involved in producing human behavior or action—motives do not stand alone. Closely related to them and significantly affecting their strength are perceptions, values, and attitudes. We are constantly subjected to many stimuli from our environment, and all of them compete for our attention. In our daily working environment there are noises, sights, sounds, smells, supervisors' instructions, memos, reports, physicians' directives, coworkers' remarks, people walking by, beepers, phones ringing, posted signs, and so on. The individual is challenged to interpret and organize the more important stimuli and respond to them appropriately.

To do so, he uses perception to screen, select, organize, and interpret the stimuli. This does not necessarily lead to an accurate portrayal of the environment, but it does create a unique picture that is influenced by the perceiver's needs, desires, values, disposition, and frame of reference. Through the process of **perceptual selectivity**, certain stimuli catch one's attention and are selected, whereas one screens out those she either does not want to bother with or finds uncomfortable.

perceptual selectivity
The process by which an individual selects which stimuli to respond to and which to screen out.

The perceptual process plays an important role in all managerial activities, including making decisions, appraising employees, communicating orally, and writing. It is important for the manager to understand the perceptual process and to realize that people perceive events, situations, and actions differently.

Perceptual organization is how an individual categorizes, groups, and fills in information systematically. Once meaning has been attached to a certain stimulus, an individual can deliver an appropriate response. Several barriers to accurate perception, however, can enter into these perceptual processes. Examples of barriers include the perceiver's frame of reference, stereotyping, the halo effect, the perceiver's biases, and perceptual defense (see chapters 5 and 19). All the perceptual processes affect a person's attitudes and behavior at work.

Attitudes and values also play a role in all behavior. Values are closely held normative standards; the individual chooses them based on personal preference. "Values carry with them an 'oughtness' component. They are frequently defined as ideas about how everyone should feel or behave" (Mitchell 1982; see also Steers 1988). Values are broader, general, more encompassing concepts than are attitudes. For example, most of us value freedom and equality; our values of equality can be translated into our attitude toward minority groups.

Attitudes can be viewed as "a predisposition to respond in a favorable or unfavorable way to objects, persons, concepts, or whatever" (Mitchell 1982; see also Steers 1988). They are the ways an individual tends to interpret, understand, or define a situation or relationship with others. Attitudes constitute one's feelings about something—likes and dislikes directed toward persons, things, situations, or a combination of all three. They are more than casual opinions, as they are heavily charged with emotional overtones. Attitudes may include feelings as well as intellectual sensibilities. They also include evaluations and value judgments. Attitudes differ in type, strength, and the extent to which they are open or hidden.

Attitudes are revealed in two ways: (1) by the individual's expressed statements or (2) by behavior. An individual may express dislike for her manager, or she may merely demonstrate this attitude by being absent excessively. Although we cannot see perceptions, values, and attitudes, their consequences can be observed in behavior.

Factors That Determine Attitudes

Attitudes are learned from prior experiences. An infinite number of factors determine and influence an individual's attitudes. One major influence is a person's biological, or physiological, makeup. Such factors as sex, age, height, race, weight, and physique are important in determining the attitudes that contribute to overall personality structure. In addition, many psychologists believe that the very early years of life are crucial to attitudinal development. Freudian psychologists (those who subscribe to the theories of Sigmund Freud), in particular, believe that early childhood is the most critical period in shaping what a person actually becomes. This theory is often referred to as childhood determinism; it maintains that such factors as feeding patterns, training patterns, and home conditions in early childhood are the primary determinants of personality structure.

Another area that influences a person's attitudes and personality is the immediate environment. Education, employment, income, and many other experiences that confront an individual as he goes through life influence who this person is today and what he eventually becomes. Furthermore, the broader culture of society influences a person's attitudes. In the United States, people generally believe in competition, reward for accomplishment, equal opportunities, and other values that are part of the democratic capitalistic society. Individuals learn from their early years to strive for achievement, think for themselves, and work hard; they learn these roads lead to success.

As the United States becomes even more of a melting pot, dominant attitudes and beliefs may be shifting. For example, some people may be willing to compromise the freedom Americans now enjoy to do essentially whatever they want and whenever they want to do it in response to heightened concerns about safety and security that arose in the aftermath of several disastrous incidents in recent years. These influencing events include the shooting at Columbine (Colorado) High School in 1999; the damage wrought by the bombs sent through the U.S. Postal Service by Theodore Kaczynski, the so-called Unabomber, in the 1970s, 1980s, and 1990s; the deliberate explosion of the Alfred P. Murrah Federal Building in Oklahoma City in 1995; the bomb that detonated in Atlanta at the 1996 Summer Olympics; and the 2001 airplane hijackings by terrorists that resulted in deadly attacks against the World Trade Center Twin Towers in New York City and the Pentagon in Washington, D.C. These events and countless other cultural factors affect a person's attitudes and thus behavior.

Attitudes and Behavior

No matter what factors have caused their development, attitudes become deep-seated attributes of the individual's makeup. They are learned and acquired through a person's life experiences, and they do not have to be rational or logical. We hold firmly to our attitudes and resist forces that attempt to interfere with them. Attitudes can change, but they change slowly. Attitudes not only exist within individuals but also are generated within groups. Often individuals accept as their own the attitudes of the group to which they belong.

As shown in Exhibit 22.1, needs and motives do not stand alone as determinants of behavior. They are also influenced by the underlying attitudes and values of a person. Indeed, we can say that values and attitudes determine the route a person takes for the satisfaction of her needs. Although the same basic needs are manifest in every person, attitudes vary greatly and affect individuals' unique responses to their needs. In other words, attitudes help determine what motivates a person to take a certain action to fulfill a certain need. For example, many people may have a strong need for achievement, but differing attitudes and values motivate them to seek fulfillment of that need through much different means. One may do this by working in a hospital, another by working in a government agency, yet another by working in a specific industry, and a fourth by teaching in a university or going into politics. Similarly one individual may find fulfillment as a cook in a nursing home's kitchen, while another may find it as a chemist in a research laboratory.

Motivation Versus Frustration

If the individual's chosen route results in goal accomplishment, his need is satisfied, the attitudes are reinforced, and the reinforcement serves as feedback for future goal setting. What happens, however, if the chosen course of action does not result in goal accomplishment? What happens when an individual wishes to pursue a certain course of action but is prevented from doing so by an external or internal circumstance?

Generally, actions that do not succeed in obtaining goals result in blocked satisfaction, frustration, and anxiety. As shown in Exhibit 22.1, feedback notifies the individual as to whether his needs are being fulfilled. The stress of negative feedback results in frustration and anxiety. People usually resolve the problems of conflict and frustration in five basic ways: (1) problem-solving behavior, (2) resignation, (3) detour behavior, (4) retreat, or (5) aggression.

Problem-solving behavior is usually the most desirable way of resolving frustration. It is advantageous if a person can look at problems objectively and base her decisions on reasoned analysis of the situation. Consider basketball superstar Michael Jordan's experience, for example: "When I got cut from the varsity team as a sophomore in high school, I learned something. I knew I never wanted to feel that bad again. I never wanted to have that taste in my mouth, that hole in my stomach. So I set a goal of becoming a starter on the varsity" (Gilbert 1999). However, many people are not capable of assessing a personal obstacle objectively and of problem solving to address frustration; it is the supervisor's duty to help the employees learn problem-solving behavior. This assistance can be initiated with nondirective interviews, as discussed in Chapter 18.

Using Non-directive Interviews to Overcome Obstacles and Conflict

Supervisors should encourage subordinates to come to them with their problems, both work and aspiration related. Conducting nondirective interviews for work-related issues shows the employee that the supervisor is willing to hear employees. The absence of such opportunities may turn minor irritations into major problems. The supervisor must realize that inherent in the managerial position is an invisible barrier between the supervisor and the subordinates. Some employees have little difficulty speaking to their supervisors, but many may be more timid. Therefore, the supervisor must make an effort to encourage those who are reluctant to reveal their thoughts. The supervisor should make sure that time is always available to listen to the subordinates. If time is not available at the moment an issue arises, the interview may be postponed for a few hours; in this way the supervisor may allow enough time and not rush through the discussion.

The principal function of the nondirective interview is to alert the supervisor as to what the interviewee really thinks and feels and what lies at the root of a particular problem such as excessive turnover, absenteeism, or complaints about work or the department. In addition, it gives the interviewee a feeling of relief and helps the subordinate develop greater insight into her own problems, often finding solutions while thinking out loud. Many sources of frustration exist within and outside the working environment, and unrelieved frustration may lead to undesirable responses, such as seeking support from the informal group leader. Another, potentially more detrimental, response is for the frustrated employee to behave badly, perhaps by being absent from work regularly or openly complaining about her employer.

For aspiration-related issues, the principles of the nondirective interview are similar. It is an opportunity for the supervisor to hear where the employee aspires to go within the organization. It is an ideal time for the supervisor to suggest different courses of action for the employee to consider, being careful not to bias or encourage one over the other. Suppose, for instance, that a licensed practical nurse (LPN) is eager to advance to a better position, but all better positions demand the registered nurse (RN) degree as a prerequisite. The LPN is frustrated because he keeps running into this obstacle and believes he is unable to find the time to become licensed as an RN. In this case, an analysis of the situation and a thorough discussion with the supervisor could encourage the LPN to obtain the RN degree through an online program in a way that does not interfere with his work schedule. This option will enable him to move up within the hierarchy of nursing services. Such a route consti-tutes intelligent problem-solving behavior.

The interview also may identify work processes or organization policies that are perceived as roadblocks to employees growing within the organiza-tion and thus leading them to consider employment opportunities outside the institution. Finally, it provides the supervisor with valuable insight into factors that motivate this employee and others to progress within their department or another unit in the organization if provided a vehicle or an opportunity to do so. This is part of the supervisor's role as a coach and mentor.

The ground rule for conducting a nondirective interview is to let the interviewee say whatever he wants to say. Conducting such an interview is more difficult than conducting a directive interview. It demands the concen-trated listening and continuous attention of the supervisor. The supervisor must exert self-control and hide her own ideas and emotions during the in-terview. She should not interrupt, argue, or change the subject. The super-visor should not express approval or disapproval even though the employee may request it. This limitation may prove exasperating to both parties, but it is essential.

In such a counseling interview, the employee must feel like he can speak openly. In all likelihood, as soon as all the negative feelings or anxieties have been expressed, the employee will start to find some favorable aspects of the same issues he had criticized earlier. When the employee is encouraged to ver-balize problems and frustrations, he may gain greater insight into these trou-bles or may arrive at an answer or a course of action that will help solve the difficulties. The employee must be permitted to work through difficulties alone, without being interrupted and advised by the interviewer.

If the problem concerns the job, work, and organization, however, the nondirective interview structure may not be appropriate. The supervisor may have to be directive so that the solution is consistent with the needs of the institution.

If the concerns are personal in nature, the supervisor should exercise great care not to give advice or become burdened with the task of running the subordinate's personal life. Most of the time the interviewee wants a sympa-thetic or empathic listener, not an adviser. The average supervisor is not equipped to provide counseling, and this is not part of the job. If necessary, the subordinate should be referred to trained specialists—for example, one of the institution's social workers or psychologists—or the organization's employee assistance program. This may be necessary when sensitive areas and deep-seated personality problems are involved. The patient–psychiatrist relationship is separate from that of subordinate and boss.

When Conflict Goes Unchecked

Some people can tolerate conflict and frustration better than others, but eventually the strain can affect anyone's performance, and conflict resolution becomes necessary. When employees do not believe they can approach their supervisor or another for guidance, they naturally resort to other alternatives. One such way to solve a conflict is by resignation. Suppose our LPN from the earlier example thinks, "What else can I do? I have to stick it out." The LPN seems resigned to his lot. This LPN will keep working for the healthcare institution but may no longer consider himself a part of it. Once an employee has given up in the face of obstacles, it is difficult to rebuild morale to the point at which institutional and departmental goals continue to be important for this person. Some employees simply stay on the job, listlessly performing their duties until they are able to retire. Such employees are usually passive and resistant to change. They are difficult for the supervisor to deal with because new ideas do not excite or stimulate them. The supervisor may try to restimulate the employee to strive either for past goals or toward some new and desirable goals that address the employee's needs. A sense of resignation in an employee usually results in her inferior performance on the job; it also can lower the morale of the department and foster a climate that is not conducive to its best performance.

Another way to solve a frustrating situation is to resort to detour behavior. With the direct way of reaching the goal barred, the employee tries to find another way to get there. Such detours, however, are often obscure and sometimes devious. For example, one kind of detour behavior is self-induced illness. Children learn early in life that being sick gives them an acceptable excuse for getting out of doing an unpleasant task. Similarly, employees often avoid conflict by inducing, many times subconsciously, painful and real physical disorders.

Retreat, or leaving the field, is a third way to meet the problems of conflict and frustration. Most people at one time or another have looked at their jobs and wished they could quit right then. They may believe that they are not getting the satisfaction they thought the position would bring, that no one realizes the difficulties involved in the job, that their supervisor does not appreciate all their efforts, and so on. Most people have such feelings sometime in their lives. In many instances an employee finds it necessary to leave the organization and find alternative employment. Whether this reaction to frustration is good or bad, however, depends on the major source of the conflict and frustration. If the major source is the employee's personality and the conflict does not stem from the working situation, leaving the field is not the right answer. In other words, if the frustration is caused by the person's own particular psychological makeup, quitting probably will not bring about the desired result. If, however, the conflict is the result of an unfavorable work situation, leaving may represent a real solution to the problem. Often it is difficult for the individual to determine whether this is the case. Of course, it is not always necessary to quit the job or move to another city to leave the field. "Leaving the field" may be displayed by daydreaming, spending a lot of time in the washroom, surfing the Internet during the workday, developing a high rate of absenteeism, resorting to alcoholism and drug abuse, or using some other form of symbolic escape.

Aggression is the fourth way in which people may meet the problem of severe frustration. Sabotage is one common form of aggressive behavior that serves as a response to frustration. Aggression not only refers to overtly hostile behavior aimed at harming other people or to hostile behavior toward inanimate objects, but also to the tendency to commit acts of aggression. This tendency may manifest itself in thoughts or words, or even in feelings that have not yet been put into words. In one situation, the staff of a dietary department used various forms of sabotage to express frustration with management: patients were served raw chicken and in some cases empty, but heated, plates. Their dissatisfaction was clear.

The supervisor should always remember that frustration and aggression are closely linked and that all aggression stems from frustration. The job of the supervisor is to see that frustration is minimized and to provide constructive outlets for it. The supervisor should try to anticipate sources of frustration and eliminate them. If this cannot be done, the supervisor should ensure that the causes of frustration are not aggravated. Often listening patiently helps to ease employee tensions, and it may enable the subordinate to seek the real source of the frustration. A supervisor's talent can be measured by her ability to accurately determine when a subordinate needs both patient listening and advice or only patient listening.

Conflicts Between Individual and Organizational Goals

A major cause of frustration arises when individual needs and goals conflict rather than coincide with those of the organization or department. Much has been written about the conflict between the individual who seeks action and independence and the climate of a bureaucratic, formalized organization that stifles a person's natural desire for freedom and self-determination. The consequences of this type of frustration are high turnover, waste, lower productivity, slowdown, lack of innovative and creative behavior, nonacceptance of leadership, and so on. The most serious consequence of a bureaucratic organization, however, is that it blocks the individual from attaining satisfaction of her needs.

Managers today are becoming more aware of these consequences and of the necessity for an organization to provide a climate that enables its employees to find personal satisfaction. In fact, the need for an appropriate organizational climate is increasing because of the rising expectations of employees. This is especially true in the healthcare field, in which organizations are confronted with ever-advancing and more sophisticated activity. The highly skilled and educated employees are primarily professionals who expect to fulfill many of their needs on the job. Because such employees tend to take high wages and appropriate fringe benefits for granted, it should be apparent that the key to long-term motivation for them rests in the satisfaction of the higher-level needs—that is, their esteem and self-fulfillment needs. It is management's duty to develop an organizational climate that produces effective motivation and satisfaction of these needs, thereby helping resolve the conflict between individual and organizational goals. Therefore, a supervisor must know the basic motivational processes because this knowledge allows her to facilitate high levels of job satisfaction and minimize conflicts.

Modifying Motivational Techniques

Flinn (2001) aptly states, "Achieving a clear understanding of human nature is an important aspect of management in the work place." For managers and staff to work together as an effective and productive unit, staff members must know how they fit into the overall scheme of the organization. Likewise managers must clearly understand how they can maximize productivity by supporting their employees through the appropriate leadership style. It is also extremely important for managers to realistically evaluate the working environment, as well as the characteristics of the task, to decide how best to deal with employees.

A supervisor today likely works with a multigenerational team or workforce (see Chapter 21 for a discussion of the generations currently in the U.S. workforce).

Clearly, the younger members of your team were raised during a time that differed substantially from that of older team members. Exhibit 22.7 depicts

EXHIBIT 22.7
Top Problems in Public Schools: 1940s Versus Late 1990s

1940	1996–1998
Talking out of turn	Drug/alcohol abuse
Chewing gum	Physical attacks/assault
Making noise	Theft and larceny
Running in the halls	Pregnancy
Cutting in line	Rape
Dress code infractions	Violence/gangs

SOURCES: Morrison (1997); Phi Delta Kappa (1998).

some of the problems encountered in schools in the 1940s through late 1990s; this list reflects changes in U.S. culture over time. A significant concern is reflected in the problems we see today by performing a simple Internet search of the terms "public," "school," and "problems": violence and shootings, physical and emotional bullying, gangs, guns, drugs, cheating and lying, and immorality.

Working with the Generations and Diversity

In Chapter 21 we discussed the challenges of managing a workforce composed of multiple generations and cultures. A great deal of change has occurred since the 1960s. Technology and telecommunications have shrunk the size of the world and altered international relations. Business has grown from these changes, and so have the perspectives of your staff. As the global economy expands, the diversity of the U.S. workforce increases accordingly. Team members from different countries and cultures have joined the American workforce and brought with them different values, attitudes, and needs.

Generation X employees grew up in a world in which access to information was relatively immediate and the ability to absorb and analyze this information was imperative. Computing technology advanced as quickly as the gen Xers were maturing. The year 1969 brought microchips, 1971 brought time-shared computers, 1973 brought microprocessors, and 1977 brought Apple personal computers. The 1980s introduced affordable laptop computers, and since that time computers have become more powerful, smaller, and cheaper. While growing up, members of Generation X were shuttled from one sporting event to another and between home and daycare by dual-career baby boomer parents. These activities taught gen Xers at least two things: (1) schedule your time wisely so you can fit everything in and (2) learn how to survive in a group, because your family is likely not around much to support you.

Furthermore, a trend toward socially conscious employment has become apparent. Current regulations recognize that workers must be given time to attend to their families and their lives. The Family Medical Leave Act, state initiatives on same-sex marriages, and similar provisions support the need for organizations to be more sensitive to worker–family requirements. Given these changes, we are seeing more and more organizations abandoning the traditional top-down, rigid, hierarchical structures. Team involvement in decision making is paramount with the growing level of specialized expertise that is needed in today's healthcare organization. Team leaders and managers must be flexible and ready to deal with changes and have available to them a group of advisers, who are often team members, to chart the course through the rapidly changing healthcare environment.

Generation Y members are not motivated by the fear of poverty, economic disasters, or international terrorism. They grew up during a time of ambitious social programs, higher taxes, and a flourishing *and* floundering economy that was being infiltrated by foreign firms. However, they are both experiencing their first economic downturn and may respond to financial incentives (see Chapter 23) in order to offset the debts of their college education and maintain their technology status. Both generations recognize that the level of security in the United States differs sharply from what prior generations experienced, and because of incidents of terrorism, they are more conscious of life-limiting odds and desire to gain the most from life and their families. This is true for medical staff members as well, with more early-career physicians looking for part-time work options in order to raise young children and preferring to be employed, rather than self-employed (Bakhtiari 2009, 15).

Generation Yers graduated from high school in the twenty-first century. They know computers, and they are and will be expert at using multimedia, networking tools, the Internet, and technology not yet developed. Not only do their music preferences differ from previous generations (as expected), but their dress also differs considerably. As far as boomers and the silent generation (1925–1945) are concerned, neither gen Xers nor gen Yers dress appropriately. To these younger generations, fashion is not used to make a statement, with generation Yers leaning toward an androgynous look. Unlike boomers and silenters, both Xers and Yers grew up on their own, as both parents worked. Many were reared in divorced and single-parent homes. This has made them independent but desirous of a "better" family atmosphere.

Graeme Codrington (2001a) suggests the leadership style most effective for generation Xers is consultative; for generation Yers (or millennials), it is grand and expansive. In fact, he predicts that Yers are being groomed to be a civic-minded, community-oriented workforce (Codrington 2001b). (See Exhibit 22.8 for a list of generational traits.) Ensman (2000) says these younger employees often seek instant gratification and certainly lack patience and an understanding of workplace fundamentals such as punctuality, terms of formal address, and workplace etiquette. Their supervisor needs to teach them these skills on the job and during their orientation.

It is anticipated that younger employees will not remain with the organization long term. The silenter trait of staying with an employer for 20, 30, or more years only to receive the traditional gold watch at retirement is not apparent with the gen X and Y employees. They will move from one job to another for better pay; a better title; more material benefits such as an office, a car, and an expense account; and more flexibility allowing a balance between work and family.

According to Ensman (2000), younger employees may voice open-ended complaints or frustrations and may not know how to address problems. He says they might be bothered by situations or acts that an older employee would shrug off, and they may appear inarticulate, gruff, whiny, or

EXHIBIT 22.8 What Makes the Generations Tick?

NAME	PERIOD	U.S. POPULATION	EVENTS AND INFLUENCES	VALUES AND CHARACTERISTICS	MANAGEMENT STYLE THEORY
Silenters	1925–1945	75 million	Depression; Pearl Harbor; WWII; radio; manufacturing advances; big band; TV; copier	"Family" values; head of household works; modest income; company loyalty; financially conservative; expect respect for their experiences	X
Baby Boomers	1946–1964	76 million	Vietnam; Watergate; Kennedy and King assassinations; Civil Rights movement; rock and roll; space travel; marijuana; hippies; women's equality	High divorce rate; career advancement; entrepreneurs; workaholics; desire material items; small families; slower economic growth affecting income, creating desire for bonuses	X/Y
Generation X	1965–1979/80	17 million	Racial integration; school bussing; rapid technology changes; floppy disk; telecom advances; both parents working; latchkey; cocaine; anti-war	Volunteer work; later-life marriages; better family life; group oriented; career minded; achievement obsessed; may still live at home; tech savvy; want to follow their own rules to get job done	Y
Generation Y (Millennials, Echo Boomers)	1980–2000+	60 million plus	Racial and ethnic diversity; economic prosperity; dual-income families; Internet; single parents; cable TV; iPods/mobile technology; street drugs; environmental disasters; terrorism; cloning; gay rights	Better family life; conservation; ecology; financial responsibility; desire meaningful work; career driven; fast track; multitaskers and tech savvy; analytical; socially conscious	Y/Z

angry. Their behavior is likely influenced by the impatience of youth and a communication style born out of e-mail—that is, informal, direct, and often grammatically incorrect. Ensman suggests that when you hear a petty complaint or criticism, explain politely and directly why the situation exists, and if it is significant, investigate it. Furthermore, he suggests dealing with younger employees' problems privately but without offering empathy; rather, address the issues with professionalism. Often the younger employees are seeking the "why" for their assignments to understand how their efforts fit into the big picture of the department. Expect that they may offer alternatives to doing the job more often that you may have experienced with boomers and silenters. All this being said, the supervisor is to be a role model; both young and mature employees will look to her for the "right" way to approach an issue. On the other hand, the supervisor needs to understand employees' needs and values to motivate them to get the job done. Some options to consider in performing this aspect of supervision appear in appendixes 22.1 and 22.2.

What's Next?

While generation Y as a defined group may still be lingering into the 2010s, there is some indication that another generation has evolved and overlaps Y, known as generation Z. Its presence as related to the workplace appeared in the late 1990s and stretches to 2012. Interestingly, mention of gen Z appears in the Australian press more than in the United States. Generation Z is known for its high dependence on mobile technology and the Internet and, therefore, less human interaction. Woodruffe (2009) likens gen Z members' bedrooms to mission control centers rather than havens of tranquility. As such, he says this generation lacks sleep, which could affect its members' receptivity to education.

They are concerned with social justice, national security, and the environment. They will have witnessed unemployment and will be picking up the tab for the government's financial rescue. They are considered the new silent generation—not because they mirror the silenters but because their main mode of communication is technology or machinery rather than human interaction. Managers may find that these multitaskers will have short attention spans, need much stimulation, pose communication challenges, be less confident than their predecessors in the workforce, and have difficulty adapting to a life without economic prosperity (Walliker 2008; Woodruffe 2009).

Temporary Workers

As stated earlier and in Chapter 17, the healthcare organization has had to become more flexible to deal with the economic and technological changes affecting the industry today. To accommodate some of this need, management has employed more part-time and temporary workers. These workers, often categorized as contingent workers, include temporary staff employed by the human resources department or through an agency, independent contractors, leased employees, and part-time employees directly hired by the organization. The American Management Association (2000) "suggests that as staffing issues become more fluid, employers are looking to these workers to provide the flexibility necessary to move their businesses quickly."

These individuals require a different set of motivators. They know they are with your organization for a relatively short period and are considered fill-in employees, so they do not feel like they are part of your team. Most individuals want to be part of the family; one measure a supervisor can take toward this end is to include them in special activities, ad hoc problem-solving groups, and events organized for the department. Notes from department or team meetings should be shared with them if they are unable to attend. Give this contingent workforce the training and resources they need. They should be assigned their own equipment and space and not be required to borrow (or beg to use) the equipment of full-time employees.

Training is essential; having to correct errors made by temporary staff after they leave is counterproductive. Moreover, these employees may be a valuable source of future full-time staff. The supervisor should build a mentoring relationship with them and learn more about their goals, interests, and skills. Some of these employees may have unique skills that you are seeking. As with all employees, these part-timers should be commended for doing a good job. They need to know that they are appreciated, and for that they will remember your facility as they move on to other organizations. Contingent workers can be your healthcare facility's best promoter in the community.

During the current economic downturn, the United States has seen a growing number of retiring baby boomers. This situation will provide an opportunity for healthcare organizations to engage those educated and talented retirees who desire part-time employment. Retirees often exhibit a high level of conscientiousness and reliability. However, these employees will require training as well and may need skill building in the use of technologies, including PCs.

Lastly, caution should be exercised when sharing company information with contingent workers that is sensitive, confidential, or not for public consumption. They may not have the loyalty of full-time, permanent employees and therefore may not use the same discretion in sharing information with friends and family.

Summary

Influencing is the managerial function in which the supervisor creates a climate that enables subordinates to find as much satisfaction as possible while getting the job done. The influencing function is particularly concerned with behavioral responses and interpersonal relations. Only by appropriately influencing will the supervisor instill the motivation in the department's employees to go about their jobs with enthusiasm and also to find personal fulfillment of their needs. Therefore, it is necessary for supervisors to understand basic motivational processes.

Motivation is the force that arouses, energizes, directs, and sustains human behavior. All human behavior is caused by unsatisfied needs. These needs eventually stimulate the formation of goals that motivate people to take certain actions. Motivation, however, is not only caused by unmet needs but also largely influenced by an individual's perceptions, values, attitudes, and entire personality.

An individual's attitudes are formed beginning in early childhood. They affect and are affected by an infinite number of factors in the person's life. Attitudes differ among generations and determine the individual route a person takes for the satisfaction of her needs. Although they vary in strength, most needs are basically the same in all people. Maslow speaks of a hierarchy of needs; in ascending order they are physiological needs, safety, social needs, esteem, and self-fulfillment. A person's level of aspiration is closely related to this hierarchy of needs. People generally move from one level to the next in Maslow's hierarchy.

McClelland focuses on describing other important human needs: achievement, affiliation, and power. Herzberg, in his two-factor approach, stresses the importance of motivators versus hygiene factors. He shows that the more important forces of employee motivation lie in factors related to work content and not work environment, or hygiene factors.

Vroom's expectancy theory espouses the belief that if one puts forth effort X and the risk is appropriately rewarded, the direct result will be Y. The individual must be willing to exert a high level of effort to reach an objective and to satisfy an individual need. Skinner's reinforcement theory ties nicely with Vroom's theory in that the reward reinforces certain behavior on the part of the employee.

A person who can understand his needs and attitudes fairly well is able to choose courses of action that result in achieving goals. Goal accomplishment serves as feedback to the individual; the need is satisfied and the underlying attitudes are confirmed. If a goal is not attained, however, conflict often sets in because action that does not succeed results in blocked satisfaction, frustration, and anxiety. Most people usually react to conflict and frustration in one of the following five ways: problem-solving behavior, resignation, detour behavior, retreat, or aggression.

It is the supervisor's duty to minimize frustrating situations, especially if they result from a conflict between individual and organizational goals. One way to minimize such conflicts is to recognize that in the work environment various factors influence the realization of an employee's expectations. Some of these factors are merely satisfiers and dissatisfiers (Herzberg's hygiene factors), whereas others are motivators and are able to fulfill the higher-level needs and goals of people.

Supervisors will be challenged in the years to come as new generations of workers join the workforce; these younger generations have attitudes and values that differ from their older coworkers. Supervisors will need to change their leadership style and approach with some of these employees to motivate them to adapt to a structured workplace; to accept ideas from their older, possibly less technology-proficient colleagues; and to contribute in a constructive manner to the objectives of the department and organization.

Note

1. In 1997, I had the special opportunity to speak with Frederick Herzberg. At that time, an earlier edition of this book cited a magazine article that referenced his work on satisfiers and dissatisfiers. Based on his guidance and permission to use his work in this book, I now use the original source, *Work and the Nature of Man*, published in 1966. Dr. Herzberg died at the age of 76 in January 2000.

Additional Reading

Christman, Corey. n.d. "Department Focus: Human Resources—From Collaboration Comes Motivation." [Online information; retrieved 4/12/10.] www.healthleadersmedia.com/content/MAG-211534/Department-Focus-Human-ResourcesFrom-Collaboration-Comes-Motivation.

APPENDIX 22.1

"One More Time: How Do You Motivate Employees?"

by Frederick Herzberg

How many articles, books, speeches, and workshops have pleaded plaintively, "How do I get an employee to do what I want him to do?"

The psychology of motivation is tremendously complex, and what has been unraveled with any degree of assurance is small indeed. But the dismal ratio of knowledge to speculation has not dampened the enthusiasm for new forms of snake oil that are constantly coming on the market, many of them with academic testimonials. Doubtless this article will have no depressing impact on the market for snake oil, but since the ideas expressed in it have been tested in many corporations and other organizations, it will help—I hope—to redress the imbalance in the aforementioned ratio.

"Motivating" with KITA

In lectures to industry on the problem, I have found that the audiences are anxious for quick and practical answers, so I will begin with a straightforward, practical formula for moving people.

What is the simplest, surest, and most direct way of getting someone to do something? Ask him? Tell him? Give him a monetary incentive? Show him? We need a simple way. Every audience contains the "direct action" manager who shouts, "Kick him!" And this type of manager is right. The surest and least circumlocuted way of getting someone to do something is to kick him in the pants—give him what might be called the KITA.

There are various forms of KITA, and here are some of them: Negative physical KITA is a literal application of the term and was frequently used in the past. It has, however, three major drawbacks: (1) it is inelegant; (2) it contradicts the precious image of benevolence that most organizations cherish; and (3) since it is a physical attack, it directly stimulates the autonomic nervous system, and this often results in negative feedback—the employee may just kick you in return. These factors give rise to certain taboos against negative physical KITA.

Negative psychological KITA has several advantages over negative physical KITA. First, the cruelty is not visible; the bleeding is internal and comes much later. Second, since it affects the higher cortical centers of the brain with its inhibitory powers, it reduces the possibility of physical backlash. Third, since the amount of psychological pain that a person can feel is almost infinite, the direction and site possibilities of the KITA are increased many times. Fourth, the person administering the kick can manage to be above it all and let the system accomplish the dirty work. Fifth, those who practice it receive some ego satisfaction (one-upmanship), whereas they would find drawing blood abhorrent. Finally, if the employee does complain, he can always be accused of being paranoid, since there is no tangible evidence of an actual attack.

Now, what does negative KITA accomplish? If I kick you in the rear (physically or psychologically), who is motivated? I am motivated; you move! Negative KITA does not lead to motivation, but to movement.

Let us consider motivation. If I say to you, "Do this for me or the company, and in return I will give you a reward, an incentive, more status, a promotion, all the quid pro quos that exist in the industrial organization," am I motivating you? The overwhelming opinion I receive from management people is, "Yes, this is motivation."

I have a year old Schnauzer. When it was a small puppy and I wanted it to move, I kicked it in the rear and it moved. Now that I have finished its obedience training, I hold up a dog biscuit when I want the Schnauzer to move. In this instance, who is motivated—I or the dog? The dog wants the biscuit, but it is I who want it to move. Again, I am the one who is motivated, and the dog is the one who moves. In this instance all I did was apply KITA frontally; I extended a pull instead of a push. When industry wishes to use such positive KITAs, it has available an incredible number and variety of dog biscuits (jelly beans for humans) to wave in front of the employee to get him to jump. But positive KITA is not motivation. If I kick my dog (from the front or the back), he will move. And when I want him to move again, what must I do? I must kick him again. Similarly, I can charge a man's battery, and then recharge it, and recharge it again. But it is only when he has his own generator that he can talk about motivation. He then needs no outside stimulation. He wants to do it.

Hygiene vs. Motivators

Let me rephrase the perennial question this way: How do you install a generator in an employee? A brief review of my motivation–hygiene theory of job attitudes is required before theoretical and practical suggestions can be offered. The theory was drawn from investigations using a wide variety of populations (including some in the communist countries). The findings of these studies, along with corroboration from many other investigations using different procedures, suggest that the factors involved in producing job satisfaction (and motivation) are separate and distinct from the factors that lead to job dissatisfaction.

Since separate factors need to be considered, depending on whether job satisfaction or job dissatisfaction is being examined, it follows that these two feelings are not opposites of each other. The opposite of job satisfaction is not job dissatisfaction but, rather, no job satisfaction; and, similarly, the opposite of job dissatisfaction is not job satisfaction, but no job dissatisfaction.

Two different needs of man are involved here. One set of needs can be thought of as stemming from his animal nature—the built-in drive to avoid pain from the environment, plus all the learned drives which become conditioned to the basic biological needs. For example, hunger, a basic biological drive, makes it necessary to earn money, and then money becomes a specific drive. The other set of needs relates to that unique human characteristic, the ability to achieve and, through achievement, to experience psychological growth. The stimuli for the growth needs are tasks that induce growth; in the industrial setting, they are the job content. Contrariwise, the stimuli inducing pain-avoidance behaviors are found in the job environment.

The growth or motivator factors that are intrinsic to the job are: achievement, recognition for achievement, the work itself, responsibility, and growth or advancement. The dissatisfaction-avoidance or hygiene (KITA) factors that are extrinsic to the job include: company policy and administration, supervision, interpersonal relationships, working conditions, salary, status, and security.

A composite of the factors that are involved in causing job satisfaction and job dissatisfaction, drawn from samples of 1,685 employees, is shown in Exhibit 1. (Refer to Exhibit 22.5.) The results indicate that motivators were the primary cause of satisfaction, and hygiene factors the primary cause of unhappiness on the job. As the lower right-hand part of the exhibit shows, of all the factors contributing to job satisfaction, 81% were motivators. And of all the factors contributing to the employees' dissatisfaction over their work, 69% involved hygiene elements.

Job Loading

In attempting to enrich an employee's job, management often succeeds in reducing the man's personal contribution, rather than giving him an opportunity for growth in his accustomed job. Such an endeavor, which I shall call horizontal job loading (as opposed to vertical loading, or providing motivator factors), has been the problem of earlier job enlargement programs. This activity merely enlarges the meaninglessness of the job. Some examples of this approach, and their effects, are:

- Challenging the employee by increasing the amount of production expected of him. If he tightens 10,000 bolts a day, see if he can tighten 20,000 bolts a day. The arithmetic involved shows that multiplying zero by zero still equals zero.
- Adding another meaningless task to the existing one, usually some routine clerical activity. The arithmetic here is adding zero to zero.
- Rotating the assignments of a number of jobs that need to be enriched. This means washing dishes for a while, then washing silverware. The arithmetic is substituting one zero for another zero.
- Removing the most difficult parts of the assignment in order to free the worker to accomplish more of the less challenging assignments. This traditional industrial engineering approach amounts to subtraction in the hope of accomplishing addition.

These are common forms of horizontal loading that frequently come up in preliminary brain storming session on job enrichment. The principles of vertical loading have not all been worked out as yet, and they remain rather general, but I have furnished several useful starting points for consideration in Exhibit 22.2.

APPENDIX 22.2

Principles of Vertical Job Loading

Principal Motivators Involved

A. Removing some controls while retaining accountability: Responsibility and personal achievement
B. Increasing the accountability of individuals for own work: Responsibility and recognition
C. Giving a person a complete natural unit of work (module, division, area, and so on): Responsibility, achievement, and recognition

D. Granting additional authority to an employee in his activity; job freedom: Responsibility, achievement, and recognition
E. Making periodic reports directly available to the worker himself rather than to the supervisor: Internal recognition
F. Introducing new and more difficult tasks not previously handled: Growth and learning
G. Assigning individuals specific or specialized tasks, enabling them to become experts: Responsibility, growth, and advancement

Steps to Job Enrichment

Now that the motivator idea has been described in practice, here are the steps that managers should take in instituting the principle with their employees:

1. Select those jobs in which (a) the investment in industrial engineering does not make changes too costly, (b) attitudes are poor, (c) hygiene is becoming very costly, and (d) motivation will make a difference in performance.
2. Approach these jobs with the conviction that they can be changed. Years of tradition have led managers to believe that the content of the jobs is sacrosanct and the only scope of action that they have is in ways of stimulating people.
3. Brainstorm a list of changes that may enrich the jobs, without concern for their practicality.
4. Screen the list to eliminate suggestions that involve hygiene, rather than actual motivation.
5. Screen the list for generalities, such as "give them more responsibility," that are rarely followed in practice. This might seem obvious, but the motivator words have never left industry; the substance has just been rationalized and organized out. Words like "responsibility," "growth," "achievement," and "challenge," for example, have been elevated to the lyrics of the patriotic anthem for all organizations. It is the old problem typified by the pledge of allegiance to the flag being more important than contributions to the country—of following the form, rather than the substance.
6. Screen the list to eliminate any horizontal loading suggestions.
7. Avoid direct participation by the employees whose jobs are to be enriched. Ideas they have expressed previously certainly constitute a valuable source for recommended changes, but their direct involvement contaminates the process with human relations hygiene and, more specifically, gives them only a sense of making a contribution. The job is to be changed, and it is the content that will produce the motivation, not attitudes about being involved or the challenge inherent in setting up a job. That process will be over shortly, and it is what the employees will be doing from then on that will determine their motivation. A sense of participation will result only in short-term movement.
8. In the initial attempts at job enrichment set up a controlled experience. At least two equivalent groups should be chosen, one an experimental unit in

which the motivators are systematically introduced over a period of time, and the other one a control group in which no changes are made. For both groups, hygiene should be allowed to follow its natural course for the duration of the experiment. Pre- and post-installation tests of performance and job attitudes are necessary to evaluate the effectiveness of the job enrichment program. The attitude test must be limited to motivator items in order to divorce the employee's view of the job he is given from all the surrounding hygiene feelings that he might have.

9. Be prepared for a drop in performance in the experimental group the first few weeks. The changeover to a new job may lead to a temporary reduction in efficiency.

10. Expect your first time supervisors to experience some anxiety and hostility over the changes you are making. The anxiety comes from their fear that the changes will result in poorer performance for their unit. Hostility will arise when the employees start assuming what the supervisors regard as their own responsibility for performance. The supervisor without checking duties to perform may then be left with little to do. After a successful experiment, however, the supervisor usually discovers the supervisory and managerial functions that he has neglected, or which were never his because all his time was given over to checking the work of his subordinates. For example, in the R&D division of one large chemical company I know of, the supervisors of the laboratory assistants were theoretically responsible for their training and evaluation. These functions, however, had come to be performed in a routine, insubstantial fashion. After the job enrichment program, during which the supervisors were not merely passive observers of the assistants' performance, the supervisors actually were devoting their time to reviewing performance and administering thorough training.

What has been called an employee-centered style of supervision will come about not through education of supervisions, but by changing the jobs that they do.

Concluding Note

Job enrichment will not be a one-time proposition, but a continuous management function. The initial changes, however, should last for a very long period of time. There are a number of reasons for this:

- The changes should bring the job up to the level of challenge commensurate with the skill that was hired.
- Those who have still more ability eventually will be able to demonstrate it better and win promotion to higher-level jobs.
- The very nature of motivators, as opposed to hygiene factors, is that they have a much longer-term effect on employees' attitudes. Perhaps the job will have to be enriched again, but this will not occur as frequently as the need for hygiene.

Not all jobs can be enriched, nor do all jobs need to be enriched. If only a small percentage of the time and money that is now devoted to hygiene, however, were given to job enrichment efforts, the return in human satisfaction and economic gain would be one of the largest dividends that industry and society have ever reaped through their efforts at better personnel management.

The argument for job enrichment can be summed up quite simply: If you have someone on a job, use him. If you can't use him on the job, get rid of him, either via automation or by selecting someone with lesser ability. If you can't use him and you can't get rid of him, you will have a motivation problem.

MORALE

Chapter Objectives

After you have studied this chapter, you should be able to do the following:

1. Discuss the supervisor's role in motivation and leadership and its bearing on the morale of subordinates.
2. Provide a basis for understanding the factors influencing morale.
3. Discuss the relationships among morale, retention, and productivity.
4. Discuss common techniques to assess and improve morale.
5. Consider the advantages and disadvantages to alternative working schedules.

Understanding the supervisor's role in motivation and leadership has much bearing on the *morale* of the subordinates. Some writers do not speak of morale of the individual but refer to job satisfaction, emphasizing the satisfaction of needs. Others stress the social aspects of groups and friendships, and some are particularly concerned with attitudes toward coworkers, the organization, and supervision. Many writers link satisfaction with the needs and attitudes of an individual, whereas morale pertains to the spirit of a group. Although this distinction is precise, it is largely academic because the factors and methods used in measuring group morale are usually the same as those used in measuring an individual's satisfaction.

Although there are many definitions for morale, a particularly useful one is to describe it as a state of mind and emotion affecting the attitudes, feelings, and sentiments of individuals and groups toward their work, environment, administration, and colleagues. Morale is the total satisfaction a person derives from the job, work group, boss, institution, and environment. "Morale pertains to the general feeling of well-being, satisfaction, and happiness of people" (Beach 1985). Parker and Kleemeier (1951) amplify this definition by stating morale is the attitude held by the individual members of a group that makes them put the achievement of group goals ahead of the achievement of personal goals. When morale is high, the employees are likely to strive hard to accomplish the objectives of the enterprise; conversely, low morale is likely to prevent or deter them from doing so.

The Nature of Morale

Supervisors often make the mistake of speaking of morale as something that is either present or absent among their employees. Morale is always present, and by itself has neither a favorable nor an unfavorable meaning. Morale can range from excellent and positive, through many intermediate degrees, to poor and completely negative. If the attitude of the subordinates is poor, the morale is also poor. If the subordinates are highly motivated to strive hard for the best possible patient care, their morale is high. Employees with high morale find satisfaction in their position in the enterprise, have confidence in their own and in their associates' abilities, and show enthusiasm and a strong desire to cooperate in achieving the healthcare organization's objectives.

One cannot order employees to have high morale. It can only be created by introducing certain conditions into the work setting that are favorable to its development. High morale is the result of good motivation, respect and dignity for the individual, realization of individual differences, good leadership, effective communication, participation, counseling, and many other practices. In other words, the state of morale reflects how appropriately and effectively the administration practices good human relations and good supervision.

The Level of Morale

Every manager, from the CEO to the supervisor, should be concerned with the level of morale in the organization. It is a supervisory function to promote and maintain the morale of the subordinates at as high a level as possible. The immediate supervisor in day-to-day contact with the employees influences and determines the level of morale more than anyone else. Raising morale to a high level and sustaining it is a long-term project and cannot be achieved solely on the basis of short-term devices such as pep talks or contests. The supervisor also will find that although good morale is slow to develop and difficult to maintain, it can change quickly from good to bad.

Bad morale can contribute to staff turnover. Turnover, as we have discussed in prior chapters, can be costly to the organization. Deloitte & Touche's special report on talent retention (2009) points to lack of job security, lack of compensation, lack of career progress, dissatisfaction with a supervisor or manager, and lack of challenges in the job as several of the top ten reasons individuals change employers. As we discussed in chapter 21, the supervisor's leadership skills affect morale as well. Organizations that win in an economic downturn are the ones that engage with employees, providing reassurance when necessary and clear direction to all, according to Hay Group (2008). Hay Group offers some basic points: provide clarity of strategic direction and pace; instill trust and confidence in your most driven, focused employees; address fundamental concerns; put people in roles suited to their skills and ambitions; and provide the tools for people to do their jobs.

One key to keeping employees is to ensure that they have been fully oriented to their new jobs and the department. The orientation is their first introduction to the culture of the department; this is where they become part of the "family." A good orientation program provides employees with enough information to do their jobs effectively and encourages an open dialogue for employees to share ideas about their assignments and work processes. Building confidence and competence in new employees pays for itself in the long run by reducing service errors or patient complaints. The program should acquaint the employees with the history of the organization, how the organization has positioned itself for the future, a clear view of how the department fits into the organization, how their jobs contribute to the department's objectives, what is expected of them, and how they may progress upward in the department. The supervisor's goal for the orientation program must be to make employees never want to leave.

No one wants to leave a positive and light-hearted environment. You can retain employees by teaching them how to do their jobs well, appreciating their input and ideas, and building high morale by keeping them happy and productive. Keeping humor in the workplace allows staff to set aside their concerns, even if momentarily, and goes a long way toward retaining employees and getting work done. Humor also reduces stress, and when staff are less stressed, they are willing to make the extra effort to achieve excellence. One way to foster a fun environment is to post appropriate jokes and stories throughout the department. Remember, the jokes should not criticize work, management, or the worker.

Morale is contagious. The higher the degree of individual satisfaction of group members, the higher is the morale of the entire group. This in turn tends to raise the overall level of morale even higher because individuals derive personal satisfaction from being in a high-morale group. Although favorable attitudes spread, unfavorable attitudes among employees spread more quickly. It seems to be human nature to forget the good quickly and remember the bad (see Appendix 23.3 later in this chapter) (Kelly 1998).

What then determines the level of morale?

Factors Influencing Morale

Because morale is a composite of feelings, sentiments, attitudes, satisfaction, well-being, and happiness, almost anything can influence the morale of the employees. Some factors are within the control of the supervisor, whereas others are not. We can divide morale determinants into two broad groups: (1) those factors that arise primarily from situations external to the institution and (2) those factors that originate mainly within the realm of the supervisor's activities. Many factors were discussed in Chapter 21; examples of both groups of factors appear in the Deloitte & Touche survey results shown in Exhibit 23.1.

External Factors

External factors affecting morale—those connected with events and influences outside the work environment and institution—are generally beyond the scope of the supervisor's control. Although they are external in origin, these factors nevertheless concern the supervisor, as everyone takes his problems to work and does not check them in the morning at the organization's door or leave them in the car. Examples of external factors are family problems or sickness, financial worries, national disasters, car troubles, or a downturn in the economy. Consider the impact on morale of those working at the local hospital when the only large employer in town, a mining company employing more than 35 percent of the town, closes, or if a large insurer's national billing office outsources its operations to India. What happens away from the job may change the employee's feelings quickly: an uplifting story on the morning news of a lost child found, an argument before leaving home, or an accident on the highway causing a long delay may set the emotional tone for the rest of the day.

In an article in *CIO Magazine*, a chief information officer offers this insight: "What you need to understand about morale is this: The mood of your employees can be brought down by external factors, such as the state of the economy, but it is your leadership skills—or lack thereof—that will tip

EXHIBIT 23.1
Decreased
Employee
Morale

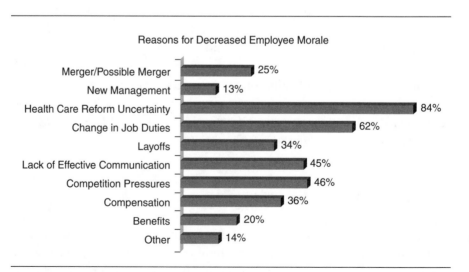

Reasons for Decreased Employee Morale

- Merger/Possible Merger — 25%
- New Management — 13%
- Health Care Reform Uncertainty — 84%
- Change in Job Duties — 62%
- Layoffs — 34%
- Lack of Effective Communication — 45%
- Competition Pressures — 46%
- Compensation — 36%
- Benefits — 20%
- Other — 14%

SOURCE: Reprinted with permission from Deloitte & Touche LLP—Human Resources Strategies Group, Member of ABC Consulting, Hospital Human Resource Survey—1995.

the morale scales one way or the other. In tough times such as these, the people you are responsible for are looking for support, leadership and reassurance. If you ignore or underestimate that need, you'll have a morale problem on your hands. Lack of communication and bad management, or lack of confidence in management, are the two biggest causes of low morale" (Kaplan 2005).

The supervisor can indirectly deal with these external factors by communicating honestly and conducting a nondirective counseling interview, as discussed in chapters 19 and 21. The supervisor should try to sense such factors; often they are reflected in the work behavior of the subordinates. If something has happened to lower an employee's morale and if the supervisor is familiar with the cause, she should try to get the employee to forget the incident as quickly as possible by supplying an antidote. One of the best ways to help an employee get past a depressing or demoralizing incident is to encourage the employee to talk about it freely. Aside from a nondirective counseling interview and keeping staff abreast of organizational changes that are being implemented, however, a supervisor can do little to counteract outside factors affecting morale.

Employee Assistance Programs

Many organizations have developed **employee assistance programs (EAPs)**. These programs are staffed by social workers and medical and counseling personnel who are trained in providing confidential, professional assistance to employees and their families. Some programs may also regularly use the services of an outside clinic or a chaplain. The purpose of the EAP is to help employees who have personal problems that may interfere with attendance and job performance; whether this counterproductive behavior is the result of work, home, or outside pressures is irrelevant. Some common problems are caused by alcoholism, drug dependency, financial worries, marriage or family difficulties, stress, and poor health. An employee can seek this support on her own, the supervisor may refer an employee to the program, or the referral might come from a medical professional or the union representative if applicable.

employee assistance programs Programs staffed by social workers and medical and counseling personnel who are trained in providing confidential, professional assistance to employees and their families.

Flexible Work Schedules and Other Alternatives

As introduced in Chapter 17, several other techniques that have become popular with organizations to help combat these external pressures, improve morale, and reduce turnover include offering flexible work hours, shared paid-time-off (PTO) banks, compressed schedules, and telecommuting opportunities. Baldiga and Doucet's (2001) study indicates that the percentage of women returning to work full time after childbirth declined from 73 percent to 61 percent between 1994 and 2000. Because a hospital's workforce is predominantly composed of women, supervisors must consider alternative work schedules for their staff. These programs speak to the employee's (male and female) need to balance external and internal needs—family time and work time. They also help to combat the stress that comes with a fast-paced world that forces us to respond instantaneously to e-mails, faxes, and electronic calendars.

Work schedules for many employees in different organizations have become more flexible. The idea is that employees should have some autonomy to adjust their work schedules to fit their lifestyles and to choose the hours they prefer to work while ensuring that a core workforce is available to attend to the department's operations. Flexible work hours allow individuals to schedule their workweek around other obligations common in dual-career families such as taking children to sporting events or aging parents to their physician appointments. According to the Society for Human Resource Management 2002 Benefits Survey, 64 percent of employers surveyed offer flexible hours (McFadden 2002). Gartner Dataquest reported in 2008 that 25 percent of workers telecommuted in 2007, and in its 2009 projections, it expected that number to hit 27.5 percent (Bright Hub 2009). Based on our prior discussions about generations X and Y, both flexible hours and telecommuting have wide appeal to younger workers.

compressed scheduling
Allowing employees to work a schedule in which more hours are worked in fewer days per week, such as 12 hours per day for 3 days.

One approach to offering flexible hours is flextime. *Flextime* enables employees to choose a schedule that fits into their off-the-job activities. It allows working parents or others with responsibilities at home to combine work with family life. Another popular work-scheduling option is the 4–10 or 3–12 arrangement, otherwise known as **compressed scheduling**. Employees choosing to work these schedules work either four 10-hour days or three 12-hour days. Often, organizations offering the 3–12 arrangement pay the employee for 40 hours of work, even though only 36 hours are worked. One concern with these extended-day schedules is that they can potentially cause fatigue, an increase in errors, and a reduction in productivity. Regardless, flexible work schedules tend to improve employee satisfaction and, in return, should contribute positively to productivity and time utilization.

telecommuting
Working from home while remaining connected to the office through telephone and computer.

Another work arrangement option, **telecommuting**, has gained popularity in many industries and is penetrating the healthcare industry. Telemedicine advances and computer and telecommunication technologies allow clinicians (physicians and specialists) to work from their home offices to serve rural and underserved areas through remote television. Organizations with electronic health records sometimes allow specialized staff members (information technology analysts, medical transcriptionists, utilization/case management staff, and coders) to telecommute. Global Telematics offers a checklist managers can use to assess whether telecommuting is an appropriate option for the department or organization. This checklist appears in Chapter 17, Exhibit 17.1.

Flexible working schedules and remote working arrangements create additional scheduling and planning challenges for supervisors. Managers must consider how to supervise staff working on different shifts and how to coordinate activities with other departments. Additionally, they should consider creating a policy and possibly a "contract" between the supervisor and employees opting for flextime or telecommuting arrangements. An example of a flextime policy appears in Appendix 23.1, and a sample telecommuting agreement is shown in Appendix 23.2. Additional telecommuting guidance, including telecommuting options, benefits and challenges, management tips, implementation considerations, a screening tool, and equipment recommendations, can be found at the website of the American Health Information Management Association (www.ahima.org) in its 2002 Practice Brief entitled "Establishing a Telecommuting or Home-Based Employee Program" by Michelle Dougherty, Rita Scichilone, and Donna Fletcher.

PTO banks permit employees to decide when and how the time is used; shared PTO banks allow employees to donate their excess time to a shared bank that can be tapped by coworkers when emergent needs arise. Both types of PTO banks allow the employee to use the excess time off accumulated to pay for hours needed to attend to personal and family matters.

Each approach allows the employee to make decisions about her work environment, a feature that can contribute to positive morale.

A more radical approach to offering alternative work schedules is that suggested by Ressler and Thompson, as reported by Belkin (2009). They propose a *results only work environment* (ROWE). Simply stated, a ROWE allows all employees to "work wherever they want whenever they want, as long as the work gets done" (Belkin 2009). Needless to say, this approach is an unlikely alternative for a healthcare facility due to specialization aspects, but it may work within a team of individuals with the same expertise and/or licensure.

Regardless of the options chosen, some caution needs to be exercised when offering these alternative work schedules. A poll reported by *USA Today* found workers expressing resentment that they must pick up the slack for coworkers who take advantage of these options; furthermore, 38 percent of the males surveyed stated that mothers get special treatment (Jones 2007). There will be naysayers regardless of the options offered, but the goal as a manager is to attempt to improve the morale of as many of the staff members as possible without compromising productivity, quality, and patient care. (An interesting, somewhat satirical, article that touches on this subject appears in Appendix 23.3.)

As long as flexible working schedules and arrangements produce good results (e.g., easier staff recruitment, better staff retention, higher morale, fewer absences, less tardiness, less dissatisfaction, better patient care), supervisors should make every effort to plan and supervise effectively to overcome these problems.

Internal Factors

Many factors that affect the morale of employees fall within the realm of the supervisor's activities. These include incentives, working conditions, and above all, the quality of supervision. When considering incentives, the first thing that comes to mind is pay. Making the work environment appealing is the responsibility of all managers. Employees want to feel important and be recognized for what they do for the organization. We have already discussed simple recognition tools such as certificates or a pat on the back for a job well done. If the organizational culture supports these techniques, it also may support the establishment of incentive plans.

Incentive plans reward employees financially. Those plans that are productivity based are commonly used in the laundry and health information departments of healthcare organizations, where output, such as pounds of laundry and lines typed, can be objectively measured. They can also be used in areas of care provision to recognize an individual's noteworthy accomplishment, such as obtaining certification in respiratory therapy or having a perfect attendance record.

Merit bonuses are a type of incentive program. These bonuses are a flat amount paid in addition to or in lieu of a salary increase. They may vary from one individual to another because they are based on an individual's performance. Some organizations offer organization-wide bonuses for staff. This may be a one-time bonus for achieving an organizational goal such as accreditation or improved patient satisfaction, or it may be a year-end distribution following favorable financial performance. Finally, incentive-type programs may be based on team performance. This type of program encourages teamwork and may promote peer pressure if a team member is slacking in her duties. A compensation survey conducted by Mercer Human Resources Consulting (2001) reported that 46 percent of healthcare providers offered short-term incentive plans. Of the hourly clinical and technical staffs, 25 to 27 percent participated in these plans. Of the plans offered, 19 to 24 percent were individual based and 12 to 14 percent were team based.

Incentive programs are similar to pay-for-performance programs (discussed in detail later in this section) and can be applied in virtually all departments. Developing a plan is not easy and must be well thought out. Management must gather data on employees' performance, track the performance for a reasonable period of time, and set an acceptable goal for the staff to pursue. The published results of an integrated incentive plan, including physicians and hospital surgical staff, demonstrated improved on-time case starts, decreased turnaround time, improved physician satisfaction, and reduced registered nurse and surgical technologist turnover; this incentive plan also recognized staff for aligning their efforts to achieve organization goals (Poole 2004).

Incentive plans do not need to be complex. In the admitting area the goal might be a reduction in registration errors; in patient financial services it could be a reduction in days in accounts receivable; and for a patient care area, it could be based on a safety issue such as a reduction in patient falls or needle sticks. Organization-wide, administration could set an incentive goal of increasing patient satisfaction based on the results of patient surveys or cost reduction without sacrificing quality or customer satisfaction.

The supervisor's role in developing an incentive plan includes setting targets that are attainable and specific and having appropriate controls in place to avoid any patient dissatisfaction. If employees do not perceive the rewards as meaningful or fair, the plan will fail. Wages are exceedingly important, but aside from wages and fringe benefits, many other aspects are essential to the employee.

Pay-for-performance (P4P) programs recognize employees for outstanding performance by tying bonus payments to the work effort of individuals who achieve defined goals or results. Employees should be involved in designing the program to facilitate their understanding of expectations, as such programs may discourage staff who are unable to achieve targets. A simple program that avoids complex formulas will be easier for staff to understand and for you to administer. Be certain to provide the tools or resources that your team will need in order to achieve the productivity levels; otherwise, they will perceive the P4P program as an unachievable management hoax, resulting in lower morale. Other concerns about P4P plans include potential for increased injuries, as workers take safety shortcuts to meet production goals, and reduction of collaboration and team work, as staff compete to be high performers (Armour 2001). To avoid these pitfalls, management should incorporate both quality and safety expectations and possibly distribute the P4P compensation based on the team's success.

pay-for-performance program
Motivation programs that tie bonus payments to achievement of goals or results.

Other programs demonstrating management's interest in the welfare of its employees are stress-reduction programs, health-risk appraisals, on-site immunization programs, on-site fitness facilities, sponsored athletics, prenatal programs, and well-baby programs. One nontraditional benefit offered to some employees is nap time during the workday. According to a poll by the National Sleep Foundation, 27 percent of adults surveyed are sleepy at work two days per week or more, 19 percent made errors at work because of sleepiness, and 2 percent sustained injury as a result of sleepiness (Gemignani 2000). Believing naps boost alertness, Google, Nike, and Virgin Active Health Club & Gyms allow employees to have midday naps (Salemme 2009). A study by NASA shows that a nap of merely 26 minutes can boost performance by as much as 34 percent (Gaebler n.d.).

However, many believe that the most important benefit an organization can offer its employees is training. It solidifies a sense of commitment between the supervisor and his employees at a time when he is most likely asking them to do more with less. According to Mercer survey, 58 percent of employers identified training and development as one of the key strategies to retaining good employees (Gross 2005).

competence
The demonstrated ability to apply knowledge and skills.

Spath (2002) notes that every supervisor is "responsible for ensuring that department personnel are competent. **Competence** is defined as the demonstrated ability to apply knowledge and skills and involves four elements: education, training, skills, and experience. To ensure that people are competent to perform their jobs, it is important they receive proper training that meets the needs of the department and the staff." Known as competency-based training, this approach focuses attention on the employee and her job. The employee benefits from better understanding of the job duties and recognizes that the organization is interested in her success. The organization benefits because the employee gains the competence needed to achieve the goals of the department.

Considerations such as job security, interesting work, good working conditions, appreciation of a job well done, skill building, chance for advancement, recognition, and prompt and fair treatment of grievances are all necessary components of a high-morale environment (see Chapter 21). Although reasonable monetary incentives may be provided and the quality of supervision is high, morale can still sink quickly if, for example, working conditions are neglected.

One change that has been highly accepted is casual day. A simple change to working conditions that permits employees to wear jeans every Friday as casual-day attire may both increase the comfort level and reduce an employee's out-of-pocket expenses for dry cleaning. More than 60 percent of human resources professionals say their organizations allow casual dress at least once a week (Perry 2000). As this practice became more prevalent, supervisors found themselves in the position of clothes cop because some employees took advantage of the casual environment. In some cases, the informal atmosphere encouraged a lax attitude toward work and an increase in flirtatious behavior (Perry 2000). Because of these circumstances, some of those same organizations have returned to a standard form of business wear, and in some organizations, the employees bucked the trend by dressing up rather than down on casual day (Perry 2000). The majority of people who work full time in an office setting have a dress code, according to a BizRate Research study, with just 26 percent allowed to don casual work attire every day. Most—64 percent—work under a business casual requirement (Armour 2005). However, we should not expect a return to the 1950s workplace attire requirement of wearing jackets and ties for men and dresses for women. The important factor is that an honest attempt is made to improve working conditions whenever possible.

Finally, recall the Hawthorne studies, discussed in Chapter 2. Morale may be affected by the simplest of issues. For example, many employees appreciate an environment that is brighter but features diffused lighting and matte surfaces to reduce glare. Less noise and warm colors may reduce stress. Thus, simply changing light bulbs and adding a coat of paint may do wonders for improving morale. In many cases, employees work under undesirable conditions and still maintain high morale as long as the supervisor has made a serious effort to correct the conditions. Rather than routinely offering a casual day that may cause lax attitudes, some managers spice up the environment with theme days, such as Hawaiian Day or Roaring Twenties Day. This occasional change likely will yield greater benefits than an every-week event.

The Supervisor's Role

Aside from these on-the-job factors, the most significant influence on morale is exercised by supervisors in their immediate, day-to-day relationships with employees. The supervisor's overall manner of supervision, direction, leadership, interpersonal skills, and general attitude more than anything else make for good or bad morale. Employees put forth their best efforts when given an opportunity to satisfy their needs through work they enjoy while helping to achieve departmental objectives. Such job satisfaction raises and keeps morale at a high level, but it can only be maintained if the supervisor tells the employees how significant their contributions are to the overall goals of the health-care organization and how their work fits into the overall effort.

Morale can also be maintained if the boss gives them a feeling of accomplishment in their work and allows them to work independently as much as possible. The supervisor who practices democratic supervision, as discussed in previous chapters, and who "practices what he preaches" is likely to reduce the undesirable features of a job and create an environment in which the employees derive genuine satisfaction from the work they do every day. In addition, the supervisor should not forget the importance of social satisfaction on the job. The employees should have an opportunity to develop friendships and work as a team, as informal groups and informal organization can make positive contributions.

Employees' morale is affected not only by what the supervisor does but also by how she does it. If the supervisor's behavior indicates a feeling of superiority to the employees or the supervisor is suspicious of the employees' motives and actions, only a low level of morale can result. The supervisor should not forget how little it takes to make one's own spirits rise or fall. A word of appreciation from the boss or administrator can change the supervisor's outlook toward the whole work setting. She will become more cheerful, and in all likelihood so will the employees.

One may think of this as a mirror effect. If the hospital vice president commends the department director on successfully completing a major project, such as publishing the annual cancer program report, the director will probably mirror the vice president's actions with those departmental supervisors who participated in accomplishing the project. The supervisors will then most likely mirror the director and share their appreciation with their line staff.

Similarly, attitudes beget similar attitudes. If the supervisor shows worry, the employees tend to follow suit. If he becomes angry, others become angry. When the supervisor appears confident in the operation of the department, employees react accordingly and believe that things are going well. This does not mean that the supervisor should only see the good side of departmental operations and refuse to acknowledge difficulties and troubles. The supervisor should show the employees that as a leader he has the situation well in hand and that if anything goes wrong, he will give them an opportunity to correct the situation and prevent it from happening again.

The Third Shift

It is not unusual for those working on the third shift to believe they are the "forgotten ones." Often they may work for weeks or months and never see the department manager because third shift typically goes home at 7 a.m. and managers traditionally start at 8 a.m. Conversely, first- and second-shift employees enjoy the opportunity to see and interact with the manager. So how does one encourage good morale on third shift?

Third shifts are inevitable for healthcare organizations. The staff on these shifts often have a greater scope of responsibility because they are "it." There is no supervisor or department manager to turn to. They must be up to date on patient care protocols, emergency practices, and regulations governing privacy and security, among other issues, so that they can apply this knowledge to decisions they make.

Recall our discussion of Maslow in Chapter 22. Every individual has needs that must be met. Often individuals work third shift because they must. These individuals may have a spouse working another shift, who, unable to afford babysitters, prefer the shift because there are fewer distractions or disruptions, or be drawn to the additional compensation associated with the shift differential. Recognizing these drivers will help you tailor your management style when communicating with third-shift staff.

A supervisor's communications with these staff likely will be conducted mostly through e-mail. To take advantage of this mode, comments may be added to e-mails that speak to their needs, which will impress upon them that you "know" them as well as those you interact with face-to-face. For example, a transcriptionist may choose to work third shift because during the day she makes and sells decorative containers. However, this start-up business is not sufficient to support her household, so she works full-time on the night shift typing for the healthcare organization. A supervisor's e-mail to her may address some new hospital security practices such as changing pass codes to the information system every six weeks rather than every six months. In the same note the supervisor might lightheartedly add, "Aren't you glad that pass codes are not required to buy your floral containers?" However, all communication should not be conducted through technological means. Occasional telephone calls to each of a supervisor's third-shift employees, inviting them to department functions, such as showers or pot luck parties, and holding department meetings on third shift promote the impression that the supervisor cares as much about them as those working on other shifts.

Himiak (2007) further suggests that in addition to communicating effectively with third-shift staff, it is important for the manager to encourage better health for these workers. Sleep and nutrition are important factors in maintaining health and thus promoting high morale. It is beneficial to keep healthy snacks around the office for those who work the third shift. Because those workers are not eating on a "normal" schedule, their diet may be affected if they eat a full meal at 6 a.m.

The Effects of Morale

The question arises as to how high or low morale affects other variables such as turnover, absenteeism, the rate of accidents, teamwork, and productivity. Much research has been done in this area, and some general conclusions can be drawn from it. For example, high morale is moderately related to lower employee turnover. The same likely holds true for a lowered rate of absenteeism. Furthermore, higher morale most likely also leads to other desirable consequences, such as fewer grievances, better mental and physical health, faster learning of new tasks, and possibly a lowered rate of accidents or care errors. The following sections consider additional consequences.

Morale and Teamwork

The term *teamwork* is often associated with morale, but the two terms do not have the same meaning. Morale applies to the attitudes of the employees in the department, whereas teamwork is the smoothly coordinated and synchronized activity achieved by a small, closely knit group of employees. Although good morale is usually helpful in achieving teamwork, it is possible for teamwork to be high and morale low. Such a situation could exist in times when jobs are scarce and when the employees put up with close and tight supervision for fear of losing their jobs. Also, teamwork may be absent even though morale is high; in such a case the employee, a solo performer, probably prefers individual effort and finds satisfaction in her own job performance.

Morale and Productivity

It is generally assumed that high morale is automatically accompanied by high productivity. Supervisors believe that as long as the morale of employees is high, their output will be correspondingly high. Moreover, some research evidence backs up the contention that there is a small but positive relationship between overall morale or job satisfaction and productivity (Beach 1985). Most supervisors also believe, based on personal experience, that a highly motivated, self-disciplined group of employees consistently does a more satisfactory job than a group whose morale is low. Therefore, supervisors should do everything possible to keep morale high so that the department's performance remains high.

However, many studies show that this general statement does not hold true in all situations. There is proof that the morale–productivity relationship can appear in many forms: low morale and high productivity, high morale and low productivity, high morale and high productivity, and low morale and low productivity. In fact, in the third quarter of 2003, the productivity of American workers grew at a rate of 9.4 percent, the best it had been since mid-1983. However, at the same time employees experienced higher levels of stress and burnout, costing the U.S. economy $344 billion a year; Harris Poll data reflected lower morale reported by 27 percent of the employees surveyed (Ceridian Corporation 2005). Level of morale depends on other factors as well, such as the economic situation, the rewards, the job market, and the mechanical pace of the job. Thus, a supervisor cannot automatically depend on the positive relationship between morale and productivity.

Assessing Current Morale

It is important for management to be familiar with the extent of job satisfaction or dissatisfaction of the employees. Much of the foregoing discussion has assumed that the level of morale is measurable, but morale cannot be measured directly. Nevertheless, suitable indirect means exist for determining the prevailing level of morale and its trends. Although some supervisors pride themselves on their ability to detect intuitively low or high morale, the wise supervisor approaches this problem more systematically in either of two ways. One approach is through observation of activities, events, trends, and changes; the other method is to administer attitude, opinion, or morale surveys. The *Journal of Accountancy* (2001) stated that when conducting a survey of employees, one of the best questions is, "What keeps you from doing your job as well as you would like to?" It not only invites employees to focus on their specific area of knowledge and expertise, it also gives them an opportunity to disclose how well they really want to do the job.

Observation
Observation involves watching people and their reactions. Although this tool is available to every supervisor, it is often not fully utilized. If the supervisor does observe the employees consciously and systematically, however, the level

HOSPITAL LAND

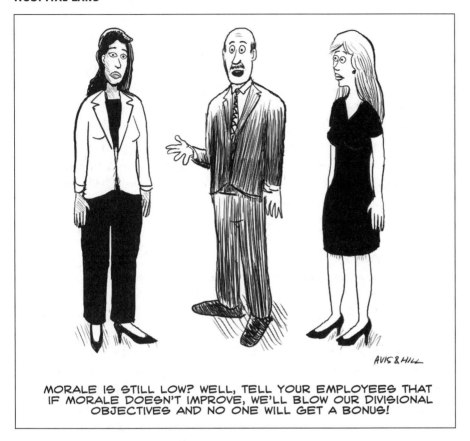

MORALE IS STILL LOW? WELL, TELL YOUR EMPLOYEES THAT
IF MORALE DOESN'T IMPROVE, WE'LL BLOW OUR DIVISIONAL
OBJECTIVES AND NO ONE WILL GET A BONUS!

of morale and major changes in it can be appraised. The manager should watch the subordinates' behavior and listen to what they have to say; he should observe their actions and notice any changes in their willingness to cooperate. The supervisor probably finds it fairly easy to recognize through observation the extremes of high and low morale. Finer means of measurement, however, may be required to differentiate among the intermediate degrees. Personal observation can be used for obvious manifestations of morale, such as a facial expression or a shrug of the shoulder, but often these signs are difficult to interpret. It is also difficult to determine how far from normal the behavior must be to indicate a shift in morale. Thus, it takes an extremely sensitive supervisor to conclude correctly from such indicators that a change in morale has occurred or is currently taking place.

Moreover, the supervisor may not be able to make the detailed observations necessary for accurate morale appraisal. Although the closeness of the day-to-day working relationship usually offers much opportunity for supervisors to become aware of morale changes, they are often so burdened with work that they do not have time to look, or if they do look, they do not actually see. At times they may even be afraid to look for fear of what they might find. Although some supervisors may realize that changes are taking place, they are frequently inclined to ignore them. Only later, after a change in the level of morale is openly manifested, will they recall the first indications and admit to noticing them but not giving them much thought.

To avoid such situations, the supervisor must take care not to brush aside indicators out of convenience. The most serious shortcoming of using observation as a yardstick to measure current morale is that when the events causing the low morale are recognized, the change has probably already occurred. The supervisor, therefore, should be extremely keen in his observation to do as much as possible to prevent such changes before they take place, or to quickly counteract them if they have already begun. The closer the supervisor's relationship with the employees, the more sensitive she is to these changes and the more quickly she can act.

Attitude Surveys

The other approach to assessing current morale is the use of attitude surveys, also called opinion or morale surveys. Many institutions use attitude surveys to find out how employees view their jobs, coworkers, benefits, wages, working conditions, quality of services, supervisors, the institution as a whole, and specific policies. Such a survey is a valuable diagnostic tool for management to assess employee problems. Administering an employee survey is like taking the pulse of the organization (York 1985). Surveys allow employees to express their feelings about their jobs. As a result, administration is aware of the general level of satisfaction in the institution and which specific areas cause dissatisfaction. The attitude survey shows employees that management is truly concerned and gives them an opportunity to vent their opinions. This in itself improves morale.

For surveys to be meaningful, however, administration must be committed to this undertaking. This means that management must be willing to invest effort, time, and money. Administration must be willing to follow through with action based on the results of the survey and be ready to communicate the major findings of the survey to the employees. Such a survey requires careful planning and professional development. Unless the institution's human resources department is large and has in-house professionals trained and experienced in giving attitude surveys, it is advisable to hire an outside consultant. This ensures that a well-designed instrument is used, with appropriate validity, reliability, sampling, and statistical methods. The employees may have more confidence having an outside consultant do the survey than having their own personnel department do it. An outside consultant could also help decide whether a standardized survey, a customized one, or a combination of the two would be most appropriate.

Administering the Survey Expressions of employees' opinions are requested in the form of answers to written questionnaires. These questionnaires must be prepared with great care and much thought. A good attitude survey measures the major variables of organizational life, such as leadership, supervision, administration, job satis-faction, job conditions and work environment, coworkers, pay, benefits and rewards, job security, advancement, and stress. The questionnaire should be written at a level appropriate for most of the employees. A cover letter from the CEO should accompany the questionnaire, encouraging the employees' participation and stressing the confidential and anonymous nature of the employees' involvement.

In a healthcare organization, attitude surveys can cover the entire organization. At times, it is appropriate to limit the survey to only one large department, such as nursing services, which usually accounts for half of all the employees. Full-scale attitude surveys should not be given in less than three-year intervals; this allows enough time to indicate significant attitude changes.

Once an institutionwide survey is decided on, the administrator and all other managers must be prepared to endure criticism because dissatisfactions are likely to be expressed. More important, management must be prepared and willing to act on the complaints once they are revealed. Until the survey is taken, management can always plead ignorance, but after a survey is conducted, everyone knows that the administration has heard about the problems causing dissatisfaction. It is hoped that some of the complaints can be adjusted; at least a serious and honest effort must now be made. If the administration is not prepared or willing to act, it is far better not to administer surveys: if management asks the employees for their input and ideas and fails to take action, the employees will avoid expressing themselves in the future.

While the types of questionnaires administered to employees vary, two general forms are used most often: objective surveys and descriptive surveys. An **objective questionnaire** (see Exhibit 23.2) asks the question and offers a choice of answers; there can be multiple choice or true-or-false questions. In **objective surveys**, the employees mark the one answer that comes closest to their feelings. In a **descriptive survey**, the question is asked, but the employees answer freely in their own words and ways. Because many employees may have difficulty expressing their opinions in writing or may not want to take the time to write out answers, the best results are usually obtained on a form that enables the employees to check the box that seems to provide the most appropriate answer for them.

The survey forms can be filled out on the job, online software, or at home. Although there are many advantages to filling out questionnaires at home, a high percentage of them are never returned. It is better to have more meaningful answers, however, even if the number of replies is smaller. Some organizations are concerned that the rate of returned surveys might be low and prefer to distribute and collect the surveys the same day during working hours. The employees complete the survey forms on the premises and on company time. This procedure is likely to maximize the number of completed surveys.

Regardless of whether questionnaires are filled out on the job or at home, care must be taken that they remain unsigned and that the replies cannot be

objective questionnaire
A questionnaire that asks questions and provides a choice of answers.

objective survey
A survey that requires the subjects to mark the answers that come closest to their feelings on the topic.

descriptive survey
A survey that allows the subjects to freely answer in their own words.

Exhibit 23.2 Employee Opinion Survey

EMPLOYEE OPINION SURVEY
Anytown Health Center
Anytown, USA

Your employer is interested in your opinions and feelings about your work. This survey is one way to obtain your input about various aspects of your work. You should answer the questionnaire items honestly and frankly because it is totally **anonymous and confidential.** No one but you will know how you answered the question items. There are four parts to this survey. After you have completed one part, proceed to the next one until you have completed all four parts. After you have finished all four parts, place this completed form in the locked box at the front of this room and return your materials to the person administering the survey.

The results of this survey will be discussed with you at a later date by your supervisor and/or area manager.

PART B

The following statements concern specific aspects of the organization and your job here. Indicate your level of agreement with each statement by filling in the bubble to the right of the statement. Possible responses are:

1 = Strongly Agree	4 = Slightly Disagree
2 = Moderately Agree	5 = Moderately Disagree
3 = Slightly Agree	6 = Strongly Disagree

For example, if you "moderately agree" with a statement, you would fill in the bubble marked ② under the column marked Moderately Agree.

Again, your answers are anonymous and confidential, so please feel free to answer honestly.

	Strongly Agree	Moderately Agree	Slightly Agree	Slightly Disagree	Moderately Disagree	Strongly Disagree
1 I am proud to work for this organization.	①	②	③	④	⑤	⑥
2 I understand how the success of my department is measured.	①	②	③	④	⑤	⑥
3 My supervisor gives me clear working instructions.	①	②	③	④	⑤	⑥
4 Efficiency is highly valued in my department.	①	②	③	④	⑤	⑥
5 My department head sets clear goals for our department.	①	②	③	④	⑤	⑥
6 Communications among shifts in this organization are good.	①	②	③	④	⑤	⑥
7 I would have to make a bad mistake to be removed from my present position in this organization.	①	②	③	④	⑤	⑥
8 Employee promotions are handled fairly in this organization.	①	②	③	④	⑤	⑥
9 Compared to similar jobs in the community, I feel that I am paid fairly.	①	②	③	④	⑤	⑥
10 The organization's top management will use the information from this survey to make improvements.	①	②	③	④	⑤	⑥
11 My department head does a good job of running this department.	①	②	③	④	⑤	⑥
12 My job is challenging enough to suit me.	①	②	③	④	⑤	⑥
13 I am satisfied with this organization's sick leave policy.	①	②	③	④	⑤	⑥
14 I am happy with my current workload.	①	②	③	④	⑤	⑥
15 My supervisor discusses my productivity with me.	①	②	③	④	⑤	⑥
16 In my department, employees are well utilized.	①	②	③	④	⑤	⑥
17 My supervisor does a good job of running my area.	①	②	③	④	⑤	⑥
18 Absenteeism is no problem in my department.	①	②	③	④	⑤	⑥

SOURCE: Management Science Associates, Inc. © 1997, Independence, MO.

personally identified. Respondents must be assured that the replies will be kept confidential. Employees are sometimes suspicious of the institution's motives, and they may respond in ways they believe the institution wants. Therefore, it is essential that no individual identification information appear on the survey. However, it may be necessary to ask the employees to identify their work group or to identify their department so management can focus its response on the source of the concern.

EXHIBIT 23.3 Employee Opinion Survey Results

MANAGEMENT SCIENCE ASSOCIATES, INC.
Measure of Organizational Health Prepared for:
Anytown Community Hospital
Anytown, USA

Norm Group: National Norms | Date of Survey: 1/97
Organization Total | Number of Respondents: 1314

Attitude Area/Question	Ind. Norm	Org. Norm	% Diff.	Very Pos. 1	Mod. Pos. 2	Slgt Pos 3	Slgt Neg 4	Mod Neg 5	Very Neg 6	# Resp.
A. JOB SATISFACTION	2.2	2.3	-2							
1. Proud to Work for Hospital	1.7	1.6	2	56%	31%	9%	2%	1%	1%	1314
2. Job Is Challenging	2.1	2.1	0	41%	32%	13%	7%	4%	3%	1310
3. Feeling of Satisfaction	2.6	2.8	-4	17%	32%	25%	12%	7%	6%	1313
4. Opportunity to Use My Abilities	2.5	2.6	-2	23%	34%	22%	11%	5%	5%	1295
B. JOB MOBILITY	3.2	3.4	-4							
1. Opportunities to Transfer	3.0	3.2	-4	13%	24%	25%	14%	11%	13%	1268
2. Chances for Advancement	3.4	3.7	-6	7%	16%	25%	23%	14%	15%	1288
C. ADMIN/SR MANAGEMENT	3.0	3.0	0							
1. Resolves Employee Complaints	3.3	3.4	-2	8%	20%	29%	19%	11%	12%	1257
2. Overall Management of Hospital	2.8	2.7	2	16%	35%	25%	13%	6%	4%	1284
3. Interest in Employees	3.2	3.2	0	14%	22%	24%	18%	11%	12%	1287
4. Communicates Hospital Objectives	2.7	2.7	0	18%	29%	30%	14%	5%	4%	1302
5. Use of Survey by Administration	2.9	3.1	-4	16%	25%	26%	13%	9%	11%	1299
D. DEPARTMENT HEAD	2.6	2.7	-2					6%		
1. Understand How Dept/Unit Success Meas.	2.5	2.7	-4	20%	34%	23%	13%	8%	5%	1303 / 1301
2. Sets Clear Goals for Department/Unit	2.6	2.7	-2	24%	28%	21%	13%	9%	6%	1305
3. Good Job of Running Department/ Unit	2.6	2.6	0	28%	28%	19%	9%		7%	
E. SUPERVISION	2.7	2.9	-4							
1. Gives Clear Instructions	2.3	2.4	-2	31%	32%	17%	9%	6%	4%	1306
2. Overall Management of Area	2.5	2.6	-2	32%	25%	16%	8%	9%	9%	1302
3. Handling Complaints	2.9	3.2	-6	20%	22%	18%	14%	9%	16%	1298
4. Administering Discipline	3.0	3.2	-4	18%	23%	20%	15%	11%	14%	1283
5. Feel Free to Tell What I Think	2.6	2.7	-2	33%	24%	16%	8%	8%	12%	1305
6. Does Not Play Favorites	3.0	3.2	-4	23%	22%	15%	12%	8%	19%	1299
7. Discusses Productivity with Me	2.7	2.7	0	28%	26%	19%	11%	8%	8%	1305
8. Communications with Employees	2.8	3.0	-4	21%	27%	19%	12%	8%	13%	1303
F. COMMUNICATIONS	3.3	3.3	0							
1. Among Departments	3.5	3.4	2	6%	19%	31%	23%	13%	8%	1289
2. Among Shifts	3.2	3.1	2	9%	29%	28%	15%	9%	8%	1251
G. PERSONNEL/HR POLICIES	3.0	2.9	2							
1. Administered Consistently	3.0	2.9	2	13%	33%	25%	14%	8%	7%	1273
2. Fairness of Promotion Policies	3.2	3.2	0	9%	27%	27%	16%	11%	10%	1273
3. Satisfied with Personnel Policies	2.7	2.6	2	16%	40%	25%	11%	5%	4%	1292
H. JOB SECURITY	2.6	3.1	-10							
1. Takes a Lot to Lose Job	2.6	3.0	-8	22%	23%	21%	14%	10%	10%	1300
2. Feeling of Security	2.7	3.2	-10	16%	25%	21%	15%	10%	13%	1307
3. I Can Be Sure of a Job	2.5	3.1	-12	20%	26%	17%	14%	11%	12%	1309

SOURCE: © 1997, Management Science Associates, Inc., Independence, MO.

Once the forms have been filled out, the results must be analyzed (see Exhibit 23.3). Even if the survey is well designed, well organized, and properly conducted, it can result in a failed opportunity if it is improperly or superficially analyzed. Proper analysis will ensure that management gets a clear picture of the results so that the real problems are addressed by action and appropriate solutions.

Analyzing the Results

A discussion of statistical approaches and concepts, such as segmenting the survey, cluster analysis, and so forth, is beyond the scope of this book. Briefly, the analysis must be thorough, and instead of simple, straight-run statistics, it should produce more meaningful interpretations. For example, the interaction of organizational and demographic variables must be examined in relation to attitudes. Instead of simply stating that 65 percent of the subordinates have frequent communication with their boss and 35 percent do not, or that 75 percent of the respondents like their jobs and 25 percent do not, it is better to state that of the 75 percent who like their jobs, 85 percent have frequent contact with their boss and 15 percent do not. Similarly, perhaps among the 25 percent who do not care for their jobs, 55 percent claim that they have infrequent communication with their superiors. The results may determine whether females are more or less satisfied than males, younger more than older employees, and so forth.

After a meaningful analysis and interpretation of the survey have been done, the results are presented to the top-level executive team. Then each executive meets with her line managers to analyze and evaluate the survey results. Plans for action to correct the problems that surfaced should be formulated in these meetings. This process then moves downward through the hierarchy, first to all supervisors and finally to the rank-and-file employees in group sessions, where the results of the attitude survey are discussed.

Besides this feedback of results, attitude surveys provide top-level administration, department heads, and supervisors with information to guide them in their overall efforts to improve morale. If the surveys reveal deficiencies, specific actions should be taken to rectify them. For example, the questionnaire may show an overwhelming interest in and need for a childcare center. This obviously is an area of dissatisfaction, and administration should take immediate action to address it. Occasionally, however, the results of initial surveys are not clear. They may raise many questions, and sometimes additional surveys are required to probe deeper. Survey techniques and analyses are becoming more and more sophisticated, and with their help management should be able to arrive at a solution to almost any morale problem that arises.

Summary

Morale is a state of mind and emotion affecting the attitudes, feelings, and sentiments of groups of employees and individuals toward their work environment, colleagues, supervision, and the enterprise as a whole. Morale is always present, and it can range from high to low. The level of morale varies considerably from day to day. Morale is contagious; favorable attitudes spread quickly, and unfavorable attitudes spread even more quickly. Achieving high morale is not the concern of just the supervisor; the employees are also interested in a satisfactory level of morale. Moreover, the effect of high or low morale is felt not only by insiders but also by outsiders such as patients and visitors.

Morale can be influenced by many factors, which can be classified into two broad groups: those factors affecting the employee's activities that arise outside the enterprise and those originating within the job environment. The supervisor can do little to directly change the effects of outside factors on the subordinates' morale, but many internal factors, such as incentives, working conditions, and quality of work life, are within the supervisor's power to control. Addressing these factors, coupled with an attentive supervisor who is willing to listen to employee concerns, can significantly raise the level of subordinates' morale. If the supervisor succeeds in maintaining high morale, good teamwork and increased productivity will likely result. Research indicates that some interesting correlations exist between morale and productivity, turnover, and absenteeism.

An astute supervisor can sense changes in the level of morale by keenly observing the subordinates, but this is difficult to accomplish. Often supervisors do not realize that a change has taken place until performance has been detrimentally affected. Attitude surveys are primarily used to find out how employees view their jobs, coworkers, wages, benefits, supervisors, working conditions, and so on. Surveys requested by management are often instituted by outside consultants or by the institution's human resources department.

Alternative work schedules may assist in retaining staff as well as satisfying needs of certain staff members. These alternative schedules may present scheduling challenges for managers, but if employee needs are met, satisfaction with the job will increase and serve as a foundation for good morale.

Surveys take the form of questionnaires submitted to the employees. Once a morale survey has been administered and properly analyzed, it is absolutely necessary that management do something about those areas of dissatisfaction that appear to contribute to low morale. It is also advisable to report the results to all those who participated and to discuss them in workshops throughout the organization to find solutions to the problems.

Additional Readings

Black, J., with D. Miller. 2008. "An Open Letter to Healthcare Leaders." In *The Toyota Way to Healthcare Excellence: Increase Efficiency and Improve Quality with Lean.* Chicago: Health Administration Press.

Collins, S. K., and K. S. Collins. 2007. "Succession Planning and Leadership Development: Critical Business Strategies for Healthcare Organizations." [Online article; retrieved 10/26/09.] www.ahraonline.org/ConfEd/Education/ 2007JanuaryFebruary1/2007JanuaryFebruary1.pdf.

Wooten, P. 1991. "Physiological Effects of Laughter." *Journal of Nursing Jocularity* 1 (3): 46–47.

APPENDIX 23.1

Sample Flex-Time Policy

The following can be used as a template for your organization if you are considering implementation of this kind of flexible work arrangement. Consider the specifics of your own organization and follow the normal review protocols used for implementation of a new policy to ensure that it meets your organizational needs and complies with all current internal policy and external legislation.

1. Policy Statement
As stated in its Policy on Equal Opportunities: "the Organization confirms its commitment to develop, maintain and support a comprehensive policy of equal opportunities in employment within the Organization." To assist in this the Organization will actively support flex-time where it is reasonable and practical to do so and where operational needs will not be adversely affected.

2. Definition of Flex-Time
Flex-time is a work schedule which allows employees to work hours that are not within the standard 8:00 AM to 5:00 PM range, while maintaining a high level of service during the organization's peak operating hours (typically 10:00 AM to 3:00 PM). With a flex-time schedule, non-exempt employees are still subject to all requirements of the Fair Labor Standards Act. Employees who are exempt from FLSA are expected to work whatever number of hours are required in order to accomplish their duties and may be permitted to set their own schedules.

3. Aims and Objectives
The Organization is committed to equality of opportunity for all its staff regardless of the number of hours worked. In order to facilitate this, the Organization may create working arrangements, in accordance with managerial interests, whereby it can widen its recruitment pool, retain the valuable skills of existing employees who no longer want to work full-time or who may want to work full-time but with an alternative schedule, and enable staff to retain career development opportunities.

4. Eligibility
Because services within each division vary, not every employee in each department will be able to work similar flex-time schedules. Therefore, supervisors will have to carefully examine the flex-time schedules which their employees request, so that they can coordinate work schedules which ensure ample employee coverage during peak hours.

5. Managing Flex-Time
It is the responsibility of the supervisor to verify and ensure performance of employees with flex-time schedules. Flex-time schedules will need to be placed in a central location so that all employees stay aware of who is covering department services.

Good relationships among everyone involved are important for a successful flex-time policy. Trust is a big factor; supervisors must feel confident that employees will not abuse the benefits that are inherent in a flex-time schedule. Flex-time is a privilege, not a right, and, if abused, can be taken away at the discretion of the supervisor.

6. Flex-Time Schedules

There are three types of flex schedules from which to choose: Peak-Hour Flex-Time, Adjusted Lunch Period, and Compressed Work Week. Once an employee signs up for a particular flex-time, the individual is expected to work that schedule in a consistent manner. However, schedules can be changed.

Peak-Hour Flex-Time: This flex-time schedule shifts daily work hours while still working an 8 hour day. For instance, instead of the normal 8–5 day, an employee could work from 7–4, 7:30-4:30, 9:00-6:00, etc. Working any arrangement of hours within an 8 hour day constitutes a valid work day. It is important to remember that the level of service must be maintained during peak hours, which are from 10:00 to 3:00. Therefore, supervisors will need to coordinate the schedules of all flex-time participants to ensure ample coverage during these hours.

Adjusted Lunch Period: This flex-time schedule allows employees to adjust the length of their lunch period, while still working an 8-hour day. An employee can take a minimum of 30 minutes and a maximum of two hours for lunch. For instance, an employee might want to go to the gym everyday from 11-1 and consequently leave work at 6:00 rather than 5:00.

Compressed Work Week: To maintain this flex-time arrangement, an employee works a full 40 hour work week in less than five days. For instance, an employee may work four 10-hour days, or on a two week rotating basis; one week employees work a regular 8–5, five day week and the next they work a compressed schedule, which is four 9-hour days and one 4-hour day.

SOURCE: Reprinted with permission of FocusForwardCoaching.com, Kirsten E. Ross, MLIR, SPHR, President. 2009.

Appendix 23.2

University of Texas Medical Branch Telecommuting Agreement

The following represents an agreement entered into by _____, and governs activities performed while telecommuting as an employee of the University of Texas Medical Branch at Galveston. This agreement is subject to approval of myself and the appropriate Vice President or Dean. All applicable institutional and departmental policies and procedures continue to apply to your employment, including the telecommuting guidelines in the University Handbook of Operating Procedures, Policy 3.5.4 on Telecommuting.

1. **Duration:** This agreement will be valid for the period of _____ beginning _____ and ending _____. This agreement, effective on the indicated conclusion date, will either be terminated or renegotiated for an additional period of time specified in the new agreement. The agreement will be reviewed at 30 days, and on a periodic basis, and based upon that review, may be cancelled by the Department by giving you thirty days notice. The employee may also cancel this agreement by giving thirty days notice.

2. **Work Location:** The employee's approved alternate workplace will be in his or her private home at _____. The employee must provide a current address and phone number where she/he can be reached at the teleworking location.

3. **Work Station:** You must have a designated, ergonomically safe work area which is primarily used for your work duties. The Department has the right to visit the remote work location to ensure it meets standards and requirements.

4. **Work hours:** Normal workweek will be 40 hours per week for full-time employees. Your schedule will be as follows:

   At UTMB location: _____

   _____

   At alternate site: _____

   _____

5. **Salary and Benefits:** UTMB agrees this arrangement is not a basis for changing employee's salary or benefits.

6. **Time and Attendance:** Attendance will be 40 hours per week for full-time employees, unless mutually agreed upon by both the Manager and the employee. Overtime and any other changes to work schedule must be approved in writing by the Manager. The method of time reporting currently used in this office will continue to be used throughout the duration of this agreement.

7. **Leave:** The employee will be required to obtain the Manager's approval before taking leave in accordance with established procedure. Unscheduled absences due to illness, or for any other reason, will be immediately reported to the office.

8. **Institution-Owned Equipment:** Equipment provided to you will be maintained by you. All institution-owned equipment will be safely returned to the Department within 48 hours if the agreement is terminated. If computer equipment is lost or stolen, employee's supervisor and Information Services

Security must be notified immediately. Equipment is to be used solely for the purpose of the employee's UTMB work duties.

9. **Liability:** Employee will be responsible for damages to UTMB's and employee's property, resulting from participation in the Telecommuting program.

10. **Reimbursement:** UTMB will not be responsible for operating costs, home maintenance, or any other incidental cost (i.e. utilities) associated with the use of the employee's residence. Costs associated with high speed internet connectivity will be at the expense of the employee.

11. **Worker's Compensation:** The employee is covered under the Worker's Compensation Law if injured in the course of performing official duties at the telecommuting location.

12. **Work expectations:** Employees are expected to at least maintain current productivity and quality levels when working at the alternate work site, and work must be of the same high caliber as presently produced. All work assignments will be completed according to work procedures mutually agreed upon between Manager and employee. Failure to meet standards of productivity and quality at any time may result in the employee having to return on site for performance improvement. Performance evaluations will take place annually, based on standard Performance Appraisal for your organization.

13. **Standards of Conduct/Compliance:** The employee agrees to adhere to UTMB standards of conduct while working at the alternate workplace. UTMB required Compliance training is to be completed within timeframes specified. Telecommuting is not an alternative to child or elder care. The employee must make appropriate arrangements for dependent care.

14. **Confidentiality/Records:** Employee will apply approved safeguards to protect patient information and institutional records from unauthorized disclosure. Telecommuting is considered official organizational business. No printing of patient health information is allowed. All papers, records and other correspondence must be safeguarded for their return to the UTMB. Records should only be destroyed in accordance with the applicable departmental Document Retention Schedule and must be shredded or returned to UTMB for approved recycling in locked bags. Computerized files and reports are considered official records and shall be similarly protected with the highest confidentiality standards.

15. **Risk Management:** Employee will be responsible for making sure telecommuting location conforms to accepted safety and human engineering standards. Work area should be secured when not occupied by employee. Employee will ensure no unauthorized access is gained to the work area or to the equipment contained therein.

16. **Amendment of Agreement:** This agreement may be amended through mutual agreement between the manager and the employee.

I have read and understand this agreement and accept its conditions.

_____   _____
Employee Signature   Date

APPROVAL:

_____   _____
Manager Signature   Date

_____
SOURCE: University of Texas Medical Center, Galveston. [Online information; retrieved 10/23/09.] http://hr.utmb.edu/hrlibrary/telecom.doc.

APPENDIX 23.3

How to Identify and Deal with "Whining Cry Baby (WCB) Syndrome"

By Chief Patrick M. Kelly, Medley Police Department

Hear it? That high-pitched, annoying, constant background noise? Maybe it's coming from the office next to yours, or from that little knot of people who have stopped to gossip in the hallway. Maybe it's even coming from—could it be?—you. One thing's for sure: It's getting louder and more persistent, and there's no getting away from it. If you can make out some of the words, they sound like: The department doesn't appreciate me. The department won't help me plan my career. Nobody ever tells me what's going on around here. The Chief is a jackass. My evaluation wasn't fair. My last raise was too long ago and too small. Everything's changing too fast, and not for the better. It's not fair. This place stinks. And the granddaddy of them all, morale is lower than it's ever been. Waaaaaaaaaaah. . . .

After discussion with many chief executive officers, in both private and public sectors, it is amply clear that Whining Cry Baby (WCB) Syndrome is alive and well. WCBs—employees suffering from WCB Syndrome—must be identified and managed effectively. Unidentified and/or poorly managed WCBs can affect organizational productivity, employee morale and motivation, customer service levels, and, most importantly, the entire organizational culture. WCBs possess many, if not all, of the following attributes.

WCB Attributes

Victim's Mentality—WCBs have acute victim's mentality. They are not responsible for their own negative behavior. Every negative outcome in their life is attributable to some other person(s) or some circumstance(s) beyond their control. When WCBs are challenged about questionable behavior, their reactions have become incredibly predictable and almost Pavlovian in nature. First, of course, the accused will deny being at fault and then, second, cleave almost immediately to the sequential steps of the "WCB's Defense:" (1) I didn't do it; (2) Okay, I did it, but it wasn't a violation of policy, or there is no written policy; (3) Well, yes, I know it was a violation of policy, but everyone else was doing it too; and besides, I was doing less of it; (4) Yes, I did it, but the means you used to catch me were inappropriate; (5) You are only picking on me because I'm (fill in the blank). These forms of rationalization work very well, because WCBs do not have to accept responsibility for anything that goes wrong in their personal and professional lives. Conversely, they take full credit for all positive outcomes or successful results they are associated with. Simply put, WCBs believe other people are totally responsible for their failures, while WCBs are totally responsible for all their successes.

Tuned into Radio Station WIFM—WCBs are tuned into What's In It For Me? (WIFM) 24 hours a day. They see themselves as the center of the universe and seldom consider how their actions impact others. This often manifests itself in their suggestions for organizational improvement, which are usually self-serving or loaded with hidden agendas. WCBs continuously assert their individual rights, even if those rights trample on the rights of others, or most importantly on what is best for the entire organization. WCBs often believe that seniority or "time in grade" should be the criteria assigned the greatest weight in personnel decisions. They often say, "I've been here the longest, so I've earned the assignment or promotion."

Apathetic—WCBs don't get involved and always approach their duties and tasks in a reactive mode. They initiate little, if any, work activity. WCBs prefer traditional policing methodologies and will often spend more time looking for ways to avoid work than simply completing the tasks as assigned. You will hear them saying, "It's not my job," "That's not in my job description," or "The only way to stay out of trouble around here is to do nothing." WCBs are usually the least productive employees. They despise community-policing initiatives and may even sabotage these proactive problem-solving efforts.

Complaining Critics—WCBs are organizational critics. They are able to identify what is wrong with everything and everyone else but spend no time assessing the individual they see in the mirror. Once WCBs complain about and/or criticize some issue or person, and place blame on it, they feverishly move to another issue. The only level of satisfaction they ever get is bringing people down to their level of anger and unhappiness. After doing this, they celebrate their hard-won battle and quickly step over the lives they have ruined.

Why Do WCBs Exist?

First, many WCBs began their behavior as children. It began with the words "Mommy and Daddy, I want . . ." and goes on and on and on. Of course, it usually takes place in public, before the largest number of strangers possible. A Kansas State University professor, who specializes in parent–child relationships, says that whining is what's called an irrelevant behavior that parents are responsible for creating. Dr. Charles Smith says, "A child whines because they have learned that kind of repetitious, aggravating behavior gets them what they want. Parents have to realize they created this behavior and now they're going to have to suffer through it."

Unfortunately, this irrelevant behavior can continue through adolescence and into adulthood. And just like the parent, the organization is responsible if this irrelevant whining behavior continues to persist. Remember basic psychology. When a person repeats a behavior pattern, that person is getting a payoff. You must avoid the old cliche, "The squeaky wheel gets the most oil." This "oil," or payoff is simply reinforcing the WCB and his or her negative, irrelevant behavior.

It is important to note that not all WCBs are genetic, or environmental as a child, but rather rookie copies who are unfortunately paired with these individuals (veteran WCBs) and thus just don't know any better.

Second, we are a society that values individuals' "rights" above all else. Psychologist Carol Tavris, in her landmark book, *Anger: The Misunderstood Emotion*, explains our tendency to whine: "The individualism of American life, to our glory and despair, creates anger and encourages its release. For when everything is possible, limitations are irksome. When the desires of the self come first, the needs of others are annoying. When we think we deserve it all, reaping only a portion can enrage." Ah, "reaping only a portion," you may say, misstates the case. WCBs don't want the whole pie, just a few more crumbs.

American organizations are simply microcosms of American society. All employees come to work with unique "individual" personalities, interests, preferences and rights. Successful employees recognize the need to balance their individual rights with the rights of the organization's internal and external stakeholders. Unfortunately, WCBs have not recognized the need to sacrifice some individual "rights" for the good of the collective organization and its customers. Those folks whom New York City behavioral scientist Deborah Bright calls "entitlists"—a polite word for WCBs—often express their outrage in passive–aggressive ways, including being chronically late or absent, stealing from the company, backstabbing coworkers or bosses, or simply withdrawing—not taking risks, not suggesting solutions, not going the extra mile—in effect just waiting around to be fired. Need we point out that these DDFO are not great career-building strategies?

Finally, our level of self-esteem affects virtually everything we think, say and do. It affects how we see the world and our place in it. It affects how others in the world see and treat us. It affects the choices we make—choices about what we will do with our lives and with whom we will be involved. It affects our ability to both give and receive praise and recognition. And, it affects our ability to take action to change things that need to be changed. WCBs, like many people in American society, suffer from low self-esteem. What separates WCBs from others suffering from low self-esteem? WCBs do not understand or have not yet accepted their low self-esteem. In fact, WCB attributes, described earlier in this article, are all manifestations of low self-esteem. They don't have time to look into the mirror objectively, because they are so busy criticizing and condemning others. Unfortunately, WCBs surround themselves with other WCBs. There is truth to the old adage, "misery loves company." WCBs commiserate with each other on a daily basis. In fact, it was from the depths of this WCB commiseration that this author broke free from the chains of this life and career-crippling syndrome.

How to Effectively Deal with WCBs

One day two frogs were playing together, hopping over each other on a park bench. Suddenly, as they neared the edge of the bench they both fell off and into a pail of milk, which was on the ground. The pail was only filled halfway, so the two frogs had a difficult time trying to get out. Eventually their commotion and cries for help drew a crowd of other frogs who gathered at the edge of the bench. When the crowd saw how hopeless their situation was, they began to jump up and down, swinging their legs and yelling, "Give up! Give up! You will never make it out! It's hopeless!" When one of the frogs in the pail saw them and heard what they were saying; he knew they were right. He didn't see the point of trying any longer, so he laid back and slowly disappeared into the pail of milk and drowned. The other frog looked up and saw the crowd jumping up and down and yelling, and this made him more determined to get out. So he started to swim around and around, faster and faster. Eventually his churning around made the milk begin to harden. He was able to get a foothold and jump out of the pail of milk and save his life.

Oh . . . by the way . . . I forgot to tell you that the second frog . . . the one that triumphed and saved his life . . . was DEAF! You see, because he was deaf, he did not hear all the negative remarks from the crowd. He saw the other frogs jumping up and down, waving and yelling to him, and he thought they were encouraging him to try harder!

The first, and most important, strategy for dealing effectively with WCBs is in this story. If you and your organization are going to succeed, you need to be like the second frog. You need to ignore the WCBs and their comments, because they will discourage you and drag you down. Getting sound advice from people who have achieved success is one thing. Listening to WCBs is another. Remember basic psychology. Ears, or people listening, is a payoff for WCBs. As long as there is an audience (payoff) for their negativity, they will continue to cry, "Waaaaaaaa. . . ." A more diplomatic way of utilizing this strategy is to become "selectively impolite." Be remote when the WCB complains. Only show interest when he or she stops complaining or says something positive.

The second strategy is to dismiss the WCB's negative comment. Say something like "You may be right," and change the subject. A leading management psychologist says that often the best way of handling something that really bothers you is not to oppose it, but to align yourself with it. This will totally confuse and disorient the WCB. Of course, it will be YOUR fault when the WCB becomes confused and disoriented.

Third, don't get flustered. If the WCB appears to enjoy upsetting you, keep your cool. Any emotional reaction from you becomes a payoff for the WCB.

Next, be direct. Tell the WCB, "Your complaining bothers me. I can't handle that kind of talk right now." Or, "It bothers me when you only talk about the negative side of things." Interestingly, as much as WCBs complain, they never seem to leave. This is because subconsciously they realize how great things really are in their current organization, or because no one else will hire them. If things are really that bad, invite them to apply elsewhere. Be cautious though; they will view this as a threat in their negative mindsets.

Fifth, jump in first. There was an office manager who had to deal with a WCB's constant complaining about her husband. One Monday morning, he asked her, "What did the MORON do to you this weekend?" Startled, she replied, "Why are you saying that about my husband?" He said he'd listened to her complaints for years and decided the man had to be a sadistic monster. She responded, "He's not that bad," and stopped complaining.

Sixth, pay attention to results. The supervisor in a printing shop said an old-time printer was always pessimistic about special printing jobs, insisting that each job was impossible. The supervisor would tell him to go ahead anyway, and in every case the job worked out. If negativity is a good employee's security blanket, let it be.

Seventh, ask for the complaints in writing. Then read them back to the WCB. Some WCBs don't know how negative they sound. Of course, many WCBs will refuse to reduce their complaints to writing, because they don't want to spend time looking for solutions. They fear formal documentation of their complaints, because then they may be asked, "How do you think we can address your complaint(s)?" This question leads to the final strategy for dealing with WCBs.

Finally, ask for clarification and empower the WCB to propose viable solutions to their complaints. Tell the WCB to describe the problem and clarify the desired outcome(s). Ask what plans the WCB has for handling the situation. Such questions will slow pathological WCBs down and force them to think about positive actions. Then again, they may respond with, "It's not my job!"

Closing Comments

One of life's greatest frustrations is dealing with WCBs who absorb your energy and drag you down. Most managers find constantly complaining, whining employees more difficult to work with than incompetent employees. "Basically, most people with positive attitudes have a negative attitude about negative attitudes," says psychologist Al Siebert, who teaches executives how to deal with difficult people on the job. "Negative people catch the blind spot of your basic optimist managerial type. These upbeat executives are very judgmental and feel negative people are defective human beings who have flawed personalities. Their position is that everything would work out if only those negative people would get an attitude transplant." Reality dictates, however, that most WCBs are not going to change as long as there are organizational "payoffs" (i.e., specialized assignments, promotions, and training opportunities) for their behavior. Eliminate rewards for inappropriate behavior and become selectively "DEAF" around WCBs, and you will become the organizational cure for "WCB Syndrome."

SOURCE: Reprinted with permission of Jeff Reh, general counsel. This article appeared in *Beretta USA Leadership Bulletin*, Sept. 1998, Vol. 3, Issue 9.

24

DISCIPLINE

Chapter Objectives

After you have studied this chapter, you should be able to do the following:

1. Define the term "discipline."
2. Discuss different techniques of administering discipline.
3. Describe different types of disciplinary actions.
4. Review the supervisor's role in disciplinary actions.
5. Outline the rights of employees in the disciplinary process.

The term "discipline" is understood in several different ways. To many, discipline (when used as a verb) carries the disagreeable connotation of punishing wrongdoers; one is often inclined to think immediately of authority enforcing obedience. But there is a positive connotation of discipline as well, one that is far more in keeping with good supervisory practices. Maintaining positive, also known as constructive, discipline (the noun form of the word) and good influence go hand in hand.

Organizational Discipline

For our purposes, *discipline* can be defined as a state of affairs or a condition of orderliness in which the members of the enterprise behave sensibly and conduct themselves according to the standards of acceptable behavior as expressed by the needs of the organization. Discipline is said to be good when the employees willingly follow the rules of the enterprise, live up to or exceed standards, and practice good self-judgment. Discipline is said to be poor when subordinates follow regulations reluctantly or refuse to follow them, violate the standards of acceptable behavior, and require constant surveillance by their supervisors. Favorable discipline thrives in an organizational climate in which management applies positive motivation, sound leadership, and efficient management.

Positive Discipline and Morale

A direct correlation exists between morale and discipline. Normally, fewer problems of a disciplinary nature arise when morale is high, and low morale tends to increase problems of discipline. While a high degree of discipline can exist in an environment of low morale—where discipline is likely controlled by fear and forcefulness—it is not usually possible to maintain a high level of morale unless there is also a high degree of positive discipline.

Self-Discipline

The best discipline is self-discipline—the human tendency to do what needs to be done. In the healthcare setting, this is doing one's share, assisting coworkers when appropriate, and subordinating some of one's own needs and desires to the standards of acceptable behavior set for the enterprise as a whole. From early childhood, people are trained to respect rules, accept orders from those legitimately entitled to issue them, and realize that all activities set limits on the behavior of the organization's members.

Experience shows that most employees want to do the right thing. Even before they start to work, most mature people accept the idea that following instructions and fair rules of conduct is a responsibility that goes with any job. Thus, most employees can be counted on to exercise a considerable degree of self-discipline. They believe in coming to work on time, following the supervisor's instructions, refraining from fights, avoiding use of inappropriate language, resisting any temptation to steal, and so forth. In other words, self-imposed discipline is based on the commitment of employees to conform to the rules, regulations, and orders that are necessary for the proper conduct of the institution.

Once the employees know what is expected of them and believe that the rules by which they are governed are reasonable, they usually observe them without problems. The supervisor must check the rules and regulations periodically to ensure they continue to be reasonable. For example, the dress codes and codes of general appearance have most certainly undergone changes in the past decade. It is unreasonable to request subordinates to comply with a dress and appearance code set up years ago that dictates that women wear dresses and men may not have facial hair. Some rules may need to be altered to address medical concerns. For example, a healthcare organization with a "no beard" policy may allow African Americans to wear beards, as some African Americans are prone to pseudofolliculitis barbae, a painful skin condition worsened by shaving.

When new rules are introduced, the supervisor must show their current rationale to the employees. For instance, short skirts may be fashionable, but they are not conducive to a nurse's appearance and movement or functioning on the job. Instead of simply outlawing short skirts, however, a rule giving nurses a choice between wearing a certain length of hemline or uniforms with long pants might be considered a more reasonable dress code. Rules regarding hair length are relevant in some job settings, as in the surgical suite, but are irrelevant in others. Because hair can compromise a state of asepsis, the supervisor, chief of surgery, infection committee, and director of patient care may need to work out rules that make hair caps mandatory for operating room personnel.

The supervisor must be alert to changing styles and mores. **Mores** are culture-driven expectations. For example, in an orthodox Jewish community, married women are expected to cover their hair and wear blouses that cover their upper body to the elbow. As noted during the discussion of cultural blindness in Chapter 21, supervisors must make certain that the rules and regulations truly respect the diverse cultures represented in the work team. Otherwise, rules are not enforceable, and many unnecessary disciplinary problems may arise.

If present, mores and **norms**—standards that regulate behavior within an organization—exert group pressure on potential wrongdoers, further reducing the need for the supervisor's disciplinary action. For example, it may be the norm in a department meeting to just listen to whatever the supervisor says and not ask questions; after the meeting, the staff will privately discuss the issues. Work groups also set norms and performance standards; for example, fellow employees are expected by the group to perform their fair share of tasks and be at work on time. Hence, group discipline reinforces self-discipline and exerts pressure on those who do not comply with group norms and standards.

Employees must also know that they have the supervisor's unqualified support as long as they stay within the ordinary rules of conduct and their activities are consistent with what is expected of them. Proper discipline is dependent on the supervisor's positive support for the right action and criticism of and punishment for the wrong action. Furthermore, the subordinate must know that failure to live up to expectations results in "punishment."

Administration cannot expect employees to practice self-discipline unless it starts at the top. Similar restrictions must be imposed on all managerial personnel to remain within the acceptable patterns of behavior: to be on time, to observe no smoking and no drinking rules, and to dress and behave in a manner commensurate with the organizational and departmental standards.

Setting an example is a key responsibility of management. The mirror effect pervades all levels of the organization if the example is displayed by all supervisors and managers. This role modeling by management can show all staff that "I only expect of you what I expect of myself." If you model poor habits (as displayed in Exhibit 24.1), your staff likely will conduct themselves similarly.

mores
Culture-driven expectations in behavior, such as the type of clothing one wears or the way one treats others.

norms
Standards that regulate behavior within an organization.

EXHIBIT 24.1

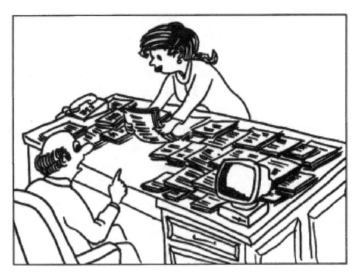

"Don't put anything there, Ms. Finkel. That spot is for my feet."

SOURCE: Reprinted from *Hospitals & Health Networks*, by permission, June 2000, © 2000, by Health Forum, Inc.

Finally, employees must be informed of expectations. Supervisors should always put policies and expectations in writing and make sure they are enforced evenhandedly. These documents should be specific, including what is not acceptable, and should not be used to discriminate. Johnson (2009) suggests that if you elect to outline a progressive disciplinary policy (discussed in a later section of this chapter), it is essential that you reserve the discretion to skip steps based on the severity of the offense. If you opt to include a defined list of potential disciplinary offenses, you also must clearly state that it is not "all inclusive" and the organization ultimately will determine when discipline is warranted.

When Discipline Is Warranted

Although the vast majority of employees exercise considerable self-discipline, a few employees in every organization occasionally fail to abide by established rules and standards even after having been informed of them. Some employees simply do not accept the responsibility of self-discipline. Also, a few unruly employees, probably because of their personality, background, and development, may find it difficult to function within policies, rules, and regulations. Common sources of disciplinary action include habitual tardiness, missed deadlines, frequent errors, and doing just enough work to get by (Spath 2006, 17).

Because the job must get done, the supervisor cannot afford to let those few get away with violations. Quick and firm action is called for to correct the situation; otherwise, the morale of the other employees in the work group will be seriously weakened. At times like this, the supervisor has to rely on the power and force inherent in the managerial position, even though she may dislike doing so. She must recognize that she is in charge of the department and is therefore responsible for discipline within it. If the supervisor does not correct the situation, some individuals who are on the borderline of being undisciplined may follow the bad example.

When administering discipline, managers should remember that the purpose is to preserve the interests of the organization and to protect the rights of the employees. Many organizations encourage a positive discipline approach. Discipline is not for the purpose of punishment or getting even with an employee. Rather, its purpose is to improve the employee's future behavior—to correct and rehabilitate, but not to injure. Discipline corrects the subordinate's breach of the rules and carries the notice of more serious consequences in the future. Discipline also serves as a warning for other people in the department. It reminds the disciplined individual's coworkers that rules exist and that violating them does not go unnoticed or without any action from the supervisor. Moreover, discipline reassures all those employees who respect the rules out of their desire to do the right thing.

The guides and checklists provided in Chapter 19, Exhibits 19.4 and 19.5, may be beneficial when delivering discipline. The interests of the organization are best served when an employee understands what is expected of him or her and complies with those expectations.

Ensuring the employee has had the proper training for and orientation to the work before applying discipline is one of the supervisor's principal duties. By doing so, the supervisor salvages a trained resource, and the organization avoids the expense of recruitment and loss of productivity resulting from a vacancy or from training a new employee.

The supervisor should administer positive discipline to motivate the employee to do what is right rather than discourage her from doing what is wrong. This is not an easy task because inherently the act of punishing a subordinate for violating a rule always presupposes that the subordinate was caught violating it. Yet many others who may have violated the same rule go unpunished because the supervisor did not catch them. This injects unfairness into the disciplinary process. Administering positive discipline is also difficult because any discipline is normally resented, and it places a strain on the supervisor–subordinate relationship. Sometimes discipline only makes the subordinate redouble her efforts not to be caught again. Nevertheless, positive discipline will generally be successful and accepted if the supervisor follows a few simple rules when taking disciplinary action. Jane Boucher's (2001) book, *How to Love the Job You Hate*, offers the advice shown in Exhibit 24.2.

Exhibit 24.2 Criticism Guidelines

If You Must Criticize Someone

Here are some suggestions for giving criticism in a way that motivates others to do a better job:

- See yourself as a teacher or coach—as being helpful. Keep in mind that you're trying to help someone improve.
- Show you care. Express your sincere concern about sharing ways the other person can boost his or her success.
- Pick the right moment to offer criticism. Make sure the person hasn't just been shaken by some incident.
- Avoid telling people they "should do such and such" or "should have done such and such." "Shoulds" make you appear rigid and pedantic.
- Avoid giving the impression that you're more concerned with seeing your recommendations put into practice than in helping the other person improve.
- Show how the person will benefit from taking the actions you suggest.
- Give specific suggestions. Being vague might only make the situation worse by creating anxiety and doubt.

Tip: Be sure you can take criticism yourself. If not, you may not be perceived as a credible source.

SOURCE: Boucher (2001). Reprinted with permission. Jane Boucher, president, Boucher Consultants, (937) 294–6960.

Taking Responsibility

Few occasions arise that force a good supervisor to take disciplinary action. When such instances do occur, the first step in addressing them is to obtain all pertinent facts. Before the supervisor does anything, he must investigate what has happened and why the employee violated the rule or failed to perform as expected. When the investigative interview is used to confront an employee about alleged acts, the skilled supervisor is observant of the employee's reactions. Reactions may expose lying and other unacceptable behavior. As Wells (2001) states, "Behaviorists tell us that lying is innate to the human species and comes about for two genetically programmed reasons: to receive rewards and/or to avoid punishment. Whether we lie depends on our calculation of the reward/punishment equation. This is called 'situational honesty.'"

In addition, the employee's past record should be checked, and all other pertinent information should be obtained before any action is taken. When the information collected indicates that disciplinary action is necessary, the supervisor is best qualified to handle the situation because she knows the employee, alleged violations, and circumstances. In addition, by being in charge of the department, the supervisor has the authority and responsibility to take appropriate action.[1] Although it may be expedient to let someone in the human resources department handle such unpleasant problems, the supervisor will not only be shirking and abdicating responsibility but also undermining her own position if this is allowed.

The same result will occur if the supervisor ignores or conveniently overlooks for any length of time a subordinate's failure to meet the prescribed standards related to, for example, use of the organization's computers for personal purposes. If such breaches are condoned, the supervisor is communicating to the rest of the employees that she does not intend to enforce the rules and regulations. Thus, the supervisor must not procrastinate in administering discipline. On the other hand, the supervisor must be careful not to take hasty or unwarranted action.

Tulgan (2007) recommends that the supervisor first review his notes from any previous one-on-one meetings with the individual. Next, he should consider his role in the employee's performance problem: is he confident he has done a thoughtful and thorough job of trying to help this person improve? Did he spell out expectations clearly? If he has done so, the confrontation should not come as a surprise to the employee.

Maintaining Control of Emotions

Whenever taking disciplinary action, the supervisor must not lose her temper. Regardless of the severity of the violation, the supervisor must not lose control of the situation and run the risk of losing the respect of the employees. If the employees do not agree with the facts on which the disciplinary action is based, the supervisor may end up arguing with the other employees over what happened. Varying eyewitness reports will only confuse the situation. In addition, public discipline humiliates the disciplined employee in the eyes of the coworkers and could cause considerable damage to the department.

This does not mean that the supervisor should face the situation half-heartedly or haphazardly. If she is in danger of losing control, however, action should be avoided until tempers have cooled down. Even if the violation is significant, the supervisor cannot afford to lose her temper. Moreover, the supervisor should follow the general rule of never laying a hand on an employee in any way. Except in emergencies, when an employee has been injured or becomes ill, or when employees who are fighting need to be separated, such a gesture could easily make matters worse.

Discipline in Private

The supervisor must make certain that all disciplinary action takes place in private, never in public. A public reprimand builds up resentment in the employee, and it may permit unrelated factors to enter the situation. For instance, if in the opinion of the other workers a disciplinary action is too severe for the violation, the disciplined employee may appear as a martyr to the rest of the group. A supervisor who is disciplining in public is bound to have his performance judged by every employee in the department. Furthermore, employees expect to be treated with the same courtesy that they extend to their supervisor. Thus, just as a supervisor expects to receive counseling in private, so should he extend the same courtesy to his subordinates. However, because of increased litigation, some organizations mandate, or encourage, the use of witnesses at disciplinary interviews. In these cases the supervisor may invite a witness to observe the counseling. Some organizations even permit the employee to invite a witness. Should this be the situation at your organization, the human resources department can outline the criteria for the use of witnesses and their roles.

Progressive Disciplinary Action

The question of which type of disciplinary action to use is answered differently in different enterprises. In recent years, however, most enterprises have accepted the idea of progressive discipline, which provides for an increase in the penalty with each new offense. First offenders get less severe penalties than do repeat offenders; those committing more serious infractions receive more severe penalties than do those committing lesser offenses. In progressive discipline, unless a serious wrong has been committed, the employee is rarely discharged for the first offense. The steps in a progressive discipline protocol generally include the following:

1. informal talk,
2. spoken warning or reprimand,
3. written warning,
4. disciplinary layoff,
5. demotion or downgrading, and
6. discharge.

disciplinary counseling
An informal conversation in which a supervisor notifies a subordinate about a problem and tries to resolve it.

These steps, presented in ascending order of severity, are suggestions; they are not the only means of disciplinary action, nor are they all necessary. Many enterprises, however, have found the progression of these disciplinary steps to be a viable approach to ensuring that the individual is provided sufficient feedback about her performance.

Informal Talk If the incident is minor and the employee has no previous record of disciplinary action, an informal, friendly talk, also referred to as **disciplinary counseling**, clears up the situation in many cases. In such a talk, the supervisor discusses with the employee his behavior in relation to the standards that prevail within the enterprise. The supervisor tries to get to the underlying reason for the undesirable behavior. If the institution has an employee assistance program, as discussed in Chapter 22, the supervisor may refer the employee to it if indications show this program can help him. At the same time, the boss will try to reaffirm the employee's sense of responsibility and reestablish the previous cooperative relationship within the department. It may also be advisable to repeat once more why the action of the employee is undesirable and what consequences it may lead to. If the supervisor later finds that this friendly talk was not sufficient to bring about the desired results, it will become necessary to take the next step, a spoken warning.

Spoken Warning or Reprimand

In the reprimand interview, the supervisor should again point out how undesirable the subordinate's violation is and how it could ultimately lead to more severe disciplinary action. Such an interview has emotional overtones, as the employee most likely is resentful for having been caught again and the supervisor may also be angry. However, the violation should be discussed in a straightforward manner as a statement of fact. In delivering the reprimand, the supervisor should not begin with a recital of how the fine reputation of the employee has now been tarnished. She also should not be apologetic but should state the case in specific terms and then give the subordinate a chance to tell his side of the story.

The supervisor should stress the preventive purpose of this disciplinary action, but the employee must be advised that such conduct cannot be tolerated. In some enterprises a record is made on the employee's personnel file that this spoken warning has taken place. The warning should leave the employee with the confidence that he can do better and will improve in the future. Some supervisors believe that such a verbal reprimand is not very effective. If it is carried out skillfully, however, many negative behaviors will be corrected at this stage.

Written Warning

A written warning is formal insofar as it becomes a part of the employee's record. Written warnings are particularly necessary in work settings in which unions exist so that the document can serve as evidence in case of grievance procedures. The written warning must contain a statement of the violation and the potential consequences. Typically, a duplicate copy of it is given to the employee, and another duplicate of the warning is sent to the human resources department so that it can be inserted in the employee's personnel record.

Disciplinary Layoff or Suspension

The next disciplinary step may be a **disciplinary layoff** or suspension. This step occurs when all previous steps have been taken and the employee has continued the offense or when a serious offense has occurred and time is required to fully investigate the issues. In the latter situation, the employee is suspended pending a final decision in the case. This device protects management as well as the employee; it gives management a chance to conduct the necessary investigation and consult higher levels of administration or the human resources department, and it provides an opportunity for tempers to cool off.

disciplinary layoff
A temporary suspension used to punish a serious infraction.

In cases of temporary suspension, the employee is told that she is suspended and will be informed as soon as possible of the disciplinary action that will be taken, if any.

When a suspension is used as described here, the suspension itself may not be punishment. If the investigation shows that there is no cause for disciplinary action, the employee has no grievance because she is allowed to return to work and will be compensated for work time missed. The obvious advantage of temporary suspensions is that the supervisor can act promptly without any prejudice toward the employee.

If, on the other hand, the penalty is disciplinary in nature, it will be considered a disciplinary layoff and the time during which the employee was suspended will not be compensated. Under such conditions, the supervisor must determine what length of disciplinary time off is appropriate. This will depend on how serious the offense is. Disciplinary layoffs typically extend over several days and are seldom longer than a few weeks. Neither temporary suspensions nor disciplinary layoffs should be used indiscriminately; these should be invoked primarily when the offense is likely to call for at least the layoff.

Some employees may not be impressed with spoken or written warnings. In these cases, employees on disciplinary layoffs may wake up to a short layoff without pay and realize that the organization is serious about enforcing the rules. In some organizations, the human resources department has a defined time frame for this type of disciplinary layoff or suspension.

There are several disadvantages to invoking a disciplinary layoff or suspension. Some enterprises do not apply this measure at all because it hurts their productivity, especially in times of labor shortages when the employee cannot be easily replaced. Also, the employee might return from the layoff in a much less pleasant frame of mind than when he left. Although most managers consider the disciplinary layoff or suspension a serious measure, some employees who frequently violate the rules may not regard it as such; they may even view a few days of layoff as a welcome break from their daily routine. While many institutions use them effectively, a number of them no longer use these measures. Instead, they move right to discharge, or they practice the new concept of discipline without punishment, discussed later in this chapter.

Demotion The usefulness of demoting an employee is seriously questioned; therefore, this disciplinary measure is seldom invoked. To demote an employee for disciplinary reasons to a lower-level, less desirable, and lower-paying job is likely to bring about dissatisfaction and discouragement. Over an extended period an employee downgrading is a form of constant punishment. The dissatisfaction, humiliation, and ill will that result may easily spread to other employees in the department. Sometimes this measure can be viewed as an invitation for the employee to quit rather than be discharged. Many enterprises avoid downgrading as a disciplinary measure just as they avoid disciplinary layoffs or the withholding of a scheduled pay increase. If so, they have to use termination of employment as the ultimate solution.

Discharge

Discharge, or corporate capital punishment, is the most drastic form of disciplinary action, and it should be reserved exclusively for the most serious offenses. Supervisors should resort to it infrequently and only after some of the preliminary steps have been taken. Alternatively, when a serious wrong has been committed, discharge should be invoked at once. For instance, when an employee uses a patient's social security number and other information to obtain a credit card or releases medical records of a celebrity to a local newspaper, immediate discharge is in order.

Discharge is costly to the organization and causes real hardship to the person who has been discharged. For the employee, discharge eliminates seniority standing, possibly some pension rights, substantial vacation benefits, pay level, and other benefits that the employee has accumulated. Discharge also makes obtaining new employment difficult for the worker. In regard to the enterprise, discharges involve serious losses and waste, including the expense of training a new employee and the disruption caused by changing the makeup of the work team. Discharge also may cause damage to the morale of the group. If the discharged employee is a member of a legally protected group, such as minorities or women, administration has to be concerned about nondiscrimination and hiring quotas.

Therefore, because of these possibly serious consequences of discharge, many organizations have removed from the supervisor the authority to fire, reserving it for higher levels in administration. In some institutions, the supervisor's recommendation to discharge must be reviewed and approved by higher administration, the human resources director, or both. In organizations where unions are present, management is concerned with possible prolonged arbitration procedures, knowing that arbitrators have become increasingly unwilling to permit discharge except for the most severe violations. Although situations may arise for which the only solution is to fire the employee for just cause, these cases are rare.

Time Element

In all of the disciplinary steps previously discussed, the time element by which the employee is held accountable is a significant factor. There is no reason to hold an indiscretion of past years against a person forever. Current practice is inclined to disregard offenses that have been committed more than a year previously if the person has reformed. For example, an employee with a poor record of tardiness starts with a clean slate if he has maintained a good record for one year. This time element varies depending on the nature of the violation.

Documentation

It is essential for the supervisor to keep detailed records of all disciplinary actions, as they have the potential of becoming the subject of further discussions, disputes, and even litigation. The burden of proof of lawful action is on the employer. The written record should cover the time of the event, details of the offense, supervisor's decision, and action taken. It should also include the reasoning involved in the decision. If at some future time the supervisor or the institution is asked to substantiate the action taken, it is not sufficient to depend on memory alone.

It is more important than ever to keep accurate, detailed personnel records because the aggrieved employee may file a lawsuit for wrongful discharge based on discrimination, harassment, or similar reasons. If a union is involved, documentation is required to justify a disciplinary measure if it is challenged by a formal grievance procedure. Regardless of any potential consequences, written documentation at the time of the event is essential for the institution and the supervisor's own records.

Other Discharge Precautions

Because the healthcare supervisor has responsibility for ensuring the security of confidential information to which an employee may have had access, when termination occurs, the supervisor must take additional steps to cease access by this individual to protected health information. These may include changing pass codes on door locks; removing the employee's access to the organization's information system; deleting employee system-access accounts; removing biometric identifiers; and retrieving keys, tokens, or other cards that allow access into the unit or organization.

The Supervisor's Dilemma

Throughout this book, the discussion has stressed the importance of the relationship of trust, confidence, and help between the supervisor and the employee. Disciplinary action is by nature painful. Therefore, despite all the restraint and wisdom with which the supervisor takes disciplinary action, it still puts a strain on the supervisor–subordinate relationship. It is difficult to impose discipline without generating resentment because disciplinary action is an unpleasant experience and puts a barrier between the supervisor and the employee. The question therefore arises as to how the supervisor can apply the necessary disciplinary action so that it is given in the least resented and most acceptable form.

The supervisor must also be concerned about equity. It is imperative that discipline be equitably applied regardless of race, sex, age, or position. Sometimes exceptions are made because the employee is the son of a "high admitter" or a neighbor of the assistant director of plant operations or the daughter of a benefactor. These are not valid reasons for exceptions. Inequitable dispensing of discipline, or for that matter, praise or assignments, because of associations unrelated to the work requirements can destroy a manager's credibility and the staff's morale more quickly than any other reason.

The "Red-Hot Stove" Approach

McGregor characterizes discipline as "the red-hot stove rule" (cited in Sayles and Strauss 1981; Strauss and Sayles 1980). Just as when one touches a red-hot stove, discipline following an infraction should be immediate, come with warning, be consistent, and be impersonal. First, the burn is immediate, and there is no question of the cause and effect. Second, there is a warning; everyone knows what happens if one touches a hot stove, especially if the stove is red from the heat. Third, the discipline is consistent; every time one touches a hot stove, one is burned. Fourth, the discipline is impersonal; whoever touches the hot stove is burned.

Immediacy
The supervisor must not procrastinate; a prompt beginning of the disciplinary process is necessary as soon as possible after the supervisor notices the violation. The sooner the discipline is invoked, the more automatic it will seem and the closer will be the connection with the offensive act. As already stated, the supervisor should refrain from taking hasty action, and enough time should elapse for tempers to cool and for assembling all the necessary facts.

In some instances the employee is clearly guilty of a violation, although the full circumstances may not be known or easy to prove. Here the need for disciplinary action is unquestionable, but some doubt may exist as to the severity of the penalty. In such cases the supervisor should tell the employee that he realizes what went on, but that some time is needed to reach a conclusion on how to settle the matter. In other cases, however, the nature of the incident makes it necessary to get the offender off the premises quickly. Some immediate action is required even if there is not yet enough evidence to make a final decision in the case.

Advance Warning
To have good discipline and ensure that employees accept disciplinary action as fair, it is absolutely essential that all employees be clearly informed in advance what is expected of them and what the rules are. There must be warning that an offense leads to disciplinary action. Some enterprises rely on bulletin board announcements to make such warnings. These cannot be as effective, however, as a section in the handbook that all new employees receive when they start working for the institution. Along with the written statements in the hand-

book, it is advisable to include verbal clarification of the rules. During the induction process shortly after new employees are hired, they should be told what is expected of them and of the consequences of not complying.

In addition to the forewarning about general rules, the employees must be told in advance how disciplinary action is taken. There are considerable doubts, however, about whether a standard penalty should be provided and stated for each offense. Should there be, for example, a clear statement that falsifying attendance records carries a one-week disciplinary layoff? Those in favor of such a list suggest that it is an effective warning device and that it provides greater disciplinary consistency. On the other hand, such a list does not permit management to take into consideration the various degrees of guilt and mitigating circumstances. In general, it is probably best not to provide a schedule of penalties for specific violations but merely to state the progressive steps of disciplinary action that can be taken. It should be clearly understood that continued violations bring about more severe penalties. Some enterprises do specify that certain serious offenses bring the penalty of immediate discharge. For most violations, however, it is unwise to spell out a rigid set of disciplinary measures.

The practice of forewarning before taking disciplinary measures also applies to rules that have not been enforced recently. If the supervisor has not disciplined anyone who violated a rule for a long time, the employees do not expect this rule to be enforced in the future. Perhaps the supervisor suddenly decides that to make a rule valid, he is going to make an example of one of the employees and take disciplinary action. Disciplinary action should not be used in this manner. Just because a certain rule has not been enforced in the past does not mean that it cannot ever be enforced; what it does mean is that the supervisor must take certain steps before beginning to enforce such a rule. Instead of acting tough suddenly, the supervisor should give the employees some warning that this rule, previous enforcement of which has been lax, will be strictly enforced in the future. In such cases it is not enough to put the enforcement notice on the bulletin board. It is essential that, in addition to a clear written warning, supplemental verbal communication be given. The supervisor must explain to the subordinates, perhaps in a departmental meeting or in an e-mail distribution to the entire team, that from the present time forward she intends to enforce this rule.

Consistency

A further requirement of good discipline is consistency of treatment. The supervisor must impose discipline at each occurrence of an offense and take the same type of disciplinary action each time. By being consistent, the supervisor sets the limit for acceptable behavior, and every individual wants to know what the limits are. Inconsistency is one of the fastest ways for a supervisor to lower the morale of the employees and lose their respect. If the supervisor is inconsistent, the employees find themselves in an environment in which they cannot feel secure, leading to anxiety and creating doubts in the employees' minds about what they can and cannot do. At times the supervisor may be tempted to be lenient and overlook an infringement. In reality, however, the supervisor is not doing the employees any favors, but rather creating a more difficult situation for all of them.

Mason Haire (1964), a well-known psychologist, compares this situation to the relationship between a motorist and a traffic police officer. He says that whenever we are exceeding the speed limit on the highway, we must feel some sort of anxiety because we are breaking the rule. On the other hand, the rule is often not enforced. We think that perhaps the police department in this location does not take the rule seriously, and we can speed a little. There is always a lurking insecurity, however, because the motorist knows that at any time the police officer may decide to enforce the rule. Many motorists think it is easier to operate in an environment in which the police are at least consistent one way or the other. The same holds true for most employees who have to work in an environment in which the supervisor is not consistent in disciplinary matters.

In addition, the supervisor faces another problem in trying to be consistent: addressing individual needs. On the one hand, the supervisor has been cautioned to treat all employees alike and to avoid favoritism, whereas on the other hand, he has been told again and again to treat people as individuals in accordance with their special needs and circumstances. On the surface these two requirements appear to contradict each other. The supervisor must realize, however, that treating people fairly does not mean treating everyone exactly the same. What it does mean is that when an exception is made, it must be considered as a valid exception by the other members of the department. The rest of the employees regard an exception as fair if they know why it was made and if they consider the reason to be justified. Moreover, the other employees must be confident that if any other employee were in the same situation, she would receive the same treatment. If these conditions are fulfilled, the supervisor has been able to exercise fair play and be consistent in discipline, and still treat people as individuals.

The extent to which a supervisor can be consistent and still consider the circumstances is illustrated as follows. Assume that three employees were engaged in surfing the Internet for a new plasma television (an inappropriate use of facility technology) at work during paid time. Conceivably the supervisor may simply have a friendly, informal talk with one employee, who just started work a few days ago. The second employee may receive a formal or written warning, as he had been warned about inappropriate use of hospital technology before. The third employee may receive a three-day disciplinary layoff because he had been involved in many previous cases of surfing, downloading games, and streaming music on hospital PCs. All three situations must be handled with equal gravity, but in deciding the penalty, the supervisor must take into consideration all circumstances.

Impartiality

Another way that a supervisor can reduce the amount of resentment and minimize the damage to future relations with the subordinates is to take disciplinary action as impartially as possible. In recalling the red-hot-stove rule, whoever touches the stove is burned, regardless of who the individual is. The penalty is connected with the act and not with the person. Looking at disciplinary action in this way reduces the danger to the personal relationship between the supervisor and the employee. It is the specific act that brings about the disciplinary measure, not the personality.

Keeping this in mind, the supervisor will be able to discuss the violation objectively, excluding the personal element as much as possible. She should take disciplinary action without being apologetic about the rule or about what she has to do to enforce it and without showing signs of anger. Additionally, as with any counseling session, the supervisor needs to be a good listener. Ask the individual why he is unwilling to comply with the rules or stated expectations. Be open minded when the employee explains. Nod occasionally to acknowledge that you hear what the employee is saying. During this dialogue, you may find that expectations require adjustment. If that is the case, be certain to tell the individual that you will evaluate his comments and follow up accordingly.

Once the disciplinary action has been taken, the supervisor must treat the employee as before and try to forget what happened. The disciplined employee will likely harbor some resentment, and the supervisor who meted out the discipline probably found doing it distasteful. Therefore, the supervisor and the employee may feel like avoiding each other for a few days. Such feelings are understandable, but it is far more advisable for the boss to find some opportunity to show her previous friendly feelings toward the disciplined employee. This is easier said than done; it takes maturity to handle discipline without hostility or guilt.

Discipline Without Punishment

Recently a number of organizations have tried to remove some of the shortcomings and resentment created by disciplinary action. In these entities it has been recognized that severe disciplinary action, such as unpaid suspension, does not cause the desired change in behavior. It has frequently been observed that no employee comes back from an unpaid suspension feeling better about herself, about the supervisor, or about the institution. While our earlier discussion on how to reduce the supervisor's dilemma is applicable in many cases, some supervisors are not satisfied with a system of discipline in which they often suffer more pain than the employee who was disciplined. Frequently the supervisor is faced with hostility, apathy, martyrdom, reduced output, a decline in trust, and an uncomfortable personal relationship with a subordinate. Some organizations, such as healthcare institutions with mostly white-collar professionals and highly educated, technology-savvy employees, have searched for a more palatable approach to discipline. An unpaid suspension for a staff pharmacist, for example, has been deemed inappropriate by many supervisors.

For all these and other reasons, many organizations have resorted to discipline without punishment, a nonpunitive approach that is a more mature, more positive, and a better way to encourage a disciplined workforce. This approach is considered a positive discipline approach by appealing to the employee's sense of responsibility and refraining from implied or spoken threats of discipline. The important feature of this concept is the decision-making leave (Campbell, Fleming, and Grote 1985). But first, let's discuss the steps that lead up to this point.

Typically, discipline without punishment includes a series of counseling sessions, starting with a meeting where the supervisor explains the rules or expectations and the rationale for them. The employee is encouraged to ask questions but is also told of the changes that are expected in her performance. Usually no record of this meeting is noted in the employee's personnel file. The second counseling meeting, which reviews the employee's performance since the first interview, is documented, and often a copy of the documentation is placed in the employee's personnel file.

When counseling discussions have not produced the desired changes, management places the person on a one-day **decision-making leave**, during which the institution pays the individual for the day to show the employer's desire to have her remain a member of the organization. This gesture removes the resentment and hostility usually produced by punitive action. The employee is instructed to return the day following the leave with a decision either to change and stay or to quit the job. Remaining with the institution is conditional on the individual's decision to solve the immediate problem and make a total performance commitment. When the employee returns to the job to announce the decision to stay, her supervisor expresses confidence in the individual's ability to live up to the requirements but also makes it clear that failure to do so will lead to dismissal (Campbell, Fleming, and Grote 1985).

decision-making leave
A temporary, paid layoff during which time an employee with a disciplinary problem considers whether to change his behavior and remain with the organization, or resign.

The decision-making leave with pay shows the individual the seriousness of the situation and offers an opportunity for cool reflection. It puts the burden on the employee and clearly represents the institution's refusal to make the employee's career decision. This nonpunitive approach forces the individual to take responsibility for future performance and behavior. The employee also realizes that she will be confronted with a tougher employer's response if she fails to meet standards. The costs connected with paying the employee for the day are far lower than those associated with disciplinary suspension without pay.

The use of decision-making leave has proved as powerful in the executive suite as on the patient care floor or in the clinical laboratory. While the approach may not be an appropriate approach for all disciplinary occurrences, the organizations that have adopted it show good results because the responsibility for action is shifted from the supervisor to the employee. Also, the time frame changes from the past to the future. Nonpunitive discipline forces the problem employee to choose: "Become either a committed employee or a former employee" (Campbell, Fleming, and Grote 1985).

Right of Appeal

Within our society's legal framework, an individual's wrongdoing is not judged by the accuser. The judge is not a party to the dispute between the accuser and the wrongdoer. In industrial and healthcare settings, however, this is not the case. The line superior decides whether a violation has occurred, how severe it is, and what the penalty should be. If a union is in place, the employee can appeal the case through a formal grievance procedure leading to binding arbitration. Nonunion organizations should also have a formal way of appealing a manager's decision because sometimes individuals in positions of authority mistreat subordinates. A system for grievances must exist that enables employees to obtain satisfaction for unjust treatment and to resolve conflict.

Following the chain of command, the immediate supervisor's boss is the one to whom such an appeal would first be directed. From there, the complaining employee can usually carry the appeal procedure through various levels, ultimately to the CEO of the organization as the final court of appeal. Unfortunately, in the contemporary organization, no system exists that serves to separate the executive functions from those functions involved in conducting a judicial review.

Great care must be taken that the right of appeal is a real right and not merely a formality. Some supervisors will gladly tell their subordinates that they can go to the next higher boss to appeal a disciplinary decision but will never forgive them if they do so. Such thinking indicates the supervisor's own insecurity in the managerial position. It is management's obligation to provide such an appeal procedure, and the supervisor must not feel slighted in the role as leader of the department when it is used. Management's failure to provide an appeal procedure may even be a chief reason employees seek recourse at local, state, or federal agencies or pursue unionization.

A supervisor must be mature to avoid perceiving some threat from appeals that go over her head. Such a situation should be handled tactfully by the supervisor's boss. In the course of an appeal, the disciplinary penalty imposed by the supervisor may be reduced or completely removed. Under these circumstances the supervisor understandably may become discouraged and frustrated because the boss has not backed her up. This usually happens in situations in which doubt remains about the actual events and the two stories do not coincide. In such cases the "guilty" employee normally goes "free." Although this is may be an unjust outcome, it is preferable to an innocent employee being punished. Just as in the U.S. legal system, where the accused is presumed innocent until proven guilty, the burden is on management to prove the employee is at fault.

Another reason for the reversal of a decision by higher-level management is that the supervisor may have been inconsistent in the exercise of discipline or that not all the necessary facts were obtained before disciplinary action was imposed. To avoid such an unpleasant situation, the supervisor must adhere closely to all that has been said in this chapter about the exercise of positive discipline. If a supervisor is a good disciplinarian, his verdict is normally upheld by the boss. Even if it should be reversed, this is still not too high a price to pay to guarantee justice for every employee. Without justice, a good organizational climate cannot exist.

Summary

Discipline is a state of affairs. If morale is high, discipline probably will be good, and little need will exist for the supervisor to take disciplinary action. A supervisor is entitled to assume that most employees want to do the right thing and that much of the discipline will be self-imposed by the employees. In order for employees to do what is right, they must know what is expected of them and what the rules are. These should be in writing. If the occasion should arise in which discipline is warranted, the supervisor must know how to take disciplinary action. There is usually a progressive list of disciplinary measures, ranging from an informal talk or an oral warning to discharge. The supervisor should bear in mind that the purpose of such disciplinary measures is not retribution or humiliation of employees. Rather, the goal is improvement in the future behavior of the subordinate and in the department's other members. Using positive discipline and discipline without punishment approaches encourages the employee to rectify his own faults without the supervisor imposing threats or inflicting harsh punishment.

Nevertheless, taking disciplinary action is a painful experience for the employee as well as the supervisor. To do the best possible job, the supervisor must ensure that all disciplinary action fulfills the requirements of immediacy, forewarning, consistency, and impartiality. Furthermore, discipline should be administered in private. The need for a good organizational climate makes necessary a system of corrective justice whereby any disciplinary action that an employee feels is unfair can be appealed.

Note

1. In all of our discussions we assume that the employees of the department do not belong to a union, and therefore no contractual obligations restrict the supervisor's authority in the realm of disciplinary action.

CONTROLLING

FUNDAMENTALS OF CONTROL AND THE CONTROLLING FUNCTION

Chapter Objectives

After you have studied this chapter, you should be able to do the following:

1. Define the managerial function of controlling.
2. Discuss different types of control systems.
3. Outline the basic requirements of a control system and steps in the control process.
4. Review the purposes of measuring and comparing performance.
5. Describe corrective-action techniques.
6. Review the basic managerial steps of setting standards, measuring performance, and taking corrective action.

Control, a term that often arouses negative connotations if it is not used properly, plays an important role in any organization. Everyone who participates in an organized activity depends on controls for effective functioning of the organization. **Controlling** is the process of checking performance against standards. Its purpose is to ensure that performance is consistent with plans and that the organizational and departmental goals and objectives are achieved. Controlling is an essential function for all managers in the organization by which they monitor performance and take corrective action when needed.

controlling
The process of checking performance against standards.

    The controlling function is closely related to the other four managerial functions, but it is most closely related to the planning function. When the manager performs the planning function, she sets the direction, goals, objectives, and policies that become standards against which performance is checked and appraised. Many of the tools discussed in Chapter 14 are used in the controlling function. If deviations are found, the manager has to take corrective action, which may entail new plans and standards. This is how planning decisions affect controls and how control decisions affect plans, illustrating the circular nature of the management process.

The Nature of Control

Although this discussion of control appears as the last part of this book, controlling is done simultaneously with the other functions. The better the manager plans, organizes, staffs, and influences, the better the supervisor can perform the controlling function, and vice versa. Controlling is often mistaken for inspection, which is a retrospective or after-the-fact activity. However, as Keister (2001) states, "four keys to achieving success in an organization include (1) having accurate measurements to indicate how well the organization is performing; (2) understanding how well other organizations (competitors as well as noncompetitors) can perform similar activities; (3) understanding why others perform better than your organization; and (4) identifying any negative discrepancy between your performance and that of another organization, and taking appropriate measures to remedy those deficiencies."

A supervisor cannot expect to have good control over the department unless he follows sound managerial principles in pursuing the other duties. Well-made plans, workable policies and procedures, a properly planned organization, appropriate delegation of authority, continuous training of employees, good instructions, and good supervision all play a significant role in the department's results. The better these requirements are fulfilled, the more effective is the supervisor's function of controlling and the less corrective action is needed.

Human Reactions to Control

Another important aspect of control is how people respond to it; as mentioned earlier, the word "control" often carries negative connotations. Previous chapters considered work and human satisfaction, tight versus loose supervision, delegation of authority, and on-the-job freedom in connection with motivation. Although controls are an absolute requirement in any organized activity, one must keep in mind that in behavioral terms control means placing constraints on behavior so that what people do in organizations is more or less predictable. Control systems are designed to regulate behavior, which implies loss of freedom, and people react negatively to loss of freedom. The amount of control determines how much freedom of action an individual has in performing the job. Complete absence of control, however, does not maximize an individual's perception of freedom because controls restrict not only a person's behavior but also the behavior of others toward her.

A certain amount of control, therefore, is essential for any organizational freedom to exist. Neither extreme of tight control nor complete lack of control brings about the desired organizational effectiveness. A balance between the two extremes, which considers the amount of decentralization in the organization, management styles, motivational factors, situation, and professional competence of the employees, is preferred. In other words, to arrive at the most desirable mixture of freedom and control, the manager must try to balance the goals of organizational effectiveness and individual satisfaction.

The Supervisor and Control

The purpose of the controlling process is to ensure that performance is consistent with plans, that plans and standards are being adhered to, and that proper progress is being made toward objectives. When supervisors set, communicate, and apply standards for performance for their staff and processes, they are exerting control. Also, controlling means correcting any deviations from these standards that may occur. At times, the supervisor may enlist experts within the organization for assistance in obtaining control information data and counsel. It is inappropriate, however, for the supervisor to expect anyone else to perform the controlling function for him.

Planning, organizing, staffing, and influencing are the preparatory steps for getting the work done. Controlling is concerned with making certain that the work is properly executed. If a supervisor is not exercising control, he is not doing a complete job of managing. Control remains necessary whenever supervisors assign duties to subordinates, as the supervisors cannot shift the responsibility they have accepted from their own superiors. In other words, a supervisor can and must assign tasks and delegate authority, but, as stated throughout this book, responsibility cannot be delegated. Rather, the supervisor must exercise control to see that the responsibility is properly carried out.

The eventual success of the department depends on the degree of difference between what should be done and what is done. Having set up the standards of performance, the supervisor must stay informed of the actual performance through observation, reports, discussion, control charts, and other devices (discussed later in this chapter). Only then can she prescribe the necessary corrections that bring about full compliance with the standards.

Anticipatory Aspect of Control

To a large degree, controlling is a forward-looking function; it has anticipatory aspects. Management is concerned with controls that anticipate potential sources of deviation from standards. Past experience and the study of past events tell the supervisor what has taken place and where, when, and why certain standards were not met. This enables management to make provisions so that future activities do not lead to these deviations. Unfortunately, the anticipatory aspect of controlling is not always sufficiently stressed, and often supervisors are primarily concerned with its corrective and reactive aspects. Deviations from standards are detected after they have occurred and are corrected, rather than anticipated, at the point of performance.

All efforts to control, whether corrective, reactive, or anticipatory, have an effect on the future. The supervisor can do little about the past. For example, if the work assigned to a subordinate for the day has not been accomplished, the controlling process cannot correct that. Some supervisors are inclined to scold the person responsible and assume that he was deliberately negligent. The good supervisor, however, looks forward rather than backward and at the same time studies the past to learn what has taken place and why. This enables her to take the proper steps to ensure corrective and ideally preventive action for the future.

Because control is a forward-looking function, the supervisor must discover deviations from the established standards as quickly as possible. Therefore, the supervisor should minimize the time lag between results and corrective action. For example, instead of waiting until the day is over, it is more advisable for a housekeeping supervisor to check at midday to see whether the work is progressing satisfactorily. Even though the morning has already passed and nothing can be done about any deviations that have occurred, monitoring progress earlier in the day can minimize the deviation and the correction to be made.

Not all anticipatory concerns relate to whether a process is completed correctly or a piece of equipment is functioning appropriately. The supervisor must consider the use, or to be more exact, the misuse of company assets. As Wells (2001, 31) states, "Sometimes, the truth isn't very pretty. Consider, for example, the American workforce. Although regarded by many as the finest in the world, it has a dark side. According to estimates, a third of American workers have stolen on the job. Many of these thefts are immaterial to the financial statements, but not all are." High-profile incidents involving executives at HealthSouth Corporation, HCA Inc., and Tenet Healthcare Corporation have led to intensified compliance and ethics monitoring programs. Stealing from the job may take many forms, including fraud, internal theft, and asset misappropriation. For example, an employee who spends an excessive amount of time sending personal e-mails when he should be working is misappropriating assets.

The inappropriate use of work time for personal business, such as surfing the Internet, is a real concern for supervisors. If the sites being visited are pornographic and other employees see them, the supervisor could have sexual harassment complaints to deal with. Some information technology departments have successfully stemmed the inappropriate use of the Internet by (1) timing out the usage period for any user, (2) restricting sites that can be visited based on site content or domain name, and (3) periodically checking the history files of the Internet user and providing reports to the area supervisor. These control techniques are both anticipatory and concurrent in nature.

However, inappropriate usage of the Internet is not the only productivity waster; there is also e-mail to contend with. E-mail is essential to communication among staff. However, according to a survey quoted in *The Sunday Oklahoman*, workers stated that they spend at least two hours a day reading and responding to e-mail (Erickson 2001). A Pew study demonstrated similar results (see Exhibit 25.1).

In addition to the loss of time it represents, e-mail fuels the grapevine and can result in inappropriate distribution of proprietary departmental or organizational information. Methods to control unwanted dissemination of information include (1) scanning the content before the e-mail is released to the Internet, (2) restricting e-mail to only individuals on an authorized list to receive messages, and (3) restricting the size of the e-mail document or not permitting attachments.

Because individuals tend to abbreviate their comments in an e-mail message, misunderstandings can arise and politically incorrect language may

EXHIBIT 25.1
Time Spent on
E-mail at Work

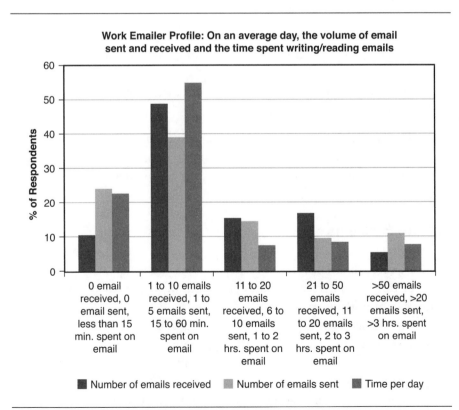

SOURCE: Reprinted with permission. Fallows, Deborah. "Work Emailer Profile." Email at Work, Pew Research Center's Internet & American Life Project, December 8, 2002. www.pewinternet.org/Reports/2002/Email-at-work.aspx.

be used. Jokes and photos sent via e-mail can be easily shared. These documents may be inappropriate and stir concerns of racism, harassment, and other complaints from employees receiving them. Furthermore, the time spent opening and discarding them is wasteful.

Lastly, and possibly most important for healthcare organizations, is the patient confidentiality concern related to e-mail. Many patient documents are electronically created and sent via e-mail to physicians and other caregivers. An employee who finds a document on a friend (or enemy) can easily transmit that document to his home e-mail account or to others who should not have access to it, thus violating the patient's privacy.

Having a written policy on Internet and e-mail usage is essential. Policy clauses may include the following (Glover 2001):

- Disclosure to employees prior to hiring and periodically thereafter that all e-mail, Internet access, and computer files are subject to monitoring
- Notification to employees that the technology provided by the organization is company property and is to be used for business purposes only
- Explanation to employees that despite the fact that they are given passwords to access the system, they should not have an expectation that the system is private
- Notification to employees about what, if any, material they are not allowed to transport into or out of the company's system, including file downloads
- A written acknowledgment of receipt from each employee of the written policy when issued and updated

The supervisor's role is to ensure each of her subordinates has read and understood the policy and to cooperate with the information technology department and others in monitoring the usage of these assets.

Control Systems

There are three different types of control systems: anticipatory (preventive or ahead of time), concurrent (in process or during the event), and feedback (reactive or after the event).

These control systems assess whether deadlines and time constraints are met (time controls), whether the appropriate amounts of inventoried parts or materials have been consumed (material controls), whether the equipment functioned properly (equipment controls), and whether the product or service was delivered at the anticipated cost (cost controls). Chapter 26 discusses how budgets are used to help management control expenses

EXHIBIT 25.2 Performance Dashboard

	Key Metrics	July, 05	Aug, 05		10 Stretch	9	8	7 - Goal	6	5	4	3	2	1	Raw Score	Weight (%)	SubTol Score
SERVICE	Emergency Dept.Sat. Mean	83.9	84.4	☺	84.5	83.9	83.3	82.7	82.2	81.7	81.2	80.7	80.2	79.5	9	0.040	0.36
	Clinic Pt Satisfac Mean (bi-annual)	88.9	88.9		91.2	90.7	90.2	89.7	88.9	88.0	87.1	86.3	85.5	84.7	6	0.040	0.24
QUALITY	Amb. Surg Pain Mean	93.0	92.6	⊗	92.1	92.0	91.8	91.6	91.1	90.6	90.1	89.6	89.1	88.6	10	0.033	0.33
	Core Measure AMI (qrtly)	92.1%	94.7%	☺	100%	96%	93%	90%	86%	83%	80%	70%	60%	50%	8	0.033	0.26
FINANCIAL	Days in AR	48.30	46.61	☺	42.00	43.00	44.00	45.00	47.00	50.00	52.00	55.00	57.00	60.00	6	0.068	0.41
	Financial Strength Index	0.99	1.30	☺	1.94	1.73	1.52	1.31	0.94	0.57	0.20	0.15	0.10	0.05	6	0.068	0.41
PEOPLE	Empl.Satisfaction (Annual)	3.72	3.72		3.80	3.77	3.74	3.72	3.67	3.62	3.57	3.52	3.47	3.42	7	0.040	0.28
	Qrtly.Emp.Satis. w Benefit pkg.	2.5	2.5		3.31	3.29	3.27	3.25	3.15	3.05	2.96	2.90	2.84	2.78	0	0.040	0.00
	Phy Recruitment (qrtly)	0.82	0.82		1.23	1.15	1.07	1.00	0.92	0.84	0.76	0.69	0.61	0.54	4	0.040	0.16
GROWTH	Cancer Center Visits	400	514	☺	455	447	440	433	428	423	417	412	407	402	10	0.027	0.27
	Births	69	81	☺	65	64	63	62	60	58	55	52	49	47	10	0.028	0.28
	Cardiac Cath Procedures	150	191	☺	156	153	151	149	144	139	135	131	127	123	10	0.027	0.27

☺ improvement since previous month   ⊗ decline since previous month   **Total Score 7.05**

	Sept	Oct	Nov	Dec	Jan	Feb	March	April	May	June	July	Goal	7
	5.12	4.56	4.93	5.31	5.31	5.21	6.27	6.08	5.31	5.9	5.2	Stretch	10

associated with services and products relative to the projected or standard expense. By their nature, budgets are financial controls. Chapter 14 discusses various quality control and performance reporting tools, such as the use of a control chart to monitor perioperative mortality or a run chart to display patient satisfaction with new menu items. However, many healthcare organizations have established dashboards or scorecards directly tied to the strategic goals established by the board of directors. According to Griffith and Alexander (2002), four major scorecard dimensions have gained acceptance in the healthcare industry: financial, internal business processes, customer, and learning and growth. An example of a healthcare organization's dashboard appears in Exhibit 25.2.

Anticipatory Controls

Anticipatory (or preventive) controls are in place before the service activity or production starts. They anticipate potential problems and prevent their occurrence. **Anticipatory control** is a proactive, not a reactive, approach whereby the supervisor previews an entire process and each related task.

The purpose of preventive controls is to anticipate and prevent mistakes by taking care of a potential malfunction in advance. For example, the

anticipatory control
A proactive approach to monitoring a process whereby a supervisor previews an entire process and each related task.

supervisor plans and arranges for regular preventive maintenance so that the equipment is operational when needed.

Other examples of anticipatory controls are policies, procedures, standard practices, and rules. These are designed so that a predetermined course of action is prescribed to prevent mistakes or malfunctioning. For example, every hospital has established detailed plans and precise procedures in case of an emergency such as a fire. Disciplinary rules dealing with staff who carry a weapon on hospital premises constitute an anticipatory control mechanism because the rules serve as a deterrent. Other examples of preventive control mechanisms are warning signals on a piece of equipment and checklists for testing procedures. Consider the extensive checklist an anesthesiologist goes through before administering anesthesia to a patient.

Concurrent Controls

concurrent controls
Controls on a process that monitor progress as it is being done, allowing corrections or adjustments to be made immediately.

Another group of control mechanisms is composed of **concurrent controls**, which help the supervisor spot problems as they occur. The purpose is to apply controls while the operations are in progress instead of waiting for the outcome. In these situations, the supervisor does not anticipate problems but monitors operations in process. For example, concurrent controls enable the supervisor to keep the quality and quantity of output standardized. Examples of concurrent control mechanisms in healthcare include simple numerical counters, automatic switches, warning alarms, and alerts, such as alerts about adverse food–drug or drug–drug interactions in sophisticated electronic health record systems. When the supervisor lacks such aids, he monitors the activities by observation and instruction. Examples of familiar concurrent control mechanisms are the fuel gauge in a car and the parking meter. Many computer software applications have concurrent controls, for example controls that require entry of data in a certain field. The software alerts the user immediately when the field is left blank so corrective action can be taken as the process is under way.

Feedback Controls

feedback controls
Control mechanisms that alert the user to discrepancies after a process is completed.

A third group of control mechanisms, **feedback controls**, alerts the supervisor after the event is completed. For example, an insurance company's benefits supervisor reviews an abandoned-call report and finds that callers abandon the "wait to speak to a customer service representative" option at the rate of 60 percent on Wednesday, but during the rest of the week the abandonment rate is under 10 percent. With this data in hand, the supervisor can implement changes to prevent future abandonment during Wednesday calls. The feedback control system is the most widely used category. The purpose of this type of control is to improve from the point of damage and to prevent any future deviation and recurrence.

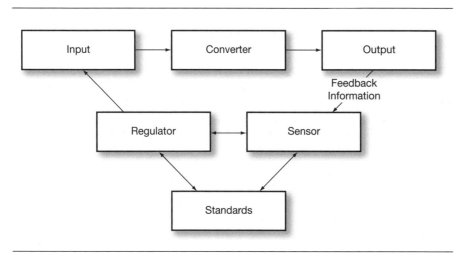

Exhibit 25.3
Closed-Loop
System of
Feedback

The Feedback Model of Control

The organizational control system can be viewed as a *feedback model*. Information on how the system is doing is obtained by the supervisor, or the sensor, who then monitors the system by comparing the actual results with the desired performance. Whenever the actual performance deviates from the standards set, the system triggers corrective action in the form of an input (see Exhibit 25.3). This **closed-loop feedback system** works the same way a thermostat in the home functions. The thermostat is set at the desired degree of temperature. Whenever the room temperature falls below or rises above that temperature, the thermostat, continuously comparing room temperature to the desired temperature, corrects the variation by turning on or shutting off the furnace or air conditioner. This type of control is known as cybernetic because it monitors and manages a process with the help of a self-regulating mechanism.

closed-loop feedback system
A feedback system that includes a self-regulating mechanism that is triggered when the process deviates from the standard.

Feedback controls are most helpful in planning process improvements. Examples of feedback controls are quality and quantity reports, opinion surveys or service surveys, and accounting reports. The quality dashboard is such a control (see Exhibit 25.2). A common human resources feedback control is the exit interview performed with employees leaving the organization (see Exhibit 25.4). The interview is performed to determine why the employee has chosen to look elsewhere for employment or to resign from her position. The feedback and information should go to the departing employee's supervisor, who in turn will translate the comments into process corrections for the remaining employees.

Because control after the fact is the least desirable control mechanism, the supervisor should make every effort to devise as many anticipatory and

Exhibit 25.4
An Exit
Interview
Form

ANYWHERE SURGI-CENTER EXIT INTERVIEW

Our human resources department is interested in your comments about your employment here. By sharing your constructive criticism, concerns, and problems encountered during your employment we will be able to plan changes to our programs, procedures, and compensation and benefit plans. Your comments are confidential, do not become part of your personnel record, and are not shared with your past supervisor.

Tell us about the position you held with our Center:

*What position did you hold? _____ Department: _____

Tell us about your new position:

* Name of the Company: _____ Position: _____

* Compensation: _____ Did this company offer any benefits or perks that were particularly appealing?_____

Please share your comments and suggestions:

* What is the principal reason for your leaving our Center?

* How do you feel about Anywhere as a place to work?

* What changes or improvements would you suggest that we should make at the Center and/or in the department where you worked?

* Were your training, skills, and experience utilized?

* Did you feel you were a contributing member of the team?

* Were your opinions or suggestions given consideration?

* Was your salary appropriate for your position and duties?

* Were you informed of promotional opportunities?

* While you were employed here, did you notice any violations of our Code of Conduct, procedures, or regulatory requirements? _____ No; _____ Yes: If so, did you discuss the situation(s) with anyone outside of the Center? _____ No; _____ Yes: _____ If so, who? _____

* If you reported these violations to someone in the Center, was the issue(s) resolved to your satisfaction? _____ Yes; _____ No: _____ Why not? _____

* Would you recommend Anywhere Surgi-Center as an employer to others?

_____ Yes; _____ No; If not, please explain: _____

*Is there anything else you would like us to know?_____

Thank you.

concurrent control mechanisms as possible. He should be able to convert many of the feedback controls into concurrent mechanisms or even into anticipatory controls with the help of up-to-date information systems and by encouraging employee involvement in problem resolution. Brainstorming is a good technique to encourage employee input. By empowering employees to take corrective action or, at a minimum, encouraging employees to contribute ideas and comments, some feedback controls become unnecessary.

The Closeness of Control

Knowing how closely to control or monitor the work of a subordinate is a real test of any supervisor's talents. The closeness of follow-up is based on such factors as the experience, initiative, dependability, and resourcefulness of the employee who is given the assignment. Giving an employee an assignment and allowing her to do the job is part of the process of delegation. This does not mean, however, that the supervisor should leave the employee completely alone until it is time to inspect the final results. Delegation also does not mean that the supervisor should watch over every detail. Rather, the supervisor must be familiar enough with the ability of the subordinate to determine accurately how much leeway to give and how closely to follow through with the control measures.

Basic Requirements of a Control System

For any control system to be workable and effective, it must fulfill certain basic requirements. Controls should (1) be understandable; (2) register deviations quickly and be timely; (3) be appropriate, adequate, and economical; (4) be somewhat flexible; and (5) indicate where corrective action should be applied. These requirements are applicable to all services in all organized activities and to all levels within the management hierarchy. They are discussed below in general terms; it would be impossible to spell out the specific characteristics of controls used in each department or service of a healthcare enterprise.

Understanding of Controls
The first requirement of a workable control system is that the control mechanisms must be understandable and fit the people involved, the tasks, and the environment. Both the manager and the subordinates must understand the data and what type of control is to be exercised. This is necessary on all managerial levels. The further down the hierarchy the system is to be applied, the less complicated it should be. Thus, the top-level administrator may use a complicated system of controls based on mathematical formulas, statistical analysis, and complex computer printouts that are understandable to them,

whereas the control system for the lower supervisory level should be less sophisticated. If the control system is too complicated, the supervisor may have to devise her own control system that fulfills the same need and can be understood by the employees as well.

Prompt Indication of Deviations from Controls

To have a workable control system, controls must indicate deviations quickly so that trends can be corrected without delay. As pointed out, controls are forward looking, and the supervisor cannot control the past. The sooner the supervisor is aware of deviations, the sooner she can take corrective action. It is more desirable to have deviations reported quickly, even if substantiated only by partial information, approximate figures, and estimates, than to wait for highly accurate information that arrives too late to be valuable. This does not mean that the supervisor should jump to conclusions or take corrective action hastily. The supervisor should be familiar enough with the job to be done, knowledgeable, and have adequate past experience to help her quickly sense when something is not progressing as planned and requires prompt supervisory action.

Appropriateness and Adequacy of Controls

Controls must always be appropriate and significant for the activity they are to monitor. Control tools that are suitable for the dietary department are different from those used in accounts payable. Even within nursing, the tools used by the director of nursing services are different from those the head nurse uses on the floor. An elaborate control system required in a large undertaking is not needed in a small department; however, the need for control still exists, only the magnitude of the control system is different. Whatever controls are applied, they must be consistent with the organizational structure so that the person with authority to act will obtain the data.

Economics of Controls

Controls must be worth the expense involved—that is, they must be economical. At times, however, it may be difficult for management to ascertain how much a particular control system is worth and how much it really costs. One important criterion might be the consequences that would follow if the controls did not exist. The nurses' control of narcotics is stringent and exact, for example, whereas no one is too concerned with close control of bandages.

Flexibility of Controls

Because all undertakings occur in a dynamic situation, unforeseen circumstances could play havoc even with the best-laid plans and standards. The control system must be built so that it remains flexible enough to keep pace with continuously changing patterns. The control system must permit change as soon as the change is required, or it is bound to fail. If the employee seems to run into unexpected conditions early in the assignment, the supervisor must

HOSPITAL LAND

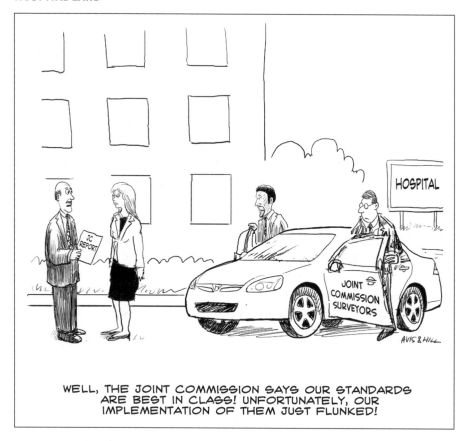

WELL, THE JOINT COMMISSION SAYS OUR STANDARDS ARE BEST IN CLASS! UNFORTUNATELY, OUR IMPLEMENTATION OF THEM JUST FLUNKED!

recognize this and adjust the plans and standards accordingly. The control system must leave room for individual judgment and changing circumstances.

Corrective Action Related to Controls

A final requirement of effective controls is that they must point the way to corrective action. It is not enough to show deviations have occurred. The system must also indicate where they have occurred and who is responsible for them. Supervisors must make it their business to know precisely where the standards were not met and who is responsible for not achieving them. If successive operations are involved, it may be necessary for the supervisor to check the performance after each step has been accomplished and before the work is passed on to the next employee or to another department.

The Supervisor's Role in the Control Function

In performing the controlling function, the supervisor must follow three basic steps. First, she sets the standards. Second, the supervisor checks and appraises performance and compares it against these standards to determine whether it meets them. Third, if standards are not met, the supervisor must take corrective action (see Exhibit 25.5). This sequence of steps is necessary for effective control. The supervisor could not possibly check and report on deviations without having set the standards in advance, and corrective action cannot be taken unless deviations from these standards are discovered.

Establishing Standards

The establishment of standards is the first step in the control process. Standards are criteria against which subsequent performance or results can be judged. Standards also are known as performance metrics. **Performance metrics** are any performance-related measurements of activity or resource utilization (Performance Co-Pilot Tutorial Glossary 2005). Standards state what should be done; they are derived from organizational goals and objectives, and they should be expressed in measurable terms. (See Exhibit 25.6.)

Occasionally, goals are established by comparing one's organization to the performance of others, which is known as **benchmarking**. (See Exhibit 25.9 later in this chapter.) Control standards can be as broad or as narrow as the level to which they apply. In planning, the CEO sets the overall objectives and goals that the healthcare center is to achieve. These overall objectives are then broken down into narrower objectives for the individual divisions and departments.

The supervisor of a department establishes even more specific goals that relate to quality, quantity, costs, time standards, quotas, schedules, budgets, and so forth. These goals become the criteria—the standards—for exercising control. Good performance measures should be linked to responsibility, customer focused, balanced, timely, credible, comparable, and simple (Henderson, Chase, and Woodson 2002). The examples of goals listed above

performance metrics
Performance-related measurements of activity or resource utilization.

benchmarking
Establishing goals by comparing performance to others.

EXHIBIT 25.5
Steps in the Controlling Process

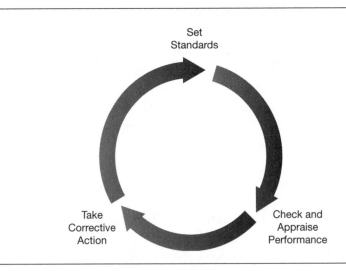

EXHIBIT 25.6
Using Metrics
to Improve
Performance in
Cash
Collections

Calculation	A	B			C	D = (B/C)*A		
Worker/Team Performance Index								
Statistic/KPI	Weight	Worker A	Worker B	Worker C	Team Avg	Worker A Pts	Worker B Pts	Worker C Pts
Stats % of Goal	15%	115%	122%	115%	117%	0.147	0.156	0.147
Payments/promises	10%	93%	90%	97%	93%	0.100	0.096	0.104
Collections per scheduled hour	35%	$825	$783	$733	$780	0.370	0.351	0.329
Average collection size	40%	$210	$190	$168	$189	0.444	0.401	0.355
	100%					1.060	1.005	0.935
						Gold Level	Silver Level	No Bonus

Calculation	A	B			C	D = (B/C)*A		
Team performance index								
Statistic/KPI	Weights	January	February	March	Team Avg	Jan PI	Feb PI	March PI
Stats % of Goal	15%	118%	115%	117%	117%	0.152	0.148	0.151
Payments/promises	10%	92%	90%	93%	92%	0.100	0.098	0.102
Collections per scheduled hour	35%	$782	$778	$780	$780	0.351	0.349	0.350
Average collection size	40%	$175	$180	$189	$181	0.386	0.397	0.417
	100%					0.988	0.922	1.020

SOURCE: Reprinted with permission from Joe Shutts, "Measuring Collections Effort Improves Cash Performance." *hfm*, September 2009. Copyright Healthcare Financial Management Association.

are tangible; other standards are intangible in nature, which, although more difficult to set and work with, must be established by healthcare institutions, especially concerning patient care.

The most common **tangible standards** are physical standards that pertain to the actual operation of a department in which goods are produced (e.g., dietary department, laundry department) or services are rendered (e.g., nursing services, nuclear medicine services). Physical standards define the amount of work to be produced within a given time span. Cost standards are also tangible standards and define direct and indirect labor costs, costs of materials and supplies used, overhead, and many other items.

These standards are quantitative and qualitative. Not only do they define, for example, how much money can be spent per patient on food, supplies, and materials for three meals a day, but they also state what quality these meals are to have in terms of nutritional value, taste, and aesthetic appeal. Likewise, standards dictate how much one pound of laundry should cost and how many pounds are to be processed in a certain time, taking into consideration the state of mechanization and automation of the laundry. Furthermore, the laundry has qualitative standards in terms of sanitation and sterilization, cleanliness of the linens, color, and absence of stains. In another example, standards specify the number of patient care personnel on a floor in relation to the severity-of-illness factor and number of patients to be cared for. Such

Tangible Standards

tangible standards
Physical standards that pertain to the actual operation of a department in which goods are produced.

standards vary depending on the time of day, the patient care unit in question (e.g., an intensive care unit versus a regular floor unit), and many other factors. Standards also exist for the patient's comfort, physical needs, and safety and for the room's cleanliness and orderliness.

Intangible Standards

intangible standards
Standards that are qualitative and subjective or based on perception.

In a healthcare facility some **intangible standards** are the organization's reputation in the community; the quality of medicine practiced; the excellence of patient care; and the degree of "tender loving care," the level of commitment to values, and the level of employee morale.

While it is impossible to express the criteria for such intangible standards in precise and numerical terms, a supervisor should not overlook the intangible achievements. Tools for appraising intangible standards include attitude surveys, questionnaires, and interviews. Although these tools are not exact, they can help determine to what extent certain intangible standards are being achieved. They also provide the manager with a sketch of the customers' expectations or perceptions of service quality.

Approaches to Establishing Standards

In setting standards, the supervisor is aided by experience and knowledge of the various jobs to be done within the department. A supervisor has a general idea of how much time it takes to perform a certain job, what resources are required, what constitutes good performance, and what is a poor job. Additionally, she has access to productivity expectations from professional associations and journals. Using her experience and these resources, the supervisor should capture data over a representative period of time to compare with what she may have assumed would be reasonable to expect. For example, if the coding supervisor intends to establish quantity and quality standards for the coders, she should collect production data for each team member along with hours worked. The data should cover several pay periods at different times of the year. Once the average production per work hour is calculated, the supervisor should determine whether the production is consistent with her experience. She can also compare that average to the performance of other comparable organizations and determine whether performance improvement initiatives should be implemented.

Motion and Time Studies

There also are more scientific and systematic ways of establishing objective standards. Work-measurement techniques help determine the amount of work an average employee should produce within a given time period. In many departments in a healthcare organization, such as housekeeping, laundry, laboratories, courier, and dietary service, this approach is worth the effort and cost. Standards determined through work-measurement techniques help the supervisor distribute the work more evenly and judge fairly whether an employee is performing satisfactorily.

The work-measurement analyses are usually assigned to an industrial engineer or outside consultant trained in conducting motion and time studies. Motion study involves an analysis of the elements of the job and of how the job is currently performed with a view to changing, eliminating, or combining certain steps and devising a method that will be quicker and easier than the current process. Often flowcharts are drawn up that analyze the steps taken in performing the job. After a thorough analysis of the motions and workflow arrangements, the engineer determines the best method for doing the job in question. For example, the workplace layout may be redesigned and hand motion processes may be revamped.

Once the best method has been designed, time studies are performed to determine the standard time required to do the job using this method. One or more qualified workers are timed with a stopwatch as they perform the prescribed work methods. Time studies are done scientifically and systematically by selecting an average employee for observation; measuring the time taken to perform the various elements of the job; applying leveling and other corrective factors; and making allowances for fatigue, personal needs, contingencies, and delays. The combined result leads to a standard time necessary to perform the job. Although this method is scientific, one must keep in mind that considerable judgment and many approximations are used to arrive at the standard time. Standard times, however, are a sound basis on which to determine objective standards. They also enable the supervisor to predict the number of employees required and the probable cost of the job to be done. In many activities outside the healthcare field, standards of this type serve as a basis for cost estimates and incentive plans.

If industrial engineers are not available, the supervisor can perform some of the studies simply by observing and timing the various operations and making the necessary adjustments previously stated. If the job to be performed in the department has never been done there before, the supervisor should try to base tentative standards on similar operations. If the new job has no similarity to any previous function, the best the supervisor can do (unless the help of industrial engineers is available) is to observe the operation while it is being performed the first few times to arrive at a standard for the new function. Sometimes the manufacturer of a new piece of equipment can provide standard data—for example, how long it will take an apparatus to perform a certain task. Regardless of the approach taken, the supervisor should attempt to align the standards established to a quality measure that gauges the employee's ability to deliver the right output, the right way, the first time, and on time (Spath 2002).

Time Ladders

Another approach to collecting data on productivity is the time ladder. This technique requires the employee to note what he does during 5-, 10-, or 15- minute increments throughout a day for several days. (See Exhibit 25.7.)

EXHIBIT 25.7

Time Ladder

TIME LADDER FOR:

Time	Activities or Duties Performed During This Period
0700	Turned on computer; went to front desk to obtain requisitions
0715	Sorted requisitions by patient floor
0730	Prepared tubes for each area/placed in phlebotomy cart
0745	same as above
0800	same as above
0815	same as above. Distributed phlebotomy carts
0830	Took break and picked up new requisitions
0845	Sorted requisitions by patient floor
0900	Prepared tubes for each area/placed in phlebotomy cart

Employees who perform the same duties maintain separate ladders. The data tell the manager the average number of units one produces in a day and the types of interference an employee encounters, as well as nonproductive time (restroom visits, breaks, and so forth). The method places the burden of data collection on the employee but requires the supervisor to validate some of the data through other techniques, such as direct observation.

Work Sampling Through Direct Observation

In the direct observation approach, supervisors periodically observe employees and note whether they are working, what they are working on, or whether they are idle or on break. The supervisor maintains a log that lists the employees along one axis and the key activities along the other. An example of an observation record form is shown in Exhibit 25.8.

Tick marks are made during each observation, representing the activity the employee is performing at the time of the observation. Each observation is usually brief (10 to 15 minutes total) depending on the number of employees in the work area, the size of the work area, and whether the supervisor must walk around to adequately observe the staff. The observations occur several times a day. This process is known as **sampling**.

Because the observation times are randomly selected, they could occur at virtually any time during the workday. After several days of the observation sampling, adequate data are compiled to indicate what percentage of the time employee X was engaged in each of her key activities. This information provides the manager with information against which to compare production data. One might expect that if Kent processes an average of 100

sampling
The process of reviewing a certain number of cases or events from the total number of cases or events. Sampling can be conducted on a randomized and nonrandom basis.

EXHIBIT 25.8 Example of Observation Record Form

**OBSERVATION RECORD FOR
HEALTH INFORMATION MANAGEMENT SERVICES**

	Jane Super-visor	Lori Tran-scriber	Tara Tran-scriber	Susan Tran-scriber	Larry File Clerk	Kent File Clerk	Kim Coder	Mel Coder	John Coder	Totals
Supervisory activities										
Technical (non-supervisory duties)										
Transcribing										
Handling transcribed work										
Filing records										
Sorting records										
Pulling records										
Coding										
Abstracting										
Idle, gone, non-productive activities										
Totals										

Date of this sampling:
Observation Times:

1.	4.	7.	10.
2.	5.	8.	11.
3.	6.	9.	12.

supply requisitions a day and Larry processes 250 a day, Larry may have a better method of doing his work. If so, the manager will want Larry to show Kent this method. Alternatively, the standard could be set at 250, and Kent would be encouraged to model Larry to achieve the standard.

Although they may not be absolutely scientific, standards are more likely to be effective if they are set with the participation of the supervisor and the subordinates instead of being handed down by a staff engineer, a manager, or an outside consultant. The purpose of any standard is to establish a specific goal for the employees to strive toward, and, as with all directives, employees are likely to be more motivated to achieve those standards in which they have had some part in developing. Furthermore, none of the above methods should be used without advising the staff in advance that the analysis is planned. Morale could be affected negatively if employees feel they are being watched and do not know why.

How to Select Strategic Standards

The number of standards or metrics that can be used to ascertain the quality and quantity of performance within a department is large and increases rapidly as the department expands. As the operations within the department become more sophisticated and complex and the functions of the department increase, it becomes more difficult and time consuming for supervisors to check against all the conceivable standards. Therefore, they need to concentrate on certain strategic standards—those that best reflect the goals.

For example, a billing manager knows which strategic points to check first. She probably checks the bill lag or accounts receivable report and makes certain that the lag between discharge and bill drop has not lengthened, the accounts receivable are within expected limits, and the lag between discharge and coding has not significantly changed. She also observes where the billing personnel are and what they are doing. Each of these areas constitutes a strategic point of control for the billing manager. Unfortunately, there are no specific guidelines on how to select these strategic control points. The peculiarities of each departmental function and the makeup of the supervisor and employees are different in each situation. Thus, only general guidelines can be suggested for selecting strategic standards.

One of the first considerations in choosing one standard as more strategic than another is timeliness. Because time is essential in control and controls are anticipatory, the earlier the deviation can be discovered, the better. This helps to correct problems early before errors begin to compound. Keeping this in mind, the supervisor can determine at what point in time and where in the process activities should be checked. For example, in the maintenance department, the strategic control point may be after a crack has been repaired but before it has been repainted.

Another consideration in choosing strategic control points is whether they permit economical observations. Earlier we noted that a control system must be worth the expense involved; it must be economical. The same applies to the strategic control points. A further consideration is that the strategic standards should allow comprehensive and balanced control. The supervisor must be aware that the selection of one strategic control point might have an adverse effect on another. Excessive control or emphasis on quantity often has an adverse effect on quality. On the other hand, if expenses are selected as a strategic control point, the quality or quantity of the output may suffer. For example, the executive housekeeper must not sacrifice quality standards that have been designed to prevent infections in order to cut expenses. All these decisions depend on the nature of the work within the department. What serves well as a strategic control point in one activity does not necessarily apply in another.

A supervisor may find it simpler to choose among many strategic control point options by identifying and prioritizing those that represent a majority of the work performed in the department (recall the Pareto Principle described in Chapter 14); those that, if not monitored, could place the department or organization at risk; and those that could affect the safety or security of the organization, its resources or assets, its staff, or its patients. For example, the following is a list of strategic control options available for the administrator of Small Town Hospital. Small Town is located in an agricultural community.

Daily
- Number of patients hospitalized
- Number of patients scheduled for surgery
- Percentage (semi-annual) of patients treated from service area zip codes
- Total admissions by physician
- Total surgeries by physician
- Cash taken in today
- Accounts receivable today
- Cleanliness of hallways and public areas
- Number of in-service sessions occurring throughout the hospital

Weekly
- Legislative action planned at the state capitol
- Current corn and cattle prices
- Openings or closures of businesses in the service area

The administrator of Small Town Hospital could monitor a number of variables as strategic control points, but many of those listed are of little value to a supervisor. However, strategic control options relevant to him, based on this list, may be knowing (1) the number of patients the hospital will serve in that day and whether there is adequate staff in his department to tend to the patients' needs or (2) the accounts receivable balance and age and cash taken yesterday. The first set of control points represents the majority of services performed, while the second set speaks to protecting the hospital's assets.

Communicating and Monitoring Standards

For control to have an effective influence on performance, the supervisor must ensure that the goals and standards are known to all the employees within the department and clarify who is responsible for their achievement so that she knows whom to contact for deviations if the results are not achieved and whom to praise if they are exceeded. After all, the supervisor is interested in having the standards and objectives reached. Only if each employee knows exactly what is expected concerning his own work can he try to achieve it. This is why the supervisor must link the standards with the individual responsibilities of each employee.

The second step in the process of control is to measure actual performance against the standards. Observing and measuring performance are ongoing activities for every manager. Work is observed, output is measured, and reports are compiled.

Some ways for a supervisor to check on and measure performance are (1) comparing performance with standards; (2) directly observing the work and personally checking on the employees; (3) measuring work in, out, and remaining to do; and (4) studying various summaries of reports and figures that are submitted to the supervisor.

Comparing As the manager observes and measures performance, it must be compared with the standards developed in the beginning of the control process. The observed performance may be higher than, the same as, or lower than the standards. In the first two situations, the supervisor obviously does not have any problems. If the performance does not meet standards, however, corrective action is required.

Because some deviation is expected in some activities, the question is how much deviation is acceptable before taking remedial action. This depends on the activity. In some activities, minor deviations may be acceptable. In other activities, such as nursing, deviations can be critical, and even a small one may not be tolerated. A common problem in many healthcare organizations is having more than one patient unit number for the same patient. This can cause havoc in health information as well as the blood bank and radiology. By developing reports to identify who is assigning new numbers to existing patients, management can determine where the problem originates. Some activities are easier to monitor and compare than others. It is the supervisor's job to develop valid performance measures to control effectively and take corrective action when necessary.

Direct Personal Observation Observation is probably the most widely used technique for measurement. There is no better way for a supervisor to check performance than by direct observation and personal contact. Personal observation is time consuming, but every manager should spend part of each day away from his desk observing the performance of the employees. For example, regular rounds are not only necessary for the head nurse; they are just as important for the director of housekeeping, the chief dietitian, and the hospital administrator.

For the supervisor, direct observations are the most effective way of maintaining close contact with employees. This opportunity for close personal observation is one of the great advantages of the supervisor's job; it is a function that the top-level administrator cannot perform to any great extent. The further removed a manager is from the front line, the less he can observe personally and the more he has to depend on reports. However, regardless of level in the management ladder, leaders should attempt to visit all areas for which they have responsibility. Also, supervisors should encourage their superiors to participate in team or department activities (e.g., Respiratory Therapy Week luncheon, promotion parties). All employees, no matter the level, like their superiors and the higher-ups to "show their faces," especially on weekends, nights, and holidays. Employees who work at these times feel left out of the mainstream activities; being given some attention during these off-hours can be a morale booster.

Whenever supervisors observe their employees at work, they should assume a questioning attitude and not a fault-finding one. Supervisors should not ignore mistakes, but the manner in which they question is essential. They should ask themselves whether there is any way they could help the employees do the job better or more easily, safely, or efficiently. They should notice the way the employee is doing the job, whether it is up to par or substandard. Such observations can verify lack of acceptable performance in specific areas, such as inadequate patient care, lack of orderliness, or sloppy work.

At times, it may be difficult to convince an employee that her work is unsatisfactory. If reference can be made to concrete cases, however, it is not easy for the subordinate to deny that the inadequacies exist. It is essential for the supervisor to make specific observations because without being specific, one cannot realistically appraise performance and take appropriate corrective action.

As stated, measuring performance through direct personal observation has some shortcomings; it is time consuming and means being away from the desk and office. Some other limitations also exist. The employee may perform well while the boss is around but drop back to a lower level of performance shortly after the boss is out of sight. Furthermore, it may be difficult to observe some of the activities at a critical time. Still, direct observation is practiced widely and is probably the best way of checking performance.

Reports

Written and oral reports are good means of checking on performance if a department operates around the clock, if it is large, or if it operates in different locations. When a department operates around the clock and one supervisor is responsible for all shifts, each day of the week, this person depends on reports to cover those shifts during which he is absent. Even with reports, the supervisor should get to work a little earlier and stay a little later in the day so that there is some overlap with the night supervisor in the morning and with the afternoon supervisor later in the day. This gives the supervisors a chance to add some spoken explanations to their written reports. Reports should be clear, complete, concise, and correct. They must be brief but still include the important details.

As the departmental supervisor checks these reports, he probably will find that many activities have been performed up to standard. The supervisor should concentrate on the exceptions—those areas in which the performance significantly deviates from the standard. Only the exceptions require the supervisor's attention. For example, in Exhibit 25.2, if the pain measurement in ambulatory surgery fell to 90 percent, management would definitely want to investigate why. In fact, if the supervisor depends on reports from the various shifts, the subordinates may have been requested not to send data on those activities that have reached the preestablished standards but to report only on those items that do not meet the standards or exceed them. In this way, the supervisor can concentrate all his efforts on the problem areas. This is known as practicing the **exception principle**. In such situations, however, a climate of trust must exist between the supervisor and subordinates so that they can freely report the deviations. Subordinates should know that the boss has full confidence in the rest of their activities even though there is no report on them.

exception principle
The practice of reporting only items that fail to meet standards, so that the respondent can focus on problem areas.

If the supervisor does depend on reports for information, it is essential that she review them immediately upon receiving them and take action without delay when needed. It is demoralizing to send reports to a supervisor who does not even read them.

The nature of healthcare activities calls for reports that are accurate, complete, and correct, especially when patient care is involved. In all other areas as well, most employees submit truthful reports, even if they are unfavorable to the employee. The supervisor must check into any matter that arises and correct any shortcomings. As long as the supervisor handles these reports constructively, stressing their honesty, the employees will continue to submit reliable reports instead of stretching the truth. The supervisor must remember the importance of upward communication; this is one opportunity to keep the channel open and flowing (see Chapter 5).

Taking Corrective Action

The third stage in the control model is taking corrective action. If there are no deviations in performance from the established standards, the supervisor's process of controlling is fulfilled by the first two steps—setting standards and checking performance. If a significant and worthwhile discrepancy or variation is found, however, the controlling function is not fulfilled until and unless the third step, appropriate corrective action, is taken. If the deviation is minor and acceptable and within a noncritical activity, it may be appropriate to do nothing except call it to the employee's attention.

The supervisor must first make a careful analysis of the facts and look for the reasons behind the deviations. This must be done before any specific corrective action can be prescribed. The supervisor must bear in mind that the performance standards were based on certain prerequisites, forecasts, and assumptions and that some of these may have been faulty or may not have materialized. A check on the discrepancy may also point out that the trouble was not caused by the employee in whose work it appeared but in some preceding activity. For instance, a patient's infection might not be caused by the nursing activities or conditions on the nursing floor, but rather by conditions or actions in the recovery room or the surgical suite. In such a situation, the corrective action must be directed toward the real source. In this case, the corrective action will emanate from the nursing director's office, assuming that the latter is the common line superior to all the departments concerned.

The supervisor might also discover that a deviation is caused by an employee who is not qualified or who has not been given the proper directions and instructions. If the employee is not qualified, additional training and supervision might help, but in other cases finding a replacement might be in order. In a situation in which directions have not been given properly and the employee was not well informed of what was expected of him, it is the supervisor's duty to explain again the standards required.

Only after a thorough analysis of the reasons for a deviation will the supervisor be in a position to take appropriate corrective action. Again, it is not sufficient merely to find the deviation; controlling means correcting the situation. The supervisor must decide what remedial action is necessary to secure improved results in the future. Corrective action may require revising the standards, having a simple discussion, giving a reprimand or other disciplinary action, transferring or even replacing certain employees, or devising better work methods. Corrective action, however, is not the final step. The supervisor must follow up by studying the effect of each corrective action on future control. With further study and analysis the supervisor may find that additional or different measures are required to produce the desired results, keep operations on line, or get them back on track.

Advisory Publications (n.d.) cautions supervisors to not assume that all deviations are the result of an employee or a team. Deviations can be the result of process flaws. Consider excessive overtime. If a supervisor notices that overtime expense is exceeding the budget or becoming excessive, she should exhaust other approaches before authorizing extra hours. Although overtime may be necessary occasionally, it can be wearing on employees, and you may find that productivity actually decreases per paid hour. As with other deviations, the supervisor should consider alternatives. If overtime is routinely used, sufficient employees may not be available to meet the work demands. Pulling together a work redesign team may identify steps or activities that have low or no value that can be eliminated, or tasks that could be automated. After these options are considered, the supervisor may determine it is better to add another full-time or part-time employee at the times that overtime is often used. The extra staff will be paid less than the direct cost of overtime. The additional person(s) can add flexibility, too. Alternatively, the team may discover the overtime only occurs during the summer months, when staff may be taking additional time off, and therefore justify hiring temporary staff to fill in for the vacancies.

The supervisor must be careful not to jump to conclusions when variations are identified and consider as many causes as possible. However, he should not take so much time in the analysis that the variation continues without any corrective action occurring.

Benchmarking

As mentioned earlier, an effective approach to improving an organization's operational performance is to identify similar organizations that seem to be performing better, visiting with the managers at those organizations, and discussing how they are able to achieve optimal performance. This process is known as benchmarking. Benchmarking allows organizations to assess their operations, become knowledgeable about competitors, and incorporate what they learn about the best practices used by these industry leaders. Tapping the wisdom of the optimally performing organization, the managers can attempt to implement the same or similar practices or processes at their own enterprise and perhaps experience some improvement in performance.

Benchmarking can begin at a macro level by comparing one's key statistics to those published by local, regional, or national organizations (see Exhibit 25.9).

Benchmarking is essentially the process of seeking best practices so that the organization remains competitive in the marketplace. Other sources of best practices are professional newsletters and journals and specialty discussion groups on the Internet. Conducting some research helps the supervisor locate organizations that closely mirror her organization and allows her to compare her institution's processes to theirs.

Benchmarking is similar to other process improvement activities. As with any activity that may require reorganizing or possibly reengineering, the customer must always be considered first, and, as noted above, the stakeholders—the employees—should always be involved in assessing the situation. According to Cashen (1999), "benchmarking is not a numbers-only exercise. Measuring the performance of best practice organizations only reveals that they are doing better in the chosen activities. Understanding the managerial and operational processes that allow the target organizations to achieve their results is necessary in order to create improvements in one's own activities. In other words, benchmarking is not about mimicking other organizations, it is about helping individuals learn new ways to think about existing problems."

Summary

Controlling is the managerial function of monitoring performance; the manager checks performance against standards and takes corrective action if deviations exist. Control is most closely related to the planning function, but it is

EXHIBIT 25.9 CMI-Adjusted Average Departmental Costs for Highest Volume Base MS-DRGs

Bed-Size Group	CMI	Routine Cost/Day	Special Care Cost/Day	Laboratory Cost/Day	Radiology Cost/Day	Inhalation Therapy Cost/Day	Med/Surg Supplies Cost/Day	Total Cost/Day
Heart failure and shock (MS-DRGs 291-292-293)								
≤ 50	1.0383	$720	$986	$137	$46	$63	$87	$1,434
51-150	1.0594	$691	$797	$128	$47	$52	$84	$1,450
151-500	1.0778	$693	$585	$118	$49	$41	$70	$1,420
500+	1.0849	$745	$538	$121	$53	$35	$61	$1,452
Simple pneumonia and pleurisy (MS-DRGs 193-194-195)								
≤ 50	1.0016	$738	$990	$104	$50	$100	$91	$1,415
51-150	1.0247	$697	$841	$109	$55	$80	$90	$1,420
151-500	1.0446	$679	$660	$105	$59	$61	$75	$1,377
500+	1.0552	$713	$661	$112	$66	$50	$67	$1,423
Chronic obstructive pulmonary disease (MS-DRGs 190-191-192)								
≤ 50	0.9292	$770	$983	$110	$42	$141	$104	$1,507
51-150	0.9399	$744	$865	$108	$47	$125	$102	$1,520
151-500	0.9511	$739	$679	$101	$51	$107	$90	$1,493
500+	0.9561	$767	$664	$105	$58	$100	$82	$1,527
Major joint replacement or reattachment of lower extremity (MS-DRGs 469-470)								
≤ 50	2.0137	$572	$675	$39	$13	$14	$1,043	$2,267
51-150	2.0415	$372	$529	$42	$16	$13	$825	$1,869
151-500	2.0438	$344	$415	$41	$16	$9	$883	$1,880
500+	2.0454	$343	$388	$40	$18	$8	$780	$1,792
Septicemia without mechanical ventilation 96+ hours (MS-DRGs 871-872)								
≤ 50	1.6257	$457	$738	$78	$37	$37	$56	$964
51-150	1.6529	$445	$669	$83	$40	$34	$58	$1,021
151-500	1.6708	$437	$548	$82	$42	$30	$57	$1,008
500+	1.6769	$466	$541	$88	$46	$26	$50	$1,045

NOTE: CMI = Case-mix index; MS-DRG = Medicare severity diagnosis-related group.

SOURCE: Reprinted with permission from William Shoemaker, "Benchmarking Tools for Reducing Costs of Care." *hfm*, April 2009. Copyright Healthcare Financial Management Association.

interwoven with all the other managerial functions as well. Control is essential in every organized activity, although in behavioral terms control means placing constraints on people. A good control system must be designed so that it brings about organizational effectiveness without infringing on individual satisfaction.

In relation to time, one can distinguish among anticipatory, concurrent, and feedback control mechanisms. There are several basic requirements for a control system to be effective. The supervisor must make sure that the subordinates fully understand the controls and that the controls are appropriate for the situation. Because control is anticipatory, a control system should be designed to report deviations as promptly as possible. Controls must also be worth the expense involved and the effort put forth. A good control system also must allow sufficient flexibility to cope with new situations and circumstances in a dynamic setting. Finally, a viable control system must clearly indicate where and why deviations have occurred so that the supervisor can take appropriate corrective action at the proper place.

In performing the controlling function, the manager should follow three basic steps: (1) set standards or metrics, (2) measure performance and compare with standards, and (3) take corrective action if necessary. In setting standards, the supervisor must be aware of both those that are tangible and those that are intangible. Many of the tangible standards can be established with the help of motion and time studies. Data collected from benchmarking activities may indicate where standards should be established and at what level. Benchmarking allows managers to build on the success of others and to avoid "reinventing the wheel."

After establishing the strategic metrics, the supervisor's function is to check and measure performance against them. In some instances, the supervisor has to depend on reports, but in most cases direct personal observation is the best means for appraising performance. If discrepancies from standards are revealed, the supervisor must take corrective action to bring activities back into line.

Additional Readings

Belkin, L. 2007. "Time Wasted? Perhaps It's Well Spent." [Online article; retrieved 11/24/09.] www.nytimes.com/2007/05/31/fashion/31work.html.

Caldwell, C., and K. Stuenkel. 2008. "Moving from Good to Best in Healthcare: Embracing Accounting in Improvements." *Healthcare Executive* 23 (3): 9–15.

Johnson, J. 2009. "Do You Know the Fair Market Value of Quality?" *Healthcare Financial Management* 63 (10) 52–60.

Kuzma, J. et al. 2004. *Basic Statistics for the Health Sciences.* New York: McGraw Hill.

Modern Times. 1936. [Motion picture.] Los Angeles: United Artists.

26

BUDGETARY AND OTHER CONTROL TECHNIQUES

Chapter Objectives

After you have studied this chapter, you should be able to do the following:

1. Define the approaches, types, and purposes of budgets.
2. Outline the role of the supervisor in preparing the budget.
3. Compare and contrast different budget models.
4. Review the function of budgets in cost containment.

Luther Halsey Gulick III (1892–1993) expanded Fayol's control function into two functions—reporting and budgeting. He described reporting as verifying progress through inspection, ensuring that things happened according to plan, and taking any corrective actions indicated. Budgeting, on the other hand, includes fiscal planning, accounting, and control (Specian 2007). The principal tool for control is the budget. A budget is a written plan expressed in figures and numerical terms, primarily in dollars and cents, that projects revenue and expenses for a specified time. It sets the financial standards to be met by the organization. The budget is the most widely used control device. Budgetary control is an effective managerial tool for all levels of leadership in all departments. For this reason, it is essential that every manager learn how to plan budgets, work within their boundaries, and use them properly for control purposes.

Of all available control devices, the budget, especially the expense budget, is probably the one the supervisor is most familiar with and has been coping with for the longest time. The supervisor's planning and controlling of financial resources for the organization's day-to-day operations is known as operations budgeting (Dunn 2008, 9–1).

As pointed out in Chapter 10, budgeting is a planning function, but its administration is part of the controlling function. Budgets are preestablished standards to which operations are compared and, if necessary, adjusted by the exercise of control. In other words, a budget is a means of control insofar as it reflects the progress of the actual performance against the plan. The budget provides information that enables the supervisor to take action, if needed, to make results conform to the plan.

The Nature of Budgeting and Budgetary Control

When all aspects of the institution's operations are covered by budgets and when all departmental budgets are consolidated into an overall budget, the enterprise practices comprehensive, or master, budgeting. Most enterprises practice **comprehensive budgeting**, which includes the overall budget for the organization and many subordinate budgets for the various divisions and departments.

Whereas the CEO and board of directors are concerned with the overall budget, the supervisor is mainly involved with the departmental budget. The term **budgetary control** refers to the use of budgets to control the department's daily operations so that they conform to the goals and standards set by the institution.

The Supervisor's Concern About Budgeting[1]

The budgeting process also has some drawbacks that management must overcome, including the following:

- *Budgeting is time consuming.* Because it is time consuming, some managers do not devote adequate time to the process. This omission must be avoided, because all parts of a budget must be sound to ensure overall effectiveness of the organization. Computerizing some aspects of budgeting can decrease the time required. Computer-generated managerial accounting reports, which provide data on actual costs and variances, often are a by-product of an organization's information system. In addition, electronic spreadsheets or more sophisticated decision support systems on departmental personal computers can be used to aid in budgeting. These data analysis products permit manipulation of budget variables without cumbersome recalculations. This is sometimes called **what-if analysis**. For example, a budget can be prepared based on volume projections, and then different levels of inflation can be programmed into the spreadsheet or decision algorithm to automatically show the effect of variable levels of inflation on the budget.
- *Budgeting is an expense in itself.* This is especially true in the case of the overly zealous manager who devotes too much time to budgeting and thus takes time away from other operational activities. For this manager,

comprehensive budgeting
The practice of establishing an organization-wide forecast of revenues and expenditures specifically defined for each operating unit within the organization.

budgetary control
The use of budgets to control the department's daily operations.

what-if analysis
Manipulating variables in a budget to see how the results change.

the budget often becomes an end in itself. Symptoms are treated as problems, and research may not be done to identify the real problems and develop solutions.

• *Sometimes management performance is evaluated only in monetary terms.* This is a case of quantity over quality. Although the bottom line is just as important to the viability of the healthcare organization as it is to the manufacturing firm, quality usually is considered to be more important. Even if a bottom-line focus is only a perception, such an attitude can negatively affect budget development and budget compliance. The manager who is overly concerned about her evaluation based on budget performance may cut corners that negatively affect the quality of care or service.

Numerical Terms in Budgeting

The budget states the anticipated results in specific numerical terms. Although the terms are ultimately monetary, at the beginning of the budget planning process not all budgets are expressed in dollars and cents. Many budgets are stated in nonfinancial numerical terms, such as labor hours, hours per adjusted patient day, quantities of supplies, operations per operating room, bills per hour, or lab tests per diagnosis-related group. Personnel budgets indicate the number of workers needed for each type of skill required, the number of hours allocated to perform certain activities, and so on. Although budgets may start out with numerical terms other than monetary values, ultimately every nonfinancial budget must be translated into dollars and cents. This is the common denominator for all activities of an organization.

Making the Budget

Making a budget, whether it is financial or nonfinancial, leads to improved planning. For budgetary purposes, it is not sufficient just to make a general statement. One must quantify, date, and state specific plans in a budget. A considerable difference exists between making a general forecast and attaching numerical values to specific plans. The figures in the budget are the actual plans that become the standard of achievement. The plans are then no longer predictions but the basis for daily operations and standards to be met.

A complete budgetary program requires the involvement of all levels of management to make serious and honest considerations. Rigorous budgetary thinking is certain to improve the quality of organizational planning. Indeed, participation by all the managers and supervisors who are affected by the various budgets is a prerequisite for their successful administration. Again, this is important because it is natural for people to resent arbitrary orders. Thus, it is imperative that all budget allowances and objectives be determined with the full cooperation of those who are responsible for executing them.

Participation in Traditional Budgeting

The supervisor's involvement in budget preparation increases the reliability, accuracy, and acceptance of the budget; the supervisor is closest to his department's activity and understands all of the elements going into the budget. He should submit a proposed budget and participate in what is commonly known as **grassroots budgeting**.

grassroots budgeting
The practice of involving operating unit managers and supervisors in the development of forecasts of expenditures and revenues for their respective units.

For example, as the fiscal year draws to a close, the supervisor of the operating rooms should sit down and gather together those figures that will make up next year's budget. The supervisor might need the assistance of his immediate line superior, in this case most likely the director of nursing services. The supervisor must gather all available information on past performance, expenses, salaries of nursing personnel, other wages, supplies, maintenance, and so forth. Then the supervisor should consider any possible new developments, such as increases in wages, increased costs of supplies, and additional personnel, before he prepares an intelligent and realistic budget. In some smaller healthcare organizations, all budgeting may be completed by the controller or even the CEO for several reasons, including to avoid budget inflation and to save line supervisors the time (because often these supervisors provide day-to-day, direct patient care services).

The full responsibility for preparing the budget does not lie with the supervisor alone. It is the administrator's and every manager's duty to work on budgets. They give the departmental supervisor information on past performance and future industry projections, which he combines with data from the controller and the accounting department. The supervisor uses this information to substantiate future estimates and proposals in a free exchange of opinions with the line superior. After both reach a certain level of agreement, the line boss conveys the overall departmental budget to higher administration.

For example, assume that the director of environmental services supervises three areas of activity: housekeeping, dietary, and plant maintenance. The supervisors of each of these three activities work out their departmental budgets and discuss and substantiate them fully with the director of environmental services. The director combines all three budgets and produces a proposed budget for the entire environmental services division. This budget is submitted and discussed with the immediate line superior. Ultimately, the final budget is adjusted and set by top-level administration, but its effectiveness is ensured because true grassroots participation has taken place.

HOSPITAL LAND

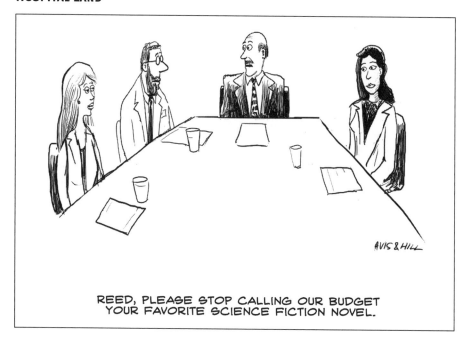

REED, PLEASE STOP CALLING OUR BUDGET
YOUR FAVORITE SCIENCE FICTION NOVEL.

Such participation does not mean that the suggestions of the supervisors should or will always prevail. A careful and thorough analysis of the figures is necessary. A full discussion should take place between the supervisor and the line superior, and the supervisor should have ample opportunity to be heard and to substantiate his case. Some subordinates are inclined to propose budgets with monetary levels they hope to achieve without too much effort. This is obviously done for self-protection and because the supervisor wants to play it safe. The supervisor rationalizes that, by setting the estimates of expenses high enough, he can be sure to stay within the allocated amount and will be praised if he does so. This, however, defeats the purpose of grassroots budgeting. In those facilities following traditional management methods, the line superior should remind the supervisor that the purpose of budget participation is to arrive at realistic budgets. The superior should explain that favorable and unfavorable variances will be carefully scrutinized and that the supervisor's managerial rating will depend on, among other factors, how realistic a budget proposal he submits.

Budgeting Approaches

Most budgets cover a period of one year. These are usually submitted at one time approximately three to four months prior to the year the budget takes effect. However, some organizations have established **rolling budget** approaches.

rolling budget
Unlike the traditional budget, which is developed for a 12-month period, the rolling budget approach starts with a base budget and continually is added to and updated for future months or segments of time.

The manager initially prepares the budget for 12 months as she would in the traditional approach. When the first month of the new budget ends, the manager projects that month's budget for the following year. As the second month of the new budget ends, the manager projects the second month for the next year, and so on. This allows budget planning to occur every month rather than in a massive flurry of work during a few weeks of the year. Alternatively, some organizations prepare the new projections every quarter.

flexible budgeting
Budgeting that is prepared with a range of potential customer levels, so that adjustments can be made throughout the year if changes in levels occur.

Another approach is **flexible budgeting**. A flexible, or variable, budget is prepared with a range of activity levels (if patient volume is x, y, or z) so that adjustments can be made throughout the year if changes in activity levels occur. In flexible budgeting, actual results are compared against the appropriate activity level. Because the flexible budget covers a range of activity, the manager can construct a new budget if actual costs are different from what was originally planned (Dunn 2005).

Although many organizations are steering away from what is known as historical or conventional budgets, they do exist. Conventional or *traditional budgeting*, discussed in more detail below, involves projections for the following year based on current expenditures and the previous annual budget. Under this approach, the amounts expended the prior year are increased by a certain inflation factor (or in some cases decreased). Another approach is **incremental budgeting**; this is often coupled with the rolling or flexible budget. Because considerable effort goes into the development of these budgets, the most critical and analytical attention by top-level management is devoted to the year-over-year increment; the base is treated as though it were already authorized and requires no review. The adjusted amounts become the manager's new budget. This approach does not consider one-time purchases and encourages managers to always spend their budgets.

incremental budgeting
Budgeting that assumes that budgeted amounts from the previous year remain set, and attention is only paid to incremental increases.

traditional budgeting
Budgeting that focuses on planned changes from the previous year's level of expenditures.

Under **traditional budgeting**, management focuses on planned changes from the previous year's level of expenditures. This method assumes that the activities making up the historical base (1) are essential, (2) must be continued, (3) are being performed effectively in a cost-efficient manner, (4) are needed more than new programs, and (5) will continue to be necessary and effective next year. Some activities meet all these criteria, but it is unrealistic to assume that all of them will. Another potential problem is wasteful expenditures. If the department incurs less cost than budgeted, the department may try to spend the money even if there is no real need. Although this is contrary to basic financial principles, the department fears losing the money if the new budget is influenced by the current level of expenditures. Another potential shortcoming arises when a department that is currently operating efficiently is faced with an across-the-board edict to cut budget amounts by a certain percentage. This cut would hurt the efficient department more than it would hurt an inefficient department.

Because of these limitations and the recent emphasis on process improvement, reengineering, and cost containment, a need for better budgeting techniques exists. **Zero-base budgeting** is a contemporary approach to budgeting. It was developed in the early 1970s in industrial settings and then was quickly introduced into state and federal government agencies. Today many major corporations are using zero-base budgeting, and more and more healthcare institutions are introducing it because of changing healthcare priorities, constrained financial resources, changing technologies, available computer capabilities, and the emphasis on cost containment in particular.

zero-base budgeting
Budgeting that ignores the previous year's budget and requires that every request for funding be justified anew.

Under zero-base budgeting, the budget for the new period ignores the previous budget; every activity submitted for funding must be justified. This approach requires substantiation and justification of each budget item from the ground up. Zero-base budgeting gives administration an opportunity to reassess all activities, departments, and projects in terms of their benefits and costs to the organization. The advantage is that each "package" has to be planned anew and costs are calculated from scratch; this avoids the tendency to look only at changes from the previous period. Ongoing programs are reviewed and have to be justified in their entirety every budget period.

Briefly, the process involves seven steps (Cleverly 1992):

1. Define the outputs or services provided by the program or departmental area, such as correspondence or transcription services by the health information department.
2. Determine the costs of these services or outputs, such as the cost for transcribing home health notes for the home health service.
3. Identify options for reducing the cost through changes in outputs or services, such as the use of an outside contract transcription service.
4. Identify options for producing the services and outputs more efficiently.
5. Determine the cost savings associated with operations identified in steps 3 and 4.
6. Assess the risks, both qualitative and quantitative, associated with the identified options of steps 3 and 4—for example, asking if the contract service will be timely.
7. Select and implement those options with an acceptable cost–risk relationship.

All budgeting systems have some limitations, and zero-base budgeting is no exception. The additional time necessary for budget preparation and the large amount of paperwork may be viewed as offsetting the benefits. However, the process takes less time as managers become familiar with it. In the long run, the benefits of zero-base budgeting seem to outweigh the additional work and expenditures involved.

Types of Budgets[1]

Three types of budgets are typically prepared in organizations. The **revenue and expense budget** is also known as the operations budget. It includes estimates of patient and nonpatient revenue as well as expenses for personnel, supplies, depreciation, interest, insurance, and so on. In this effort, the supervisor uses volume estimates to project revenues and expenses.

The **capital budget** is a plan that shows the major assets to be purchased, anticipated purchase dates, and funding sources for those purchases. It is supported by cost–benefit analyses and priority assignments that may be used to rank projects if cash or financing is inadequate to invest in all projects. The supervisor may be asked to sit on a capital expenditure committee to help assign priorities to the various projects and items requested. Often items requested are submitted on a capital request form—the organization's policies dictate when a form must be used—and this is usually linked to a dollar amount. The form varies from organization to organization; however, it often includes a description of the item requested, the cost, the source of the cost estimate, the estimated life of the item for depreciation purposes, and an indication of whether any other departments may be affected by the item. (See Exhibit 26.1.)

The last common budget is the **cash budget**, which is a projection of cash balances at the end of each month throughout the budget year. It is prepared by projecting when the billed charges for revenues during one period will be paid (in cash). This budget not only determines when cost-containment measures may be imperative but also whether capital items, budgeted or not, can be purchased.

Preparing the Budget

A long-standing approach to preparing and selling a budget is the *three Ps approach*: preapproach, proof, and publication (Lindo 1981).[2]

Preapproach
1. Identify demands for your services. Determine who your customers are and assess whether they are growing in number or declining. Are there other potential new customers?
2. Evaluate your facility's economic climate. Discuss this with peer supervisors, other departments, the fiscal director, and so on.
3. Locate internal competition for funds. Consider those departments that are providing similar services or planning to do so.
4. Establish a set of realistic budget expectations. If the patient activity (e.g., number of encounters, surgeries, days) is declining 10 percent, do not submit a budget requesting 15 percent more resources.

EXHIBIT 26.1 Capital Request Form

ANYWHERE HEALTH CENTER	**EQUIPMENT REQUEST**
PROJECT DATA SHEET—COSTS	**YEAR 2009**

I. IDENTIFICATION:
    Cost Center Name: Health Information Management

    Cost Center Number: 8910

EQUIPMENT CLASSIFICATION:
Replacement: N
Addition: X
Regulatory Agency Requirement: N

II. DESCRIPTION:
    Epson Stylus (per C. Dante's recommendation) similar to the one purchased for Security.

III. JUSTIFICATION:
    As the Director performs more duties related to charting/graphing results of RAC activities, CORE Measure results, and other managerial documents, the need for a color printer becomes greater. The printer need not be a high-speed printer, but should have good color printing capabilities.

IV. COST INFORMATION:
    Capital Expense
    (A) List Price of Equipment: $400.00
    (B) Freight Costs:
    (C) Installation Costs:
    (From Worksheet III)
Capitalized Cost (A+B+C): $400.00

    (D) Less: Trade-In Value: (N/A)
    (Year purchased:)

Final Estimated Cost: $400.00

Effect on Annual Operating Expenses

(A) Depreciation:
    Capitalized Cost/Useful Life
    $400.00/5 = $80.00
(B) Maintenance Contract:
(C) Additional Supply Cost: $100.00
(D) Staff Training: _____
    (Inc. travel, etc.)
Total Direct Expense (A+B+C): $180.00

V. APPROVALS:
    Engineering Department: _____ Date: _____
    Information Systems: _____ Date: _____
    Department Head: _____ Date: _____
    Administration: _____ Date: _____

SOURCE: Reprinted with permission from *Finance Principles for the Health Information Manager*, 2nd ed. St. Louis, MO: First Class Solutions, Inc.

---

5. Always start your budget preparation a year in advance. Do not wait until the notice arrives on your desk to begin data collection and budget preparation.

Proof

1. Provide details and sources for your budget estimates.
2. Present past performance. How well have you achieved budget expectations in the past? How successful have you been in implementing new programs and reaching the goals planned?

3. Analyze and present applicable trend data that support the activity levels projected. Remember to use written comments and graphs to enhance comprehension of your presentation.
4. Discuss the current status of prior programs implemented and/or goals assigned.
5. Prioritize new programs and/or services being proposed so you are ready, if asked to do so, to eliminate some programs and/or services proposed.

Publication

1. Once the budget is approved, summarize for your supervisor the new and ongoing key authorized programs.
2. Update the status of each of these on a regular basis, no less often than quarterly. Try to discuss your report in person as well as provide a written report to your superior.
3. Identify in your quarterly updates any enhancements being considered to the approved or ongoing programs that may appear in the next budget.
4. Well in advance of the next budget notices, meet with your superior to discuss planned enhancements or new programs being considered and to begin the preapproach process.

Using the guidance of these three phases allows the supervisor to stay ahead of others competing for funds and ensures that her boss is kept informed throughout the year.

Other Budget Considerations

Budget Director and Budget Committee

A team of staff accountants, headed by a budget director, the controller, or the CFO, may assist the supervisor in the budgeting process. This team, serving in an advisory capacity, can provide the line managers with advice and technical assistance and may even prepare the initial budget letter, budget instructions and packet of forms, and data, which are sent to all managers, but it should not prepare the actual budgets. Once all budgets have been approved by the designated superiors, the budget department staff will put the various budget estimates together in final form so that top-level administration can submit it to the board.

Some institutions also have established a budget committee that serves in an advisory and supportive capacity in coordinating the various budgets. In this instance the budget committee clearly performs a staff function. This must be distinguished, however, from those budget committees to which the board has delegated the line function of setting, rather than just coordinating, the budget. In this situation the budget committee considers all departmental budget estimates and requests, including expenses and capital expenditures, and makes the final decisions. In large institutions, there may be subcommittees of the budget committee, for example, the capital expenditure committee. This form of budget committee has ultimate line authority and responsibility for determining the budget instead of a single person such as the institution's top-level administrator or executive director. The budget is approved by the committee. If budget revisions and changes are requested, it is also up to the budget committee to allow or disallow them. Several arrangements are possible within these two extremes as to where the final authority for the overall budget rests. Usually the budget needs the authorization of the CEO, the finance committee of the board, and eventually the board of directors.

Length of the Budget Period

Although the length of the budget period may vary, most healthcare enterprises choose one year. This period is then broken down into quarters, and many institutions even divide it by months at the time of the original budget preparation. This is usually referred to as periodic budgeting.

Healthcare institutions also typically have budgets extending over a longer term, such as three or five years. These budgets usually cover such items as capital expenditures, research programs, and expansions. Long-term or long-range budgets of this nature are used for projecting major capital needs (such as replacing the roof or acquiring a picture archiving and communication system). The supervisor is asked to project capital needs for the department over a given period (three to five years, possibly more). These needs are evaluated by senior management and, as appropriate given the long-range strategic plan of the organization, compiled into the long-term capital budget. These budgets are planning, not controlling, tools. For most healthcare organizations it is difficult to plan much beyond five years because healthcare is so heavily regulated and the regulations vary greatly, depending on elected officials and the economy.

Flexibility of the Budgetary Process

The supervisor should keep in mind that budgets are merely tools for management and not a substitute for good judgment. Also, care should be taken not to make budgets so detailed that they become cumbersome. Budgets should always allow the supervisor enough freedom to accomplish the best objectives of the department. There must be a reasonable degree of latitude and flexibility. In fact, one of the most serious shortcomings of budgeting is the danger of inflexibility. Although budgets are plans expressed in numerical terms, the supervisor must not be led to believe that these figures are absolutely final and unalterable. Enlightened management teams build into the budgetary program a degree of flexibility and adaptability so that the institution can cope with changing conditions, new developments, and even incidents of human error and miscalculation. Flexibility should not be interpreted to mean, however, that the budget can be changed with every whim or that it should be taken lightly.

Nevertheless, if operating conditions have appreciably changed and there are valid indications that the budget cannot be followed in the future, a revision of the budget is in order. Such circumstances may be caused by unexpected events, new legislation, unanticipated wage increases, or large fluctuations in demand. Consider, for example, the budget of the nuclear medicine department, in which activities have been increasing constantly because of new applications and technology breakthroughs. Revenues derived from this service are increasing rapidly at the same time. It would be absurd to expect the supervisor of this department to stay within the budgeted figures for salaries and supplies if growth is significantly in excess of the budgeted volume. If the department is expected to respond and supply the increased demand for this service, the budget must be altered. In such a case the old budget has become obsolete; unless provisions are available to make the budget flexible, it will lose its usefulness altogether.

Budget Review and Revision

Increasing attention has been given to ways of ensuring budget flexibility to avoid the danger of rigidity and obsolescence. Most enterprises achieve this by conducting periodic budget reviews and revisions. The budget is reviewed at regular intervals of one, two, or three months. In meetings between the departmental supervisor and the line superior, performance data are checked and compared with the budgeted figures, and the supervisor is called on to explain the causes for any variations. A thorough analysis must then be made to discover the reasons for the deviation from the budgeted amount; this may lead to budget revisions or other corrective measures.

An unfavorable variation by itself does not necessarily require a budget change; it must be studied and explained. The supervisor of nuclear medicine in the earlier example will not have any difficulties proving the need for an upward budget revision. In some organizations such a revision can be made on the departmental level, whereas in other institutions it must be carried up to the CEO or even the board's budget committee. If the deviations are of sufficient magnitude, it is advisable to make the necessary revisions no matter how high up in the hierarchy they have to go or how much work they may involve. If the variation is minor and it has been explained and justified, it may be more expedient to let it go instead of revising the entire budget.

No matter what decision is made, regular budget reviews and revisions seem to be the best way of ensuring the flexibility of the budgetary process. They prevent the budget from being viewed as a straitjacket and allow the supervisor to consider it a living document and a valuable tool for control purposes.

Budgets and Human Relations Issues

Budgets necessarily represent restrictions, and for this reason subordinates generally resent budgets. Often subordinates take a defensive approach to budgets, one acquired through painful experience. Many times the subordinates become acquainted with budgets only as a barrier to spending, or the budget is blamed for failure to get or give a raise in salary. Moreover, in the minds of many subordinates the word "budget" has become associated with miserly behavior rather than with planning and direction.

The line manager's job is to correct this erroneous impression by pointing out that budgeting is a disciplined approach to resolve or prevent many problems and is necessary to maintain standards of performance. The budget must be presented as a planning tool and not as a pressure device.

Avoiding unnecessary pressures over the budget presupposes that a good working relationship exists between the supervisor and the immediate superior. This in turn rests on clear-cut organizational lines and a thorough understanding that the line managers are responsible for control. Effective use of budgetary procedures depends on the administration's attitudes toward the entire budgetary process. Only with the planning-tool view will a supervisor believe that whatever can be done without a budget can be done much more effectively with a budget.

Cost Controls

Healthcare providers have been under continuous, unrelenting pressure to keep healthcare expenditures from spiraling. It is safe to predict that the drive to control costs will increase even more because of pressures from government agencies for pricing transparency; legislators seeking ways to support the cost of healthcare reform; insurers attempting to offset catastrophic healthcare costs; and purchasers of healthcare, such as large corporations, managed care organizations, and even individuals, using information provided by such organizations as the Leapfrog Group and Healthgrades to assess morbidity and cost. In such an environment, control of costs is an ongoing problem for everyone from the CEO to the supervisor.

Cost control, also referred to as cost awareness, cost consciousness, or cost containment, should be viewed as a significant part of the supervisor's daily job. Supervisors must strive for cost consciousness with consistency. Sporadic cost-cutting efforts seldom have lasting results. Because cost awareness is an ongoing issue, the supervisor must set definite numerical objectives and make plans for containing cost. Priorities must be clarified without infringing on the quality of healthcare; this is difficult to achieve, especially if more sophistication in patient care is accompanied by general escalation of prices and wages.

cost control
The practice of consistently monitoring and managing costs.

To succeed in cost containment, it is essential to involve the medical staff as well as the employees of the department and make them realize that ultimately their actions will bring about results. Recall our discussion in Chapter 14 about alternatives to downsizing and in Chapter 20 about communicating change. Medical staff members, especially surgeons, can have a significant impact on the cost of surgery when prosthetics and specialized instruments are required. Therefore, the physicians must be pulled into the cost-containment discussions. Sometimes this is accomplished through a medical staff committee charged with establishing clinical pathways. All employees should consider cost consciousness as a part of their job. Most physicians and employees will help cut costs and reduce waste, especially if the results of their efforts are fed back to them. Most workers are not deliberately wasteful. Many physicians and employees can make valuable suggestions and contributions to cost effectiveness. The supervisor should welcome all suggestions, investigate each one, and not fault anyone for not having thought of these changes before. Cost awareness should be an ongoing challenge in everyone's daily job and be a part of every employee's annual performance review as well as the biennial credentialing review.

Allocation of Costs

Every supervisor must see that his department contributes financially to the operation of the institution. However, supervisors must realize that in a healthcare center, just as in all other organized activities, some departments are revenue producing, and others are not. Clearly, the operating rooms and pharmacy services produce revenue, but these patient care departments could not function without the services provided by departments such as housekeeping, dietary services, health records, laundry, and administration. Although these are not revenue-producing departments, their costs must be carried if the healthcare facility is to function on a fiscally sound basis. As part of the Medicare-required cost-reporting function, hospitals must allocate costs of the non-revenue-generating departments to those patient care departments that do produce revenue. How are the costs of the non-revenue-producing departments allocated to the revenue-producing departments? The supervisor has no control over this portion of a department's expenses, which can make the difference between ending up with a departmental surplus or with a deficit.

A detailed discussion of the various methods of cost analysis, the contribution margin approach, and other bases for allocations is beyond the scope of this book. However, the supervisor should have a general understanding of the bases on which a department is being charged for these various expenditures. In reality she is powerless to influence the costs allocated to the department, but she should be able to readily understand the direct expenses (e.g., wages, salaries, supplies, materials) and some indirect expenses (e.g., Social Security and workers' compensation taxes) charged to the department. The supervisor also should know that the department is charged with maintenance expenses on the basis of work orders, telecommunications expenses based on the number of telephone lines, and so forth.

The overall financial performance of a department is greatly affected by how allocations for other expenditures are made—for example, administrative expenses, operation of the plant, depreciation, intern and resident service costs, in-service education, and interest expenses. Although all this is determined higher up in the administrative hierarchy, the supervisor should obtain some information on the basis of the allocation and an explanation of how it is done. The healthcare institution will try to select a basis of distribution that is fair to all departments and is feasible from an accounting point of view. Understanding this cost allocation enables the supervisor to better understand how a department's budget may not turn out as well as expected, despite the effective work of the manager and her employees.

Additional Controls

The supervisor's controlling function is closely related to and goes on simultaneously with all other managerial functions. Throughout this book many subjects are discussed as part of a particular function; now their meaning as an aid in the system of control can also be shown.

In Chapter 9, standing plans, such as policies, procedures, methods, and rules, are discussed. At this point in the book, they can also be viewed as anticipatory control devices. These tools are established with the intention that they will be followed and that they work out as preventive controls. If they are violated, the supervisor, using feedback control, must take the necessary corrective action; in some cases disciplinary measures may be necessary.

We discuss positive discipline and disciplinary measures in Chapter 24 as a component of the influencing function. In the controlling context, this topic can be viewed as a preventive and reactive control technique. If a rule has been violated, the supervisor must invoke disciplinary measures, which is synonymous with taking corrective action and sending a message to the employees about proper behavior on the job.

On various occasions, we have discussed management by objectives (MBO), an agreement between the subordinate and the supervisor concerning a measurable performance objective to be achieved and reviewed within a given time period. This concept includes aspects of control. After mutually agreed on objectives have been set, results are evaluated in light of these standards, and, if necessary, shortcomings are corrected.

Performance appraisal systems, the process of formally evaluating performance and providing feedback for performance adjustments, are discussed in Chapter 19. This process can also be viewed as part of the organizational control system. Although performance evaluation measures are presented with the staffing function, they can now be regarded as a feedback control technique in the managerial control system.

These are just a few examples, taken from discussions in previous chapters, of the various managerial control functions. They show how closely related the controlling function is to all the other functions and confirm the statement that the better the supervisor plans, organizes, staffs, and influences, the better she can perform the controlling function.

Summary

Budgeting is planning, whereas working with the budget and budget administration fall into the manager's controlling function. Budgets are plans expressed in numerical terms, which ultimately are reduced to dollars and cents as the common denominator used in the final analysis. Budgets are also preestablished standards to which the operations of the department are compared and, if necessary, adjusted by the exercise of control. Of all control devices, the budget (primarily the expense budget) is the one most widely used and thus the one with which supervisors should be most familiar.

Because the supervisor is responsible for adhering to the departmental budget, he must play a significant role in its preparation. Budget making is a line responsibility shared by the supervisor and the direct line superior. Ultimately, all budgets are submitted to and approved by top-level administration, but it is essential that lower-level managers participate in making their own budgets and have sufficient opportunity to be heard and substantiate their cases.

Zero-base budgeting is a relatively new approach to budgeting. Under traditional budgeting, management's attention is primarily focused on planned changes from the previous year; under zero-base budgeting every activity and budget item must be substantiated and justified from scratch. For a budget to be a live document, the budgetary process must be flexible. There must be frequent periodic budget reviews within the normal one-year budgeting period and provisions for budget revision. Such provisions lessen the human relations problems that budgetary controls often cause.

In addition to budgetary controls, the supervisor should be aware of other costs that influence the overall performance of the department. Here the supervisor is concerned with how the expenditures of the non-revenue-producing departments in a healthcare institution are allocated to those departments that do produce revenues. The bases of these allocations can often make the difference between showing a departmental surplus and operating at a loss. Supervisors also play an important role in cost containment. Cost awareness, or cost consciousness, should be an ongoing consideration and part of the supervisor's daily activities.

Throughout this book, we stress the close relationship between the controlling function and the other managerial functions. Many of the managerial duties and activities discussed previously can now be viewed as additional controls, including policies and procedures, disciplinary measures, MBO, and performance appraisals. The most widely used control device, however, remains the budget and budgetary procedures.

Notes

1. This section is adapted from Chapter 9 of *Finance Principles for the Health Information Manager*, 2nd ed., by Rose T. Dunn (First Class Solutions, 2008).
2. Reprinted with permission of David K. Lindo, PhD, chief financial officer, Jobview, LLC, and author of more than 200 articles on financial management, cost control, and performance evaluation.

Additional Reading

White, K. R., and J. R. Griffith. 2010. "Human Resources Management." In *The Well-Managed Healthcare Organization*, 7th ed., chapter 11. Chicago: Health Administration Press.

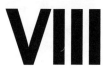
VIII

LABOR RELATIONS

27

THE LABOR UNION AND THE SUPERVISOR

Special thanks to Marc J. Leff, Esq., vice president, Human Resources, Maimonides Medical Center, Brooklyn, New York, for his update to this chapter.

Chapter Objectives

After you have studied this chapter, you should be able to do the following:

1. Review the history of collective bargaining and labor-related legislation.
2. Discuss the content of a typical labor contract.
3. Outline areas of concern for the supervisor.
4. Differentiate the role of the supervisor and the shop steward in organized labor environments.

Although labor unions have lost membership, declining from 20.1 percent of all U.S. workers in 1983 to 12.4 percent in 2008, they are still an influential part of the workforce. As of 2008, about 16.1 million employees were represented by unions, of which 6.5 percent were healthcare workers. Healthcare union membership grew by 1.5 percent from 2007 to 2008 (Bureau of Labor Statistics 2009a). Therefore, it is essential for supervisors to be familiar with the role labor unions play in the workplace to work with them properly.

Collective bargaining gained its major legal basis in 1935 with the enactment of the National Labor Relations Act, also known as the Wagner Act, which guaranteed workers the right to bargain collectively with their employers. In 1947, the Wagner Act was amended by the Labor-Management Relations Act, also known as the Taft-Hartley Act. By the late 1950s, union membership rose to nearly 30 percent. In 1959 the Labor-Management Reporting and Disclosure Act, sometimes referred to as the Landrum-Griffin Act, was added. In 1974, these laws were extended to cover most healthcare institutions.

collective bargaining
The practice of bargaining for better pay and working conditions as a group, rather than individually.

The union movement was primarily a blue-collar campaign because there were more blue-collar workers in the United States labor force than white-collar workers (Bureau of Labor Statistics 2009b). Since the middle 1950s, however, the number of people in white-collar occupational categories and in service industries has surpassed the blue-collar sector. As of 2004, 7.9 million union members represent white-collar employment, while 7.6 million represent blue-collar employment (Bureau of Labor Statistics 2009b). With this change, labor unions have made inroads in representing business services (e.g., computers), retail trade, finance, healthcare, government, and other sectors. A number of unions or employee associations have become the bargaining agents for teachers, college professors, nurses, airline pilots, doctors, and various other white-collar workers. However, it is beyond the confines of this book to discuss the details of labor laws or give the full history of the union movement in the United States.

The Nuances of Unions

There is little doubt that the introduction of a union or an employee association into a hospital or healthcare facility may be a trying experience for the supervisors, as well as for the CEO. It may bring with it tension, during which time finding constructive solutions to problems may be difficult. The issues, claims, and counterclaims are on everyone's mind and are present in the workplace, the parking lot, and even the local news media. The verbal battle may even escalate into work slowdowns or stoppages. If the employees vote to join a union, managers are likely to believe that they have lost a battle and that their employees and union representatives have been victorious. It will take time for the ill feelings created during the organizing campaign to disappear.

However, the union and the administration must learn to work together. Every manager must accept the fact that the labor union is a permanent force in our society. Every manager must realize that the union, just as any other organization, has the potential for either advancing or disrupting the common effort of the institution. It is in the self-interest of the administration to create a labor–management climate that directs this potential toward constructive ends. There is no simple or magic formula, however, for cultivating a favorable climate that will result overnight in cooperation and mutual understanding between the union and management. It takes wisdom and sensitivity from every manager of the organization, from the administrator to the supervisor, to demonstrate in day-to-day relations that the union is respected as a responsible part of the institution.

In this effort to create and maintain a constructive pattern of cooperation between the healthcare institution and the union, the most significant player usually is the supervisor of a department. Supervisors, more than anyone else, feel the strongest impact of the new situation because they make the largest number of decisions concerning unionized employees. The supervisor is the person in day-to-day employee relations who makes the labor agreement a living document, for better or for worse. An article in *Textile World* discussed the movement away from unions and preference for cooperative labor–management committees. Of the 2,408 manufacturing employees polled, 63 percent opted for the committees, while only 22 percent chose unions. The survey also found that workers complained of a lack of participation in decisions and acknowledged the importance of management cooperation in achieving their goals (Morrissey 1995). Others during the 1990s (Finkelstein 1998; Miller and Zeller 1991) identified the critical factors that would lead to a successful labor–management council or collaboration effort. Based on the foundation of nearly two decades of success through this approach, President Obama signed an executive order in December 2009 creating labor–management forums to improve delivery of government services (White House 2009).

Supervisors are often unsure as to how they should behave during an organizing campaign and after the election when the union arrives on the scene. The supervisor should realize that the subordinates usually decide for a union not because they were gullible or naive or because the union used deceit or strong-arm methods but primarily because some of their major needs were not satisfied on the job. The supervisor should approach the union professionally and try to build a satisfactory relationship.

The supervisor should have received information and training in the fundamentals of collective bargaining and in the nature of labor agreements from the human resources department. This is essential for the development of good labor relations. The supervisor is involved in two distinct phases of labor relations: (1) the inception of unionization and (2) the day-to-day administration of the union agreement, which includes disciplining, scheduling, and reviewing performance of employees. Although the supervisor is primarily concerned with the second phase of relations with the union, she also plays a role in the first.

Unionization and Labor Negotiations

As soon as supervisors learn that union-organizing activities are starting, this information should be passed on to higher administration and the director of human resources. (Often administration has already learned of such a campaign through other channels.) This information enables the organization to plan its strategy, usually with the help of legal counsel. Supervisors should be aware of a number of legal restrictions that must be observed during the union-organizing efforts. The following remarks are of a very general nature; supervisors should receive more detailed instruction from their administrators and lawyers.

Labor laws restrict what managers, including supervisors, are permitted to say and do during this critical period. Administration should provide supervisors with information on the dos and don'ts to follow during a union-organizing campaign (see Exhibit 27.1). Generally, supervisors should not make any statements in reference to unionization that could be construed as a promise if the union fails or as a threat if the union is successful. Supervisors

EXHIBIT 27.1 Dos and Don'ts for Managers and Supervisors During a Union-Organizing Campaign

Do

1. Tell employees that the organization does not believe that they need union representation.
2. Answer employees' questions about organizational policies and discuss the union campaign issues.
3. Tell employees that if they join the union, they are expected to pay union dues and fees.
4. Assure employees that, with or without the union, management is going to continue to try to make the organization a good place to work.
5. Explain to employees that the organization will recognize the union and bargain in good faith if the majority of the employees really want it but that any improvements in wages and benefits are negotiable and not automatic.
6. Administer appropriate disciplinary action or terminate any employee who threatens or coerces other employees, whether for or against the union.
7. Request outside union officials to leave facility property if they try to solicit employees there.
8. Remind employees to vote if there is a union election. A majority of those who actually vote will determine whether there is a union.

Don't S.P.I.T.

S: Spy on employees or conduct surveillance of any kind to determine the level of union sentiment.

P: Promise anything. You should not do anything to suggest that you are soliciting grievances.

I: Interrogate anyone. Asking questions about union sympathies or union activity is an unfair labor practice under the law.

T: Threaten, coerce, or intimidate any employee because of her union activity.

SOURCE: Adapted from Abdelhak et al. 1996. *Health Information: Management of a Strategic Resource*. Philadelphia, PA: W. B. Saunders Co. Reprinted by permission.

Note: In addition to the above, Marc Leff recommends that supervisors do not handle, touch, review, or accept union authorization cards and do not initiate one-on-one conversations on the subject of union representation.

should not question their employees privately or publicly about organizing activities. When asked, supervisors can express their opinions about unionization in a neutral manner, if this is possible, without having the answer interpreted as a threat or promise. The safest approach, however, is for the supervisors to avoid discussing opinions with employees in the office.

Usually an election conducted by the National Labor Relations Board determines the outcome of the organizing campaign. If the union loses the election, the employees do not have a union for the immediate future. If the union wins, management has to recognize the union as the bargaining agent and begin negotiations in good faith. However, this is subject to change if President Obama signs the Employee Free Choice legislation. It is believed that this legislation will take away rights from those employees who do not desire a union (Sherk and Kersey 2009). Ritter (2009) summarizes the changes that this legislation will bring, including the following: signing of signature cards using Internet means and other approaches may not be conducted by secret ballot; a secret ballot election will no longer be required; bargaining for the initial contract must begin within ten days of the election, and if an agreement is not reached within 90 days, either side may request mediation and the arbitrator's decision will be binding for two years; and stiffer penalties will be imposed for employer violations of the process while there will be *no* change in penalties for union violations.

On the surface, the supervisor does not appear to be significantly involved in the negotiations of a labor agreement. As stated earlier, the period during which a union first enters a department of a healthcare organization is usually trying and filled with tension. Emotions run high, and considerable disturbance can result. Under such conditions, it is understandable that the delicate negotiations of a union contract are carried out primarily by members of top-level administration, probably assisted by legal counsel.

Because a committee of employees may be participating in these negotiations, a direct line of communication exists to the other employees of the healthcare institution, but not necessarily to the supervisor. In fact, the supervisor often is less well informed about the course of negotiations than the employees. Therefore, the administrator must see that the supervisor is fully advised as to the progress and direction the negotiations are taking. In addition, the supervisor should be given an opportunity to express opinions on matters brought up during the negotiations. In other words, even though top-level management is representing the institution at the negotiating sessions, supervisors should be able to express their views through them, because ultimately it is the supervisor who bears the major responsibility for fulfilling the contract provisions.

The same necessity exists whenever renegotiations of the labor agreement take place. At that time, top-level administration should consult with the supervisors to determine how specific provisions in the contract have worked out and what changes in the contract the supervisors would like to have made. Both the administrator and the supervisors must realize that although the supervisors do not actually sit at the negotiating table, they have much to do with the nature of the negotiations. Many of the demands made by the union during the negotiations have their origin in the day-to-day operations of the department. Often the most difficult questions to be solved in the bargaining process stem from the relationship that the supervisors have with their employees.

To supply valuable information, the supervisor must know what has been happening in the department and have facts to substantiate her statements. This points to the value of documentation—that is, keeping good records of disciplinary incidents, productivity, leaves, promotions, and so forth. The supervisor should also be alert to problems that should be called to the administration's attention so that in the next set of negotiations these matters may be worked out more satisfactorily. It is in the interest of both the union and the institution to have as few unresolved problems as possible. If problems do arise, however, it is the supervisor's responsibility to see that the administration is aware of them at the time of contract negotiations.

Content of the Agreement

management rights clause
The clause in a labor agreement that gives management the authority to manage the workforce.

Once administration and the union have agreed on a labor contract, this agreement will be the basis on which both parties must operate. Virtually all collective bargaining agreements are constructed with what is called a **management rights clause**. That clause usually gives management broad authority to manage the workforce. All other provisions in the contract are exceptions to that authority. Because the supervisor is now obligated to manage the department within the overall framework of the labor agreement, she must have complete knowledge of its provisions and how they are to be interpreted. The supervisor can cause disagreements between the union and the healthcare institution by failing to live up to the terms of the agreement. Thus, the content of the union contract must be fully explained to and understood by the supervisor.

A good way to present such explanations is at a meeting arranged for top administration and all the supervisors, which is usually chaired by the human resources or labor relations director. The purpose of the meeting is to brief the supervisors on the content of the labor contract, giving them an opportunity to ask questions about any part they do not understand. Copies of the contract and clarification of the various clauses may be furnished to the supervisors so that they may study them in advance. Because no two contracts are alike, however, it is impossible to pinpoint specific provisions that the supervisor should explore. Normally all contracts deal with matters such as union recognition, management's rights, union security, wages, conditions and hours of work, overtime, vacations, holidays, leaves of absence, seniority,

HOSPITAL LAND

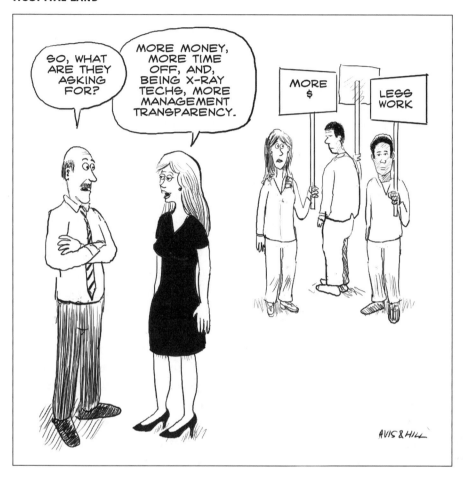

promotions, and similar terms and conditions of employment. Almost certainly there are also provisions concerning complaint and grievance procedures and arbitration. In addition, many other provisions are likely to be peculiar to each institution.

Besides the need to familiarize the supervisors with the exact provisions of the contract, it is important for the administrator to explain to them the philosophy of top-level administration in reference to general relations with the union. The supervisors should understand that the intention of the administration is to maintain good working relations with the union so that organizational objectives can be achieved in a mutually satisfactory fashion. The CEO should clarify that the best way to achieve good union–management relations in a hospital or any other institution is by effective contract administration. The experts in the human resources or labor relations department have a great deal to do with effective contract administration, but much still depends on how the supervisor handles the terms of the contract on a day-to-day basis.

The supervisors must bear in mind that the negotiated contract was carefully and thoughtfully debated and finally agreed on by both parties. Thus, it is not in the interest of successful contract administration for the supervisors to try to "beat the contract," even though they may think they are doing the institution a favor. The administrator must make it clear that to achieve satisfactory cooperation, supervisors may not construct their own contractual clauses or interpret clauses in their own way. Once the agreement has been reached, supervisors should not attempt to change or circumvent it.

If the administrator fails to familiarize the supervisors with the provisions and spirit of the agreement, they should insist on briefing sessions and explanations before they apply the clauses of the contract in the daily working situation of the department. The advent of the labor contract does not change the supervisor's job as a manager. The supervisor must still perform the managerial functions of planning, organizing, staffing, influencing, and controlling. There is no change in the authority delegated to the department head by the administrator or in the responsibility the supervisor has accepted. The significant change is that the supervisor must now perform the managerial duties within the framework of the union agreement. She still has the right to require the subordinates to carry out orders and the obligation to get the job done within the department. Certain provisions within the union agreement, however, are likely to influence and even limit some activities, especially within the areas of job assignments, disciplinary action, and dismissal. In many instances, these provisions of the contract undoubtedly make it more challenging for the supervisor to be a good manager. The only way to meet the challenge is for the supervisor to improve her own managerial ability as well as her knowledge and techniques of good labor relations.

Applying the Agreement

It is in the daily application of the labor agreement that the real importance of the supervisor's contribution appears. The manner in which the day-to-day problems are handled within the framework of the union contract makes the difference between positive labor–management relations and a situation filled with unnecessary tensions and bad feelings. At best, a union contract can only set forth the broad outline of labor–management relations. To make it a positive instrument of constructive relations, the contract must be supported by appropriate and intelligent supervisory decisions. It is the supervisor who interprets management's intent by everyday actions. In the final analysis, the supervisor, through decisions, actions, and behavior, really gives the contract meaning and life.

In many instances, the supervisor may expand on some of the provisions of the contract when interpreting and applying them to specific situations. In so doing, the supervisor sets precedents that arbitrators pay heed to when deciding grievances that come before them. Almost all labor agreements have a grievance procedure leading to arbitration. An **arbitrator** is an independent outside person selected by the union and management to make a final and binding decision in a grievance that the parties involved are unable to settle themselves.

It is impossible for the administrator and the union to draw up a contract that anticipates every possible situation in employee relations and specifies exact directives for dealing with them. Therefore, the individual judgment of the supervisor becomes very important in handling each particular situation. This again illustrates the significance of the supervisor's influence on the interpretation of the labor agreement.

As a representative of administration, any error in the supervisor's decision making is the administration's error. The immediate supervisor has the greatest responsibility for seeing that the clauses of the agreement are carried out appropriately. This includes the supervisor's duty to ensure that the employees comply with the provisions, just as supervisors have to operate within them. Therefore, the administrator must realize how significant a role the supervisor plays in the contract administration. Likewise, it is just as essential for the supervisor to realize how far reaching his decisions and actions can become.

Problem Areas

The supervisor is likely to run into difficulties in the administration of a labor agreement in two broad areas. The first covers the vast number of complaints that are concerned with single issues, such as those involving a particular disciplinary action; assignment of work; distribution of overtime; and questions about promotion, transfer, and downgrading. In each situation, the personal judgment of the supervisor is of great importance. As long as the contract provisions are met, the supervisor should feel free to deal with grievances as she sees fit. She must make certain, however, that the actions are consistent and logical even though they are made on the basis of personal judgment rather than on specifically documented rules.

The second area of difficulty in contract administration covers those grievances and problems in which the supervisor is called on to interpret a clause of the contract. The supervisor is placed in a situation in which he must carry out the generalized statement of the contract but finds that it is subject to varying interpretations. In such instances, he would be wrong to handle the problem without consulting the human resources department first. Whenever an interpretation of the contract is at issue, any decision is likely to be long lasting. Such a decision may set a precedent that the institution, the union, or even an arbitrator would want to make use of in the future. By referring these situations to human resources, management ensures that the contract is interpreted consistently throughout the healthcare organization.

Therefore, if interpretation of a clause is in doubt, the question should be brought to the attention of the human resources director. Although the

arbitrator
An independent outside person selected by the union and management to make a final and binding decision in a grievance that the parties involved are unable to settle themselves.

supervisor may have been well indoctrinated in the meaning, philosophy, and clauses of the contract, his perspective is probably not broad enough to make a potentially precedent-setting interpretation. Because the supervisor did not attend the bargaining meetings, he cannot know the intent of the parties or the background of this provision.

The Supervisor's Right to Make Decisions

In non-precedent-setting situations and in the daily administration of the labor agreement, the supervisor, as a member of management, has the right and even the duty to make a decision. The union contract does not abrogate management's right to decide; the union does, however, have a right to grieve.

For example, the supervisor's job is to maintain discipline, and if disciplinary action is necessary, she can take action without discussing it with the union's representative. The supervisor should understand that usually there is no duty to negotiate, and she should not set any precedent of determining together with the union what the supervisor's rights are in a particular disciplinary case. Of course, before any disciplinary measures are taken, a prudent supervisor will examine all the facts in the case, fulfill the preliminary steps of decision making, and think through the appropriateness of the action. This process is more fully discussed in Chapter 28.

In a few cases, the union contract will call for consultation or advance notice before the supervisor can proceed. Advance notice or consultation, however, does not mean agreement or negotiation on the final decision. Repercussions or protests from the union can still occur, although prior communication on anticipated action can prevent them. In any event, the right to decide on day-to-day issues of contract administration still rests with the supervisor and not with the union.

The Supervisor and the Shop Steward

shop steward
A union representative who usually is also an employee of the healthcare facility.

The supervisor probably has the most union contact with the **shop steward**, who is the first-line official of the union and is sometimes referred to as union representative or delegate. The union representative is not the same as a union business agent or business representative; these are normally full-time union officials who are employed and paid by the local or national union. At times, the supervisor is also required to interact with them.

The shop steward normally remains an employee of the healthcare facility and is subject to the same regulations as every other employee. He is expected to put in a full day's work for the employer, regardless of having been selected by fellow workers to be their official spokesperson with both the institution and the union. This obviously is a difficult position, as the shop steward has to serve two masters. As an employee, he must follow the supervisor's orders and directives; as a union official, though, he has responsibilities to coworkers.

Just as individuals vary in their approach to their jobs, shop stewards vary in their approach to their positions. Some are unassuming; others are overbearing. Some are helpful and courteous, whereas others are difficult. Unless special provisions exist, the shop steward's rights are the same as those of any other union member. Moreover, the shop steward is subject to the same regulations regarding quality of work and conduct as the other employees of the department. However, shop stewards are entitled to time off from their job responsibilities to conduct union business, such as representing employees at grievances.

The role of the shop steward depends considerably on the makeup of the individual and the philosophy of the union. The supervisor should always remember that the shop steward is an employee of the organization and should be treated as such. The supervisor should also remember, however, that the shop steward is the representative of the other employees; in this capacity, he learns quickly what the other employees are thinking and what is being said in the grapevine. Thus, the supervisor will come to understand and take advantage of the fact that the dual role can make the shop steward a good liaison between management and employees.

Although shop stewards perform a number of union functions, such as promoting political causes and other union agenda items, the supervisor should realize that the shop steward's most important responsibility concerns employees' complaints and grievances. The shop steward's job is to bring such complaints and grievances before the supervisor. The supervisor's job is to settle them to the best of his ability, using the grievance procedures described in great detail in every union contract. Throughout these procedures, discussed more fully in Chapter 28, the supervisor represents management and the shop steward represents the employees for the union.

In most cases, the shop steward sincerely tries to redress the aggrieved employee by winning a favorable ruling. At times, however, the supervisor may be under the impression that she is out looking for grievances merely to stay busy. Supervisors should keep in mind that the union has a legal responsibility to represent the employee, even if they believe the discipline that the supervisor administered was just. Employees can sue the union for failure to provide proper representation. The shop steward does have a political assignment, and it is necessary to assure the employees that the union is working on their behalf. The shop steward must be able to convince the employees that they can rely on him, and therefore on the union, to protect them. On the other hand, an experienced shop steward knows that normally real grievances are settled. He or she sees no need to look for complaints that do not have a valid background and would be rightfully turned down by the supervisor.

Most unions ensure that the shop steward is well trained to present the complaints and grievances so that they can be carried to a successful conclusion. The shop steward understands the content of the contract, management's obligations, and employees' rights. Before presenting a grievance, the shop steward should determine such matters as whether the contract has been violated, the employer acted unfairly, the employee's health or safety has been jeopardized, and so forth. In grievance matters, management has the obligation to prove its actions were not in violation of the contract between the union and the healthcare facility. The shop steward will challenge the management decision or action, and the supervisor must justify what she has done.

Because the shop steward's main interest is in the union, at times this may antagonize the supervisor. In some instances, it will be difficult for the supervisor to keep a sense of humor and remain calm. Often the supervisor also will have difficulty discussing a grievance with a shop steward on an equal footing because the shop steward is a subordinate within the working situation. When assuming the role of shop steward, however, the position as representative of the union members gives him equal standing to the supervisor. The supervisor should always bear in mind that the shop steward's job is political and legal and as such carries certain weight. At the same time, the supervisor should understand that a good shop steward keeps any supervisor on the alert and forces her to be a better manager.

Employee-Friendly Legislation

As noted earlier, regulations are under review by the Obama administration. Ritter (2009) states that already several employee-friendly acts have been enacted, including the following:

- The Lily Ledbetter Fair Pay Act provides that unlawful discrimination occurs when a discriminatory compensation decision is adopted or an individual is affected by the application of a discriminatory compensation decision, including wages, benefits, and other compensation. The act also eliminates the statute of limitations.
- Consolidated Omnibus Budget Reconciliation Act (COBRA) provisions of the American Recovery and Reinvestment Act provide for an employer subsidy of 35 percent of COBRA premiums for "involuntarily" terminated employees.
- Whistle-blower protection is included in the economic stimulus package and provides significant protection against retaliation to employees who report abuses concerning their employer's use of stimulus monies and applies exclusively to nonfederal employers.
- The proposed Working Families Flexibility Act would require all employers, even nonunion employers, to negotiate employee requests

relating to the number of hours the employee is required to work, the times when the employee is required to work, and where the employee is required to work. This includes the "14 and 14 rule," which requires an employer to act upon an employee's request for changed work hours, schedule, or location within 14 days.

- The Family Friendly Workplace Act would amend the Fair Labor Standards Act by authorizing private employers to provide compensatory time off to employees at a rate of 1.5 hours per hour of employment for which overtime compensation is required. There is an accrual maximum of 160 hours.

A proposed Executive Order, as outlined by Ritter (2009), includes the requirement to post notices advising employees of their right to organize under the National Labor Relations Act and removing President George W. Bush's language regarding the employees' right not to organize and right to protest the use of nonunion member dues. In addition to the above, a host of other acts related to union processes are being considered.

Supervisors should be attentive to these and other regulations that have been approved and ask their human resources liaison to keep them up to date on any changes and implications they may have for current management practices.

Summary

Approximately 12 percent of the labor force in the United States are members of an employee association or a labor union. Because unions are attempting to represent more and more employees from the service industries, it is essential that supervisors in healthcare undertakings are familiar with some basic aspects of labor union relations.

The supervisor's role in the union relations of a healthcare facility cannot be minimized. Although the supervisor is not normally a member of the management team that sits down with union negotiators to settle the terms of the labor contract, she does play an important indirect role in this meeting. Many of the difficulties and problems discussed at a negotiating meeting can be traced back to the daily activities of the supervisor. At best, the union contract resulting from the negotiations can set forth only the broad outline of labor–management relationships. It is the day-to-day application and administration of the agreement that makes the difference between harmonious labor relations and a situation filled with unnecessary tensions and bad feelings.

The supervisor is the person who, through daily decisions and actions, gives the contract real meaning. She must therefore be thoroughly familiar with the contents of the contract and with the general philosophy of management toward the union. She must understand the difficult and important political and legal role of the union shop steward, who serves in a dual capacity as a regular employee and as the representative of the union members. In grievance cases, the supervisor must learn to regard the shop steward as an equal, as one who is trained to present the complaints of union members as effectively as possible. The shop steward will challenge management's decisions, and the supervisor must justify them. Although at times it may be difficult to keep a balanced perspective, the supervisor should always remember that an alert shop steward can force her to be a better manager.

Additional Readings

Malvey, D. 2010. "Unionization in Healthcare – Background and Trends." *Journal of Healthcare Management*, 55 (5): 154-7.
Stickler, K. B. 2009. "Unions in Healthcare: How to Preserve and Defend Your Organization in the Face of Organizing Activities." Audioconference, Chicago, February 22.

28

HANDLING GRIEVANCES

Special thanks to Marc J. Leff, Esq., vice president, Human Resources, Maimonides Medical Center, Brooklyn, New York, for his update of this chapter.

Chapter Objectives

After you have studied this chapter, you should be able to do the following:

1. Define the term "grievance."
2. Differentiate between the roles of the shop steward and the supervisor in responding to a grievance.
3. Review the process of handling a grievance.

A grievance can be defined as a complaint that usually results from a misunderstanding, a misinterpretation, an alleged violation of a provision of the labor agreement, or discipline of an employee. This complaint has been formally presented to management by the union. Almost all union contracts contain provisions for a grievance procedure. The first step of the procedure begins at the departmental level—with the supervisor or the manager and the shop steward. If the grievance is not settled there, it can be appealed to the next higher level of management; at this point usually a chief steward or a business agent of the union will enter the grievance process. Union contracts typically provide for an appeal to the human resources director.

The grievance procedure usually sets a time limit in which each step is to be completed. If the dispute cannot be settled by the first two or three steps to the mutual satisfaction of both parties, the agreement usually has an arbitration provision. This means that the issue may be submitted to an impartial outsider—an *arbitrator*. After hearing testimony and evidence, the arbitrator renders a final decision, which is binding on both parties.

In a unionized setting, one of the supervisor's most important duties is to make certain that most complaints and grievances are properly disposed of during the first step of the grievance procedure. Most organizations require that supervisors consult with a labor relations specialist in the human resources department when handling complaints. This is important because many complaints could have organization-wide implications, such as discrimination and equal employment opportunity issues.

The supervisor is not shirking responsibility or admitting ignorance by consulting with specialists in the human resources department. In some organizations, management even has conferred on the labor relations staff (a division of the human resources department) the final authority to adjudicate grievances, as discussed in Chapter 11.

The following discussion is based on an organizational setup in which the human resources and labor relations experts are in a strictly staff-level position and the initial formal authority and responsibility to handle grievances rest with the line supervisor. In every unionized organization, line supervisors know that handling grievances is part of their job and that resolving them takes judgment, tact, and often more patience than comes naturally to most people.

Supervisors should not feel threatened by grievances. They may think that too much of their time is spent discussing complaints and grievances instead of getting the job done in the department. They may also believe that they perform more as labor lawyers than as supervisors. Supervisors should realize, however, that higher management regards the skill in handling grievances to be an important index of supervisory ability. The number of grievances that arise within a department is considered an indication of the state of employee–management relations.

A fine distinction can be made between the terms "complaint" and "grievance." From the supervisor's point of view, a *grievance* means a complaint that has been formally presented either to the supervisor as a management representative or to the shop steward or any other union official. The supervisor must learn to distinguish between those grievances that are admissible and those that are gripes and merely indicate that the employee is unhappy or dissatisfied. In every case, the supervisor should listen carefully to what the employee has to say to decide what action can be taken to correct the situation.

The Shop Steward's Role

As discussed briefly in Chapter 27, the *shop steward* (or union delegate) is usually the spokesperson for the employee in a grievance procedure. A grievance can be the result of a disciplinary action taken against an employee after the supervisor has made a thorough investigation of the incident. The union has a legal obligation to fairly represent an employee at a grievance hearing. Failure to do so could lead to a lawsuit by a union member against the union (considered as a duty of fair representation violation). The shop steward is familiar with the labor agreement and has been trained to present the employee's side of the grievance. What should the supervisor do if an employee approaches him without having consulted the shop steward? In such a case, it is appropriate for the supervisor to listen to the employee's story to see if it involves the union or may be of interest to it. However, the supervisor must be careful not to violate the **Weingarten Rule**, which states that if a supervisor is meeting with an employee

Weingarten Rule
A rule that states that if a supervisor is meeting with an employee and the result of that meeting could be discipline, the employee must have the ability to have a union delegate or representative present.

and the result of that meeting could be discipline, the employee must have the ability to have a union delegate or representative present (ATU 2008). If the contract or the union appears to be involved, the supervisor should call in the shop steward to listen to the employee's presentation. Although it is unlikely that a union member would present a grievance without the shop steward, the supervisor must notify the shop steward if this happens.

Similarly, if the shop steward submits a grievance on behalf of the employee without that employee present, the supervisor should listen carefully and with understanding. It is always preferable, however, to listen to complaints when both the shop steward and the complaining employee are present. Nothing can keep the supervisor from speaking directly to the employee unless it is part of an investigation, which falls under the Weingarten Rule. An employee may be represented by the union at an investigatory interview with her supervisor when the employee reasonably believes that the interview may lead to a disciplinary action (ATU). The hospital must negotiate any issue that is a term and condition of employment with the union as the employee's legal representative. If the shop steward is not present, the supervisor should take great care not to give the impression that he is undermining the shop steward's authority or relationship with the union members. There should always be free and open communication between the supervisor and the shop steward, even though the shop steward's job is to represent employees and to fight hard to win their cases.

The Supervisor's Role

One of the supervisor's primary functions is to attempt to dispose of all grievances at the first step of the grievance procedure. Part of the supervisor's job, usually with help from staff in the labor relations department, is to explore fully the details of the grievance, deal with the problems brought out, and try to settle them. To achieve prompt and satisfactory adjudication of grievances at this early stage, the supervisor should observe the following points in dealing with the grievance procedure.

Being Available
The supervisor must be readily available to the shop steward and to the aggrieved employee. Availability does not only mean being physically present. It also means being approachable and ready to listen with an open mind. The supervisor must not make it difficult for a complaining employee to see him. It is not necessary for him to stop immediately what he is doing, but every effort must be made to set a time as quickly as possible for the first discussion. An undue delay could be interpreted by the employee and the union as managerial stalling, indifference, or resentment.

Hospital Land

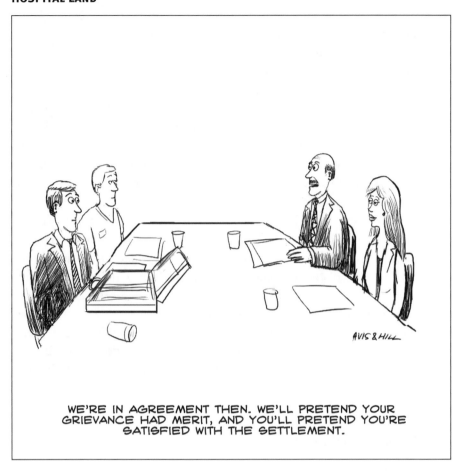

WE'RE IN AGREEMENT THEN. WE'LL PRETEND YOUR
GRIEVANCE HAD MERIT, AND YOU'LL PRETEND YOU'RE
SATISFIED WITH THE SETTLEMENT.

Listening

The discussions earlier in the book about communication (see Chapter 5)
and interviewing (see Chapter 18) are applicable to the grievance procedure
as well. When a complaint is brought to the supervisor, the shop steward and
the employee should be given the opportunity to present their case fully.
Sympathetic listening by the supervisor is likely to minimize hostilities and
tensions during the settlement of the case. The supervisor must know how
to listen well. He must give the shop steward and the employee a chance to
say whatever is on their minds. If they believe that the supervisor is truly listening to them and that fair treatment will be given, the complaint will not
loom as large to them in the presentation of the problem. Halfway through
the discussion, the complaining employee may even realize that she does not
have a true complaint at all. Also, sometimes the more a person talks, the
more likely she is to make contradictory and inconsistent remarks, thus weak-
ening the argument. Only an effective listener will be able to catch these inconsistencies and use them to help resolve the case. Frequently supervisors

are so preoccupied with defending themselves or trying to justify their points of view that they simply do not listen.

Having Emotional Control

The supervisor must take great care not to get angry at the shop steward or the employee. The shop steward's job and legal responsibility is to represent the employee even when she knows that the grievance is not valid. In such a situation, the supervisor's job is to point out objectively that the grievance has no merit. The supervisor cannot expect the shop steward to do this because she must serve as the employee's spokesperson at all times. Sometimes a union deliberately creates grievances to keep tensions elevated. Even this situation must not arouse the anger of the supervisor. If the supervisor does not know how to handle such occurrences successfully, he should discuss the matter with higher management and experts in the labor relations or human resources department.

If arguments, tempers, and emotional outbursts run high and make good communication difficult, the supervisor may want to terminate the meeting and reschedule it. He must use caution not to participate in a shouting match.

Defining the Problem

Often the shop steward and the employee are not sufficiently clear in their presentations. It is then the supervisor's job to summarize clearly what has been presented and make certain that everyone understands the problem that must be resolved. Sometimes the complaint merely deals with the symptoms of the problem. The supervisor must know how deeply to delve to get at the root of the situation. It is necessary to define the employee's complaint and the extent of the problem precisely to determine whether a grievance is valid under the contract. Once the real problem is clarified and handled properly, it is unlikely that similar grievances will come up in the future.

Obtaining the Facts

All the facts should be obtained as quickly as possible to arrive at a solution to the problem and a successful adjudication of the grievance. The supervisor can probably get most of the facts by asking the complaining employee pertinent questions. He must ascertain who or what caused the grievance, where and when it happened, and whether unfair treatment was involved. He must also determine whether any connection exists between the current grievance and other grievances. The supervisor must further determine if there are witnesses and get written statements from all parties, including the complainant and the employee who may be disciplined, before drawing a conclusion. No fair investigation can be complete without getting a written statement from both sides of an issue.

Although it sometimes may be tempting to avoid dealing with the grievance by claiming a need to search for more facts, the supervisor must not do so. Furthermore, the information gathered in this investigation should be shared with the union, for several reasons. First, the union has a legal right to the information. Second, the more facts the union has, the less likely it is to pursue the grievance. If patient-sensitive information or protected health information is collected in the investigation, the supervisor should contact the human resources staff for guidance. He must make a decision on the basis of those facts that are available and that can be obtained without undue delay.

Sometimes, however, it is impossible to gather all the information at once; therefore, the grievance cannot be settled immediately. In this case, the supervisor must inform the aggrieved employee and the shop steward. If they see that the supervisor is working on the problem, they are likely to be reasonable and wait for an answer to be given at a specified future date.

Having Familiarity with the Contract and Consultation

After having determined the facts, the supervisor must ascertain whether the grievance is legitimate in the context of the contract. As mentioned earlier, a grievance is usually not a grievance in the legal sense unless provisions of the labor contract have been violated or administered inconsistently. Therefore, it is necessary to check the provisions in the contract when any reference to a violation is made. If the supervisor has any question about this, she should consult with someone in the human resources or labor relations department or with higher management. Provisions in the labor agreement may not be clearly stated, and a question may exist about whether a certain provision in the contract is applicable at all. In such a situation, the complaining employee should be told that additional clarification in reference to the agreement is needed and that the answer will be delayed for a few days.

Respecting Time Limits

Usually the grievance procedure sets a time limit within which the grievance must be answered. The supervisor must see that all grievances are settled as promptly and justly as possible. Postponing a judgment in the hope that the complaint disappears is courting trouble and more grievances. Moreover, an unnecessary postponement is unfair because the employee and the shop steward are entitled to know the supervisor's position as quickly as the facts can be obtained.

Speed is definitely important in the settlement of grievances, but not if it will result in unsound decisions. If a delay cannot be avoided, the aggrieved parties must be informed. Waiting for a decision is bothersome to everybody concerned. In such a situation, it may be a good idea to put the grievance in writing and sign it so that the parties involved do not forget the details.

Adjudicating Grievances

Part of the supervisor's job is to try to resolve all grievances, preferably at the first step of the grievance procedure. As already pointed out, this is included in the managerial aspects of the supervisory function. It is far better to settle a minor issue at this stage than to allow it to escalate into a major issue. The only cases that should be referred to higher levels of management are those that are unusual, that require additional interpretation of the union contract's meaning, that contain problems that have not shown up before, that involve broad policy considerations, or in which disciplinary action was taken inappropriately.

In the adjudication of grievances, the supervisor must ensure that the rights of management are protected and that the policies and precedents of the institution are followed. If the supervisor must deviate from previous adjudications, she must explain the reasons to the employee and the shop steward. The supervisor must make certain that both of them fully understand that this exception does not set a precedent. In such cases, the supervisor is obliged to have his actions reviewed and approved by higher-level administration, the human resources department, or both before informing the parties involved.

Consistency of Action

The supervisor must check previous settlements and make certain that the current intended decision is consistent with past decisions, the institution's policy, and the labor agreement. The supervisor should avoid making an exception, because exceptions are likely to become precedents. In adjudicating grievances, the supervisor must consider not only what effect the adjudication will have in that instance but also its implications for the future. Whenever the supervisor settles a grievance, the possibility exists that the settlement will show up as part of the labor contract in following years. Also, if the case goes to arbitration, the arbitrator is likely to look for precedents, consider them almost as binding as the labor agreement, and use them as a valid basis for the final decision.

Consequences of the Settlement

Providing a Clear Answer

The supervisor must answer the grievance in a straightforward, reasonable manner that is perfectly clear to the aggrieved party. The answer must not be phrased in language that the aggrieved party cannot understand, regardless of whom the judgment favors. If the supervisor rules against the employee, the employee is that much more entitled to a clear, straightforward reply stating the reasons for the decision. Although the employee may disagree with such a reply, at least it will be understood.

Clarity is even more necessary if the supervisor has to reply to the grievance in writing. In that case, the answer must be restricted to the specific complaints involved, the words used must be appropriate, and any reference to a particular provision of the labor agreement or to the organization's rules must be clearly cited. Unless required, a written reply should not be rendered. If such a reply is required under the labor agreement, however, it is appropriate for the supervisor to discuss all the implications with higher management or with the human resources department so that a properly worded reply is given.

Nonunionized Organizations

Many healthcare facilities have implemented grievance procedures regardless of whether the facility has a union. Grievances need to be heard by management in a timely fashion to avoid the possible introduction of a third party and to ensure staff concerns are heard and given appropriate attention. To avoid the potential introduction of a third party, human resources departments in many facilities have developed detailed procedures that allow for (1) first-level supervisors to investigate and attempt to remedy concerns, (2) an appeal(s) process, and (3) an ad hoc committee of peers and management to hear and recommend final action. Each step has an associated time frame to ensure timely response to the complainant.

Record Keeping

It is essential for the supervisor to keep records and documents whenever a grievance decision is made. If the employee's request is satisfied, this decision may become a precedent. If the complaint cannot be settled in the first step, this grievance probably will go further, possibly to arbitration or to a government agency or litigation, as in cases of discrimination. The case will certainly go to higher levels of management, and the supervisor should not defend the action by depending on memory. Diligent recording of the facts, reasoning, and decisions should be available.

Good records are an absolute necessity because the burden of proof is on the supervisor and management in disciplinary actions. Management has the right to discipline, but only for good or just cause. Management has the right to decide, but the union has the right to submit a grievance. Whenever the employee or the union maintains that the supervisor has violated the agreement or has administered its provisions in an unfair or inconsistent manner, the supervisor must defend the action. Without good records and documentation, this is often difficult, if not impossible.

Summary

The labor agreement sets forth a broad, general outline of labor–management relationships. This outline must be fulfilled with intelligent supervisory decisions. Occasions to make such decisions arise mainly in the settlement of grievances. Indeed, the proper adjudication of grievances is one of the important components of the supervisory position. Whenever the supervisor settles grievances, the labor contract is referred to and interpreted. The settlements may have far-reaching implications because they set precedents. Much of what the union will discuss at the next contract negotiations originates with day-to-day supervisory decisions. If a grievance should go to arbitration, the impartial arbitrator will also attach great importance to precedents set by the supervisor.

Often it is not so much what the contract says that counts, but how it has been interpreted by management's frontline representative—the supervisor. This shows how important a role the supervisor plays in the adjudication of grievances and how necessary it is to gain considerable skill in the use of adjudication techniques. In most organizations, specialists in labor relations are involved in arriving at the appropriate settlement.

To apply adjudication techniques appropriately, the supervisor should always be available, listen carefully, and behave professionally. The supervisor must learn to define the problem, obtain the facts, and draw on her thorough knowledge of the contract. It is also important to avoid unnecessary delays and settle grievances at an early stage. Moreover, the supervisor must be fair in all decisions, protecting the rights of the institution and respecting the content and spirit of the agreement. The supervisor also must keep good records, give clear replies, and, above all, remain consistent.

Historically, unions have developed because management responded to the needs of their workforce inappropriately. Today unions are established for similar reasons, or at least because employees perceive a lack of attention to their needs on the part of management. Supervisors manage a variety of resources, but their most productive, costly, and visible resource is the employee. Effective management yields high quality, high productivity, and high morale. Recognizing that employees are inherently good and desire the facility to succeed makes the management of other resources (such as money, materials, and machinery) much easier.

EMERGING INFLUENCES IN HEALTHCARE

Chapter Objectives

After you have studied this chapter, you should be able to do the following:

1. Recognize the many different forces affecting healthcare and healthcare management today.
2. Apply traditional management principles to address a rapidly changing healthcare environment.

The Force of Change

The healthcare industry is in a state of flux as a result of mergers, de-mergers, bankruptcies, overzealous regulations, technology leaps, staffing shortages, high consumer demand, a poor economy, and increasingly educated consumers. All of these issues, and many more, affect how a supervisor manages her department, structures her workplace, and achieves her goals.

This chapter examines the issues on the horizon and highlights those that will present management challenges. Up until now, the book has discussed relatively traditional approaches to the roles of management—planning, organizing, staffing, influencing, and controlling. However, the successful supervisor can take the theories explored in this book and apply them to the new challenges ahead. For our ninth edition, we discuss some challenges for the future. They are categorized by occupation, consumer satisfaction, technology and medicine, economics, regulations, staff, communication, and quality.

Changing Occupations

In the coming years, half of college seniors will be working in jobs that do not exist today (Sena 2005). According to the U.S. Census Bureau, there were 2,076,000 railroad workers in 1920; they number only 125,000 today. Conversely, today we have 319,000 medical technicians whereas in 1910, there were none (Long Island Association, n.d.; Bureau of Labor Statistics 2009). As the United States became more industrialized, occupations were created and eliminated (Federal Reserve Bank of Dallas 1992).

Our aging baby boomers will place a strain on today's healthcare system. Forty percent of today's 50-year-old women will live to be 100. Although healthcare professionals are specializing in many areas, geriatrics is not one of them. The United States will need 36,000 geriatricians by 2030, but it has fewer than 7,600 today (American Geriatric Society 2010). Fewer than half of the medical schools in the United States incorporate geriatrics into their undergraduate curriculum (National Center for Policy Analysis 2005).

While occupational opportunities are unfolding in an era of technological advances and diversity, the federal government's Health Resources and Services Administration has concluded that staffing shortages, especially in the nursing and pharmacy areas, will become critical. Analysts now are projecting a nationwide shortage of almost 100,000 physicians, as many as 1 million nurses, and 250,000 public health professionals by 2020 (U.S. Department of Health and Human Services 2010). Nursing vacancies are projected to be at 20 percent by 2020 (U.S. Department of Health and Human Services 2001) (see Exhibit 29.1). But the nurse and pharmacist shortages are only part of the story. Less publicized, but equally important, is the shortage of other healthcare professionals. Hospitals nationwide report vacancy rates of 18 percent for radiology technicians, 12 percent for laboratory technologists, and 9 percent for housekeeping and maintenance staff. Every healthcare worker is an integral part of the healthcare system, and a shortage in any area creates problems for every other classification of worker (AFT 2004). College students are not entering the healthcare profession, possibly because of the high caseloads, long hours, or alternating shifts or because there are so many other,

EXHIBIT 29.1

National Supply and Demand Projection for FTE Registered Nurses, 2000 to 2020

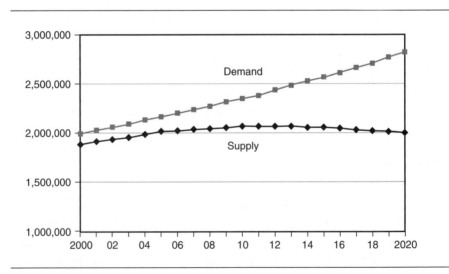

Note: FTE = full-time equivalent.

SOURCE: U.S. Department of Health and Human Services (2002).

more glamorous, less stressful options available to today's youth. Healthcare management needs to aggressively promote this career option and provide work-site considerations that address the negative aspects of the job.

Changing Consumers and Satisfaction

The baby boomers are now in their late 50s and 60s and will continue to be the most powerful consumers of healthcare. They also are well educated, technology savvy, and demanding of service. They are taking care of their aging parents and overseeing the healthcare delivered to that generation. Ensuring customer satisfaction with the services a healthcare organization's staff and facility provide today is paramount in tying the boomers to the facility for future healthcare services. Training staff in customer service techniques must be a component of every orientation program. Although person-to-person skills are important, training in telephone, PC, and e-mail skills and etiquette should not be ignored. Skill building in explaining the psychology that governs upset customer behavior, implementing strategies for successful customer encounters, and understanding attitudes and actions should be included in the training program. Healthcare providers need to remember that customers today—patients as well as their relatives—are living in a fast-paced, but litigious, world. They expect answers and explanations that they understand, and they expect them both now. Delays of any kind may be perceived as maneuvers to hide information from them, leaving consumers potentially angry and certainly dissatisfied.

Today's consumer is much more health conscious and "health literate." Abundant websites offer health information and facility-specific comparative data to the public; no longer must individuals rely on the physician office visit to learn about their conditions or determine at which hospital to be treated.

Consumers are seeking "quality care" (see Exhibit 29.2), for which each consumer has her own definition. In an effort to inform customers about institution and physician quality, entities such as the Centers for Medicare & Medicaid Services, through its Hospital Compare database; HealthGrades; and the Leapfrog Group have increased transparency of service outcomes and developed comprehensive benchmarking and performance measurement programs.

In response, facilities can demonstrate their interest in providing quality and ensuring customer satisfaction by addressing disease outcomes, participating in community health projects, and surveying consumers. Organizations are encouraged to seek quality recognition awards by participating in quality measurement programs such as the Malcolm Baldrige National Quality Award program. The Baldrige criteria include an established culture and processes

EXHIBIT 29.2

What Is the
New
Healthcare
Consumer
Looking For?

"Patients aren't basing their decisions on medical technology or the adequacy of staffing on a nursing station. They base their decisions on things they feel qualified to judge: the room; the food; how hard it was to find a parking place; whether or not the people are smiling and friendly; the admission process; the questions they are asked and the answers they get to their questions. Those things do not necessarily have anything to do with the quality of medical care, but they are the way that healthcare providers are being evaluated.

"It seems that the new healthcare consumers simply assume that members of the healthcare fraternity will do their best to cure their ills and fix what is broken. They evaluate care and base their buying decision on the way they are treated. In a sense, it's not the care, it's the *caring*, that new consumers have on their minds."

—Dawn M. Gideon

SOURCE: Used with permission from Transition Management Group.

that will sustain quality outcomes and are repeatable to consistently produce quality results (Cohen 2008). Leaders within their departments should seek to proactively make critical decisions that will help ensure services are delivered at the highest quality level. Sometimes good team players are reluctant to assert themselves because they do not wish to offend another manager by identifying a process that could be enhanced or they just wish to protect their self-interests. But these same supervisors should not be surprised when they are overlooked for promotions, raises, and requests for additional resources (Cohen 2008). As discussed in Chapter 25, benchmarking metrics should be developed to evaluate and improve supervisors' performance. The metrics should be shared with their staff so that they can gauge the success of their team as well.

As for employees, the old adage "seeing is believing" may work for or against a healthcare organization. Employees who see and believe resources are being properly channeled toward replacing and updating technology, hiring qualified workers, and staffing patient care areas at the appropriate level feel more positive about the quality of care delivered in their institution. These staff promote to friends and neighbors the advances that the organization is making in technology, patient satisfaction, outcomes, and other crucial areas. Employees who are disgruntled about any of these issues may discuss widely with friends and neighbors the management shortfalls by pointing to medication errors, unexpected deaths, safety issues, and so forth. Supervisors must seriously consider employee concerns and discontent and recognize that they serve as a barometer of consumer satisfaction with the organization.

Changing Technology and Medicine

A new wave of technology and medicine is on the horizon. Cloning, genetic mapping, and tissue engineering are creating the ability to design humans in the future. Although this may be considered radical thinking today, in two decades or less, the use of stem cells to treat conditions such as spinal cord damage, multiple sclerosis, Alzheimer's disease, and baldness may be commonplace. A new industry of "genetaceuticals" will combine genetic research and drug therapies. Alternative medicine using herbal remedies, acupuncture, biofeedback, and other methods will grow and be a viable supplement, if not an alternative, to traditional treatment options.

Myoelectric sensors will read impulses from nerves to trigger movements and actions of prosthetic devices. Spring-like mechanical struts in prosthetic legs allow them to outperform their biological counterparts, and there are complex electronic knees and feet that contain narrow artificial intelligence (Saenz 2009b). Prosthetic hands have made great strides with robotic advancements such as Deka's Luke Arm. Dean Kamen, inventor of the Segway scooter and head of Deka, helped design the electronic arm to fit the needs and desires of modern amputees. The Luke Arm went into clinical trials in the summer of 2009 and could become the prosthetic limb of choice for U.S. soldiers returning from Iraq and Afghanistan (Saenz 2009c). Add to this the advances in nerve-control research. Consider the rehabilitative advantages that Ambient Corporation, makers of the Audeo—a device that reads nerve impulses in the neck to help people speak and even control an electronic wheelchair—will provide for people suffering from diseases such as amyotrophic lateral sclerosis (ALS, or Lou Gehrig's disease), which erode muscle control over time (Saenz 2009a), or for athletes who sustain spinal cord injuries. These new technologies will change the way physical and occupational therapists teach their patients how to adapt to the loss of a limb and paralysis.

Access to specialists will be facilitated by electronic health records; health information exchanges through community, system, and regional health information networks; and other technology. After all, not long ago providing healthcare services via satellite was considered unlikely, and yet today telemedicine is commonplace. Telehealth depends on sophisticated information system technology that cuts across campuses and geography and provides immediate access to critical patient care information and expert healthcare guidance from specialists across the world. It is not unrealistic to assume that in the next decade patients may not leave their homes for primary medical care.

With the 2009 American Recovery and Reinvestment Act's (ARRA) mandate to enhance health information exchange, medical care will come from remote terminal connections to home computers, capture data from health monitoring devices, and use sources currently in homes to analyze a patient's bodily functions. Currently, in Japan the Intelligence Toilet II is proving that a toilet can record and analyze important data, such as weight, body mass index, blood pressure, and blood sugar levels. This information is sent to the patient's computer via WiFi and can help him, with the guidance of a trained physician, monitor health and provide early detection for some medical conditions. Graphs on the patient's desktop PC will show whether glucose levels and urine temperatures have been fluctuating. These trends can help diabetics time their insulin shots and women track their hormone levels (Saenz 2009d).

Health information exchange will support biosurveillance monitoring to identify suspicious complaint patterns in a localized area, which may signal the need for further investigation, or to report a disease outbreak or bioterrorism event. Some experts believe the deployment of biosurveillance networks is a precursor to a national health information network (Goedert 2007) whereby data reporting would satisfy ARRA-proposed meaningful use criteria that providers must demonstrate to obtain funding for electronic health record systems.

The days have passed when physicians believed they "knew it all." Many now seek advice from other consultants and have online access to the latest findings on drugs, treatments, and other medical advances. With patient needs becoming more complex, sophisticated medical knowledge, including human understanding and published data, and diagnostic equipment must be linked with sophisticated technology systems. Robotics in the operating room and rolling along hospital corridors have become a reality. Surgeons no longer need to touch the patient during heart bypass surgery, which, according to reports, is easier for the surgeon to perform and less traumatic for the patient to experience (Lanfranco et al. 2004). Imaging technology has advanced to the stage where surgeons are using micro-instrumentation to correct defects in the unborn fetus.

As healthcare costs in the United States rise, patients, with the encouragement of their insurance firms, will seek quality healthcare services overseas. Known as **medical tourism**, this phenomenon saw an estimated 750,000 Americans travel abroad for care in 2007, a number expected to increase to 6 million by 2010 (Fried 2009, 6). UnitedHealth Group, which insures more than 70 million Americans, has already moved to make Bumrungrad International Hospital in Bangkok an in-network facility. When Aetna, with 37 million members, bought the overseas insurer Goodhealth Worldwide last year, Aetna's CEO explained the move by saying that globalized surgery is "an important emerging trend." The company has already started a pilot program to send patients abroad for hip and knee replacements (Portfolio.com 2009). Medical tourism also appeals to foreign patients seeking specialty care available in the United States. New forms of telemedicine will enable broader application of virtual medical tourism. Diagnoses and some forms of treatment may be facilitated by the Internet and associated distance-traversing technologies (Fried 2009, 5). At the same time, essentially every hospital is coping with staff shortages. In a world where there is virtual parity in educational preparation for many health specialties and where organizations are seeking foreign

medical tourism
The practice of seeking medical care in a foreign country because of cost savings, quality, expertise, or other reasons.

patients, it may be appropriate for managers to recruit from foreign sources to fill their staffing voids as well as to be able to understand the cultural differences of and communicate with foreign patients (Fried 2009, 7).

Supervisors who are managing technology will require staff to be technologically proficient. Fortunately, many of today's youth (Generations X and Y and millennials) have grown up during a time when technology was prevalent and do not fear using it. Patient information will be available electronically both within a healthcare organization and through health information exchanges among associated healthcare organizations, facilitating patient care in a healthcare system, across a region, and across oceans. Access authorization to patient information will be facilitated by using ATM-like devices to accommodate our mobile citizens. Robotic systems for delivering medications and other materials for the lab, pharmacy, and central supply will replace existing human courier systems. Robots work 24 hours a day, 7 days a week and require no sick or vacation time. The need for file clerks, technicians, and couriers will diminish. Management will need to decide if people in these roles will be displaced, retrained, or terminated.

Security will be heightened because of the accessibility of sensitive data. Thus, we should expect higher surveillance levels, more rigorous card access systems, biometrics, and other similar approaches to control who has access to what, when, and where. Some employees may find biometric approaches distasteful or possibly in conflict with their religious or cultural mores. The supervisor will be required to address these concerns.

Changing Economics

Healthcare leadership has been balancing declining reimbursement against the rising cost of care for underinsured and uninsured populations, and Congress's fervor for healthcare reform may force organizations to reconsider their structures, affiliations, and service offerings. Seventy-five million adults—42 percent of the under-65 population—had either no insurance or inadequate insurance in 2007, up from 35 percent in 2003 (Schoen et al. 2008). This condition has created rising bad debt and charity rates for healthcare organizations. Adding to the reimbursement dilemma are several regulatory changes, including the self-reporting of hospital-acquired conditions (HACs), which will result in lower reimbursement or no reimbursement for treating the HAC. This regulation has prompted changes in patient care protocols, additional surveillance of patients who are prone to injury such as the elderly, and additional precautionary measures prior to surgery and other procedures.

Another significant change related to healthcare economics is implementation of the ICD-10 coding system update slated for 2013. The International Classification of Diseases, Tenth Revision, is the first major coding classification change in more than 30 years in the United States. It will provide payers and governmental agencies with much more specificity on the conditions being treated to identify HACs and epidemiological concerns, and it will facilitate payers' ability to profile providers to gauge their outcome performance and adjust reimbursement based on those outcomes. Finally, it signals the possibility of a new prospective payment system that will pay for an entire episode of care to a single healthcare entity that will have the responsibility of paying other providers that participated in the episode, thus paving the way for closed networks of providers at all levels tied to a single healthcare facility. Such changes will require managers to educate their staff on documentation requirements, accurate data entry, data analysis, and of course, process improvements to address unexpected patient outcomes.

Mergers, once thought to be the cure-all for providing cost-effective healthcare to a region, have had relatively high failure rates in major cities. Instead of reducing costs, mergers often created a new layer of management, resulting in increased and often nondirect patient care costs. The merger of University of California, San Francisco and Stanford University medical centers added nearly 1,000 employees to the combined organization. This new layer was seen by some as nothing more than additional bureaucracy stifling the actual delivery of healthcare. However, J. P. Morgan forecasts a wave of consolidations that will eliminate the weaker facilities and create large, multistate systems that can withstand regional economic crises on the strength of their diversity, rationalize capital spending with systemwide service line planning, and strategically offer clinical programs to achieve market share (Bush 2009). When mergers failed to yield the cost savings anticipated, outsourcing gained acceptance with healthcare organizations, and payers outsourced to on- and offshore business services, including claims processing, utilization management, collections, transcription, radiology reading, coding, and information systems management.

As mergers, closures, and outsourcing occur, supervisors will have to respond to grapevine rumors predicting budget cutting, downsizing, and other staff apprehensions. Morale is likely to deteriorate. Following the guidance discussed in previous chapters, incorporating regular, truthful, and complete communication into the culture will be imperative. Furthermore, encouragement of staff to voice their fears will serve as a buffer between them and a union organizer, especially when healthcare union membership is growing. Listening and empathizing will be a supervisor's best attributes. The first-line supervisor will be the agent who will make sense of, unite, and transmit the organization's culture (Valentino 2004).

Changing Policies and Regulations

The number of organizations that have some part in regulating healthcare organizations is astonishing. Exhibit 29.3 identifies several of these organizations, but does not include those that healthcare facilities voluntarily invite to evaluate their activities, such as the National Committee on Quality Assurance, the

International Organization for Standardization, the Malcolm Baldrige National Quality Award program, and the Healthcare Facilities Accreditation Program. It also does not reflect new entities such as Recovery Audit Contractors, Medicare Administrative Contractors, Medicaid Integrity Contractors, and other relatively new external review agencies. Supervisors will continue to enforce security, privacy, safety measures, error prevention, documentation enhancement, and process improvement in compliance with the many regulations imposed on healthcare organizations, and they likely will need to accomplish this demand with fewer staff. Delegation and team empowerment may be necessities rather

EXHIBIT 29.3 Who Regulates Hospitals?

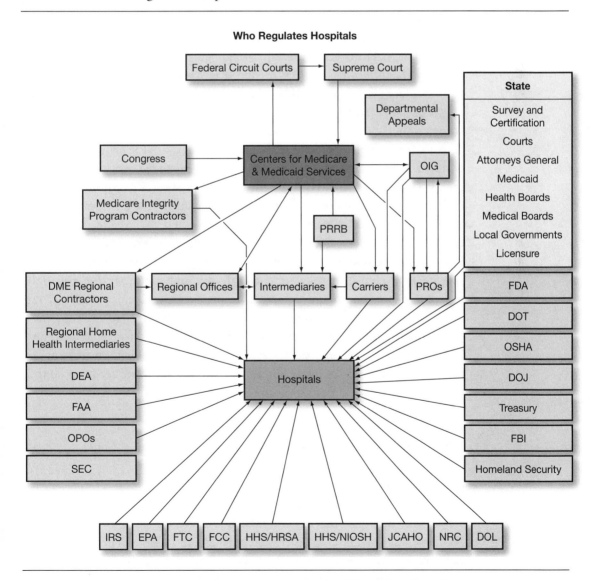

SOURCE: Reprinted from *AHA News*, Vol. 36, No. 21, by permission, May 29, 2000, © 2000, by Health Forum, Inc.

than options for tomorrow's managers to fulfill all the requirements in this regulated environment.

Among the several regulations mentioned in earlier chapters, the impact of ARRA may be the most far reaching. The act provides funding for the advancement of electronic health records and imposes penalties for their absence, provides for educational programs to enhance the health information technology skills of the healthcare workforce, heightens awareness of privacy and security measures and increases penalties for violating them, expands the role of consumers in their healthcare choices, and increases the amount of data about patients and providers that will be accessible to the federal and state governments.

Beyond ARRA are a variety of bills and amendments looming that, if passed, will affect the way supervisors direct their staff (see Chapter 25) and will increase demands for pricing transparency, requiring healthcare organizations to publicly post their charges for services. Immigration status monitoring will be heightened, with the federal government's E-Verify program allowing organizations to check an employee's status. In an effort to increase patient safety, managers should anticipate that states will increasingly require credentials for staff who previously were permitted to perform jobs following completion of on-the-job training.

Accountability of tax-exempt healthcare entities for providing services to those who cannot pay will continue with expanded disclosure requirements. Governmental and private insurer audits of services to uncover fraud and payments for unnecessary care will increase due to the favorable results of the Recovery Audit Contractors for Medicare and the Medicaid Integrity Contractors for Medicaid. Beyond the requirements of the Deficit Reduction Act enacted in 2006, mandates likely will surface that require management to repeatedly remind its employees, medical staff, and contractors of their obligation to report any billing or service improprieties, which in turn may encourage employees or others to become whistle-blowers to seek *qui tam* compensation. Department managers will be responsible for keeping administration informed of any regulatory changes that will affect departments or the organization and for increasing staff communication and feedback so that they realize that the supervisors are acting on the issues identified.

Changing Staff Issues

Goldsmith (2007) predicts a "workforce tsunami" in healthcare's future, meaning that critical workforce shortages will cause catastrophic gaps in care. His prediction has merit, as the current U.S. healthcare system, powered by baby boomers, is aging. The average age of registered nurses is 47, 38 percent of physicians are over age 50, and the entire senior management cadre of most hospitals and health systems are nearing retirement. The U.S. Department of Health and

HOSPITAL LAND

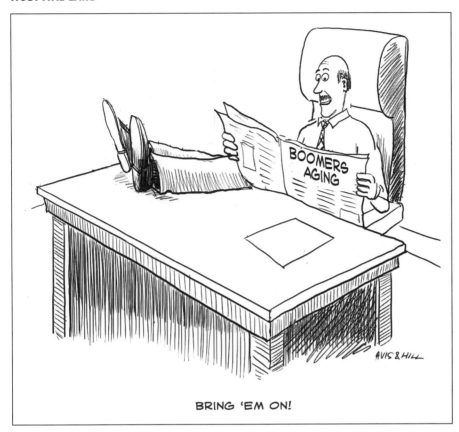

BRING 'EM ON!

Human Services (2010) anticipates that by 2020 there will be a shortage of 1 million nurses and 100,000 physicians. This human resources crisis is not cyclical, and incremental productivity improvements will not close the gap. Managers must focus on retention of skilled workers by redesigning jobs to retain older workers to fill the gaps while allowing them sufficient leisure time and time to deal with family obligations and by redesigning jobs to reduce stress and turnover.

Specialization will continue. A new title in nursing is surfacing—clinical nurse leader (CNL). CNLs are master's-prepared nurses who assume accountability for healthcare outcomes for a specific group of clients through application of research-based information to design, implement, and evaluate client care plans (Begun, Tornabeni, and White 2006). Other professions are following suit. Securing education, even in the most sophisticated fields, is easier through distance learning programs. New positions will be created, such as clinical documentation improvement specialists, taking nurses out of bedside positions and placing them in clinical support roles.

As discussed in an earlier chapter, Generation Y workers are seeking positions with greater flexibility, including fewer working hours and more telecommuting, to accommodate their personal, community service, and social needs. With several recent stories of shooting sprees at healthcare facilities, supervisors will be challenged to recruit employees and, once hired, retain them by ensuring that the workplace is safe and secure and does not need modifications. These conditions may lead more managers to consider tailoring work and work settings to align with the employees' life interests.

Obviously, these approaches cannot work for all healthcare staff because someone must stay at the facility to care for patients. Recruiting and retaining bedside and facility-based staff will be more difficult than before. In response, supervisors may need to involve their patient care staff in rethinking how work is done. In addition, they may turn to audio and video conferencing and conduct what-if brainstorming scenarios with staff to build a more efficient and effective patient care environment and one that is more rewarding to the staff. Borrowing models from other industries will help identify options that fit in healthcare.

Workforce diversity will create unique situations for a healthcare facility, including language and cultural differences and communication concerns. It is hard to tell an employee what is expected of her if she does not speak the same language as the supervisor, both metaphorically and literally. Similarly, patients are encountering the same frustrations if they cannot communicate to healthcare providers in a language that is mutually understood. Supervisors may find the need to send staff members to special training courses to teach them to speak, read, and write in English. Meanwhile, the diversified labor pool may prove to be advantageous and an alternative to hiring translators to meet the needs of patients who speak a language other than English.

Other challenges that may confront supervisors in the future include developing employee safety programs. Gun sales keep going up, some of which is attributed to anticipated tightening of gun control and some to concerns about terrorism and the increasingly tough economic times (Ritter and Rosenberg 2009). Coworker dating issues may surface as well. With people spending the bulk of their time at work, it is not surprising that Cupid may set up shop in your department. Some human resources departments now require that a "love contract" be executed to provide guidelines for dating or romantically involved coworkers, especially those in executive-level positions (Ritter 2009; Gardner 2008). American with Disabilities Act modifications in 2008 broaden the definition of and offer greater protection to individuals with disabilities. Managers will likely see a dramatic increase in employees' requests for workplace accommodations and a potential spike in litigation (Ritter and Alkhas 2009).

Finally, ethics, ethical issues, and ethical compliance will continue to be a central focus for administration. Employees, boards, and the public will expect the highest ethical conduct from healthcare leaders and employees, and patients will be encouraged to report any action they consider to be to the contrary. Supervisors should monitor their ethical position regularly to be able to answer the question, "Why shouldn't we do what is right and moral?" Ethical dilemmas, such as those involved in the Terri Schiavo case, in which family members, healthcare providers, and the public battled over her right to life or death; the effect of fertility failures such as the birth of octuplets to Nadya Suleman, a single, unemployed woman who already had six young children; and the progress of stem cell research and how stem cells will be used, will surface more frequently as technology, rather than human organs, keeps people alive and will be further complicated by the battle between right-to-life groups and right-to-die organizations. Supervisors will be faced with these issues and the burdens they place on those who serve the patient directly. Guiding staff effectively through these challenges will be paramount.

Changing Communication Methods

In the last five years the use of social networking sites has exploded. The 2008 presidential election campaign saw dramatic increases in contributions based in part on the use of sites such as Twitter, Facebook, LinkedIn, and Ning because of the appeal of these sites to Generation X and Generation Y. Retailers and businesses seek a presence on these sites to coax purchases, groom fellowship, and meet customers where they are. Blogs continue to be popular. Individuals prefer those social networking sites and blogs that allow them to state their position on topics, share information with others, and link to others with similar preferences. For management, however, the use of these sites by staff may result in lower productivity as employees check in routinely for updates from friends. Additionally, blogs may create public relation nightmares if disgruntled employees post their perception of a change and others throughout the world jump in to voice their opinions. Clearly, communication approaches supported by these technologies are different from those used in the past, with less face-to-face interaction and visual feedback.

Changing Our Cost Structure Through Collaboration to Achieve Quality

Healthcare has faced great challenges from rising costs for talented labor, state-of-the-art technology, and new facilities to meet the changing population demographics and demands for access. To deal with the rising costs, labor considered nonessential has been eliminated, perks have been cut, debt has grown, and prices have been increased. Even as this chapter is written, the U.S. Congress is voicing its concern with the cost of healthcare. One of the additional readings (see Chapter 14) selected for this edition discusses the value of quality. Does quality care cost any more than poor care? One answer may be that quality care ultimately costs less because errors add cost to healthcare.

Errors are not intentional. They are the result of lack of orientation, lack of processes that provide for the second check, haste, excessive workloads, and leadership that fails to put in place quality control mechanisms to avoid errors. When organizations fail to put quality first, consumers find out when they review the organizations' publicly displayed performance profiles. Improving performance will require collaboration from the entire healthcare team to find more efficient protocols, more effective tools (prostheses, drugs, diagnostic tests, etc.), and more patient-friendly communication approaches. After 20 years, the Malcolm Baldrige National Quality Award continues to set the gold standard for organizational excellence. The "journey" to prepare to apply for the award has been described as a strategic diagnostic analysis of the organization's leadership systems (Goonan and Muzikowski 2008). Healthcare providers must deploy their limited resources to conduct such an analysis—at the department level and at the overall organization level—to improve care for patients and simultaneously enhance the organization's bottom line.

Achieving these goals will require collaboration, trust, and mutual respect between clinicians and organizational leadership (Boehler et al. 2009). Otherwise, costs will continue to rise and regulators will force organizations to address the costs. Management's overall approach must encourage participation. An approach championed by Clay Sherman, known as the "uncommon leader" method, requires employees to look at operations and suggest ideas for improvements in four categories: best people, high quality, low cost, and customer satisfaction. Workers must generate ideas to score well on annual reviews. Most employees want to make a difference where they work, and this is their opportunity to do it. As employees at all levels continue to step up, organizations will survive reimbursement cuts and the recession (Thrall 2009). As David Walker, former U.S. comptroller general, said, "It's better to control your own destiny. It's better to try to make changes proactively and on your own initiative rather than to be forced to change based upon rules that are dictated by others" (*Healthcare Financial Management* 2009).

A Final Word

Supervisors have a challenging job in any organization but particularly in healthcare, where the product of the organization can result in life or death. As a summary to this book, Appendix 29.1 includes a list of the potential pitfalls that supervisors face daily. May you be successful in your career.

APPENDIX 29.1

First-Time Management Blunders

by Danny Pancho

It's a heady feeling to finally get that new title, but fresh-faced managers will do well to bone up on the skills set and mind frame crucial to a successful transition from being one of the boys to becoming The Boss.

So you have finally gained that much-coveted position—you are now a manager. But if you think you have it made, think again. Like Humpty Dumpty, many a new manager has suffered a great fall, largely due to missteps and miscues in climbing the high wall of success.

So how do you avoid becoming one of the casualties of managerial unpreparedness? How do you ensure a smooth and successful transition? Here are a few tips:

Think like a manager. Many dewy managers encounter transition difficulties because they retain their rank-and-file mentality. They should be prepared to make the necessary mindset switches to cope with the higher responsibilities.

- Have the perspective of an eagle, not an ant. See the forest, not the trees— Your thinking should now take on a broader perspective. Evaluate the effect of your actions or decisions not only on your unit, but on the whole organization. Your problem solving approach should now be strategic rather than merely straightforward. (You'll learn that sometimes, it may be necessary to lose a battle to win the war.) You should begin steering a course along the company's vision.
- Analyze deeply if you have the time, but decide quickly when needed—One weakness of new managerial appointees, especially those fresh from graduate business school, is a tendency to be wishy-washy. After going through endless case studies in school, they have become so good at analyzing situations that they tend to develop analysis paralysis. They cannot decide without first making a thorough study.

    A manager must have enough self-confidence to size up situations quickly, and then, even with the barest of information available, make hard and fast decisions when called for. You must learn to develop your "gut feel" and to rely on it at crunch time.
- Think ahead: be proactive, not reactive—Often, new managers are so afraid of failure that they defer making risky decisions, waiting instead for things to come to a head and then reacting to them. A good manager is one who trains himself or herself to look ahead, weigh all possible scenarios, decide on the most probable outcome and proact accordingly.

- Be organizationally aware—Understand how the organization works—its systems, situations, pressures, culture, etc.—and how these factors combine to influence your unit. Also, study how your own unit impacts on the other components of the organization.

  A newly promoted purchasing manager I once knew paid a dear price for not heeding this advice. To win his subordinates over, he solicited assistance from the suppliers in treating them to an excursion. His objective was laudable, but his method was questionable. He violated the organization's stand against soliciting from suppliers and stirred envy in other departments. The resulting fallout was so bad that he had to leave the company.

Behave like a manager. Another managerial pitfall is failing to act appropriately. You should know that, as a manager, you are a company role model, expected to act in a certain manner reflective of your stature in the organization.

- Integrity is very important—As a role model, you must maintain and promote social, ethical and organizational norms in conducting your internal and external business activities. Bear in mind that you now represent the company inside and outside its walls, and how you behave reflects on the company.

  There was once a marketing service officer who was good at his job and was promoted to manager. Part of his new function was to manage the agency promo girls assigned to different department stores. Unfortunately, he found these pretty ladies so alluring that he was soon into relationships with some of them, and rumors of these liaisons eventually reached the higher echelon. Unable to fire him due to lack of solid proof, they decided to transfer him to a far-flung post where his reputation could do no harm. He ended up resigning from the company.

- Be a leader, not a boss—A few years back, I encountered a situation where the Engineering Department, once performing well, suddenly became a problem area. It turned out that the people had a beef against the newly promoted engineering manager. Some of their feedback: "Mabuti pa noong `bisor siya, ang bait. Nang maging manager, naging mayabang!" "Grabe maka-utos.Ora-orada! Pag di agad nasunod, nagagalit." ("It was better when he was supervisor. As manager, he has become swell-headed!" "He's too bossy. He wants things done at once, and gets angry otherwise.")

  Several coaching sessions with the manager and a teambuilding workshop with his staff were conducted, and the situation was rectified.

  To be an effective manager, you should be a leader, not a boss. You must earn your subordinates' respect, not demand it. You must also delegate properly rather than give orders. You must be sensitive to their needs and assist them when the situation demands it. And most of all, develop them to be better employees, because your success depends on their success.

Work like a manager. Your new post will necessitate a change in work style and a sturdy stomach to withstand the increased pressure.

- Observe flexible work hours—A manager cannot afford to be tardy or even knock off early. Otherwise, you will have a difficult time enforcing time discipline among your subordinates.

Also, do not observe a regular "eight-to-five" routine simply because you are not paid overtime. Remember that your performance is no longer measured in work hours, but in work output. Oftentimes, this calls for putting in long and hard hours, especially if you have deadlines to meet.

- Learn to live under pressure and to avoid burnout—The major reason why the engineering manager mentioned earlier developed staff problems was his difficulty in coping with pressure. He wanted to prove himself so badly that he took on more jobs than he could possibly handle, and the demands of these simply overwhelmed him. As a result, he vented his exasperation on his hapless subordinates.

   Learn to prioritize your tasks based on their perceived importance to the organization or, equally important, to your boss. Tackle the big ones immediately and try to squeeze in the small tasks afterward. If you fill a container with sand, there is no way you can add the pebbles and stones anymore. But put in the stones first, and you can push the pebbles between the gaps, and then squeeze sand into whatever gaps still remain.

   Master the art of pacing yourself and conserving your energy for the long grind ahead. It is useless to expend all your energy at the start, only to falter at the end because you've run out of gas.

   Finally, learn to handle pressure. You should be able to tolerate stress and relieve it in a manner acceptable to the people around you. There are many articles and self-help books that can teach you how to do this.

- Be tenacious but resilient—As a manager, you should be determined to succeed. Stay on course until you have achieved your objective, or until it is no longer reasonably attainable. However, be resilient as well. You are not Superman and should expect some disappointments and failures along the way. But you should be able to handle these setbacks well and maintain your effectiveness.

There are many more expectations from you as a manager than can be mentioned in this article. Your success will depend on how well you cope with these expectations. Most important, however, is that you learn to think out of the employee box and acknowledge that you still have a lot to learn to become an effective manager. Adopt this frame of mind, and you are halfway there.

SOURCE: Courtesy of JobStreet.com Philippines, Inc. http://ph.jobstreet.com/employers/mot13.htm.

GLOSSARY

Alderfer's ERG Model: A motivation model based on three levels—existence, relatedness, and growth.

anticipatory control: A proactive approach to monitoring a process whereby a supervisor previews an entire process and each related task.

appealed policy: A policy established as an exception to an existing policy. The appealed policy may be for a single instance or special circumstance or may apply to a subset of the organization.

appraisal interview: An interview that may take on characteristics of both directive and nondirective interviews. Usually designed to discuss an employee's strengths and weaknesses.

arbitrator: An independent outside person selected by the union and management to make a final and binding decision in a grievance that the parties involved are unable to settle themselves.

assessment center: A method of evaluating in-house candidates for promotion to management. Assessment centers include a battery of exercises and activities that allow observers to evaluate the management prospects of those seeking promotion.

attrition: The practice of not replacing employees who leave.

authority: The right to direct others and to give orders.

authority acceptance theory: The belief that a leader's authority originates at the bottom of the organizational pyramid and is determined by his subordinates' willingness to comply with it.

autocratic supervision: A management style based on Theory X, i.e., that involves little participation by subordinates in the decision-making process.

behaviorally anchored rating scales (BARS): An assessment method that combines elements from the critical incidents and graphic rating scale assessments.

benchmarking: Establishing goals by comparing performance to others.

benchmark jobs: Jobs that are similar in every healthcare organization, such as dietitian and housekeeper.

borrowed servant doctrine: The doctrine that a hospital employee is under the direct supervision of a physician when the employee is aiding the physician. In this case, respondeat superior liability falls on the physician, not the institution.

boss-imposed time: Time used by an individual to accomplish items required by the boss.

budgetary control: The use of budgets to control the department's daily operations.

business intelligence: The use of information to improve business decisions.

capital budget: The budget that shows the major assets to be purchased, anticipated purchase dates, and funding sources for those purchases.

capitation: A system that pays physicians, or healthcare organizations, a fixed monthly amount for each individual in a plan, regardless of whether they are treated or not.

captain of the ship doctrine: The doctrine that a surgeon directly supervises all personnel assisting an operation; thus respondeat superior liability falls on the surgeon, not the institution.

cash budget: A projection of cash balances at the end of each month throughout the budget year.

center of excellence: A department chosen by the healthcare organization to receive special attention and resources, such as cardiology or oncology. Centers of excellence are sometimes called "institutes."

central tendency: The tendency to appraise all employees as roughly average.

chaos theory: The theory that the world is unorganized and events are unpredictable; thus, managers must recognize that events cannot always be controlled.

charismatic authority: Authority stemming from the personal qualities of an individual.

circular chart: An organizational chart that depicts the various levels in concentric circles rotating around the top-level administrator, who is at the hub of the wheel.

closed-loop feedback system: A feedback system that includes a self-regulating mechanism that is triggered when the process deviates from the standard.

coercive power: Power based on fear.

collaboration: The act of individuals working together to achieve a common goal.

collective bargaining: The practice of bargaining for better pay and working conditions as a group, rather than individually.

committee: A formal group with defined purposes and relationships within an organization.

comparative standards: An assessment method that compares employees to other employees in the department.

competence: The demonstrated ability to apply knowledge and skills.

comprehensive budgeting: The practice of establishing an organization-wide forecast of revenues and expenditures specifically defined for each operating unit within the organization.

compressed scheduling: Allowing employees to work a schedule in which more hours are worked in fewer days per week, such as 12 hours per day for 3 days.

concentrated mass offensive: A strategy of pulling together all resources and taking sudden, radical action to quickly solve a problem.

concurrent controls: Controls on a process that monitor progress as it is being done, allowing corrections or adjustments to be made immediately.

conformance quality: A level of work outcome that meets the minimum standard.

consultative supervision: A type of supervision based on the assumption that employees are eager to do a good job, have the motivation to perform their best, and are capable of doing so. Also called *participative, democratic*, and *permissive supervision*.

content theory: The theory that individuals are motivated by needs. Also called *need theory*.

controlling: Checking performance against standards.

coordination: The linking together of the activities in the organization to achieve the desired results.

corporate negligence: The doctrine that a corporation, in this case a hospital, is legally responsible for actions of associated individuals, even non-employees.

cost control: The practice of consistently monitoring and managing costs.

critical access hospital: A designation that allows a hospital to receive Medicare reimbursement based on its actual costs, which is generally more than typical Medicare reimbursement. The designation was designed to help hospitals in underserved areas.

critical incidents assessment: An assessment method in which the supervisor focuses on specific behaviors that separate effective from ineffective performance.

critical success factors (CSFs): Sub-goals of a plan. CSFs are monitored during performance management to measure progress of the overall plan.

cultural blindness: The practice of ignoring differences in culture and assuming that all employees are the same.

decision-making leave: A temporary, paid layoff during which time an employee with a disciplinary problem considers whether to change his behavior and remain with the organization, or resign.

decisional role: A supervisor's behavior that uses information to make decisions.

delegation of authority: The act of a superior granting authority on some level to a subordinate.

departmentalization: The process of grouping various activities into natural units by logical arrangements.

descriptive survey: A survey that allows the subjects to freely answer questions in their own words.

diagonal coordination: Coordination that cuts across organizational arrangements, ignoring positions and levels.

directive interview: A structured interview between a supervisor and employee in which the interviewer knows beforehand the goals, objectives, and areas of discussion.

disciplinary counseling: An informal conversation in which a supervisor notifies a subordinate about a problem and tries to resolve it.

disciplinary layoff: A temporary suspension used to punish a serious infraction.

discussional meeting: A meeting in which the leader encourages other members to participate.

doctrine of charitable immunity: The legal concept that the assets of charitable organizations, such as non-profit hospitals, will not be jeopardized by lawsuits.

downward communication: Communication that flows down the hierarchy of an organization, such as when a vice president tells a line supervisor about a new initiative, and the line supervisor tells her employees.

E-Discovery Rules: Part of the Federal Rules of Civil Procedure that pertain to access to electronic patient records for parties to a civil lawsuit.

employee assistance program: Programs staffed by social workers and medical and counseling personnel who are trained in providing confidential, professional assistance to employees and their families.

employment interview: An interview between a supervisor and prospective employee designed to determine if the prospective employee is a good fit for the position, and vice versa. Also called a *pre-employment interview.*

empowerment policies: Policies that sanction in advance decisions made by subordinates, as long as they stay within the policy guidelines.

environmental assessment: A comprehensive analysis of conditions inside and outside an organization, ranging from politics to finances.

exception principle: The principle that some decisions faced by an individual are beyond his scope of authority and must be referred to his superior. Also the practice of reporting only items that fail to meet standards, so that the respondent can focus on problem areas.

experiential decision making: The practice of making decisions based on experience.

extender role: The role of an employee who takes on tasks or projects for a manager who cannot do all the work himself.

external alignment: Aligning salaries within an organization with salaries of similar positions outside the organization, but within the surrounding community.

fee-for-service: A system that pays physicians based on the number of services they perform.

feedback control: A control mechanism that alerts the user to discrepancies after a process is completed.

flexible budget: A budget that is prepared with a range of potential customer levels, so that adjustments can be made throughout the year if changes in levels occur.

flextime: Scheduling that allows employees to modify their personal schedule to fit their off-the-job activities.

force-field analysis: An approach to overcoming resistance to change that involves openly discussing the pros and cons of a planned change.

formal authority theory: The belief that authority originates at the top of an organization and is delegated downward from superiors to subordinates.

4 Es approach: A technique to engage subordinates in planning for changes that involves engagement, empathy, education, and enlistment.

free-rein leadership: A leadership approach that assumes that individual employees are self-motivated and perform well with minimum supervision. Also called *laissez-faire leadership.*

functional authority: Authority given to individuals with expertise in specialized areas and limited to particular situations. For example, a hospital's safety officer may be given the authority to send ambulances away from the emergency department—something he normally would not have the authority to do—if he feels the emergency department is dangerously overcrowded.

Gantt chart: A chart featuring horizontal bars, each representing the time allotted for a different task of given project. Seen together, the bars reveal tasks that can be done simultaneously contrasted with those that must be done sequentially.

general supervision: Supervision that provides goals in broad terms, with the expectation that the employees will decide how to reach those goals.

grapevine: The informal channel of communication in an organization.

graphic rating scale: An assessment method that uses a list of performance factors that the supervisor uses to rate employee performance.

grassroots budgeting: The practice of involving operating unit managers and supervisors in the development of forecasts of expenditures and revenues for their respective units.

grooming: The process of preparing an individual to take on more authority and responsibility.

group deliberation: The practice of discussing issues among all members of a committee.

groupthink: The result of allowing group discussion to be dominated by a desire to find group concurrence on a conclusion, even if facts point to another conclusion.

halo effect: A circumstance in which an interviewer bases an applicant's potential for job performance on one or two characteristics and allows this impression to color all the other factors. Can also be seen in performance appraisals, when high or low marks are given on an entire appraisal because of high or low marks on one aspect of the appraisal, even if other aspects of the appraisal do not deserve the high or low marks.

Herzberg's Two-Factor Motivation-Hygiene Theory: The theory that workplace factors can be divided into two categories, those that do not motivate (hygiene factors) and those that do (motivators).

horizontal chart: An organizational chart that reads from left to right, stressing functional relationships more than hierarchical levels.

horizontal communication: Communication across departments or among peer managers, departments, and coworkers in charge of different activities.

horizontal coordination: Coordination between departments on the same organizational level, such as between the emergency department and the radiology department.

hospital acquired: An adjective describing an injury or infection that occurred due to negligence by a healthcare facility.

hospitalist: A physician who practices solely in a hospital instead of in private practice, and who is employed by the hospital.

housestaff: Physicians who serve in a hospital during their internship or fellowship.

human resources management: The management, including planning, of the staffing function.

imposed policy: A policy created to comply with outside factors, such as accrediting requirements.

incremental budgeting: Budgeting that assumes that budgeted amounts from the previous year remain set.

informational meeting: A meeting in which the leader presents information and facts, usually with limited discussion from other members.

informational role: A supervisor's behavior that ensures that information is received and processed.

intangible standards: Standards that are qualitative and subjective or based on perception.

internal alignment: The alignment of salaries of positions within a department, relative to the monetary value of the positions. That is, paying people who are equally valuable approximately equal pay.

interpersonal role: A supervisor's behavior, such as relationships with other supervisors, that links all managerial work.

inverted pyramid chart: An organizational chart featuring the chief administrator on the bottom and others farther up. This chart expresses the idea that the superiors support those who report to them.

job analysis: A study of the jobs within an organization to document the activities, tools used, and working conditions of each position.

job description: A document that describes the duties and responsibilities of a position.

job evaluation: A method of determining the relationships between pay rates and the relative monetary value of jobs within a department.

job specialization: Breaking down a task into smaller parts, and having each part or step of the task performed by a different individual.

job specification: A document that identifies the minimum acceptable qualifications of a person in a given position.

kaizen (or kaizen blitz): A Lean term for rapidly trying out improvements in processes.

language barrier: A hindrance to communication that occurs when a person speaks in a manner another person is unfamiliar with. A language barrier can exist when the two literally speak different languages, or if they speak the same language but use different terminology or style.

liability: The potential of a lawsuit.

line authority: Formal authority granted by an organization to a supervisor.

line organization: The organizational structure built on a straight chain of command from the top of an organization to the bottom.

line personnel: Employees with direct responsibility to ensure goals are achieved through their subordinates. Line personnel may be advised by staff personnel, but line personnel make the decisions.

management by objective (MBO): A management system in which managers and subordinates set goals and use progress toward those goals as measures of success. Developed by Peter Drucker.

management engineer: An individual who uses data and analytics to improve processes.

management rights clause: The clause in a labor agreement that gives management the authority to manage the workforce.

managerial authority: The legal or rightful power of a manager to act or direct others.

managerial functions: Functions that must be performed by a supervisor for him to be considered a true manager.

Maslow's Hierarchy of Needs: A motivation model that involves levels of needs, from basic physiological needs to the need for self-actualization.

matrix organization: An organizational structure that adds cross-departmental connections to a traditional vertical organization. These connections may unite departments for special projects or products or services that span several geographic areas. In a matrix organization, employees often report to more than one superior.

McClelland's Achievement Theory: The theory that individuals are motivated by their needs for affiliation, achievement, and power.

mechanistic organization: An organization whose structure is characterized by high specialization, extensive departmentalization, narrow spans of control, many rigid rules and regulations, a limited information network, and authority vested in a few higher-level executives.

medical tourism: The practice of seeking medical care in a foreign country because of cost savings, quality, expertise, or other reasons.

mentor: An individual who helps a subordinate establish goals and a path to achieve them.

method: A standing plan that details one single part of a procedure.

micromanaging: The practice of directing every detail of a subordinate's action.

mores: Culture-driven expectations in behavior, such as the type of clothing one wears or the way one treats others.

motivation: The process affecting the inner needs or drives that arouse, move, energize, direct, channel, and sustain human behavior.

negligence: An action or non-action that results in an injury by an individual who is not acting as a "reasonably prudent person" would under the same circumstances.

nominal group technique: A method to allow all members of a group to have equal voice in discussions.

nondirective interview: An unstructured interview between a supervisor and an employee, often used to discuss a problem or grievance. Also called a *counseling interview*.

non-programmed decisions: Decisions pertaining to situations for which no standard solutions or protocols exist.

norms: Standards that regulate behavior within an organization.

objective questionnaire: A questionnaire that asks questions and provides a choice of answers.

objective survey: A survey that requires the subjects to mark the answers that come closest to their feelings on the topic.

offshoring: Using an outsourcing contractor who uses labor from countries other than the United States.

open architecture system: A system that allows different, nonproprietary systems from a variety of manufacturers to work well together.

operations research: The use of mathematical models, analytical methods, or structured inquiry to analyze a complex situation and identify the optimal approach to the situation.

organic structure: An organizational structure in which jobs tend to be general; few rules and regulations exist; communication is vertical, diagonal, and horizontal; and the organization is highly adaptive and flexible and encourages decentralized decision making by the employees.

organizational design: A process involving decisions about such things as work or job specialization, departmentalization, chain of command, span of control, and centralization or decentralization.

organizational structure: The formal arrangement of jobs in an organization.

ostensible agency: An organization that appears to employ an individual, even if it does not actually employ that individual.

outsourcing: Contracting with a third party to handle some aspect of an organization's work.

Pareto Principle: The principle that states that 80 percent of results are caused by 20 percent of causes.

parity principle: The concept that individuals who are given responsibility for a function must be given enough authority to carry out that function.

pay-for-performance program: Motivation programs that tie bonus payments to achievement of goals or results.

perceptual selectivity: The process by which an individual selects which stimuli to respond to and which to screen out.

performance appraisal: A formal system of measuring, evaluating, and influencing an employee's job-related activities.

performance development plan: A plan to facilitate correction of weaknesses identified during a performance appraisal.

performance management (PM): The process of monitoring the implementation and effectiveness of a plan.

performance metrics: Performance-related measurements of activity or resource utilization.

PESTHR analysis: An acronym that stands for Political, Economic, Social, Technological, Human resource, and Regulatory forces. These are all elements of an environmental analysis.

Pike Place Fish Market model: A motivational model based on the practices at a popular fish market in Seattle where employees perform for customers to show how much they enjoy their work.

plaintiff: The individual or entity that sues another.

planning horizon: The length of time for which a manager should plan.

policies: Standing plans that express an organization's general response to a problem or situation.

positional authority: Authority of a superior over a subordinate.

power: The ability to influence others or get others to act in a certain way.

primary care: Initial physician contact, such as in an emergency room, clinic, or physician's office.

procedure: Repeat-use plans that lead toward achievement of an organization's goals. Procedures explain the actions required to comply with policies.

process theory: The theory that individuals are motivated by equity and expectancy, i.e., that they expect equal compensation and treatment (equity) and that they will be rewarded for their effort (expectancy).

productivity standards: Reasonably achievable quantitative and qualitative expectations based on relevant data, benchmarks, or industry metrics.

program: A single-use plan with a complex set of activities to reach a specific major objective.

programmed decisions: Decisions that pertain to repetitive, structured, and routine problems that have fixed answers and standardized operating procedures, methods, rules, and regulations.

project: A single-use plan that is smaller in scope than a program, and may be undertaken within an overall program.

project evaluation and review technique (PERT): A planning tool that ensures complex projects are completed on time.

pro re nata (PRN): Latin term that means "as needed." Used to identify healthcare workers who work only as needed, rather than on regular shifts.

prospective payment system: A system that pays physicians and healthcare organizations a fixed amount for every episode of care. For example, treatment for a particular injury is reimbursed at a flat rate regardless of the length of stay in the hospital or the number of physician visits related to the injury.

quality of kind: A level of work outcome that exceeds customer expectations.

qui tam: A provision of the Federal Civil False Claims Act that allows a private citizen to file a suit in the name of the U.S. government.

rational authority: Authority based on law, procedures, and rules.

reciprocity: A tactic that involves giving a colleague something in return for something. Also called *you scratch my back and I'll scratch yours.*

recruitment: The process of attracting and seeking a pool of applicants from which to choose a qualified candidate.

reengineering: A reorganization process in which leadership determines the best way to accomplish its tasks, regardless of how those tasks were accomplished in the past.

referent power: Power based on the personal attraction of an individual or the desire of other people to be like that person.

repeat-use plans: Plans that can be used whenever a situation arises that is similar to the situation the plan was originally created for.

requirements quality: A level of work outcome that meets customer expectations.

respondeat superior: The legal doctrine by which an employer is responsible for the actions or omissions of its employees.

revenue and expense budget: The traditional budget that includes estimates of revenue and expenses. Also called the *operations budget.*

reward power: Power based on the ability to distribute something of value.

role theory: The concept that when employees receive inconsistent expectations and little information, they experience role conflict, which leads to stress, dissatisfaction, and ineffective performance.

rolling budget: Unlike the traditional budget, which is developed for a 12-month period, the rolling budget approach starts with a base budget and continually is added to and updated for future months or segments of time.

rule: A statement that forbids or requires a certain action or inaction.

sampling: The process of reviewing a certain number of cases or events out of the total number of cases or events. Sampling can be conducted on a random or nonrandom basis.

scalar chain: The line of vertical authority relationships from superior to subordinate. Also called the *chain of command.*

scientific decision making: The practice of making decisions based on quantitative data.

secondary care: Patient care provided by specialists who do not normally have first contact with a patient, such as urologists or dermatologists.

selection: The process of choosing from a pool of applicants.

self-actualization: Realizing one's potential.

self-appraisal: A self-rating by an employee, which provides a supplemental source of appraisal input.

self-imposed time: Time used by an individual to accomplish items she originates herself.

semantics: The study of language, particularly the multiple meanings of words and phrases and how they are used in the context of messages.

shop steward: A union representative who usually is also an employee of the healthcare facility.

similar-to-me tendency: The tendency of supervisors to rate employees whose attitudes resemble their own higher than otherwise deserved.

single-use plans: Plans for nonrecurring situations.

Six Sigma: A combination of reengineering principles and quality improvement approachs that focuses on delivering defect-free services and products.

skills inventory: A list of skills an individual possesses, regardless of whether the skills are applicable to the person's job.

Skinner's Reinforcement Model: The theory that behavior can be controlled through the use of rewards.

span of management: The scope of supervision, or the number of people who report to a particular manager.

staff authority: Authority that resides in those with certain expertise who counsel or assist those with line authority. People who work in the accounting department, for example, may have staff authority and advise the department managers on financial matters.

staff personnel: Employees who specialize in specific duties or areas of expertise, but who generally do not make important decisions impacting the organization.

staffing: The managerial function concerned with the procurement and maintenance of human resources.

status position: One of four positions vis-à-vis the informal organization. These are the informal leader, members of the primary group, members on the fringe of the group, and those outside the fringe.

subordinate-imposed time: Time spent dealing with subordinates, such as with counseling, evaluating, and providing direction.

succession planning: Preparing employees to take on new assignments within or outside of the current department.

SWOT analysis: An examination of the Strengths, Weaknesses, Opportunities, and Threats an organization faces.

system-imposed time: Time used by an individual to support peers and cooperate with the organization.

tactical approaches: Short-term actions leading toward goals.

tangible standards: Physical standards that pertain to the actual operation of a department in which goods are produced.

telecommuting: Working from home or another off-site location while remaining connected to the office through telephone and computer.

tertiary care: Highly sophisticated and specialized inpatient care, normally in a healthcare facility that specializes in that type of care, such as a heart institute.

Theory X: A theory that employees perform best under supervision that involves close control, centralized authority, authoritarian practices, and minimal participation of the subordinates in the decision-making process.

Theory Z: A management approach that is based on lifetime employment, slow promotion paths, consensual decision making, collective responsibility, and informal controls. Theory Z assumes workers want to build strong relationships with their colleagues.

360-degree feedback: An assessment method that incorporates feedback from all of an employee's coworkers, including superiors, peers, and subordinates. Also called *multisource* or *multi-rater feedback*.

timesizing: A cost-cutting technique that involves employees' taking unpaid time off, or using accrued vacation time.

tort: An action or omission of action that results in injury to another.

traditional authority: Authority that arises from the subordinates' belief in social order.

traditional budgeting: A budgeting process that focuses on planned changes from the previous year's level of expenditures.

traditional structure: The most common form of organization design, in which hierarchical relationships develop vertically, and each employee reports to one superior.

transfer: A reassignment of an employee to another job of similar pay, status, and responsibility.

unity of command: The principle that states that each employee has a single immediate supervisor, who in turn is responsible to her immediate superior, and so on along the chain of command.

upward communication: Communication that flows up the hierarchy, such as when a nurse tells the nursing shift supervisor about a problem with a patient.

value statement: A statement that defines what an organization holds important.

vertical chart: An organizational chart that shows the different levels of the organization in a step arrangement in the form of a pyramid.

vertical coordination: Coordination between different levels of an organization, such as between the CEO and a vice president.

vicarious liability: The concept that one party may be held responsible for the actions of another even though the original party was not involved in the act.

virtual position: A job held by an employee who works offsite.

Vroom's Expectancy Model: The theory that people act in a certain way because they anticipate that the behavior will achieve the outcome or goal desired.

wage survey: A survey that collects data on wages paid in the community for similar key jobs in similar or related enterprises.

Weingarten Rule: A rule that states that if a supervisor is meeting with a union employee and the result of that meeting could be discipline, the employee must have the ability to have a union delegate or representative present.

what-if analysis: An analysis involving manipulation of variables in a budget to see how the results change.

work specialization: Breaking down a job into smaller, more specialized tasks.

zero-base budgeting: A budgeting process that ignores the previous year's budget and requires that every request for funding be justified anew.

REFERENCES

Abdelhak, M., S. Grostick, M. A. Hanken, and E. Jacobs. 1996. *Health Information: Management of a Strategic Resource.* Philadelphia, PA: Saunders.

Accountemps. 2008. "TGI . . . TUESDAY? Second Day of the Week Remains Most Productive, Survey Shows." [Online news release; created 2/7/08; retrieved 1/26/09.] www.accountemps.com/PressRoom?id=2121.

Advisory Publications. n.d. "A Tight Overtime Policy Provides Good Financial Control." *Financial Management Strategies for Medical Offices.* Conshohocken, PA: Advisory Publications.

AICPA. 2004. "Golden Business Ideas." *Journal of Accountancy* 197 (1): 112.

Aldag, R. J, and T. M. Stearns. 1991. *Management,* 2nd ed., 696. Cincinnati, OH: South-Western Publishing Co.

Allen, G. 2000. *Supervision.* Denton, TX: RonJon Publishers.

Allen, J. M., and M. D. Wircenski. 2005. "Training Older Learners: Issues for the New Millennium." [Online article; updated 7/1/05; retrieved 3/8/09.] www.cps.unt.edu/natla/age_shr/trainolder.html.

Alliance for Non-Profit Management. 2009. "What Are the Key Concepts and Definitions in Strategic Planning?" [Online information; retrieved 2/17/09.] www.allianceonline.org/content/index.php?pid=172.

Altman, S., E. Valenzi, and R. M. Hodgetts. 1985. *Organizational Behavior: Theory and Practice.* New York: Harcourt Brace Jovanovich, Inc.

Amalgamated Transit Union. 2008. "The Weingarten Rule." [Online information; retrieved 11/29/09.] www.atu19.org/Documents/weingarten_ rule.htm.

American Federation of Teachers. 2004. "Empty Hallways: The Hidden Shortage of Healthcare Workers." [Online article; retrieved 12/6/09.] www.aft.org/pubs-reports/healthcare/Empty-Hallways.pdf.

American Geriatrics Society. 2010. "Frequently Asked Questions About Geriatricians." [Online information; retrieved 12/06/09.] www.americangeriatrics.org/news/geria_faqs.shtml#2.

American Health Information Management Association. 1999. "Pre-Employment Testing." *Journal of AHIMA* 70 (4): 54.

American Hospital Association–McKesson. 2009. *Quest for Quality Prize 2009.* Chicago: Health Forum.

American Management Association. 2000. "Growing Use of Temporary Workers Driven by Employers' Needs for Flexibility." *Snelling Report* (Nov.): 3.

Anderson, C. 2001. "The Two Countries That Invented the Industrial Revolution." [Online article; retrieved 02/08/06.] www.darex.com/new/articles/brittool.html.

Appold, K. 2007. "Effective Delegation." *Advance for Health Information Professionals* 17 (16): 19.

———. 2006. "Keeping Your Workplace on Course." *ADVANCE for Health Information Professionals* 19 (21): 21–22.

Armour, S. 2005. "Dust Off Those Ties and Pumps: Dress Codes Gussy Up." *USA Today*, Oct. 26, 1B.

———. 2001. "Firms Find Pitfalls in Pay-for-Performance Programs." *USA Today*, July 5, B-1.

Atchison, T. 2005. *Leadership's Deeper Dimensions: Building Blocks to Superior Performance*. Chicago: Health Administration Press.

——— 2004. *Followership: A Practical Guide to Aligning Leaders and Followers*. Chicago: Health Administration Press.

Atchison, T. A., and K. J. McDonagh. 2007. "CEO Boot Camp." Presented at the American College of Healthcare Executives Congress on Healthcare Leadership, New Orleans, March.

Bacal, R. 2009. "Understanding Informal Leaders in an Organization (and Benefiting from Them)." [Online article; retrieved 3/2/09.] www.work911.com/leadership-development/articles/informalleadersunderstanding.htm.

Baker, A. 2005. "Growing Talent Is Everybody's Business." *Journal of Accountancy* 200 (3): 91.

Bakhtiari, E. 2009. "Time for Dr. NeXt." *Health Leaders* XII (7): 14–22.

Baldiga, N. R., and M. S. Doucet. 2001. "Special Report. Having It All: How a Shift Toward Balance Affected CPAs and Firms." [Online article; retrieved 2/13/02.] www.aicpa.org/pubs/JOFA/may2001/news_sr.htm.

Barker, J. 1993. *Paradigms: The Business of Discovering the Future*, 15–18. New York: Harper Business.

Barnard, C. I. 1989. *Management*, 4th ed., edited by R. Krietner, 281. Boston: Houghton Mifflin Co.

———. 1956. *The Functions of the Executive*, 163. Cambridge, MA: Harvard University Press.

Barry, R., A. C. Murcko, and C. E. Brubaker. 2002. *The Six Sigma Book for Healthcare: Improving Outcomes by Reducing Errors*. Chicago: Health Administration Press.

Batalden, P., D. Leach, and G. Ogrine. 2009. "Knowing Is Not Enough— Executives and Educators Must Act to Address Challenges and Reshape Healthcare." *Healthcare Executive* 24 (2): 68.

Batchelor, E. 2008. "Setting Aside Two Hours for Staff Keeps the Interruptions in Check." *Medical Office Manager* 22 (9): 2.

Beach, D. S. 1985. *Personnel: The Management of People at Work*, 5th ed, 307. New York: Macmillan.

Beckham, D. 2005. "The Right Questions." *Hospitals and Health Networks* [Online article; created 9/23/05; retrieved 1/16/09.] www.hhnmag.com/hhnmag_app/jsp/printer_friendly.jsp?dcrPath=HHNMAG/PubsNewsArticle/data/050920HHN_Online_Beckham&domain=HHNMAG.

Begun, J., J. Tornabeni, and K. White. 2006. "Opportunities for Improving Patient Care Through Lateral Integration: The Clinical Nurse Leader." *Journal of Healthcare Management* 51 (1): 19–25.

Belkin, L. 2009. "Flexible Work in a Recession." [Online article; retrieved 0/23/09.] http://parting.blogs.nytimes.com/2009/10/02/flexible-work-in-a-recession/htm.

Bennis, W., and J. Goldsmith. 2003. *Learning to Lead*. Cambridge, MA: Basic Books.

Blanton, W. H. 2009. "Organizing and Authority." [Online lecture notes; retrieved 2/13/09.] http://faculty.etsu.edu/blanton/Organizing%20lecture_8.ppt.

Boehler, R., D. Hardesty, E. Gonzales, and K. Kasnetz. 2009. "The Business Case for Quality." *Healthcare Financial Management* 63 (10): 62–66.

Bolster, C. J. 2007. "Take This Job and Love It." *Healthcare Financial Management* 61 (1): 57.

Boothby, S. 1998. "The Three Cs Make Outsourcing an 'In' Thing for Many Hospitals." *AHA News* (Sept. 7): 5.

Boucher, J. 2001. *How to Love the Job You Hate*, 163–66. Nashville, TN: Thomas Nelson.

The Bowen Center for Study of the Family. 2008. "Bowen Theory." [Online information; retrieved 11/19/08.] www.thebowencenter.org/pages/theory.html.

Box, T. A., T. A. West, L. R. Watts, and M. L. Whisman. 1999. "Learning Organizations: Panacea or Partial Answer?" *Academy of Strategic and Organizational Leadership Journal* 3 (2): 57–58.

Bradley, B. 2005. Quote. [Online information; retrieved 02/21/06.] www.insightquotes.com/l.html.

Branden, N. n.d. BrainyQuote.com. [Online information; retrieved 5/4/10.] www.brainyquote.com/quotes/quotes/n/nathanielb163773.html.

Brett, J., K. Behfar, and M. C. Kern. 2006. "Managing Multi-cultural Teams." *Harvard Business Review* 84 (11): 84–91.

Bright Hub. 2009. "Telecommuting Trends in the 2009 Economy." [Online article; retrieved 10/23/09.] www.brighthub.com/office/home/articles/22829.aspx.

Burns, T., and G. M. Stalker. 1961. *The Management of Innovation*. London: Tavistock.

Bush, H. 2009. "Take a Deep Breath and Brace Yourself." *Hospitals and Health Networks* 83 (1): 22–26.

Business Knowledge Source. 2010. "Continuous Process Improvement: The Kaizen Approach." [Online article; retrieved 3/7/10.]

http://businessknowledgesource.com/manufacturing/continuous_process_improvement_the_kaizen_approach_extended_entry_026152.html.

California HealthCare Foundation. 2005. "Health Affairs: 25 Percent of U.S. Workers Will Be Uninsured in 2013." [Online report; retrieved 10/6/05.] www.chcf.org/print.cfm?itemID=109910&currentURL=http://www.chcf.org//topics.

Campbell, D. N., R. L. Fleming, and R. C. Grote. 1985. "Discipline Without Punishment—At Last." *Harvard Business Review* (July–August): 162–78.

Campbell, R. J. 2008. "Change Management in Health Care." *The Health Care Manager* 27 (1): 23–39.

Cashen, L. H. 1999. "Benchmarking for Competitive Improvement." *QualityResource* 18 (5): 15.

Catholic Healthcare West. n.d. "Environment." [Online information; retrieved 4/9/10.] www.chwhealth.org/Who_We_Are/Environment/index.htm.

Center for Health Affairs. 2005. "Industry Brief: Is Inefficiency Ailing the Healthcare System?" [Online information; retrieved 10/6/05.] http://chanet.org/Inefficiencies_in_Healthcare.pdf.

Centers for Disease Control and Prevention. 2008. *Health, United States, 2008.* [Online report; retrieved 1/8/09.] www.cdc.gov/nchs/hus.htm.

Ceridian Corporation. 2005. "The Flip Side of Productivity." [Online article; retrieved 9/29/05.] www.ceridian.com/myceridian/article/printerfriendly/1,2723,11337–53923,00.html.

Chandler, A. D., Jr. 1962. *Strategy and Structure: Chapters in the History of the American Industrial Enterprise.* Cambridge, MA: The MIT Press.

Cherrington, D. J. 1991. *The Management of Human Resources,* 3rd ed., 2–3. Boston: Allyn & Bacon.

Clark, C. S., and S. E. Krentz. 2006. "Avoiding the Pitfalls of Strategic Planning." *HFM* 60 (11): 64–65.

Cleverly, W. O. 1992. *Essentials of Health Care Finance,* 3rd ed., 299. Rockville, MD: Aspen.

Coburn, T. 2009. "How to Talk about Layoffs." *CFO* 25 (2): 44–51.

Codrington, G. 2001. "Defining Characteristics of Generations." [Online information; retrieved 2/21/06.] www.youthpastor.com/lessons/index.cfm/124.pdf?fuseaction=viewdoc&L=124.

———. 2001. "Definitive Influences on Today's Youth." [Online information; retrieved 1/2/01.] http://home.pix.za/gc/gc12/genx/thesis/ch1.htm.

Cohen, K. R. 2008. "Measuring What Matters—How to Make Changes for Sustainable Success." [Online article; retrieved 12/8/09.] www.nxtbook.com/nxtbooks/naylor/AHHQ0408/index.php?startid=28#/28.

Colonna, J. 2005. "Why Teams Matter in Healthcare: 7 Characteristics Define Successful Teams." *Healthcare Purchasing News* [Online article; retrieved 7/26/09.] http://findarticles.com/p/articles/mi_m0BPC/is_7_29/ai_n14735111/pg_4/?tag=content;col1.

Commins, J. 2009. "HCA's Next Leaders Are in the Pipeline." *Health Leaders* 12 (5): 54.

Connecticut Post. 2005. [Online article; retrieved 2/11/06.] http://www1.va.gov/vasafety/page.cfm?pg=678

Contino, D. S. 2004. "Leadership Competencies: Knowledge, Skills, and Aptitudes Nurses Need to Lead Organizations Effectively." *Critical Care Nurse* 24 (3): 52–64.

Controller Magazine. 1997. "Outsourcing and the Bottom Line." Special Report. *Controller Magazine* (Nov.): 4.

Cornish, E. 2005. "Special Report: Trends and Forecasts for the Next 25 Years." In *The Futurist,* 7–8. Bethesda, MD: World Future Society.

Coughlin, C. M. 2000. "Show Your Stuff." *Today's Dietitian* 3 (3): 20.

Covey, S. R. 1989. *The Seven Habits of Highly Effective People.* New York: Simon & Schuster.

Cowen, M., L. Halasyamani, D. McMurtrie, D. Hoffman, T. Polley, and J. Alexander. 2008. "Organizational Structure for Addressing the Attributes of the Ideal Healthcare Delivery System." *Journal of Healthcare Management* 53 (6).

Darling v. Charleston Community Memorial Hospital, 33 Ill. 2d 326, 211 N.E. 2d 253, 14 A.L.R. 3rd 860 (1965), cert. denied, 383 U.S. 946 (1966).

Davis, B. L., L. W. Hellervik, C. J. Skube, S. H. Gebelein, L. A. Stevens, and D. G. Lee. 2000. *Successful Manager's Handbook,* 6th ed. Minneapolis: Personnel Decisions International.

Davis, R. 1951. [Online article; retrieved 9/19/05.] www.aviation.sosu.edu/salluisi/avia3133/chapter-6-notes.pdf.

Deloitte. 2009. "Managing Talent in a Turbulent Economy—Keeping Your Team Intact." [Online article; retrieved 10/23/09.] www.deloitte.com/view/en_US/us/Services/additional-services/Talent-Human-Capital-HR/article/882be382ed8c3210VgnVCM100000ba42f00aRCRD.htm.

Deloitte & Touche. 1996. "Interview with Michael Hammer." In *Health Care Review.* Washington, DC: Deloitte & Touche, LLP.

———. 1996. "Facts and Fallacies About Reengineering: A Change Agent at a Critical Time in Health Care History." In *Health Care Review,* 2. Washington, DC: Deloitte & Touche, LLP.

Deming, W. E. 1994. *The New Economics,* 116. Cambridge, MA: Massachusetts Institute of Technology.

———. 1986. *Out of the Crisis.* Cambridge, MA: Massachusetts Institute of Technology, Center for Advanced Engineering Study.

Department of Justice. 2008. "News Release: More than $1 Billion Recovered by Justice Department in Fraud and False Claims in Fiscal Year 2008." [Online information retrieved 12/29/08.] www.usdoj.gov/criminal/npftf/pr/press_releases/2008/nov/11-10-08_frd-fls-clam-fy08.pdf.

Dessler, G. 1998. *Management, Leading People and Organizations in the 21st Century.* Upper Saddle River, NJ: Prentice Hall.

Dessler, G., and F. Stark. 2004. *Principles and Practices for Tomorrow's Leaders*, 154–161. Upper Saddle River, NJ: Prentice Hall.

Dichter, J. R. 2003. "Teamwork and Hospital Medicine: A Vision for the Future." *Critical Care Nurse* 23: 8–11.

Dlugaz, Y. D. 2004. "Six Sigma Adds New Dimension to Quality Management." *Journal of Healthcare Quality* 26 (5): 2, 46.

Doran, D., A. S. McCutcheon, M. G. Evans, K. MacMillan, L. McGillis, D. Pringle, S. Smith, and A. Valente. 2004. "Impact of the Manager's Span of Control on Leadership and Performance." [Online article; retrieved 9/18/05.] www.chsrf.ca/final_research/ogc/doran2_e.php.

D'Oro, R. 2008. "Former Alaska Hospital Worker Shoots 2 Ex-Supervisors, Kills 1, Before Fatally Shot by Police." [Online report; retrieved 12/5/08.] www.startribune.com/templates/Print_This_ Story?sid=35155629.

Drayton, W. n.d. Think Exist.com. [Online information; viewed 2/21/06.] http://en.thinkexist.com/quotes/william_drayton/.

Dreachslin, J. L. 2007. "The Role of Leadership in Creating a Diversity-Sensitive Organization." *Journal of Healthcare Management* 52 (3): 151–52.

Drucker, P. 1954. *The Practice of Management*. New York: HarperCollins Publishers.

Duffy, C. 2006. "Managing Meetings." *Journal of Accountancy* 201 (4): 62.

Dunn, R. 2005. *Finance Principles for the Health Information Manager*, 2nd ed. St. Louis, MO: First Class Solutions.

Dychtwald, K. 2009. "The Longevity Revolution: Healthy Aging or Tithonus's Revenge?" *Futurescan: Healthcare Trends and Implications 2009–2014*, 9. Chicago: Health Administration Press.

Dye, C. F., and A. N. Garman. 2006. "Energizing." In *Exceptional Leadership: 16 Critical Competencies for Healthcare Executives*, 120. Chicago: Health Administration Press.

The Economics Press, Inc. 1999. "Plan for Success." *Better Supervision* 738: 3–4.

Ensman, R. G., Jr. 2000. "Working with Young Employees." *ADVANCE for Health Information Professionals* 10 (19): 57.

———. 1999. "Delegation: Pick the Strategy That's Right for You." *ADVANCE for Health Information Professionals—Online Edition*. [Online information; retrieved 2/12/06.] http://health-information. advanceweb.com/common/editorialsearch/searchresult.aspx?FN=p32 .html&AD=7/19/1999 &CR=true.

Equal Employment Opportunity Commission. 2002. "Enforcement Guidance: Reasonable Accommodation and Undue Hardship Under the Americans with Disabilities Act." [Online information; retrieved 5/4/10.] www.eeoc.gov/policy/docs/accommodation.html#general.

Erickson, P. B. 2001. "Study Shows E-mail Eating Up Workdays." *The Sunday Oklahoman*, July 1, 1–C.

Fayol, H. 1949. *General and Industrial Management*. Trans. C . Storrs. London: Pitman.

Federal Reserve Bank of Dallas. 1992. "The Churn—The Paradox of Progress." [Online report; retrieved 12/29/01.] www.dallasfed.org/htm/pubs/pdfs/anreport/arpt92.pdf.

Feldman, D. C. 1984. "The Development and Enforcement of Group Norms." *Academy of Management Review* 9 (1): 47–53.

Fiedler, F. E. 1967. *A Theory of Leadership Effectiveness.* New York: McGraw-Hill.

———. 1965. "Engineer the Job to Fit the Manager." *Harvard Business Review* 43(5).

Finkelstein, M. 1998. "A Start-Up Guide for Worksite Labor Management Committees in the United States." [Online information; retrieved 5/7/10.] www.newunionism.net/library/workplace%20democracy/Start%20up%20Guide%20for%20Labor-Management%20Committees%20in%20the%20US%20-%201998.doc.

Finnegan, R., and M. Amatayakul (eds.). 1990. *Medical Record Management,* 9th ed., 678. Berwyn, IL: Physicians' Record Company.

Flinn, W. P. 2001. "The Theory XY&Z of Management Theory." [Online article; retrieved 2/9/01.] http://fsosvr.arizona.edu/dickportfolio/dissertation/ToFile/xyz.htm.

Fontaine, M. 2009. "Crisis Leadership: It's a Question of Style?" *The Hay Group Leader* 10 (February).

Frankel, H. L., W. B. Crede, J. E. Topal, S. A. Roumanis, M. W. Devlin, and A. B. Foley. 2005. "Use of Corporate Six Sigma Performance-Improvement Strategies to Reduce Incidence of Catheter-Related Bloodstream Infections in a Surgical ICU." *Journal of the American College of Surgeons* 201 (3): 349–58.

French, J. P., Jr., and B. Raven. 1960. "The Bases of Social Power." In *Group Dynamics*, edited by D. Cartwright and A. Zander, 607–23. New York: Harper and Row.

Fried, B. J. 2009. *The Globalization of Healthcare: Obstacles and Opportunities*, 4–8. Chicago: Health Administration Press.

Gaebler, A. n.d. "Napping at Work." [Online article; retrieved 10/25/09.] www.gaebler.com/Napping-At-Work.htm.

Gardner, M. 2008. "Office Romance? First, Sign a Contract." [Online article; retrieved 12/5/09.] www.csmonitor.com/2008/0211/p13s01-wmgn.html? page=2.

Garman, A., and J. L. Tyler 2004. "Development and Validation of a 360-Degree-Feedback Instrument for Healthcare Administrators." *Journal of Healthcare Management* 49 (5): 306–21.

Garner, B. D. 1999. *Black's Law Dictionary,* 7th ed.. St. Paul, MN: West Group Publishing.

Gee, E. P. 2000. "Leaner Is Greener." *Journal of Healthcare Management* 45 (3): 151–54.

Geldart, W. 1999. "Management Challenges for the 21st Century—A Review." [Online information; retrieved 11/18/08.] http://tap3x.net/EMBTI/j6drucker.html.

Gemignani, J. 2000. "American Workers Are Sleep Deprived." [Online article; retrieved 6/4/10.] www.findarticles.com/cf_dls/m0903/5_18/62276351/ p1/article.jhtml.

Gilbert, R. 1999. *Bits & Pieces*. Fairfield, NJ: Economics Press.

Glover, R. H. 2001. "Monitoring of Employee's Use of Company-Owned Technology and the Privacy Issues It Creates in the Workplace." Gardner, Carton & Douglas Client Memorandum. *Technology and HR Law* (June): 4–5.

GOAL/QPC. 1988. *The Memory Jogger: A Pocket Guide of Tools for Continuous Improvement*. Methuen, MA: GOAL/QPC.

Goedert, J. 2007. "The Biosurveillance Evolution." *Health Data Management* 15 (2): 50–54.

Golden Business Idea. 2005. "Drucker on Motivation." *Journal of Accountancy* 200 (11): 19.

Goldsmith, J. 2007. "Baby Boomers and the Health System: It's the Workforce Stupid!" *FutureScan: Healthcare Trends and Implications 2007–2012*, 10–12. Chicago: Health Administration Press.

Goonan, K., and J. Muzikowski. 2008. "Baldrige: Myths and Realities." *Hospitals and Health Networks* 82 (5): 84–85.

Graham, B. B. 2001. "Rediscover Work Simplification." [Online article; retrieved 9/17/05.] www.worksimp.com/articles/rediscover %20work %20simplification.htm.

Graham, P. (ed.). 1995. *Mary Parker Follett Prophet of Management*. Washington, DC: Beard Books.

Graicunas, V. A. 1937. "Relationship in Organization." In *Papers on the Science of Administration*, edited by L. Gulick and L. F. Urwick, 183–87. New York: Columbia University's Institute of Public Administration.

Gratto Liebler, J., and C. R. McConnell. 2004. *Management Principles for Health Professionals*, 4th ed., 166. New York: Jones & Bartlett.

Griffith, J. R., and J. A. Alexander. 2002. "Measuring Comparative Hospital Performance." *Journal of Healthcare Management* 47 (1): 42.

Grimes, S. 2008. "BI at 50 Turns Back to the Future." [Online article; accessed 5/10/10.] http://intelligent-enterprise.informationweek.com/showArticle.jhtml;jsessionid=5MIKIBREUXYC1QE1GHRSKH4ATMY32JVN?articleID=211900005.

Gross, S. 2005. "2005/2006 US Compensation Planning: Executive Overview." [Online video presentation; retrieved 10/25/09.] www.dppl.com/mercercompensationsurvey.

Haire, M. 1964. *Psychology in Management*, 2nd ed., 74. New York: McGraw-Hill.

Hamilton, I. 1921. *The Soul and Body of an Army*, 229. London: Hamilton.

Hanke, J. 1998. "The Psychology of Presentation Visuals." *Presentations* 12 (5): 42–51.

Hartner, K. 2007. "Generational Diversity in the Workplace." *ADVANCE for Health Information Professionals* 17 (24): 28.

Hay Group. 2008. "Clarity of Direction Prevents Defection." [Online article; retrieved 11/19/08.] http://newsweaver.co.uk/haygroupglobal/index000276521.cfm.

Healthcare Financial Management. 2009. "Reduce Costs First, then Expand Coverage." Interview with David Walker. *Healthcare Financial Management* 63 (10): 45–50.

Healthcare Financial Management Association. 2009. *HFMA's Healthcare Finance Outlook—2009*, 4, 7. Westchester, IL: HFMA.

———. 2000. "Number of Hospitals Dipped Below 6,000 in 1999." CFO Forum Mailing, 3. Westchester, IL: HFMA.

HealthGate Compass. 2007. "No End in Sight for Committee Overload as Quality Improvement Programs and Technology Implementation Surge Ahead." [Online article; retrieved 2/25/10.] www.community.icontact.com/p/healthgate/newsletters/compass/posts/healthgate_compass_no_end_ in_ sight_for_committee_overload.

Henderson, D. A., B. W. Chase, and B. M. Woodson. 2002. "Performance Measures for NPOs." *Journal of Accountancy* 193 (1): 63.

Herzberg, F. 1987. "One More Time: How Do You Motivate Employees?" *Harvard Business Review* 65 (5): 87–96.

———. 1966. *Work and Nature of Man.* Cleveland, OH: World Publishing.

Himiak, L. 2007. "Keeping the Third Shift Happy." *Advance for Health Information Professionals* 17 (3): 18–20.

Hoffman, H. F. 2005. "Organizations Through the Eyes of a Project Manager." [Online article; retrieved 08/31/05.] www.tcicampus.net/userfolder/hhoffman/MOT.

Hofmann, P. B. 2004. "Why Good People Behave Badly." *Healthcare Executive* 19 (2): 40–41.

Holiday Inn Express Navigator. 2000/2001. "Talkin' 'Bout My Generation." *Holiday Inn Express Navigator*, 10.

Holt, D. H. 1990. *Management Principles and Practices,* 2nd ed., 116. Englewood Cliffs, NJ: Prentice Hall.

Holzschu, M. 2001. "Here's What Makes Job Reviews Successful—and Also Why They Fail." *Law Office Administrator* (Jan.): 5.

Homans, G. C. 1950. *The Human Group.* New York: Harcourt Brace Jovanovich, Inc.

Huitt, W. G. 1998. "Maslow's Hierarchy of Needs." [Online information; retrieved 2/24/01.] http://chiron.valdosta.edu/whuitt/col/regsys/maslow.html.

Integrated Publishing. 2009. "Authority and Power." [Online article; retrieved 2/12/09.] www.tpub.com/content/advancement/14144/css/14144_67.htm.

Jackson, K. 2004. "Employee Retention in an Era of Shortages—It's All About Leadership." *For the Record* 16 (18): 30–31.

Jamison, B., and M. O'Connor. 2002. "Road Warriors and Virtual Employees." *Advance for Health Information Professionals* 12 (6): 25.

Jeffords, R., M. Scheidt, and G. M. Thibadoux. 2000. "Securing the Future." *Journal of Accountancy* 189 (2): 49.

Jennings, A. T. 2000. "Hiring Generation X." *Journal of Accountancy* 189 (2): 55.

Johnson, E. 2009. "Dusting Off the Employee Handbook." [Online article; retrieved 3/6/09.] www.workforce.com/archive/feature/26/13/95/index_printer.php.

Jones, D. 2007. "Poll Finds Resentment of Flextime." [Online article; retrieved 10/23/09.] www.usatoday.com/money/workplace/2007-05-10-flex-time-usat_ N.htm.

Journal of Accountancy. 2001. "The Best Survey Question." *Journal of Accountancy* 191 (2): 120.

———. 2000. "Golden Business Ideas." *Journal of Accountancy* (July): 124.

Jusinski, L. 2007. "Connecting with Generation Y." *ADVANCE for Health Information Professionals* 17 (20): 17.

Kaplan, S. 2005. "What to Do When Morale Is Low." [Online article; retrieved 9/28/05.] www.cio.com/archive/050102/morale.html.

Katz, D. M. 2008. "What's Wrong with the Kids?" *CFO* 24 (2): 65.

Katz, R. L. 1974. "Skills of an Effective Administrator." *Harvard Business Review* 52 (5): 90–102.

Keister, J. 2001. "Benchmarking: Healthcare's Invaluable Measuring Stick." *For the Record* 13 (26): 19.

Kelleghan, K. M. 1999. "Use Memos for Clear, Concise Communication." *Office Hours* 408: 1.

Kelly, P. M. 1998. "How to Identify and Deal with 'Whining Cry Baby (WCB) Syndrome'." *Beretta USA Leadership Bulletin* 3 (9).

K&L Gates. 2006. "Electronic Discover Law." [Online blog; retrieved 2/7/10.] www.ediscoverylaw.com/2006/12/articles/news-updates/ediscovery-amendments-to-the-federal-rules-of-civil-procedure-go-into-effect-today/.

Knowels, S. "Son, Ex-Husband Speak About O'Fallon Murder Victim." [Online report; created viewed 11/17/08.] Fox 2, St. Louis. www.myfoxstl.com/myfox/pages/Home/Detail?contentId=7875693&version=6&locale=EN-US&layoutCode=TSTY&pageId=1.1.1.

Kohn, L. T., J. M. Corrigan, and M. S. Donaldson (eds.) 2001. *To Err Is Human: Building a Safer Health System.* Washington, DC: National Academies Press.

Kotter, J. 1996. *Leading Change*, 21. Cambridge, MA: Harvard Business School Press.

Kouzes, J. and B. Posner. 2003. The Leadership Challenge. San Francisco, CA: Jossey-Bass.

Lakein, A. 1989. *How to Get Control of Your Time and Your Life*, 11. New York: Signet.

Lanfranco, A. R., E. Andres, M. D. Castellanos, J. P. Desai, and W. C. Meyers. 2004. "Robotic Surgery: A Current Perspective." *Annals of Surgery* 239 (1).

Larkin, T. J., and S. Larkin. 1994. *Communicating Change—Winning Employee Support for New Business Goals*, xii. New York: McGraw Hill Professional.

Law Office Administrator. 2001. "Positive Discipline: How to Turn Up the Heat Without the Usual Threats." *Law Office Administrator* 5.

Lawrence, P. R., and J. W. Lorsch. 1969. *Organization and Environment: Managing Differentiation and Integration*. Homewood, IL: Richard D. Irwin, Inc.

———. 1967. *Organization and Environment*. Cambridge, MA: Harvard University Press.

Leadership-Tools.com. n.d. "Cultural Diversity in the Workplace: Strength in Diversity!" [Online article; retrieved 10/17/09.] http://jobfunctions .bnet.com/abstract.aspx?docid=176794.

Lenaz, M. P. 2004. "Added Value in Health Care with Six Sigma." *Managed Care Interface* 17 (6): 50–51, 54.

LeTourneau, B. 2004. "Communicate for Change." *Journal of Healthcare Management* 49 (6): 354–57.

Levin, L. S. 2004. "Aligning the Stars: Creating Dialogue within Healthcare Teams." *Healthcare Executive* 19 (2): 17.

Lewin, K. 1947. "Frontiers in Group Dynamics: I. Concept, Method and Reality in Social Sciences; Social Equilibria and Social Change." *Human Relations* 1: 5–41.

Lindo, D. K. 1981. "How to Increase Your Budget." *Journal of Administrative Management* (Oct.): 28–40.

Lippitt, M. 1987. "The Managing Complex Change Model." Enterprise Management, Ltd.

Longest, B. B. 1998. "Managerial Competence at Senior Levels of Integrated Delivery Systems." *Journal of Healthcare Management* 43 (2): 115–32.

Long Island Association. n.d. "Destruction and Creation." President's Letter. [Online information; retrieved 2/23/06.] www.longislandassociation.org/ presidents_arch.cfm?num=Pres2346111106&old=Pres5905150228.

Mackenzie, K. 2008. "The CEO as Mentor." *Health Leaders* XI (7): 51–52.

Mager, R. F. 1999. *What Every Manager Should Know About Training*, 2nd ed., 52, 68. Atlanta, GA: Center for Effective Performance Press.

Maier, N. P. R. 1983. "Assets and Liabilities in Group Problem Solving: The Need for an Integrative Function." In *Perspectives on Business in Organizations*, 2nd ed., edited by J. R. Hackman, E. E. Lawler III, and L. W. Porter, 385–92. New York: McGraw-Hill Book Co.

Markovitz, D., and N. Giangrande. "Make Every Minute Count." *Journal of Accountancy* 202 (6): 28.

Marriner-Tomey, A. 2004. *Guide to Nursing Management and Leadership*, 7th ed. St. Louis, MO: Mosby.

Massachusetts Nursing Association. 2005. [Online report; retrieved 2/11/06.] www.massnurses.org/News/2005/04/ massnurse7.htm.

McClellan, B. 2008. *The Care Digest.* [Online blog; retrieved 3/1/09.] http://caredigest.blogspot.com/2008/06/economic-downturn-affects-local.html.

McClelland, D. C., J. W. Atchison, R. A. Clark, and E. L. Lowell. 1953. *The Achievement Motive.* New York: Appleton-Century-Crofts.

McClelland, D. C., and D. H. Burnham. 1976. "Power Is the Great Motivator." *Harvard Business Review* (March/April): 100–10.

McConnell, C. R. 1993. *The Healthcare Supervisor*, 212. New York: Jones & Bartlett Publishers.

McFadden, J. 2002. "Companies Offer Flex-Time to Attract and Retain Employees." [Online article; retrieved 10/23/09.] www.bizjournals.com/albany/stories/2002/12/16/focus2.html.

McGregor, D. 1985. *The Human Side of Enterprise*, chs. 3 and 4. New York: McGraw-Hill Book Co.

McNamara, C. 1999. "Brief Overview of Contemporary Theories in Management." [Online article; retrieved 02/08/06.] www.managementhelp.org/library/mgmnt/cntmpory.htm.

Medical Officer Manager. 2001. "Finding the Right Job Candidate." *Medical Officer Manager* 14 (5): 6–8.

———. 2000. "Motivating Staff to Do More than the Minimum." *Medical Office Manager* 14 (8): 9.

Mercer Human Resources Consulting. 2001. "Healthcare Trends and Commentary—An Annual Check Up," 6–8. [Online article; viewed 4/22/06.] www.imercer.com/us/mercercommentary/healthcaretrendscommentary.pdf.

Miles, R. E. 1978. *Theories of Management: Implications for Organizational Behavior and Development.* New York: McGraw-Hill.

Miller, R. W. and F. A. Zeller. 1991. "Critical Factors in the Successful Development of an Area Labor-Management Committee." *Employee Responsibilities and Rights Journal* 4 (3): 215–230.

Mintzberg, H. 1973. *The Nature of Managerial Work*, 55–58. New York: HarperCollins Publishers.

Mitchell, T. R. 1982. *People in Organizations*, 2nd ed., 127–28. New York: McGraw-Hill.

Molpus, J. 2009. "Care Team Architecture." *Health Leaders* 12 (10): 20–26.

Morrison, J. L. 1997. "Future Scan 2000 and Beyond." [Online presentation; retrieved 4/12/10.] http://horizon.unc.edu/projects/presentations/Wfs/index-2.html.

Morrissey, J. A. 1995. "Manufacturing Employees Believe Unions Ineffective." *Textile World* 146 (12): 63.

Mowll, C. A. 1989. "Controlling the Patient Accounting Department." *Healthcare Financial Management* 43 (10): 90.

Munson, R. 1992. *Intervention and Reflection: Basic Issues in Medical Ethics*, 4th ed. Belmont, CA: Wadsworth Publishing Company.

Myers, V. 2007. "Recruitment and Retention of a Diverse Workforce: Challenges and Opportunities." *Journal of Healthcare Management* 52 (5): 290.

National Assessment of Adult Literacy. 2006. "Health Literacy of America's Adults: Results of the National Assessment of Adult Literacy (NAAL)." Washington, DC: National Assessment of Adult Literacy.

National Center for Education Statistics. 2009. [Online information; retrieved 3/10/09.] www.nces.ed.gov/naal/estimates/index.aspx.

———. 1998. "Violence and Discipline Problems in U.S. Public Schools: 1996–1997." [Online information; retrieved 10/06/05.] http://nces.ed.gov/pubsearch/pubsinfo.asp?pubid =98030.

National Center for Policy Analysis. 2005. "Where Have All the Geriatricians Gone?" [Online article; retrieved 9/2/05.] www.ncpa.org/newdpd/dparticle.php?article_id=2201.

National Institute of Standards and Technology. 2009. "Baldridge National Quality Program" [Online information; retrieved 3/22/10.] www.quality.nist.gov/.

National Right to Read Foundation. 2005. [Online information; retrieved 9/11/05.] www.nrrf.org/essay_Illiteracy.html#thegrimstatistics.

Nelson, B., and P. Economy. 1996. *Managing for Dummies*. Foster City, CA: IDG Books Worldwide.

Neuborne, E. 1997. "Companies Save, But Workers Pay." *USA Today* February 25, 2B.

Nickols, F. 2000. "Strategy Is . . . a Lot of Things." [Online article.] http://home.att.net~nickols/articles.htm.

Nielsen, D. M., M. D. Merry, D. Martin, P. M. Schyve, and M. Bisognano. 2004. "Can the Quality Gurus' Concepts Cure Healthcare?" *Quality & Healthcare*, supplement to *Hospitals & Health Networks* (Sept.): 1–12.

NIOSH. 2002. "Violence: Occupational Hazards in Hospitals." [Online report; retrieved 4/21/06.] www.cdc.gov/niosh/pdfs/2002-101.pdf.

Noffsinger, R., and S. Chin. 2000. "Improving the Delivery of Care and Reducing Healthcare Costs with the Digitization of Information." *Journal of Healthcare Information Management* 14 (2): 29.

Nowack, K. 2007. "Why 360 Degree Feedback Doesn't Work and What to Do About It." Presentation at the 2007 ASTD International Conference and Expedition. Atlanta, GA.

Oak, J. C. 2005. "Accepting Vendor Gifts." *Healthcare Executive* 20 (4): 32.

OfficeTeam. 1999. "Do You Hear What I Hear? Survey Finds Poor Communication Devours Seven Work Weeks Per Year." Press Release, Sept. 3. Menlo Park, CA: OfficeTeam.

O'Leary, G. 2009. "What Is a Progressive View of Leadership?" *CORO Connections Newsletter* 2 (1).

Oncken, W., Jr., and D. L. Wass. 1974. "Management Time: Who's Got the Monkey?" *Harvard Business Review* (Nov.–Dec.): 75–80.

Orlitzky, M., F. Schmidt, and S. Rynes. 2003. "Corporate Social and Financial Performance: A Meta-analysis." *Organization Studies* 24 (3): 403–41.

Osborn, A. F. 1963. *Applied Imagination*, 3rd ed., 151–63. New York: Charles Scribner's Sons.

Osland, J., D. Kolb, I. Rubin, and M. Turner 2006. *Organizational Behavior: An Experiential Approach*, 8th ed., 519. Upper Saddle River, NJ: Prentice Hall.

Ouchi, W. G. 1981. *Theory Z: How American Business Can Meet the Japanese Challenge*. Reading, MA: Addison-Wesley Publishing Co.

Ouchi, W. G., and A. M. Jaeger. 1978. "Type Z Organization: Stability in the Midst of Mobility." *Academy of Management Review* (April): 305–14.

Parker, P. 2008. *Arises: Webster's Quotations, Facts and Phrases*, p. 266. San Diego, CA: ICON Group International.

Parker, W. E., and R. W. Kleemeier. 1951. *Leadership in Management*, 96. New York: McGraw-Hill.

Passell, J. S., and D. Cohn. 2008. "U.S. Populations Projections: 2005–2050." [Online report; retrieved 6/4/10.] http://pewhispanic.org/files/reports/85.pdf

Peckron, D., and M. Herbst 2006. "Process Improvements Boost Quality and Physician Satisfaction at Christian Hospital." [Online article; retrieved 6/4/10.] www.shawresources.com/artprocess_

Performance Co-Pilot Tutorial Glossary. 2005. [Online information; retrieved 10/4/05.] http://pcp4cgl.sourceforge.net/turorial/glossary.html.

Perra, B. M. 2001. "Leadership: The Key to Quality Outcomes." *Journal of Nursing Care Quality* 15 (2): 68–73.

Perry, B. 2000. "Companies Rethink Casual Clothes." *USA Today*, June 27, 1A–2A.

Peters, T. 2001. "Rule #3: Leadership Is Confusing as Hell." [Online article; retrieved 4/9/10.] www.fastcompany.com/online/44/rules.html.

Petree, J. 2001. "Part 1: History of Chaos Theory." [Online article; retrieved 12/12/01.] www.wfu.edu/petrejh4/HISTORYchaos.htm.

Pfiffner, J. M., and F. P. Sherwood. 1960. *Administrative Organization*. Upper Saddle River, NJ: Prentice-Hall.

Phi Delta Kappa. 1998. "The 30th Annual Phi Delta Kappa Gallup Poll of the Public's Attitudes Toward the Public Schools." [Online information; retrieved 10/06/05.] www.pdkintl.org/kappan/kp9809-3.htm.

Pollard, D. 2005. "Meeting of Minds." [Online blog; accessed 3/10/10.] http://blogs.salon.com/0002007/stories/2005/11/18/theIdealCollaborativeTeamAndAConversationOnTheCollaborativeProcess.html.

Poole, D. 2004. "Incentives as Tools to Improve Efficiency." [Online article; viewed 4/26/06.] www.IndState.edu/mary/gradpapers/orstudy.doc.

Porter, M. E., J. W. Lorsch, and N. Nohria. "Seven Surprises for New CEOs." *Harvard Business Review* 82 (10): 62.

Portfolio.com. 2009. "The Future of Health Care: Outsourcing the Patient." [Online article; retrieved 12/6/09.] www.portfolio.com/views/columns/dual-perspectives/2009/03/03/Outsourcing-the-Patient/.

Power, D. J. 2007. "A Brief History of Decision Support Systems, Version 4.1." [Online article; retrieved 7/10/08.] www.dssresources.com.

Prenda, K. M., and S. M. Stahl. 2001. "The Truth About Older Workers." *Business and Health* 19 (5): 30–37.

PriceWaterhouseCoopers. 2005. "Cost of Caring: Key Drivers of Growth in Spending on Hospital Care." [Online information; retrieved 8/30/05.] www.aha.org/aha/press_room-info/content/PwCcostsReport.pdf.

Pritchett, P. 1996. *Resistance,* 1. Dallas, TX: Pritchett & Associates, Inc.

Purcell, T. 2001. "Strategic Planners Lead the Pack." *Journal of Accountancy* 192 (Dec.): 27.

Quicken Company. 2000. "CCH Business Owner's Toolkit." [Online newsletter] www.quicken.com/small_business/ cch/text/?article=P05_0001.

Ramsey, R. D. 2005, "Interpersonal Conflicts." *SuperVision* 66 (4): 14–17.

Rauber, C. 2009. "Kaiser Wins Kudos for Its Workplace Diversity Efforts." [Online article; retrieved 3/17/10.] www.bizjournals.com/sanfrancisco/stories/2009/03/16/newscolumn3.html.

Rice, B. 1984. "Square Holes for Quality Circles." *Psychology Today* (Feb.): 17.

Ritter, D. B. 2009. "Legal Update—Change Is On the Way: The New Administration's Impact on Labor and Employment Law." Audio conference, Chicago, June 9.

———. 2009. "Should Dating Co-workers Sign a 'Love Contract'?" [Online article; retrieved 12/8/09.] www.ngelaw.com/news/pubs_detail .aspx?ID=978.

Ritter, D., and N. Alkhas. 2009. "Employee Protections Broadened Under the ADA: Employers Should Be Prepared." [Online article; retrieved 12/8/09.] www.ngelaw.com/news/pubs_detail.aspx?ID=953.

Ritter, D., and S. Rosenberg. 2009. "Is 'Bring Your Gun to Work Day' Coming? Protecting Your Workplace from Gun Violence." [Online article; retrieved 12/8/09.] www.ngelaw.com/news/pubs_detail.aspx?ID=1029.

Robbins, S., R. Bergman, I. Stagg, and M. Coulter 2006. *Foundations of Management,* 2nd ed., *9.* Sydney: Pearson Education Australia.

Roberts, T. 2006 "Coaching Managers Through Their Conflicts" *Management Services* 49 (4): 16–18.

Robinson, D. 2005. "Management Theorists: Thinkers for the 21st Century?" *Training Journal* (Jan.): 32.

Rosenstein, B. 2008. "A Management Classic That's So Useful It's Back Again, Updated." *USA Today,* September 2, 9B.

Roussel, L., R. Swansburg, and R. Swansburg. 2006. *Management and Leadership for Nurse Administrators*, 4th ed. New York: Jones & Bartlett Publishers.

Saenz, A. 2009. "Audeo Lets You Talk or Control Wheelchair with Your Thoughts." [Online article; retrieved 12/7/09.] http://singularityhub.com category/bionic-body/.

———. 2009. "Bionic Limbs with Artificial Intelligence." [Online article; retrieved 4/21/10.] http://singularityhub.com/2009/08/27/bionic-limbs-with-artificial-intelligence/.

———. 2009. "Deka's Luke Arm in Clinical Trials: Is It the Future of Prosthetics?" [Online article; retrieved 12/7/09.] http://singularityhub .com/category/bionic-body/.

———. 2009. "Smart Toilets: Doctors in Your Bathrooms." [Online article; retrieved 12/6/09.] http://singularityhub.com/2009/05/12/smart-toilets-doctors-in-your-bathroom/.

SAIC. n.d. "Glossary." [Online information; retrieved 10/29/09.] www.investors.saic .com/glossary.cfm.

Salemme, N. 2009. "Workers Dare to Dream of Naptime." [Online article; retrieved 10/25/09.] www.news.com.au/business/business-smarts/workers-dare-to-dream-of-naptime/story-e6frfm9r-1225783856604.

Sayles, L. R., and G. Strauss. 1981. *Managing Human Resources*, 2nd ed., 129. Englewood Cliffs, NJ: Prentice-Hall.

Schein, E. H. 1996. "Leadership and Organizational Culture." In *The Leader of the Future*, edited by F. Hesselbein, M. Goldsmith, and R. Beckhard, 69. San Francisco: Jossey-Bass.

Schoen, C., S. R. Collins, J. L. Kriss, and M. M. Doty. 2008. "How Many Are Underinsured? Trends Among U.S. Adults, 2003 and 2007." [Online article; retrieved 12/6/09.] www.commonwealthfund.org/Content/Publications/In-the-Literature/ 2008/Jun/How-Many-Are-Underinsured—Trends-Among-U-S—Adults—2003-and-2007.aspx.

Scott, G. 2009. "Teamwork—A Focus on Internal Customers Can Lead to Satisfied Patients." *Healthcare Executive* 24 (2): 46.

Seeley, M., and G. Hargreaves. 2003. *Managing in the Email Office*, 5. Oxford, UK: Butterworth-Heinemann.

Sena, J. 2005. "Managing Sustainable Change." Seminar. St. Louis, MO, September 14.

Sherk, J., and P. Kersey. 2009. "How the Employee Free Choice Act Takes Away Workers' Rights." [Online article; retrieved 11/29/09.] www.heritage.org/research/Labor/bg2027.cfm.

Siegel, J. 2004. "Mending Your Meetings." *Southwest Airlines Spirit* 13 (3): 48–49.

Simon, H. A. 1997. *Administrative Behavior: A Study of Decision-Making Processes in Administrative Organizations*, 4th ed. New York: The Free Press.

Singer, I. D. 1999. "Work-Life Benefits Can Lighten the Load." *Business & Health* 17 (10): 25.

Sinha, R. n.d. "Key Factors of Multicultural Team Management & Leadership." [Online article; retrieved 10/17/09.] http://ezinearticles.com/?Key-Factors-of-Multicultural-Team-Management/Leadership&id=293829.

Sisk, H. L. 1977. *Management and Organization*, 3rd ed. Cincinnatti, OH: South-Western Publishing Company Snelling Report. 1998. The Skilled Workforce Shortage: A Growing Challenge to the Future Competitiveness of American Manufacturing. Dallas, TX: Snelling.

Solovy, A. 2001. "All the Right Moves." *Hospitals and Health Networks* 75 (3): 30.

Spath, P. 2006. "Confronting the Problem Employee." *For the Record* 18 (18): 16–20.

———. 2002. "Don't Overlook the Human Side of Process Improvement." *For the Record* 14 (20): 21–24.

———. 2002. "Productivity and Quality in the HIM Department." *For the Record* 14 (11): 30.

———. 2002. "Upgrade Skills with Competency-Based Training." *For the Record* 14 (2): 21–22.

———. 2001. "Applying the Pareto Diagram to HIM." *For the Record* February 5, 23–24.

Specian, M. 2007. "POSDCORB." [Online information; retrieved 11/26/09.] http://polt906f07.wikispaces.com/POSDCORB.

Steers, R. M. 1988. *Introduction to Organizational Behavior*, 3rd ed. Glenview, IL: Scott, Foresman & Co.

Stefl, M. E. 2008. "Common Competencies for All Healthcare Managers: The Healthcare Leadership Alliance Model." *Journal of Healthcare Management* 53 (6): 364–65.

Stern, S. 2009. "Time for Managers to Stand and Deliver." *Financial Times* (January 23: 3).

Stine, S. 2008. "Managing Millenials: Part I." [Online document; accessed 2/2/10.] http://hrhero.com/hl/articles/2008/04/04/managing-the-millennials-part-1/.

Strauss, G., and L. R. Sayles. 1980. *Personnel: The Human Problems of Management*, 4th ed, 221. Englewood Cliffs, NJ: Prentice-Hall.

Sullivan, E. J., P. J. Decker, and S. Hailstone. 1985. "Assessment Center Technology: Selecting Head Nurses." *The Journal of Nursing Administration* (May): 13–18.

Taylor, F. 1911. *Principles of Scientific Management*. New York: Harper Bros.

Thom, R. 1975. *Structural Stability and Morphogenesis*. Reading, MA: W.A. Benjamin, Inc.

Thomas, E. C. 2002. "The Challenges of Cutback Management." *Public Policy & Practice* [Online article; retrieved 10/4/05.] http://ipspr.sc.edu/ejournal/cutbackmanage.asp.

Thrall, T. 2009. "Employees Generate Recession-Busting Ideas." *Hospitals and Health Networks* 83 (6): 22.

Torres, E. J., and K. L. Guo. 2004. "Quality Improvement Techniques to Improve Patient Satisfaction." *International Journal of Health Care Quality Assurance* 17 (6): 334–38.

Toussaint, J. 2009. "Why Are We Still Underperforming?" *Frontiers of Health Services Management* 26 (1): 27–32.

Tulgan, B. 2007. *It's Okay to Be the Boss.* New York: HarperBusiness, 134–35.

UCLA Health System. n.d. "Cultural Diversity and Health Care." [Online PowerPoint presentation; retrieved 10/17/09.] http://hr.healthcare.ucla .edu/Download/Cultural%20Diversity%20and%20Health%20Care.ppt.

Urwick, L. F. 1956. "The Manager's Span of Control." *Harvard Business Review* (May–June): 39–47.

U.S. Bureau of Labor Statistics. 2009. *Occupational Outlook Handbook 2008–2009 Edition: Rail Transportation Occupations.* [Online information; retrieved 12/06/09.] www.bls.gov/oco/ocos244.htm.

———. 2009. "Table 10. 30 Occupations with the Largest Number of Total Job Openings."[Online table; modified 12/11/09; retrieved 2/9/10.] www.bls.gov/news.release/ecopro.t10.htm

———. 2009. "Union Affiliation of Employed Wage and Salary Workers by Occupation and Industry." [Online information; retrieved 11/29/09.] www.bls.gov/news.release/union2.t03.htm.

———. 2009. "Union Members Summary." [Online information; retrieved 11/29/09.] www.bls.gov/news.release/union2.nr0.htm.

———. 2008. "Career Guide to the Industry, Healthcare." [Online information; retrieved 11/18/08.] www.bls.gov/oco/cg/cgs035.htm.

———. 2008. "Nonfatal Occupational Injuries and Illnesses Requiring Days Away from Work, 2007." [Online report; created 11/20/08; retrieved 1/18/09.] www.bls.gov/news.release/osh2.nr0.htm.

U.S. Department of Health and Human Services. 2010. "Health Workforce Studies." [Online report; retrieved 12/6/09.] http://bhpr.hrsa.gov/ healthworkforce/default.htm.

———. 2002. "Reports: Projected Supply, Demand and Shortages of Registered Nurses, 2000–2020. [Online report; retrieved 10/6/05.] http://bhpr.hrsa .gov/healthworkforce/reports/rnproject/default.htm.

———. 2001. "National Sample Survey of Registered Nurses—March 2000. Preliminary Findings, February 2001." [Online report; retrieved 2/21/01.] www.bhpr.hrsa.gov.

———. 2000. "The Pharmacist Workforce: A Study of the Supply and Demand for Pharmacists." Washington, DC: U.S. Department of Health and Human Services.

U.S. Department of Labor. 2000. *Testing and Assessment: An Employer's Guide to Best Practices.* Washington, D.C.

U.S. Department of Labor Occupational Safety and Health Administration. 2009. "Guidelines for Preventing Workplace Violence for Health Care & Social

Service Workers." [Online information; retrieved 1/18/09.] www.osha.gov/Publications/OSHA3148/osha3148.html.

U.S. Department of Health and Human Services. 2010. "Health Workforce Studies." [Online information; retrieved 5/19/10.] http://bhpr.hrsa .gov/healthworkforce/default.htm.

Valasquez, M. G. 1988. *Business Ethics Concepts and Cases,* 2nd ed. Englewood Cliffs, NJ: Prentice Hall.

Valenstein, P. N., R. Souers, and D. S. Wilkinson. 2004. "Staffing Benchmarks for Clinical Laboratories: A College of American Pathologists Q-Probes Study of Staffing at 151 Institutions." *Archives of Pathology and Laboratory Medicine* 129 (4): 467–73.

Valentino, C. L. 2004. "The Role of Middle Managers in the Transmission and Integration of Organizational Culture." *Journal of Healthcare Management* 49 (6): 393.

Von Bertalanffy, L. 1951. *General System Theory: A New Approach to Unity of Science.* Baltimore, MD: Johns Hopkins Press.

Vroom, V. H., and P. W. Yetton. 1973. *Leadership and Decision Making.* Pittsburgh, PA: University of Pittsburgh Press.

Walliker, A. 2008. "Get Ready, Here Comes Generation Z." [Online article; retrieved 10/21/09.] www.news.com.au/story/0,23599,23270333-3,00.html.

Walonick, D. S. n.d. "Organizational Theory and Behavior." [Online information; retrieved 2/17/09.] www.survey-software-solutions.com/walonick/ organizational-theory.htm.

Walton, M. 1986. *The Deming Management Method.* New York: The Putnam Publishing Group.

Washington State Department of Labor and Industries. 2006. "Workplace Violence in Health Care Settings." [Online information; retrieved 4/22/06.] www.lni.wa.gov/Safety/Topics/AtoZ/WPV/wpvhealthcare.asp.

Watson, W. 2000. *HFMA Wants You To Know.* Westchester, IL: Healthcare Financial Management Association.

Weber, M. 1985. "The Three Types of Legitimate Rule." *Berkeley Journal of Sociology* 4: 3–10.

———. 1974. *The Theory of Social and Economic Organizations,* edited by T. Parsons, 324–63. New York: Oxford University Press.

Wells, J. T. 2001. "Enemies Within." *Journal of Accountancy* 192 (6): 31–33.

———. 2001. "A Fish Story—Or Not?" *Journal of Accountancy* 190 (4): 114–17.

West Publishing. 1979. *Black's Law Dictionary,* 5th ed. St. Paul, MN: West Publishing.

White House. 2009. Office of Press Secretary. "Executive Order: Creating Labor-Management Forums to Improve Delivery of Government Services. December 9, 2009." [online document; viewed 5/7/10.] www.whitehouse .gov/the-press-office/executive-order-creating-labor-management-forums-improve-delivery-government-servic.

Wickline v. State of California, 239 Cal. Rptr. 810 (Ct. App. 1986) review granted, 231 Cal. Rptr. 560 (1986), review dismissed, remanded, ordered published 239 Cal. Rptr. 805 (1987).

Williams, J. 2007. "Follow the Leader." *Healthcare Financial Management* (Jan.): 51.

Witt, J. D. 1996. "How to Implement Changes from Your QI Team." *Occupational Health Management* 6 (7): 77–78.

Woodard, T. D. 2005. "Addressing Variation in Hospital Quality: Is Six Sigma the Answer?" *Journal of Healthcare Management* 50 (4): 226.

Woodruffe, C. 2009. "Still in the Making." [Online article; retrieved 10/21/09.] www.trainingjournal.com/generation.pdf.

Word Web Online. 2006. "Noun: Team." [Online information; retrieved 2/12/06.] www.wordwebonline.com/en/TEAM.

York, D. R. 1985. "Attitude Surveying." *Personnel Journal* (May): 70–73.

Young, D. 2004. "Six Sigma Black-Belt Pharmacist Improves Patient Safety." *American Journal of Health System Pharmacist* 61 (19): 1988, 1992, 1996.

Zarowin, S. 2005. "Overcome the Seduction of Consensus." *Journal of Accountancy* 199 (3): 116.

———. 2004. "How to Make Meetings More Productive." *Journal of Accountancy* 197 (1): 112.

Zatz, D. A. 2004. "Organizational Development Toolpack." [Online information; retrieved 02/08/06.] www.toolpack.com.

Zuckerman, A. 2005. *Healthcare Strategic Planning,* 2nd ed. Chicago: Health Administration Press.

———. 2000. "Creating a Vision for the Twenty-First Century Healthcare Organization." *Journal of Healthcare Management* 45 (5): 298.

———. 1998. *Healthcare Strategic Planning: Approaches for the 21st Century,* 37. Chicago: Health Administration Press.

INDEX

ABOUT THE AUTHOR

Rose T. Dunn, MBA, RHIA, CPA, FACHE, FHFMA, has been in healthcare management for more than 30 years. She started her career as the director of health information management services at Barnes Hospital immediately following graduation from Saint Louis University. She was later promoted to vice president. After 13 years at Barnes, Dunn became the assistant vice president in Metropolitan Life Insurance Company's HMO subsidiary. Following this position, Dunn served as the chief financial officer of a dual-hospital system. In 1988, Dunn started a consulting firm, First Class Solutions, Inc.^{sm}, which has now grown to serve health providers and third-party payer clients nationwide. She is the chief operating officer of First Class Solutions, Inc.^{sm} based in Maryland Heights (St. Louis), MO.

During her 30-year career, Dunn has had more than 200 articles published, is a sought-after public speaker on a variety of healthcare subjects, and has authored books on release of information, finance, productivity, process improvement, and management. She has served as a faculty member at the University of Minnesota's Health Administration Program, teaching finance; at Saint Louis University's School of Business, teaching management; and at Stephens College's Health Information Management Program, teaching legal and ethical issues, management, and finance.

Dunn is active in several professional organizations including the Healthcare Financial Management Association (HFMA), American College of Healthcare Executives (ACHE), American Institute of Certified Public Accountants (AICPA), and American Health Information Management Association (AHIMA). She is a past president of AHIMA and a recipient of AHIMA's highest award, the Distinguished Member award. In 2008, she was recognized by AHIMA with its Legacy Award. Dunn holds fellowship status in AHIMA.

Dunn was one of the youngest individuals to receive the prestigious President's Award from Saint Louis University, from which she received her bachelor of science (summa cum laude) and master's (cum laude) degrees.